To the alumni, present students, and future students
of Temple University School of Pharmacy

■

Brief Contents

Contents

Preface

The genesis of *Frequently Prescribed Medications: Drugs You Need to Know* began at the Temple University School of Pharmacy as a resource for students to prepare for their "Top 200 Exam," an exam focused on the highly pertinent facts of frequently prescribed medications that all third-professional-year students must pass before beginning the fourth professional year. Before writing earlier versions of this text, faculty at Temple reviewed many other books, flashcards, and resources but found none to be optimal references for our students' needs. Many books were extraordinarily detailed or did not emphasize important information clearly and concisely, and important drugs were not included. For the past 12 years at Temple, we have used versions of this text, and students and faculty have found *Frequently Prescribed Medications* to be a very helpful resource. This *Second Edition* expands on the Temple in-house versions by including key points for each drug and drug class as well as review questions.

We hope that this text will serve as a useful reference for healthcare students and professionals of various disciplines as they learn the most frequently used medications in clinical practice.

New to the *Second Edition*

In creating this second edition of *Frequently Prescribed Medications: Drugs You Need to Know*, we reviewed the current usage patterns of medications available in the United States. In doing so, 98 new drugs were added to this edition as well as a new chapter titled "Biologic and Immunologic Agents." All aspects of each drug and drug class were updated to include new dosage forms, dosing schedules, side effects, drug interactions, and new indications. Pregnancy categories and Rx or OTC designations also have been added to every drug in this revised edition. All controlled substances are designated as Schedule 2 through 5 as appropriate. All drugs and drugs classes have been expanded, and more descriptive mechanism of action information has been included. Finally, 30 new review questions were added to every chapter.

Acknowledgments

We are indebted to the many clinicians and faculty who have assisted in developing and revising *Frequently Prescribed Medications: Drugs You Need to Know, Second Edition* into its final version. We would like to thank all of the section editors and authors. We would also like to thank the following people, as, without their assistance, earlier versions of this text could not have been written (in alphabetical order): Joseph Boullata, PharmD, BCNSP; Ina Calligaro, PharmD; Christine Fitzgerald, PharmD; Steven Gelone, PharmD; Karissa Kim, PharmD, CACP; Olga M. Klibanov, PharmD; Tanya Knight-Klimas, PharmD, CGP, FASCP; Nisha Mehta, PharmD; Christina Ruggia-Check, PharmD; Patrick Scoble, PharmD; Joel Shuster, PharmD, FCCP; and Sarah Slabaugh, PharmD, RD.

Abbreviations Used in the Text

5-HT$_3$ receptors	Serotonin subtype-3 receptors		HCTZ	Hydrochlorothiazide
ACE	Angiotensin converting enzyme		HDL	High-density lipoprotein
ACE-I	Angiotensin converting enzyme inhibitor		HGB	Hemoglobin
ADHD	Attention deficit hyperactivity disorder		HIT	Heparin-induced thrombocytopenia
AIDS	Acquired immune deficiency syndrome		HIV	Human immunodeficiency virus
ALT	Alanine aminotransferase		HMG-CoA	Hydroxymethylglutaryl-coenzyme A
aPTT	Activated partial thromboplastin time		HPA	Hypothalamic-pituitary-adrenal axis
ARB	Angiotensin receptor blocker		IBS	Irritable bowel syndrome
ARDS	Acute respiratory distress syndrome		IM	Intramuscular
AST	Aspartate aminotransferase		INR	International normalized ratio
BAS	Bile acid sequestrant		IOP	Intraocular pressure
BMT	Bone marrow transplant		IV	Intravenous
BPH	Benign prostatic hyperplasia		LDL	Low-density lipoprotein
BZD	Benzodiazepine		LFT	Liver function test
CABG	Coronary artery bypass graft		LMWH	Low molecular weight heparin
CBC	Complete blood count		MAO	Monoamine oxidase
cGMP	Cyclic guanosine monophosphate		MAOI	Monoamine oxidase inhibitor
CHF	Congestive heart failure		MDI	Metered-dose inhaler
CKD	Chronic kidney disease		MI	Myocardial infarction
ClCrest	Estimated creatinine clearance		MOA	Mechanism of action
CNI	Calcineurin inhibitors		MRI	Magnetic resonance imaging
CNS	Central nervous system		NG tube	Nasogastric tube
COPD	Chronic obstructive pulmonary disease		NLO	Nasolacrimal occlusion
COX-2	Cyclooxygenase-2		NMS	Neuroleptic malignant syndrome
CPK	Creatine phosphokinase		NNRTI	Non-nucleoside reverse transcriptase inhibitor
CrCl	Creatinine clearance			
CRF	Chronic renal failure		NRTI	Nucleoside reverse transcriptase inhibitor
CTZ	Chemoreceptor trigger zone		NSAID	Nonsteroidal anti-inflammatory drug
CVA	Cerebrovascular accident		NTE	Not to exceed
CYP	Cytochrome P450		OTC	Over the counter
DHA	Docosahexaenoic acid		PBPC	Peripheral blood progenitor cell collection
DIC	Disseminated intravascular coagulopathy		PCI	Percutaneous coronary intervention
DKA	Diabetic ketoacidosis		PCP	*Pneumocystis carinii* pneumonia
DNA	Deoxyribonucleic acid		PDE5	Phosphodiesterase type 5
DVT	Deep vein thrombosis		PE	Pulmonary embolism
EKG	Electrocardiogram		PI	Protease inhibitor
EPA	Eicosapentaenoic acid		PPARα	Peroxisome proliferator activated receptors
EPS	Extrapyramidal symptoms		PPI	Proton pump inhibitor
FAP	Familial adenomatous polyposis		PUD	Peptic ulcer disease
FDA	U.S. Food and Drug Administration		RA	Rheumatoid arthritis
G-CSF	Granulocyte colony-stimulating factor		RDA	Recommended dietary allowance
GERD	Gastroesophageal reflux disease		RNA	Ribonucleic acid
GFR	Glomerular filtration rate		SCN	Severe chronic neutropenia
GI	Gastrointestinal		Scr	Serum creatinine
HCT	Hematocrit		SJS	Stevens-Johnson syndrome

SLE	Systemic lupus erythematosus	TLC	Therapeutic lifestyle changes
SSRI	Selective serotonin-reuptake inhibitor	TMJ	Temporomandibular joint
SUB-Q	Subcutaneous	TNF	Tumor necrosis factor
TCA	Tricyclic antidepressant	TPA	Tissue plasminogen activator
TG	Triglyceride	UFH	Unfractionated heparin
TIA	Transient ischemic attack	VLDL	Very low density lipoprotein

FDA Pregnancy Category Definitions

Category A: Adequate and well-controlled studies have failed to demonstrate a risk to the fetus in the first trimester of pregnancy (and there is no evidence of risk in later trimesters).

Category B: Animal reproduction studies have failed to demonstrate a risk to the fetus and there are no adequate and well-controlled studies in pregnant women.

Category C: Animal reproduction studies have shown an adverse effect on the fetus and there are no adequate and well-controlled studies in humans, but potential benefits may warrant use of the drug in pregnant women despite potential risks.

Category D: There is positive evidence of human fetal risk based on adverse reaction data from investigational or marketing experience or studies in humans, but potential benefits may warrant use of the drug in pregnant women despite potential risks.

Category X: Studies in animals or humans have demonstrated fetal abnormalities and/or there is positive evidence of human fetal risk based on adverse reaction data from investigational or marketing experience, and the risks involved in use of the drug in pregnant women clearly outweigh potential benefits.

Contributors

Editors

Michael A. Mancano, PharmD
Chair, Department of Pharmacy Practice
Clinical Professor of Pharmacy Practice
Temple University School of Pharmacy
Philadelphia, Pennsylvania

Jason C. Gallagher, PharmD, BCPS
Clinical Associate Professor of Pharmacy Practice
Temple University School of Pharmacy
Philadelphia, Pennsylvania

Contributing Authors

Michael C. Barros, PharmD, BCPS, BCACP
Clinical Assistant Professor of Pharmacy Practice
Temple University School of Pharmacy
Clinical Pharmacist, Heart Failure/Transplant
Temple University Hospital

Neela Bhajandas, PharmD
Clinical Assistant Professor of Pharmacy Practice
Temple University School of Pharmacy
Clinical Pharmacist, Pulmonary and Critical Care
Temple University Hospital

Jane F. Bowen, PharmD, BCPS
Assistant Professor of Clinical Pharmacy
Department of Pharmacy Practice and
    Pharmacy Administration
Philadelphia College of Pharmacy, University of the Sciences

Rachel Clark-Vetri, PharmD, BCOP
Clinical Professor of Pharmacy Practice
Temple University School of Pharmacy
Clinical Oncology/Palliative Care Pharmacist
Temple University Cancer Center

Deborah DeEugenio-Mayro, PharmD, BCPS, CACP
Clinical Associate Professor of Pharmacy Practice
Temple University School of Pharmacy
Clinical Pharmacist, Ambulatory Internal Medicine
Temple Group Practice

Carol Holtzman, PharmD, MSc
Clinical Assistant Professor of Pharmacy Practice
Temple University School of Pharmacy
HIV Pharmacotherapy Specialist
Temple Comprehensive HIV Program

Susan Kent, PharmD, CGP
Clinical Assistant Professor of Pharmacy Practice
Temple University School of Pharmacy
Clinical Pharmacist, Ambulatory Care
HealthLink Medical Center

Donna Leverone, PharmD
Clinical Assistant Professor of Pharmacy Practice
Temple University School of Pharmacy
Clinical Pharmacist, Internal Medicine
Fairmount Primary Care Center

Patrick McDonnell, PharmD
Clinical Professor of Pharmacy Practice
Temple University School of Pharmacy
Clinical Pharmacy Consultant
Jeanes Hospital

Nima M. Patel, PharmD, BCPS
Clinical Professor of Pharmacy Practice
Temple University School of Pharmacy
Ambulatory Care Clinical Pharmacist
Department of Medicine
Temple University Hospital

Mirza Perez, PharmD, BCPS
Clinical Associate Professor of Pharmacy Practice
Temple University School of Pharmacy
Clinical Pharmacist, Ambulatory Internal Medicine
Temple University Hospital

Talitha Pulvino, PharmD, BCPS
Clinical Assistant Professor of Pharmacy Practice
Temple University School of Pharmacy
Clinical Pharmacist, Temple University
    General Internal Medicine

Charles Ruchalski, PharmD, BCPS
Clinical Professor of Pharmacy Practice
Temple University School of Pharmacy
Stroke Prevention Clinic
Temple University Hospital
Department of Neurology

Christina Rose, PharmD, BCPS
Clinical Assistant Professor of Pharmacy Practice
Temple University School of Pharmacy
Clinical Specialist in Critical Care
Temple University Hospital

Jamila Stanton Seibel, PharmD, BCPS
Pharmacy Coordinator
Aurora Sinai Medical Center

Anna M. Wodlinger Jackson, PharmD, BCPS (AQ Cardiology)
Clinical Consultant Pharmacist
Inova Fairfax Hospital

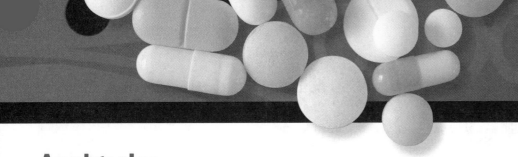

Analgesics

Rachel Clark-Vetri, PharmD, BCOP

MISCELLANEOUS ANALGESICS

Introduction

Two commonly used analgesics fall into categories of their own and are discussed here. Acetaminophen, one of the most commonly used analgesics, as well as antipyretics, is generally well tolerated but noted for its hepatotoxicity when given in doses exceeding daily recommendations. Butalbital combinations are most frequently used to treat headaches.

Mechanism of Action for the Drug Class

Acetaminophen inhibits brain prostaglandin synthesis, leading to analgesic and antipyretic activity. Butalbital is a barbiturate that depresses the sensory cortex and motor activity, producing sedation and drowsiness. Caffeine increases cAMP and acts as a vasoconstrictor and CNS stimulant. The combination is commonly used to treat headaches.

Members of the Drug Class

In this section: Acetaminophen, butalbital with caffeine and acetaminophen
Others: Butalbital with caffeine; butalbital with caffeine, acetaminophen, and codeine

◉ Acetaminophen

Brand Names

Tylenol, Paracetamol, Ofirmev (injectable), various others

Generic Name

Acetaminophen

OTC

Injection: Rx only

Dosage Forms

Tablet (oral, chewable, disintegrating, and extended-release), capsule, gelcap, elixir, solution, suspension, suppository, injection

Usage

Mild pain such as headaches and arthritis pain,* fever,* combined with other analgesics for moderate to severe pain*

Pregnancy Category B (Oral) and C (Injection)

Dosing

- Usual dose:
  - 500–650 mg PO every 4–6 hours as needed
  - Maximum adult dose: 4 g/day and 3 g/day for chronic use
- IV:
  - < 50 kg: 15 mg/kg every 6 hours or 12.5 mg/kg every 4 hours
    - Maximum single dose: 750 mg
    - Maximum daily dose: 75 mg/kg/day
  - > 50 kg: 650 mg every 4 hours or 1,000 mg every 6 hours
    - Maximum single dose: 1,000 mg
    - Maximum daily dose: 4 g/day
- Children:
  - Age > 12 years: Refer to adult dosing
  - Oral:
    - 10–15 mg/kg per dose every 4-6 hours as needed
    - Do not exceed 5 doses in 24 hours
  - IV:
    - 15 mg/kg every 6 hours or 12.5 mg/kg every 4 hours
    - Maximum single dose: 15 mg/kg
    - Maximum daily dose: 75 mg/kg
  - Rectal: < 12 years 10–20 mg/kg every 4–6 hours as needed

---

* Throughout the text, an asterisk (*) is used to indicate the most common uses of a drug.

- Renal impairment:
  - CrCl 10–50 mL/min: administer every 6 hours
  - CrCl < 10 mL/min: administer every 8 hours
- Hepatic impairment: Limit to 2 g/day in chronic alcoholics and avoid chronic use

Adverse Reactions: Most Common

Nontoxic at therapeutic doses

Adverse Reactions: Rare/Severe/Important

Hepatotoxicity with excessive dosing

Major Drug Interactions

Drugs Affecting Acetaminophen
- Carbamazepine: May increase the risk of hepatotoxicity
- Ethanol use: > 3 drinks/day may increase risk of hepatotoxicity
- Isoniazid: May increase the risk of hepatotoxicity
- Phenytoin: May increase the risk of hepatotoxicity

Acetaminophen's Effect on Other Drugs
Warfarin: Increased anticoagulant effect

Contraindications

Hypersensitivity to acetaminophen or any component of the formulation; severe hepatic impairment or severe active liver disease

Essential Monitoring Parameters

Signs of hepatoxicity, including dark urine, abdominal pain, and elevated liver function tests

Counseling Points

- Report unresolved pain or fevers to your healthcare provider
- Use weight-based dosing in children
- Adults: Do not exceed 4 g/day; less than 3g/day for chronic dosing
- Shake suspension well before pouring
- Extended-release products must be swallowed whole, not chewed or crushed

Key Points

- Adherence to maximum daily dose recommendations is important to avoid hepatotoxicity
- Many OTC cold and pain products and opioid analgesic combinations contain acetaminophen, and patients should be warned to avoid inadvertently overdosing on acetaminophen by taking them in excessive combinations.
- Careful consideration should be taken when measuring out a pediatric dose from a liquid formulation to ensure correct dosing
- Acetaminophen is the preferred analgesic during pregnancy and breastfeeding

◉ Butalbital with Caffeine and Acetaminophen

Brand Names
Fioricet, Zebutal, Dolgic Plus

Generic Names
Butalbital, acetaminophen, caffeine

Rx Only
Class III controlled substance

Dosage Forms
Tablet, capsule, oral liquid

Usage
Relief of tension or muscle contraction headaches*

Pregnancy Category C

Dosing
- Initial:
  - 1–2 tablets or capsules (or 15–30 mL solution) every 4 hours
  - Do not to exceed 6 tablets or capsules (or 180 mL solution) daily
- Renal dosage adjustment: Caution using in severe impairment
- Hepatic dosage adjustment: Caution using in severe impairment

Adverse Reactions: Most Common

Drowsiness, depression, nervousness, insomnia, nightmares, nausea

Adverse Reactions: Rare/Severe/Important

Hallucinations, hypotension, respiratory and CNS depression, tachycardia, hepatotoxicity (exceeding acetaminophen dosing recommendations)

Major Drug Interactions

Drugs Affecting Butalbital with Caffeine and Acetaminophen
- CNS depressants: May enhance the adverse/toxic effect of other CNS depressants
- Ethanol use: > 3 drinks/day may increase risk of hepatotoxicity
- Isoniazid: May increase the risk of hepatotoxicity

Butalbital with Caffeine and Acetaminophen's Effect on Other Drugs
Increases the metabolism of calcium channel blockers, contraceptives, corticosteroids, cyclosporine, disopyramide, doxycycline, tricyclic antidepressants, voriconazole, warfarin

Contraindications

Hypersensitivity to butalbital, acetaminophen, caffeine, or any component of the formulation; porphyria

Counseling Points

- Report unresolved headache to your healthcare provider
- Do not use more than the recommended daily dose

Key Point

Many OTC cold and pain products contain acetaminophen; increased risk of hepatotoxicity when taken with butalbital, acetaminophen, and caffeine combinations

ANALGESICS, NARCOTICS

Introduction

Narcotic analgesics are common medications used for moderate and severe pain. Given by a variety of different routes of administration and effective for both nociceptive and neuropathic pain symptoms, narcotics are controlled substances with a risk of abuse and diversion.

Mechanism of Action for the Drug Class

Act as μ-opioid receptor agonists, altering the perception and response to pain centrally and peripherally. Tramadol and tapentadol also inhibit the reuptake of norepinephrine, which modifies the ascending pain pathway, in addition to being μ-agonists. Buprenorphine is a μ-agonist with weak κ-antagonist activity. Butorphanol and nalbuphine are both partial agonists of μ- and κ-receptors. The variability of receptor affinity and activity produces varying degrees of analgesia among the agents. Fentanyl, hydromorphone, methadone, morphine, and oxycodone are the strongest opiate analgesics discussed in this section.

Contraindications of the Drug Class

Severe respiratory disease or depression, including acute asthma (unless patient is mechanically ventilated); paralytic ileus

Members of the Drug Class

In this section: Buprenorphine, fentanyl, hydromorphone, methadone, morphine, oxycodone, tramadol, tapentadol
Others: Alfentanil, buprenorphine, butorphanol, codeine, hydrocodone, levorphanol, meperidine, nalbuphine, opium tincture, oxymorphone, pentazocine, remifentanil, sufentanil

◉ Buprenorphine

Brand Names

Buprenex, Butrans, Subutex

Generic Name

Buprenorphine

Rx Only

Class III controlled substance

Dosage Forms

Injection, transdermal patch, sublingual tablet

Usage

Moderate to severe pain,* opioid dependence,* opioid withdrawal in heroin-dependent hospitalized patients

Pregnancy Category C

Dosing

- Usual dose: 0.15–0.6 mg every 4–8 hours as needed
- Acute pain: 0.3 mg IM or IV every 6–8 hours as needed
- Chronic pain: transdermal patch; opioid-naïve: Initial 5 μg/hour applied once every 7 days; may titrate with a minimum interval of 72 hours up to a maximum patch dose of 20 μg/hr applied once every 7 days. Patients receiving daily dose of 30–80 mg of oral morphine equivalent may be initiated at 10 μg/hour applied once every 7 days.
- Opioid dependence: Sublingual tablets; day 1: 8 mg; usual range 12–16 mg/day during induction with a target dose of 16 mg/day for maintenance
- Opiate withdrawal in heroin-dependent hospitalized patients (unlabeled use): IV 0.3–0.9 mg every 6–12 hours

Adverse Reactions: Most Common

Sedation, hypotension, dizziness, nausea, vomiting, headache, respiratory depression (IV), constipation, application site rash (patch)

Adverse Reactions: Rare/Severe/Important

Respiratory depression, QTc prolongation, hepatotoxicity, severe allergic reactions

Major Drug Interactions

Drugs Affecting Buprenorphine

- CNS depressants (including alcohol): Increase sedation and dizziness
- CYP3A4 inhibitors and inducers: Alter buprenorphine's metabolism
- Drugs that can potentially cause QTc prolongation: May increase the risk of arrhythmias
- MAO inhibitors: May increase sedation

Contraindications

Contraindications to the transdermal patch: Management of mild, acute, or intermittent pain; management of pain requiring short-term opioid analgesia; management of postoperative pain

Counseling Points

- Avoid excessive alcohol use
- May cause drowsiness and impair your ability to operate machinery
- May cause constipation requiring laxatives
- May cause physical or psychological dependence with prolonged use
- Notify your healthcare provider if pain is unrelieved
- Do not place direct heat (i.e., heating pads) on patch
- Report any allergic reactions
- Never cut the transdermal patches
- Rotate patch sites on arms, chest, and back; apply to hairless, dry area
- Keep any used and unused patches away from children

Key Points

- The combination of buprenorphine and naloxone is preferred over buprenorphine monotherapy for maintenance treatment of opioid dependence
- Patch doses of 20 µg/hr are associated with increased risk of QT interval prolongation
- Buprenorphine can lower seizure threshold and cause seizures in patients at risk
- Prescribers must be certified in the REMS program to prescribe the tablets and transdermal patch
- Transdermal patch should not be used for postoperative or acute pain
- Avoid use if suspected paralytic ileus
- Avoid use within 14 days of a MAO inhibitor

◉ Fentanyl

Brand Names

Actiq, Duragesic, Fentora, Sublimaze, Onsolis, Lazanda

Generic Name

Fentanyl

Rx Only

Class II controlled substance

Dosage Forms

Transdermal patch, buccal tablets, buccal film, buccal lozenge, nasal spray, sublingual spray, injection

Usage

Severe pain*

Pregnancy Category C

Dosing

- Initial dose:
  - Transdermal patch: 12.5–25 µg/hour every 72 hours
  - Buccal: 200 µg every 3 hours as needed
  - IV:
    - Single dose: 25–100 µg
    - Infusion: 1 µg/kg per hour
- Maintenance dose: Titrate to response; usual basal rate < 50 µg/hr IV
- Maximum dose: Usually 4 patches for the transdermal system (limited by skin surface area); no maximum dose based on efficacy
- Epidural:
  - Single dose: 25–100 µg
  - Continuous infusion: 25–100 µg/hour
- Intrathecal: 5–25 µg/dose
- Nasal and sublingual spray: Initial 100 µg/dose/spray

Adverse Reactions: Most Common

Constipation, nausea, vomiting, sedation, dizziness, xerostomia, pruritus (histamine release), skin rash (transdermal)

Adverse Reactions: Rare/Severe/Important

Hallucinations, hypotension, respiratory and CNS depression

Major Drug Interactions

Drugs Affecting Fentanyl

- Amphetamines: Increase analgesic effects
- Antipsychotic agents: Enhance hypotensive effects
- CNS depressants (including alcohol): Increase sedation and dizziness
- MAO inhibitors: Serotonin syndrome
- Strong and moderate inhibitors of CYP3A4: Decrease metabolism

Fentanyl's Effect on Other Drugs

CNS depressants: Additive respiratory and CNS depressant effects

Counseling Points

- Wear for 72 hours; then replace with a new patch
- Rotate the application sites of the transdermal system to reduce skin irritation
- Takes 12 hours for onset of effect of the transdermal system
- Never cut patches
- Avoid direct heat on the patches
- Abrupt discontinuation of fentanyl may result in an abstinence syndrome
- Avoid excessive alcohol use
- May cause drowsiness and impair your ability to operate machinery
- May cause constipation requiring laxatives
- May cause physical or psychological dependence with prolonged use
- Notify your healthcare provider if pain is unrelieved
- A new prescription is required for any refill

Key Points

- Fentanyl has a shorter half-life than other opiates in its class
- Avoid use within 14 days of using an MAO inhibitor
- Do not wear transdermal patches during MRI
- Fever and heat can increase absorption of fentanyl
- Transmucosal products should only be used for breakthrough for chronic cancer pain
- When converting patients to fentanyl patch from another narcotic, use a recommended equivalent dose
- Do *not* use buccal and transdermal fentanyl in narcotic naïve patients or for acute and postoperative pain
- Use preservative-free solution for epidural and intrathecal use
- All physicians prescribing the buccal formulations must be registered in REMS program.
- The transmucosal products have specific disposal instructions.

◉ Hydromorphone

Brand Names
Dilaudid, Exalgo

Generic Name
Hydromorphone

Rx Only
Class II controlled substance

Dosage Forms
Liquid oral, immediate-release tablet, extended-release tablet, injection, suppository

Usage
Moderate to severe pain,* antitussive

Pregnancy Category C

Dosing
- Children:
  - Oral: 0.03–0.08 mg/kg per dose every 4 hours as needed
  - IV, IM, SUB-Q: 0.015 mg/kg per dose every 3–4 hours as needed
  - Antitussive dose: 0.5 mg every 3–6 hours
- Initial adult dose:
  - Oral: 2–4 mg every 4 hours as needed
  - SUB-Q, IV, IM: 0.2–0.6 mg every 2–4 hours as needed
  - Epidural: 1–1.5 mg bolus; 0.04–0.4 mg/hour
- Maintenance adult dose:
  - Oral: 2–8 mg PO every 3–4 hours as needed
  - IV, SUB-Q continuous range: 0.1–0.5 mg/hour
  - Rectal: Every 4 hours
  - Oral, IV, SUB-Q: No maximum dose; titrate to response
  - Extended-release: 8–64 mg PO every 24 hours in opioid-tolerant patients only

Adverse Reactions: Most Common
Constipation, nausea, vomiting, sedation, dizziness, xerostomia, pruritus (histamine release)

Adverse Reactions: Rare/Severe/Important
Hallucinations, agitation, respiratory and CNS depression

Major Drug Interactions
Drugs Affecting Hydromorphone
CNS depressants: Increase sedation and dizziness

Hydromorphone's Effect on Other Drugs
- CNS depressants: Additive effect
- MAO inhibitors, SSRIs: Serotonin syndrome

Counseling Points
- May cause drowsiness and impair your ability to operate machinery
- May cause constipation, requiring laxatives
- Avoid alcohol use
- May cause physical or psychological dependence with prolonged use
- After prolonged use, abrupt discontinuation of hydromorphone may result in an abstinence syndrome
- Notify your healthcare provider if pain is unrelieved
- The extended-release tablets must be swallowed whole
- A new prescription is required for any refill

Key Points
- Very soluble in injectable form; useful for continuous pump and epidural or intrathecal administration
- Use only preservative-free solution for the epidural and intrathecal route
- All prescribers of Exalgo, extended-release hydromorphone, must be registered in the REMS program and an FDA-approved patient medication guide must be given every time it is dispensed

◉ Methadone

Brand Names
Methadose, Dolophine

Generic Name
Methadone

Rx Only
Class II controlled substance

Dosage Forms
Tablet, dispersible tablet, injection, oral solution

Usage
Severe pain,* detoxification for opiate addiction* (as part of a program)

Pregnancy Category C

Dosing

- Severe pain:
  - Initial dose:
    - Oral: 5 mg every 6–8 hours
    - IV: 2.5–10 mg every 8–12 hours
  - Maintenance dose: 15–60 mg daily in divided doses
  - Maximum dose: No maximum dose; titrate to response; no ceiling effect
- Addiction:
  - Initial dose: 20–30 mg single daily dose
  - Maintenance: 40–120 mg single daily dose
- Renal dosage adjustment: If CrCl < 10 mL/min, reduce dose 50–75%
- Hepatic dosage adjustment: Avoid in severe hepatic dysfunction

Adverse Reactions: Most Common

Constipation, nausea, vomiting, sedation, dizziness, xerostomia, pruritus (histamine release)

Adverse Reactions: Rare/Severe/Important

Hallucinations, hypotension, respiratory and CNS depression, ECG changes; QT interval prolongation

Major Drug Interactions

Drugs Affecting Methadone

- CNS depressants: Increase sedation and dizziness
- Nonnucleoside reverse transcriptase inhibitors (NNRTIs) and protease inhibitors (PIs): Reduce methadone levels
- CYP3A4 inducers: Reduce methadone levels
- CYP3A4 inhibitors: Increase methadone levels
- St. John's wort: Decreases methadone levels
- Grapefruit juice: Decreases absorption

Methadone's Effect on Other Drugs

- CNS depressants: Additive respiratory and CNS depressant effects
- QTc-prolonging agents: Additive risk of ventricular arrhythmias
- Stavudine and didanosine: Decrease bioavailability

Counseling Points

- Abrupt discontinuation of methadone may result in an abstinence syndrome
- Avoid excessive alcohol use
- May cause drowsiness and impair your ability to operate machinery
- May cause constipation, requiring laxatives
- May cause physical or psychological dependence with prolonged use
- Notify your healthcare provider if pain is unrelieved
- A new prescription is required for any refill

Key Points

- May prolong QT interval and increase risk for torsade de pointes. Patients should be evaluated for risk. ECG monitoring may be necessary within 1 month of initiation and annually.

- When converting patients to methadone from another narcotic, use a calculated equivalent dose, which is dependent on the daily equivalent dose of morphine
- Accumulation can occur with extended use because of the long half-life
- Monitor for sedation with extended use
- Discontinue slowly after prolonged use
- It is unlawful to dispense methadone for addiction maintenance without a license
- Methadone administration for opioid addiction is permitted during inpatient care, when the patient was admitted for any condition other than concurrent opioid addiction, to facilitate the treatment of the primary admitting diagnosis

◉ Morphine

Brand Names

Astramorph, Avinza, Kadian, MS Contin, Oramorph, Roxanol, various others

Generic Name

Morphine

Rx Only

Class II controlled substance

Dosage Forms

Immediate- and sustained-release tablets, injection, oral solution, suppository

Usage

Moderate to severe pain*

Pregnancy Category C

Dosing

- Children:
  - Oral: 0.2–0.5 mg/kg per dose every 4 hours as needed
  - IV, IM, SUB-Q: 0.1–0.2 mg/kg per dose every 2–4 hours as needed. Usual maximum: 15 mg/dose
  - IV, SUB-Q continuous:
    - Sickle cell or cancer pain: 0.025–2 mg/kg per hour
    - Postoperative pain: 0.01–0.04 mg/kg per hour
- Initial adult dose:
  - Oral:
    - Immediate release: 10–30 mg PO every 4 hours as needed
    - Controlled release: 15–30 mg PO every 12 hours (opioid naive)
  - SUB-Q, IV, IM: 2.5 mg–10 mg every 2–4 hours as needed
  - IV, SUB-Q continuous: 0.5–1 mg/hour
  - Epidural: 5 mg

- Maintenance adult dose:
  - Oral controlled-release: Usual range 60–200 mg/day in divided doses
  - IV, SUB-Q, IM: 10 mg every 4 hours as needed
  - IV, SUB-Q continuous range: 0.5–10 mg/hour up to 80 mg/hour
  - Rectal: 10–20 mg every 4 hours
- Maximum dose:
  - Oral, IV, SUB-Q: No maximum dose; titrate to response
  - Epidural: 10 mg/24 hours
- Renal dosage adjustment:
  - CrCl 10–50 mL/min: Reduce dose 25%
  - CrCl < 10 mL/min: Reduce dose 50%
  - Dialysis: Administer 50% of normal dose

Adverse Reactions: Most Common

Constipation, nausea, vomiting, sedation, dizziness, xerostomia, pruritus (histamine release)

Adverse Reactions: Rare/Severe/Important

Hallucinations, hypotension, respiratory and CNS depression

Major Drug Interactions

Drugs Affecting Morphine

- Alcohol can disrupt the extended-release characteristic of Avinza
- CNS depressants increase sedation and dizziness

Morphine's Effect on Other Drugs

- CNS depressants: Additive effect
- MAO inhibitors: May cause serotonin syndrome
- SSRIs: May cause serotonin syndrome

Contraindications

MAO inhibitor use (concurrent or within 14 days)

Counseling Points

- May cause drowsiness and impair your ability to operate machinery
- May cause constipation, requiring laxatives
- Avoid alcohol use
- May cause physical or psychological dependence with prolonged use
- After prolonged use, abrupt discontinuation of morphine may result in an abstinence syndrome
- Do not crush or chew the controlled-release products
- Notify your healthcare provider if pain is unrelieved
- A new prescription is required for any refill

Key Points

- Avoid use within 14 days of using an MAO inhibitor
- Contraindicated in paralytic ileus
- Avoid in patients with increase intracranial pressure, such as with head trauma
- The equivalent oral dose is three times more than the IV dose

- Controlled-release products should not be used to treat acute postoperative pain
- Use preservative-free solutions for epidural and intrathecal use

◉ Oxycodone

Brand Names

OxyContin, OxyIR, Roxicodone

Generic Name

Oxycodone

Rx Only

Class II controlled substance

Dosage Forms

Capsule, oral liquid, oral concentrate, immediate- and controlled-release tablets

Usage

Moderate to severe pain*

Pregnancy Category C

Dosing

- Initial dose:
  - 5–15 mg PO every 4–6 hours as needed
  - 10 mg extended-release PO: Every 12 hours (opioid naive)
- Maintenance extended-release dose: 20–160 mg PO every 12 hours
- Maximum dose: No maximum dose; titrate to response
- Pediatric dose (6–12 years): 1.25 mg PO every 6 hours as needed

Adverse Reactions: Most Common

Constipation, nausea, vomiting, sedation, dizziness, xerostomia, pruritus (histamine release)

Adverse Reactions: Rare/Severe/Important

Hallucinations, hypotension, respiratory and CNS depression

Major Drug Interactions

Drugs Affecting Oxycodone

CNS depressants: Increase sedation and dizziness

Oxycodone's Effect on Other Drugs

- CNS depressants: Additive effect
- MAO inhibitors: May cause serotonin syndrome
- SSRIs: May cause serotonin syndrome

Counseling Points

- May cause drowsiness and impair your ability to operate machinery
- May cause constipation requiring laxatives
- Avoid alcohol use

- May cause physical or psychological dependence with prolonged use
- After prolonged use, abrupt discontinuation of oxycodone may result in an abstinence syndrome
- Do not crush or chew the controlled-release products
- Notify your healthcare provider if pain is unrelieved
- A new prescription is required for any refill

Key Points

- Commonly found in combination products with acetaminophen and ibuprofen
- Only available in oral formulations
- Controlled-release products should not be used to treat acute postoperative pain
- Deaths due to overdose have been reported due to misuse/abuse after crushing the sustained-release tablets

⊙ Tapentadol

Brand Names

Nucynta, Nucynta ER

Generic Name

Tapentadol

Rx Only

Class II controlled substance

Dosage Forms

Tablet, extended-release tablet

Usage

Moderate to severe pain*

Pregnancy Category C

Dosing

- Acute pain: 50–100 mg every 4–6 hours as needed; maximum daily dose on day 1 of 700 mg/day and 600 mg/day on subsequent days
- Chronic pain: Extended-release 50 mg PO every 12 hours initially, up to a maximum of 500 mg/day; may titrate every 3 days
- Moderate hepatic impairment: Decrease immediate-release dosing to 50 mg every 8 hours or extended-release to 50 mg every 24 hours
- Severe renal impairment: Use not recommended
- Severe hepatic impairment: Use not recommended

Adverse Reactions: Most Common

Sedation, hypotension, dizziness, nausea, vomiting, constipation, pruritus

Adverse Reactions: Rare/Severe/Important

Serotonin syndrome, seizure, respiratory depression

Major Drug Interactions

Drugs Affecting Tapentadol

- Alcohol may enhance the CNS depressant effect and increase absorption of extended-release product
- CNS depressants may increase the sedation
- MAO inhibitors, TCAs, and SSRIs may increase the risk of seizures and serotonin syndrome
- Naloxone may induce a seizure

Tapentadol's Effect on Other Drugs

CNS depressants: Additive respiratory and CNS depressant effects

Contraindications

Use of MAO inhibitors within 14 days

Counseling Points

- May cause drowsiness and impair your ability to operate machinery
- May cause constipation requiring laxatives
- Avoid alcohol use
- May cause physical or psychological dependence with prolonged use
- After prolonged use, abrupt discontinuation may result in an abstinence syndrome
- Do not crush or chew the extended-release products
- Notify your healthcare provider if pain is unrelieved
- A new prescription is required for any refill

Key Points

- Only available in oral formulations
- Extended-release products are not intended for the management of acute or postoperative pain
- An FDA-approved patient medication guide must be given every time it is dispensed
- May be confused with tramadol
- Use caution in patients with a seizure history

⊙ Tramadol

Brand Names

ConZip, Rybix ODT, Ultram, Ultram ER, Ultracet

Generic Name

Tramadol

Rx Only

Dosage Forms

Immediate-release tablet, orally disintegrating tablet, extended-release tablet; Ultracet is a combination with acetaminophen

Usage

Moderate* to severe pain, neuropathic pain

Pregnancy Category C

Dosing

- Initial dose: 50 mg PO every 4–6 hours as needed
- Maintenance dose: 50–100 mg every 4–6 hours as needed
- Maximum dose: 400 mg/day; 300 mg/day extended-release products
- Hepatic dosage adjustment: 50 mg immediate-release PO every 12 hours
- Renal dosage adjustment: 50–100 mg immediate-release PO every 12 hours (maximum: 200 mg/day)

Adverse Reactions: Most Common

Sedation, dizziness, constipation, nausea and vomiting, somnolence, euphoria/dysphoria

Adverse Reactions: Rare/Severe/Important

Hypotension, seizures at ≥ 500 mg/day (discontinuation)

Major Drug Interactions

Drugs Affecting Tramadol

- Carbamazepine: Decreases tramadol levels
- MAO inhibitors, TCAs, and SSRIs: May increase the risk of seizures and serotonin syndrome
- Naloxone: May induce a seizure

Tramadol's Effect on Other Drugs

CNS depressants: Additive respiratory and CNS depressant effects

Counseling Points

- Extended-release tablets must be swallowed whole
- May cause drowsiness
- Abrupt discontinuation may result in withdrawal symptoms

Key Points

- Serotonin syndrome or seizures can occur when combined with antidepressants
- Use with caution in patients with a seizure history
- Tramadol has the potential for abuse
- It is *not* a controlled substance
- May be confused with tapentadol, Toradol, or trazodone

NARCOTIC/NON-NARCOTIC COMBINATIONS

Introduction

Narcotic combinations are common agents prescribed for management of moderate pain. The nonopioid is most commonly ibuprofen or acetaminophen, which works as a coanalgesic. The side effects of the individual components must be considered. These drugs are classified as controlled substances and have the risk of abuse and diversion.

Mechanism of Action for the Drug Class

The narcotic component binds to opioid μ-receptors, altering the perception and response to pain. The non-narcotic analgesic inhibits brain prostaglandin synthesis.

Contraindications of the Drug Class

Significant respiratory depression (in unmonitored settings), acute or severe bronchial asthma, hypercapnia, paralytic ileus

Members of the Drug Class

In this section: Codeine/acetaminophen, hydrocodone/acetaminophen, hydrocodone/ibuprofen, oxycodone/acetaminophen
Others: Pseudoephedrine/hydrocodone/chlorpheniramine

⊙ Codeine/Acetaminophen

Brand Names

Capital and Codeine, Tylenol 2, Tylenol 3, Tylenol 4, Tylenol with Codeine

Generic Name

Codeine/acetaminophen

Rx Only

Tablets: Class III controlled substance
Solution: Class V controlled substance

Dosage Forms

Tablet, oral solution

Usage

Mild to moderate pain,* antitussive

Pregnancy Category C

Dosing

- Children: 0.5–1 mg codeine/kg per dose every 4–6 hours *or*
  - 3–6 years: 5 mL every 6 hours of elixir
  - 7–12 years: 10 mL every 6 hours of elixir
  - > 12 years: 15 mL every 4 hours of elixir

- Adult:
  - Antitussive: 15–30 mg codeine every 4–6 hours
  - Pain: 30–60 mg codeine every 4–6 hours
  - Maximum dose: 4,000 mg of acetaminophen component/day (2,000 mg in chronic alcoholics)
- Renal dosage adjustment:
  - CrCl 10–50 mL/min: Reduce dose 25%
  - CrCl < 10 mL/min: Reduce dose 50%
- Hepatic dosage adjustment: Limit acetaminophen component to < 2 g/day and avoid in cirrhosis patients

Adverse Reactions: Most Common

Constipation, nausea, vomiting, sedation, dizziness, xerostomia, pruritus

Adverse Reactions: Rare/Severe/Important

Hallucinations, hypotension, respiratory and CNS depression, hepatotoxicity (exceeding acetaminophen dosing recommendations)

Major Drug Interactions

Drugs Affecting Codeine/Acetaminophen

- CYP2D6 inhibitors: Prevent conversion of codeine to its active metabolite morphine
- CNS depressants: Increase sedation and dizziness
- Ethanol use: > 3 drinks/day may increase risk of hepatotoxicity
- Isoniazid: May increase the risk hepatotoxicity

Codeine/Acetaminophen's Effect on Other Drugs

- Warfarin: Increased anticoagulant effect
- CNS depressants: Additive effects

Counseling Points

- May cause drowsiness and impair your ability to operate machinery
- May cause constipation, requiring laxatives
- Avoid alcohol use
- May cause physical or psychological dependence with prolonged use
- After prolonged use, abrupt discontinuation may result in an abstinence syndrome
- Notify your healthcare provider if pain is unrelieved

Key Points

- Differences in individual metabolism means that some patients will not convert codeine to its active form, necessitating the use of other agents; others may be ultrarapid metabolizers of codeine, producing higher levels of morphine and leading to more numerous or intense adverse effects
- Caution during breastfeeding; use lowest possible effective dose
- Controlled substance
- Do not exceed acetaminophen daily dosing recommendations

◉ Hydrocodone/Acetaminophen

Brand Names

Lorcet, Lortab, Norco Vicodin, Zydone, various others

Generic Name

Hydrocodone/acetaminophen

Rx Only

Class III controlled substance

Dosage Forms

Tablet, capsule, oral solution

Usage

Moderate pain*

Pregnancy Category C

Dosing

- Children: < 50 kg; 0.1–0.2 mg/kg per dose hydrocodone component every 4–6 hours
- Usual adult dose: 1–2 tablets every 4–6 hours or 5–10 mL elixir every 4–6 hours
- Maximum dose: 4,000 mg of acetaminophen component/day (2,000 mg in chronic alcoholics)

Adverse Reactions: Most Common

Constipation, nausea, vomiting, sedation, dizziness, xerostomia, pruritus (histamine release)

Adverse Reactions: Rare/Severe/Important

Hallucinations, hypotension, respiratory and CNS depression, hepatotoxicity (exceeding acetaminophen dosing recommendations)

Major Drug Interactions

Drugs Affecting Hydrocodone/Acetaminophen

- CNS depressants: Increase sedation and dizziness
- Ethanol use: > 3 drinks/day may increase risk of hepatotoxicity
- Isoniazid: May increase the risk hepatotoxicity

Hydrocodone/Acetaminophen's Effect on Other Drugs

- Warfarin: Increases anticoagulant effect
- CNS depressants: Additive effect

Counseling Points

- May cause drowsiness and impair your ability to operate machinery
- May cause constipation, requiring laxatives
- Avoid alcohol use
- May cause physical or psychological dependence with prolonged use
- After prolonged use, abrupt discontinuation may result in an abstinence syndrome
- Notify your healthcare provider if pain is unrelieved

Key Points
- Schedule III controlled substance
- Do not exceed acetaminophen daily dosing recommendations

◉ Hydrocodone/Ibuprofen

Brand Names
Ibudone, Reprexain, Vicoprofen

Generic Name
Hydrocodone/ibuprofen

Rx Only
Class II controlled substance

Dosage Form
Tablet

Usage
Moderate pain*

Pregnancy Category C

Dosing
- Usual adult dose: 1 tablet every 4–6 hours
- Maximum dose: 5 tablets per day

Adverse Reactions: Most Common
Constipation, nausea, vomiting, sedation, dizziness, xerostomia, pruritus (histamine release), dyspepsia

Adverse Reactions: Rare/Severe/Important
Hallucinations, hypotension, respiratory and CNS depression, edema, renal impairment, GI bleeding or ulcers, increased blood pressure

Major Drug Interactions
Drugs Affecting Hydrocodone/Ibuprofen

CNS depressants: Sedation and dizziness

Hydrocodone/Ibuprofen's Effect on Other Drugs
- Anticoagulants: Enhanced anticoagulation
- Antihypertensives: Decreased effects
- Aspirin: Increased bleeding
- CNS depressants: Additive effects
- Lithium: Increased concentration
- MAO inhibitors and SSRIs: Serotonin syndrome

Contraindications
Asthma, urticaria, or allergic-type reactions to aspirin or other NSAIDs; perioperative pain in the setting of coronary artery bypass graft (CABG) surgery

Counseling Points
- May cause drowsiness and impair your ability to operate machinery
- May cause constipation, requiring laxatives
- Avoid alcohol use
- May cause physical or psychological dependence with prolonged use

- After prolonged use, abrupt discontinuation may result in an abstinence syndrome
- Notify your healthcare provider if pain is unrelieved

Key Points
- Schedule III controlled substance
- Do not exceed daily dosing recommendations

◉ Oxycodone/Acetaminophen

Brand Names
Endocet, Percocet, Roxicet, Tylox

Generic Name
Oxycodone/acetaminophen

Rx Only
Class II controlled substance

Dosage Forms
Capsule, caplet, tablet, oral liquid

Usage
Moderate or severe pain*

Dosing
- Initial dose:
  - Tablets: 1–2 tablets every 4–6 hours
  - Oral solution: 5–10 mL oral solution every 4–6 hours
- Maximum dose: 3,000 mg acetaminophen/day (2,000 mg/day in chronic alcoholics)

Major Drug Interactions
Drugs Affecting Oxycodone/Acetaminophen
- CNS depressants: Increase sedation and dizziness
- Ethanol use: > 3 drinks/day may increase risk of hepatotoxicity
- Isoniazid: May increase the risk hepatotoxicity

Oxycodone/Acetaminophen's Effect on Other Drugs
- Warfarin: Increases anticoagulant effect
- CNS depressants: Additive effect

Counseling Points
- May cause drowsiness and impair your ability to operate machinery
- May cause constipation, requiring laxatives
- Avoid alcohol use
- May cause physical or psychological dependence with prolonged use
- Notify your healthcare provider if pain is unrelieved
- A new prescription is required for any refill

Key Points
- Multiple combinations of oxycodone/acetaminophen are available in various strengths. Prescriptions and orders for this drug must include the strength desired.
- Schedule II controlled substance
- Do not exceed acetaminophen daily dosing recommendations

NONSTEROIDAL ANTI-INFLAMMATORY DRUGS, SELECTIVE COX-2 INHIBITORS

Introduction

The selective COX-2 inhibitor celecoxib is commonly used for mild pain syndromes, such as arthritis, with the benefit of a lower incidence of GI ulcers than nonselective NSAIDs. Its use is complicated by a small but significant increase in cardiovascular events such as stroke and myocardial infarction. Although celecoxib has less GI toxicity than nonselective NSAIDs, many of the same warnings, adverse effects, and counseling points apply.

Mechanism of Action for the Drug Class

Inhibits prostaglandin synthesis by decreasing the activity of the enzyme COX-2, which results in decreased formation of prostaglandin precursors. COX-2 inhibitors do not appear to block COX-1 as extensively as nonselective NSAIDs, decreasing their toxicity to the GI mucosa.

Members of the Drug Class

Celecoxib

◉ Celecoxib

Brand Name

Celebrex

Generic Name

Celecoxib

Rx Only

Dosage Form

Capsule

Usage

Relief of the signs and symptoms of osteoarthritis,* ankylosing spondylitis, juvenile idiopathic arthritis (JIA), and rheumatoid arthritis*; management of acute pain; treatment of primary dysmenorrhea

Pregnancy Category C (Prior to 30 Weeks Gestation) and D (≥ 30 Weeks Gestation)

Dosing

- Osteoarthritis: 200 mg/day PO as a single dose or in divided doses twice daily
- Ankylosing spondylitis:
  - Initial dose: 200 mg/day PO as a single dose or in divided doses twice daily
  - If no effect after 6 weeks, may increase to 400 mg/day
  - If no response following 6 weeks of treatment with 400 mg/day, consider discontinuation and alternative treatment
  - Canadian labeling: Recommended maximum dose of 200 mg/day

- Rheumatoid arthritis: 100–200 mg PO twice daily
- Acute pain or primary dysmenorrhea:
  - Initial dose: 400 mg, followed by an additional 200 mg if needed on day 1
  - Maintenance dose: 200 mg twice daily as needed
- Renal dosage adjustment: Avoid in advanced renal disease
- Hepatic dosage adjustment: Reduce 50% in moderate impairment; not recommended in severe impairment

Adverse Reactions: Most Common

Nausea, GI ulcers, peripheral edema, hypertension, headache, diarrhea

Adverse Reactions: Rare/Severe/Important

GI ulcers, bleeding, and perforation; thrombosis, including MI and stroke; renal toxicity; exfoliative dermatitis; Stevens-Johnson syndrome; toxic epidermal necrolysis; fulminant hepatitis; liver failure; acute renal failure

Major Drug Interactions

Drugs Affecting Celecoxib

- Antacids: Decrease absorption of celecoxib
- Corticosteroids: Increase GI side effects
- Ethanol: Increased GI irritation
- Fluconazole: Can increase concentrations of celecoxib

Celecoxib's Effect on Other Drugs

- ACE inhibitors and angiotensin II receptor blockers: Decrease antihypertensive effect and increase renal toxicity
- Anticoagulants: Increase bleeding risk
- Aspirin: Increases bleeding risk; diminishes cardioprotective effect
- Cyclosporine: Increases cyclosporine levels
- Diuretics: Decreased effects
- Lithium: Increased concentrations

Contraindications

Hypersensitivity to celecoxib, sulfonamides, aspirin, and other NSAIDs; perioperative pain in the setting of coronary artery bypass graft (CABG) surgery

Counseling Points

- Be informed about signs and symptoms of GI bleeding
- Take with food if GI upset occurs
- Report any abnormal swelling or bleeding to your healthcare provider
- Call your healthcare provider if your pain does not improve
- This medicine can increase your cardiovascular risk

Key Points

- Use with caution in patients with fluid retention, congestive heart failure, renal insufficiency, or hypertension

- Use of NSAIDs can compromise renal function. Renal toxicity is more likely to occur in patients with impaired renal function, dehydration, heart failure, liver dysfunction, those taking diuretics and ACE inhibitors, and the elderly. Monitor renal function closely. Not recommended for use in patients with advanced renal disease.
- Black box warning: Increased risk for thrombosis, stroke, and myocardial infarction
- Elderly are at increased risk for GI ulcers, CNS effects, and renal toxicities
- Patients with hypersensitivity reactions to sulfonamides (especially nonantibiotic sulfonamides) should avoid celecoxib

- Patients with "aspirin triad" (bronchial asthma, aspirin intolerance, rhinitis) may be at increased risk of hypersensitivity. Do not use in patients who experience bronchospasm, asthma, rhinitis, or urticaria with NSAID or aspirin therapy.
- GI events may occur at any time during therapy and without warning. Use caution with a history of GI disease (bleeding or ulcers); concurrent therapy with aspirin, anticoagulants, and/or corticosteroids; smoking; use of alcohol; and the elderly or debilitated patients.
- Celecoxib does not inhibit platelets or prolong bleeding time

NONSTEROIDAL ANTI-INFLAMMATORY DRUGS

Introduction

Nonsteroidal anti-inflammatory drugs (NSAIDs) are commonly used for mild pain symptoms. They possess both anti-inflammatory and antipyretic effects. The use of these agents is complicated by their GI side effects and cardiovascular risks. Ibuprofen and naproxen are two agents in the class that are available OTC and found in many common cold and headache formulations. NSAIDs have many characteristics in common, and they are listed here. Agent-specific characteristics are listed with the individual agents.

Mechanism of Action of the Drug Class

Inhibit prostaglandin synthesis by decreasing the activity of COX enzymes 1 and 2, resulting in decreased formation of prostaglandin precursors associated with inflammation and pain

Adverse Reactions for the Drug Class: Most Common

Nausea, gastritis, abdominal cramps, GI ulcers, peripheral edema, hypertension, diarrhea

Adverse Reactions for the Drug Class: Rare/Severe/Important

GI perforation and bleeding, renal toxicity, acute renal failure, angioedema, bronchoconstriction, asthma, rash, tinnitus, hearing loss

Major Drug Interactions for the Drug Class

Drugs Affecting NSAIDs
- Corticosteroids: Increased GI side effects
- Ethanol: Increased GI irritation

NSAIDs' Effects on Other Drugs
- ACE inhibitors and angiotensin II receptor blockers: Decrease antihypertensive effect
- Anticoagulants: Increase bleeding risk

- Antiplatelet therapy: Increases bleeding risk
- Beta blockers: Diminish effect
- Digoxin: Increase level
- Diuretics: Diminish diuretic effect
- Heparin: Increases anticoagulant effect
- Warfarin: Enhances anticoagulant effect
- Lithium: Increased concentrations, possible toxicity

Contraindications for the Drug Class

Hypersensitivity to aspirin or NSAIDS, peptic ulcer disease, perioperative pain with coronary artery bypass graft (CABG) surgery

Counseling Points for the Drug Class

- Be aware of the signs and symptoms of GI bleeding
- Take with food if GI upset occurs
- Report any abnormal swelling or bleeding to your healthcare provider
- Call your healthcare provider if your pain does not improve
- This medicine can increase your cardiovascular risk (except aspirin, which is cardioprotective)

Key Points for the Drug Class

- Use with caution in patients with fluid retention, congestive heart failure, renal insufficiency, or hypertension. They are not contraindicated in these disease states, but they may worsen them in some situations.
- Use of NSAIDs can compromise existing renal function. Renal toxicity can occur in patients with impaired renal function, dehydration, heart failure, liver dysfunction, those taking diuretics and ACE inhibitors, and the elderly. Monitor renal function closely.
- May increase risk for thrombosis, stroke, and myocardial infarction
- Elderly patients are at increased risk for GI ulcers, CNS effects, and renal toxicities

- Patients with "aspirin triad" (bronchial asthma, aspirin intolerance, rhinitis) may be at increased risk of hypersensitivity. Do not use in patients who experience bronchospasm, asthma, rhinitis, or urticaria with NSAID or aspirin therapy.
- GI events may occur at any time during therapy and without warning. Use caution with a history of GI disease (bleeding or ulcers), concurrent therapy with aspirin, anticoagulants, and/or corticosteroids, smoking, use of alcohol, the elderly or debilitated patients. The concurrent use of proton pump inhibitors or histamine-2 antagonists may reduce the risk of GI ulcers in high-risk patients.

Members of the Drug Class

In this section: Aspirin, diclofenac, etodolac, ibuprofen, indomethacin, ketorolac, meloxicam, nabumetone, naproxen
Others: Diflunisal, fenoprofen, flurbiprofen, ketoprofen meclofenamate, mefenamic acid, oxaprozin, piroxicam, sulindac, tolmetin

◉ Aspirin

Brand Names
Bayer, Bufferin, Ecotrin, Excedrin, various others

Generic Name
Aspirin

OTC

Dosage Forms
Enteric-coated, buffered, chewable, and controlled-release tablets; gum; suppository

Usage
Treatment of mild to moderate pain,* inflammation, and fever; prevention and treatment of MI,* acute ischemic stroke,* and transient ischemic episodes*; management of rheumatoid arthritis, rheumatic fever, osteoarthritis, and gout (high dose); adjunctive therapy in revascularization procedures (CABG,* PTCA, carotid endarterectomy*), and stent implantation*

Pregnancy Category
No formal category, but it is contraindicated except for low doses

Dosing
- Adults:
  - Antiplatelet indications: 50–325 mg daily
  - Pain and inflammation:
    - Oral: 325–650 mg every 4–6 hours up to 4 g/day
    - Rectal: 300–600 mg every 4–6 hours up to 4 g/day
- Pediatrics:
  - Analgesic and antipyretic: Oral, rectal: 10–15 mg/kg/dose every 4–6 hours, up to a total of 4 g/day

- Anti-inflammatory:
  - Initial: 60–90 mg/kg per day PO in divided doses
  - Maintenance: 80–100 mg/kg per day PO in divided doses every 6–8 hours
- Severe renal and hepatic impairment: Avoid use

Adverse Reactions: Rare/Severe/Important
Reye's syndrome (children)

Major Drug Interactions (in addition to those of the class)
Drugs Affecting Aspirin
- Ginkgo biloba: Increases antiplatelet effect
- Other NSAIDs: Increase bleeding risk

Aspirin's Effect on Other Drugs
- ACE inhibitors: Diminish the antihypertensive effect
- Anticoagulants: Increase bleeding risk

Contraindications
Hypersensitivity to salicylates, other NSAIDs, or any component of the formulation; nasal polyps; inherited or acquired bleeding disorders (including factor VII and factor IX deficiency); do not use in children (< 16 years of age) for viral infections (chickenpox or flu symptoms), with or without fever, due to a potential association with Reye's syndrome

Counseling Points
- High-dose aspirin should only be used short term for pain
- Report any signs of bruising or bleeding, nausea, or vomiting to your healthcare provider
- Do not use aspirin with a strong vinegar-like odor
- Take with food or milk

Key Points
- Do not use in children during viral infections due to the potential for Reye's syndrome, a rare but life-threatening disorder associated with aspirin use during viral infections
- Contraindicated during pregnancy and in patients with bleeding disorders
- Aspirin therapy should be stopped 1 week prior to surgery to reduce bleeding risk unless otherwise indicated by physician

◉ Diclofenac

Brand Names
Flector, Pennsaid, Solaraze, Voltaren

Generic Name
Diclofenac

Rx Only

Dosage Forms

Capsule, tablet, delayed-release enteric tablet, extended-release tablet, topical gel, topical solution, transdermal patch, ophthalmic solution

Usage

Acute treatment for mild to moderate pain,* dysmenorrhea,* osteoarthritis,* rheumatoid arthritis,* ankylosing spondylitis, postoperative inflammation following eye surgery, actinic keratosis, migraine

Pregnancy Category

- Topical gel 3%: Category B
- Oral, ophthalmic, or topical gel 1%, topical solution, topical patch: Category C
- Oral or topical solution ≥ 30 weeks gestation: Category D

Dosing

- Analgesia: 50 mg PO three times daily
- Primary dysmenorrhea: 150–200 mg PO daily in divided doses
- Rheumatoid arthritis and osteoarthritis:
  - 150–200 mg/day in divided doses
  - Extended-release: 100–200 mg daily
- Ankylosing spondylitis: Delayed-release tablet 100–125 mg/day in four to five divided doses
- Migraine: Oral solution 50 mg as a single dose at the time of migraine onset
- Topical gel 1%:
  - Upper extremities: 2 g to affected area four times daily
  - Lower extremities: 4 g to affected area four times daily
- Topical patch: 1 patch daily to painful site
- Topical solution: Apply 40 drops four times daily to each affected knee
- Cataract surgery: Instill 1 drop ophthalmic solution into affected eye four times daily beginning 24 hours after cataract surgery and continuing for 2 weeks
- Corneal refractive surgery: Instill 1–2 drops ophthalmic solution into affected eye within the hour prior to surgery, within 15 minutes following surgery, and then continue four times daily for up to 3 days

Contraindications

Hypersensitivity to bovine protein (capsule formulation only)

◉ Etodolac

Brand Name
Lodine

Generic Name
Etodolac

Rx Only

Dosage Forms

Tablet, capsule, extended-release tablet

Usage

Acute treatment for mild to moderate pain,* osteoarthritis,* rheumatoid arthritis*

Pregnancy Category C

Dosing

- Acute pain: 200–400 mg every 6–8 hours as needed, maximum dose of 1,000 mg/day
- Rheumatoid arthritis, osteoarthritis:
  - Immediate-release formulation: 400 mg twice daily or 300 mg two to three daily or 500 mg twice daily (doses > 1,000 mg/day have not been evaluated)
  - Extended-release formulation: 400–1,000 mg once daily
- Children (6–16 years) for juvenile rheumatoid arthritis: 400–1,000 mg daily depending on weight using extended-release product
- Dosing in renal impairment: Avoid use in severe impairment

Counseling Points

- Be aware of the signs and symptoms of GI bleeding
- Take with food if GI upset occurs
- Report any abnormal swelling or bleeding to your healthcare provider
- Call your healthcare provider if your pain does not improve
- This medicine can increase your cardiovascular risk

◉ Ibuprofen

Brand Names
Motrin, Caldolor, NeoProfen, Advil, Motrin, Excedrin IB, Haltran, Ibuprin, Midol 200, Nuprin, Pamprin IB, Trendar, Uni-Pro

Generic Name
Ibuprofen

OTC and Rx (Injection)

Dosage Forms

Tablet, chewable tablet, caplet, oral infant drops, oral suspension, injection

Usage

Acute treatment for mild to moderate pain,* acute treatment for gout,* osteoarthritis*, rheumatoid arthritis, antipyretic, dysmenorrhea,* patent ductus arteriosus, ankylosing spondylitis, cystic fibrosis

Pregnancy Category C

Pregnancy category D after ≥ 30 weeks gestation

Dosing

- Adults:
  - Inflammatory disease: 400–800 mg PO three to four times a day; maximum 3.2 g/day
  - Analgesia/pain/fever/dysmenorrhea: 200–400 mg PO every 4–6 hours (maximum daily dose: 1.2 g, unless directed by physician; under physician supervision, daily doses ≤ 2.4 g may be used)
  - Analgesic IV: 400–800 mg every 6 hours as needed (maximum: 3.2 g/day)
  - Antipyretic IV: Initial dose of 400 mg, then every 4–6 hours or 100–200 mg every 4 hours as needed (maximum: 3.2 g/day)
  - Analgesic, antipyretic OTC labeling: 200 mg PO every 4–6 hours as needed (maximum: 1,200 mg/24 hours)
  - Migraine OTC labeling: 2 capsules or tablets at the onset of symptoms (maximum: 400 mg/24 hours)
- Children:
  - Antipyretic for ages 6 months to 12 years:
    - Temperature < 102.5°F (39°C): 5 mg/kg PO
    - Temperature > 102.5°F (39°C): 10 mg/kg PO given every 6–8 hours
    - Maximum daily dose: 40 mg/kg/day
  - Juvenile idiopathic arthritis (JIA): 30–50 mg/kg every 24 hours PO divided every 8 hours; start at lower end of dosing range and titrate upward (maximum: 2.4 g/day)
  - Analgesic: 4–10 mg/kg PO every 6–8 hours
  - Chronic (> 4 years) cystic fibrosis (unlabeled use): Twice-daily PO dosing adjusted to maintain serum concentration of 50–100 µg/mL has been associated with slowing of disease progression in younger patients with mild lung disease
  - Patent ductus arteriosus: IV ibuprofen lysine (NeoProfen): Infants between 500–1,500 g and ≤ 32 weeks gestational age should receive initial dose of ibuprofen 10 mg/kg, followed by two doses of 5 mg/kg at 24 and 48 hours. Dose should be based on birth weight.

Adverse Reactions: Most Common

Infant injection: Skin irritation, intraventricular hemorrhage, hypocalcemia, hypoglycemia, anemia, sepsis, apnea

Adverse Reactions: Rare/Severe/Important

Injection: Electrolyte imbalances, hemorrhage

Contraindications

Ibuprofen injection: Preterm infants with untreated proven or suspected infection; congenital heart disease where patency of the PDA is necessary for pulmonary or systemic blood flow; bleeding (especially with active intracranial hemorrhage or GI bleed); thrombocytopenia; coagulation defects; proven or suspected necrotizing enterocolitis (NEC); significant renal dysfunction

Key Point

Patients should be well hydrated prior to the administration of IV ibuprofen

◉ Indomethacin

Brand Names

Indocin, Indocin SR

Generic Name

Indomethacin

Rx Only

Dosage Forms

Capsule, extended-release capsule, injection, suspension, suppository

Usage

Pain and inflammation associated with rheumatoid disorders, moderate to severe osteoarthritis,* acute gout,* acute bursitis/tendonitis, ankylosing spondylitis, patent ductus arteriosus*

Pregnancy Category C

Dosing

- Initial: 25–50 mg two to three times daily; sustained-release capsules should be given one to two times daily; maximum dose 200 mg daily
- Inflammatory/rheumatoid disorders (use lowest effective dose):
  - Oral, rectal: 25–50 mg/dose two to three times a day; maximum dose is 200 mg/day
  - Extended-release capsule: Should be given once or twice a day (maximum dose: 150 mg/day). In patients with arthritis and persistent night pain and/or morning stiffness, may give the larger portion (up to 100 mg) of the total daily dose at bedtime.
- Bursitis/tendonitis, oral, rectal:
  - Initial dose: 75–150 mg/day in three to four divided doses
  - Extended-release: One to two divided doses
  - Usual treatment: 7–14 days
- Acute gouty arthritis, oral, rectal: 50 mg three times daily until pain is tolerable, then reduce dose; usual treatment < 3–5 days
- Patent ductus arteriosus (pediatric-only indication): 0.2 mg/kg IV followed by two doses depending on postnatal age

Adverse Reactions: Most Common

Infant injection: Skin irritation, intraventricular hemorrhage, hypocalcemia, hypoglycemia, anemia, sepsis, apnea

Adverse Reactions: Rare/Severe/Important

Injection: Electrolyte imbalances, hemorrhage

Contraindications

- Suppositories: History of proctitis or recent rectal bleeding
- Neonates: Necrotizing enterocolitis, impaired renal function, active bleeding, thrombocytopenia, coagulation defects, untreated infection, congenital heart disease where patent ductus arteriosus is necessary

◎ Ketorolac

Brand Names

Toradol, Sprix, Acular, Acuvail

Generic Name

Ketorolac

Rx Only

Dosage Forms

Tablet, injection, nasal spray, ophthalmic solution

Usage

Short-term management of moderate-to-severe acute pain,* postoperative pain,* ocular itching due to seasonal allergies, ocular pain, ocular surgery inflammation (ophthalmic)

Pregnancy Category

- Oral, injection, or ophthalmic: C
- Nasal after ≥ 30 weeks gestation: D

Dosing

- Acute pain:
  - IM: 60 mg as a single dose or 30 mg every 6 hours (maximum daily dose: 120 mg)
  - IV: 30 mg as a single dose or 30 mg every 6 hours (maximum daily dose: 120 mg)
  - Oral: 20 mg, followed by 10 mg every 4–6 hours; do not exceed 40 mg/day; oral dosing is intended to be a continuation of IM or IV therapy only
  - Geriatric:
    - ◆ IM: 30 mg as a single dose or 15 mg every 6 hours (maximum daily dose: 60 mg)
    - ◆ IV: 15 mg as a single dose or 15 mg every 6 hours (maximum daily dose: 60 mg)
- Nasal spray:
  - One spray in each nostril every 6–8 hours up to four times daily
  - Adults < 50 kg or ≥ 65 years of age: One spray in one nostril up to four times daily
- Seasonal allergic conjunctivitis (relief of ocular itching): Instill 1 drop (0.25 mg) of ophthalmic solution four times daily
- Inflammation following cataract extraction: Instill 1 drop (0.25 mg) ophthalmic solution to affected eye(s)

four times daily beginning 24 hours after surgery; continue for 2 weeks
- Pain following corneal refractive surgery: Instill 1 drop of ophthalmic solution four times daily as needed to affected eye for up to 4 days

Contraindications

Severe renal impairment, recent or history of GI bleeding or perforation, use before major surgery, suspected or confirmed cerebrovascular bleeding, labor and delivery, breastfeeding

Key Points

- Use lowest effective dose and limit use to 5 days to decrease the risk of ulcers
- Prolonged use may lead to renal toxicity

◎ Meloxicam

Brand Name

Mobic

Generic Name

Meloxicam

Rx Only

Dosage Forms

Tablet, oral suspension

Usage

Osteoarthritis,* rheumatoid arthritis,* juvenile rheumatoid arthritis

Pregnancy Category C

Pregnancy category D ≥ 30 weeks gestation

Dosing

- Adults: 7.5 mg daily up to 15 mg daily
- Children: 0.125 mg/kg per day; maximum dose 7.5 mg daily
- Renal dosage adjustment:
  - Use not recommended in patients with severe impairment
  - No adjustment for mild to moderate impairment

◎ Nabumetone

Brand Name

Relafen

Generic Name

Nabumetone

Rx Only

Dosage Form

Tablet

Usage

Osteoarthritis,* rheumatoid arthritis*

Pregnancy Category C

Dosing

- 1,000 mg/day; maximum 2,000 mg daily
- Renal dosage adjustment:
  - Moderate impairment of CrCl 30–49 mL/min: Initial 750 mg up to 1,500 mg/day
  - Severe impairment of CrCl < 30 mL/min: Initial 500 mg up to 1,000 mg/day

◉ Naproxen

Brand Names

Aleve, Anaprox, Midol, Naprosyn, Pamprin

Generic Name

Naproxen

OTC and Rx

Dosage Forms

Tablet, capsule, controlled-release tablet, enteric-coated tablet, gelcap, suspension

Usage

Acute treatment for mild to moderate pain,* acute treatment for gout, osteoarthritis,* rheumatoid arthritis, bursitis, tendonitis, dysmenorrhea,* fever, migraine headaches

Pregnancy Category C

Dosing

- Gout, acute: Initial 750 mg PO, followed by 250 mg every 8 hours until attack subsides
- Migraine, acute (unlabeled use): Initial 500–750 mg PO; an additional 250–500 mg may be given if needed; maximum: 1,250 mg in 24 hours
- Pain (mild to moderate), dysmenorrhea, acute tendonitis, bursitis: Initial 500 mg PO, then 250 mg every 6–8 hours; maximum: 1,250 mg/day naproxen base
- Rheumatoid arthritis, osteoarthritis, and ankylosing spondylitis: 500–1,000 mg/day in two divided doses; may increase to 1.5 g/day of naproxen base for limited time period
- OTC labeling for pain/fever: 200 mg naproxen base every 8–12 hours; if needed, may take 400 mg naproxen base for the initial dose; maximum: 400 mg naproxen base in any 8- to 12-hour period or 600 mg naproxen base over 24 hours

---

REVIEW QUESTIONS

1. Which of the following agents can be used as an analgesic and antipyretic but does not possess any anti-inflammatory activity?

   a. Acetaminophen
   b. Butalbital
   c. Codeine
   d. Meloxicam

2. Acetaminophen is available in which of the following dosage forms?

   a. Tablet, liquid
   b. Tablet, liquid, suppository
   c. Tablet, liquid, gelcap, suppository, extended-release
   d. Tablet, liquid, gelcap, suppository, extended-release, injection

3. Which of the following is the analgesic of choice during pregnancy?

   a. Ibuprofen
   b. Codeine
   c. Acetaminophen
   d. Butorphanol

4. Acetaminophen has a maximum daily dosing because of which of the following adverse effects?

   a. Gastrointestinal bleeding
   b. Renal toxicity
   c. Hepatic toxicity
   d. Neurotoxicity

5. Fioricet, a combination product used for headaches, contains which of the following?

   a. Butalbital
   b. Butalbital, aspirin
   c. Butalbital, caffeine
   d. Butalbital, caffeine, acetaminophen

6. Which of the following is the maximum dose of Fioricet per day?

   a. 4 tabs
   b. 6 tabs
   c. 8 tabs
   d. 10 tabs

7. Which of the following is both a μ-agonist and an inhibitor of norepinephrine uptake?

   a. Tapentadol
   b. Butorphanol
   c. Buprenorphine
   d. Methadone

8. Which of the following is true regarding buprenorphine?

   a. It is a Class II controlled substance.
   b. It is only available as oral tablets.
   c. It is indicated for moderate to severe pain and opioid dependence.
   d. It is safe and effective for pregnant patients.

9. Butrans should be limited to a maximum dose of 20 μg/hr because of the risk of which of the following?

   a. Sedation
   b. Respiratory depression
   c. QTc prolongation
   d. Constipation

10. Which of the following would be an appropriate use of fentanyl patches?

    a. Acute postoperative pain
    b. Sickle cell crisis
    c. Chronic cancer pain
    d. Labor and delivery pain

11. Which of the following is true regarding fentanyl?

    a. Short-acting buccal fentanyl can only be prescribed by physicians registered in the REMS program.
    b. It is available only in transdermal and injectable forms.
    c. It is a Class III controlled substance.
    d. It has a longer half-life than other narcotics in its class.

12. Which of the following would be an appropriate dose and frequency for fentanyl transdermal?

    a. 25 μg/hr patch changed daily
    b. 50 μg/hr patch changed every 48 hours
    c. 75 μg/hr patch changed every 72 hours
    d. 10 μg/hr patch changed every 48 hours

13. Which of the following is a brand name of a buccal fentanyl product?

    a. Onsolis
    b. Duragesic
    c. Sublimaze
    d. Lazanda

14. Which of the following would an appropriate starting dose of hydromorphone in an adult?

    a. 20 mg PO every 4 hours as needed
    b. 4 mg PO every 4 hours as needed
    c. 64 mg PO daily
    d. 10 mg/hr IV continuous infusion

15. Which of the following is true of methadone?

    a. Any physician can prescribe methadone for opiate addiction.
    b. Methadone has a short half-life.
    c. Methadone is a Schedule II narcotic.
    d. Methadone should not be used for pain.

16. Which of the following monitoring parameters are recommended for methadone?

    a. ECG
    b. Echocardiogram
    c. EEG
    d. EMG

17. Which of the following is true regarding morphine?

    a. It requires no dose adjustment for severe renal impairment.
    b. It is only available in oral and injectable forms.
    c. It can cause constipation, dizziness, and itching.
    d. The extended-release products are recommended for acute pain.

18. Which of the following is a common brand name of extended-release oxycodone?

    a. Roxanol
    b. Opana
    c. OxyContin
    d. Percocet

19. Which of the following is true of oxycodone?

    a. It is a Class III controlled substance.
    b. It is pregnancy category D.
    c. It is available as an injection.
    d. It can cause psychological dependence with prolonged use.

20. Ketorolac is available in which of the following dosage forms?

    a. Tablet, capsule, injection, nasal spray
    b. Tablet, injection, nasal spray
    c. Tablet, injection, nasal spray, ophthalmic solution
    d. Tablet, capsule, injection, nasal spray, ophthalmic solution

21. Which of the following includes all the available dosage forms for tramadol?

    a. Immediate-release tablet
    b. Immediate-release tablet, extended-release tablet
    c. Immediate-release tablet, extended-release tablet, liquid
    d. Immediate-release tablet, extended-release tablet, orally disintegrating tablet

22. Which of the following is *false* with regard to tramadol?
    a. It is indicated for neuropathic pain.
    b. It can increase seizure risk with concurrent use of antidepressants.
    c. The dose should be reduced in cases of renal impairment.
    d. It is a controlled substance.

23. Which of the following narcotics is also commonly used as an antitussive?
    a. Tapentadol
    b. Codeine
    c. Morphine
    d. Hydrocodone

24. Which of the following brand name products contains hydrocodone and acetaminophen?
    a. Ultracet
    b. Percocet
    c. Norco
    d. Tylenol 3

25. Which of following will decrease the conversion of codeine to its active metabolite?
    a. CYP2D6 inducers
    b. CYP2D6 inhibitors
    c. CYP3A4 inducers
    d. CYP3A4 inhibitors

26. Ultrarapid metabolizers of codeine will have which of the following?
    a. No benefit from codeine
    b. Higher levels of morphine
    c. Lower levels of morphine
    d. Less analgesia from the codeine

27. Hydrocodone daily dosing is limited because of which of the following?
    a. It is a poor analgesic.
    b. It can cause seizures at higher doses.
    c. It has a acetaminophen or ibuprofen dosing limit.
    d. It has the potential for addiction.

28. The brand name drug Tylox contains which of the following?
    a. Oxycodone/ibuprofen
    b. Oxymorphone/acetaminophen
    c. Oxycodone/acetaminophen
    d. Hydrocodone/acetaminophen

29. Compared to naproxen, celecoxib has a lower incidence of which of the following adverse events?
    a. Renal toxicity
    b. Elevated blood pressure
    c. Peripheral edema
    d. Gastrointestinal ulcers

30. Which of following is an appropriate dose of celecoxib for osteoarthritis?
    a. 50 mg twice daily
    b. 100 mg twice daily
    c. 200 mg twice daily
    d. 400 mg twice daily

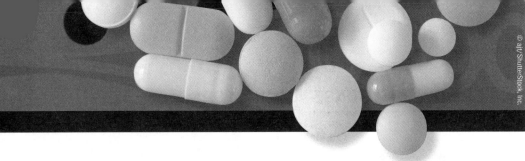

Antidiabetic Agents

Charles Ruchalski, PharmD, BCPS

BIGUANIDES

Introduction

For newly diagnosed patients with type 2 diabetes, the biguanide metformin is the drug of choice for initial therapy, adjunctive to diet and exercise. Metformin is contraindicated in certain patients to prevent lactic acidosis, a rare but serious side effect (approximately 0.03 cases per 1,000 patient-years, with approximately 0.015 fatal cases per 1,000 patient-years). It is often used in combination with other oral antidiabetic agents and/or insulin in patients who do not reach glycemic goals on those therapies. HbA1c reductions with metformin are generally between 1.5% and 2%.

Mechanism of Action for the Drug Class

Biguanides improve glucose tolerance by lowering both basal and postprandial plasma glucose. They decrease hepatic glucose production and intestinal absorption of glucose and improve insulin sensitivity by increasing peripheral glucose uptake and utilization through the activation of adenosine monophosphate-activated protein kinase (AMPK).

⊙ Metformin

Brand Names

Fortamet, Glucophage, Glucophage XR, Glumetza, Riomet

Generic Names

Metformin, metformin extended-release

Rx Only

Dosage Forms

Tablet, extended-release tablet, oral solution

Usage

Type 2 diabetes mellitus,* polycystic ovary syndrome, antipsychotic-induced weight gain

Pregnancy Category B

Dosing

- Initial dose: 500 mg twice daily with morning and evening meals, 850 mg once daily with a meal, or 500 mg extended-release once daily with a meal
- Maintenance dose: 2,000–2,550 mg daily in divided doses or 2,000 mg extended-release once daily (2,500 mg daily with Fortamet)
- Renal dosage adjustment: Not recommended in patients with renal dysfunction (see Contraindications below)

Adverse Reactions: Most Common

Diarrhea, vomiting, dyspepsia, flatulence, metallic taste, weight loss

Adverse Reactions: Rare/Severe/Important

Lactic acidosis, megaloblastic anemia

Major Drug Interactions

Drugs Affecting Metformin

- Alcohol potentiates the effect on lactate metabolism
- Cimetidine increases plasma concentrations (use alternative H2 blocker)
- Iodinated contrast media can lead to acute renal failure and metformin toxicity

Contraindications

Renal disease (males: SrCr ≥ 1.5 mg/dL; females: SrCr ≥ 1.4 mg/dL), decompensated heart failure, acute or chronic metabolic acidosis, active liver disease

Counseling Points

Discontinue immediately and promptly notify healthcare practitioner if unexplained myalgia, malaise, hyperventilation, or unusual somnolence occur because these are symptoms of lactic acidosis

Key Points

Temporarily withhold in patients undergoing radiologic procedures involving the parenteral administration of iodinated contrast media because it may result in acute alteration of renal function. Do not restart for at least 48 hours or until renal function appears adequate.

---

* Throughout the text, an asterisk (*) is used to indicate the most common uses of a drug.

DI-PEPTIDYL PEPTIDASE-4 INHIBITORS

Introduction

Di-peptidyl peptidase-4 inhibitors inhibit the breakdown of active GLP-1 to inactive GLP-1 through the inhibition of the enzyme DPP-4. Active GLP-1 is released from the alpha cells of the pancreas in response to food intake. GLP-1 plays a role in regulating blood glucose by increasing the secretion of insulin from the pancreas in a glucose-dependent manner. GLP-1 also helps regulate glucagon secretion and decreases hepatic glucose production. These drugs are used as monotherapy as an adjunct to diet and exercise or in combination with other oral antidiabetic agents in patients who do not reach glycemic goals. Average HbA1c reductions are between 0.7% and 1%.

Mechanism of Action for the Drug Class

Inhibition of DPP-4 enhances the activity of active GLP-1, thus increasing glucose-dependent insulin secretion and decreasing levels of circulating glucagon and hepatic glucose production

Members of the Drug Class

In this section: Sitagliptin
Others: Linagliptin, saxagliptin

◉ Sitagliptin

Brand Name
  Januvia

Generic Name
  Sitagliptin

Rx Only

Dosage Form
  Tablet

Usage
  Type 2 diabetes mellitus

Pregnancy Category B

Dosing
  - 100 mg once daily with or without food
  - Renal dosage adjustment:
    - 50 mg once daily: CrCl ≥ 30 to < 50 mL/min
    - 25 mg once daily: CrCl < 30 mL/min

Adverse Reactions: Most Common

Nasopharyngitis, nausea, diarrhea, vomiting, hypoglycemia, weight loss

Adverse Reactions: Rare/Severe/Important

Acute pancreatitis, rash (Stevens-Johnson syndrome)

Major Drug Interactions

Sitagliptin's Effect on Other Drugs
Digoxin: Increased levels

Counseling Points

Discontinue immediately and promptly notify healthcare practitioner if unexplained persistent nausea and vomiting occur (signs of acute pancreatitis)

INSULIN

Introduction

The hormone insulin is endogenously released from the beta cells of the pancreas. Patients with type 1 diabetes mellitus have an absolute deficiency of insulin; patients with type 2 diabetes mellitus may also have decreased production of endogenous insulin. Type 1 diabetics require insulin as a lifelong treatment. Insulin is commonly used in type 2 diabetic patients as either adjunct therapy to oral antidiabetic agents or as monotherapy as the disease progresses. Various substitutions on the insulin molecule and other modifications have led to multiple types of insulin. They are characterized and administered based on their pharmacodynamic and pharmacokinetic characteristics, such as onset, peak, and duration of action. The various types of insulin are classified as rapid-acting, short-acting, intermediate-acting, or long-acting insulin.

Mechanism of Action for the Drug Class

Insulin lowers blood glucose by stimulating peripheral glucose uptake, especially in skeletal muscle and fat, and by inhibiting hepatic glucose production

Usage for the Drug Class

Type 1 diabetes mellitus,* type 2 diabetes mellitus,* hyperkalemia, diabetic ketoacidosis*/diabetic coma

Dosing for the Drug Class

  - Initial dose: 0.5–1 unit/kg per day SUB-Q (high interpatient variability)

- Maintenance dose: Adjust doses to achieve premeal blood glucose levels of 70–130 mg/dL
- Renal dosage adjustment:
  - CrCl 10–50 mL/min: Administer 75% of normal dose
  - CrCl < 10 mL/min: Administer 25–50% of normal dose; monitor closely

Adverse Reactions for the Drug Class: Most Common
Hypoglycemia (anxiety, blurred vision, palpitations, shakiness, slurred speech, sweating), weight gain

Adverse Reactions for the Drug Class: Rare/Severe/Important
Severe hypoglycemia (seizure/coma), edema, lipoatrophy or lipohypertrophy at injection site

Major Drug Interactions for the Drug Class
Drugs Affecting Insulin (Decreased Hypoglycemic Effect)
- Acetazolamide
- Diuretics
- Oral contraceptives
- Albuterol
- Epinephrine
- Phenothiazines
- Asparaginase
- Estrogens
- Terbutaline
- Corticosteroids
- HIV antivirals
- Thyroid hormones
- Diltiazem
- Lithium

Drugs Affecting Insulin (Increased Hypoglycemic Effect)
- Alcohol
- Fluoxetine
- Anabolic steroids
- Lithium
- Beta blockers
- Sulfonamides
- Clonidine

Contraindications for the Drug Class
Severe hypoglycemia; allergy or sensitivity to any ingredient of the product

Essential Monitoring Parameters for the Drug Class
Fasting blood sugar (70–130 mg/dL)

Counseling Points for the Drug Class
- Follow a prescribed diet and exercise regularly
- Rotate injection sites to prevent lipodystrophy
- Insulin requirements may change during times of illness, vomiting, fever, and emotional stress
- Wear diabetic identification

- Insulin stored at room temperature will be less painful to inject compared to refrigerator-stored insulin
- Mild episodes of hypoglycemia may be treated with oral glucose or carbohydrates

Members of the Drug Class
In this section: Insulin glulisine, insulin lispro, insulin NPH, insulin (R), insulin glargine, insulin detemir, insulin aspart Various mixtures also are available

◉ Insulin Glulisine
Brand Names
Apidra, Apidra SoloStar

Generic Name
Insulin glulisine (rapid-acting insulin)

Rx Only

Dosage Form
Injection 100 units/mL (10 mL vial and 3 mL cartridge for pen use)

Pregnancy Category C

Dosing
- Administer SUB-Q 15 minutes before or immediately after starting a meal
- May be administered by continuous subcutaneous infusion (insulin pump)

◉ Insulin Lispro
Brand Names
Humalog, Humalog KwikPen

Generic Name
Insulin lispro (rapid-acting insulin)

Rx Only

Dosage Forms
Injection 100 units/mL (10 mL vial and 3 mL cartridge for pen use)

Pregnancy Category B

Dosing
- Administer SUB-Q 15 minutes before or immediately after starting a meal
- May be administered by continuous subcutaneous infusion (insulin pump)

⊙ Insulin NPH

Brand Names
Humulin N, Novolin N

Generic Name
Insulin NPH (intermediate-acting insulin)

OTC

Dosage Forms
Injection, suspension, 100 units/mL (10 mL vial and 3 mL cartridge for pen use)

Pregnancy Category B

Dosing
- NPH should only be mixed with regular insulin
- Draw regular insulin into the syringe first, then add the NPH insulin to the syringe

⊙ Insulin Regular

Brand Names
Humulin R, Novolin R

Generic Name
Insulin regular (short-acting insulin)

OTC

Dosage Forms
Injection 100 units/mL (10 mL vial and 3 mL cartridge for pen use)

Pregnancy Category B

Dosing
- Administer SUB-Q 30 minutes before a meal
- May be administered by continuous subcutaneous infusion (insulin pump)
- Caution: A concentrated 20 mL vial containing 500 units/mL is available

⊙ 70% NPH and 30% Regular Insulin Mixture

Brand Names
Humulin 70/30, Novolin 70/30

Generic Name
70% NPH and 30% regular insulin mixture

OTC

Dosage Forms
Injection, suspension, 100 units/mL (10 mL vial and 3 mL cartridge for pen use)

Pregnancy Category B

Brand Name
Humulin 50/50

⊙ 50% NPH and 50% Regular Insulin Mixture

Generic Name
50% NPH and 50% regular insulin mixture

OTC

Dosage Forms
Injection, suspension, 100 units/mL (10 mL vial and 3 mL cartridge for pen use)

Pregnancy Category B

⊙ 75% Intermediate-Acting Lispro Suspension and 25% Rapid-Acting Lispro Solution

Brand Name
Humalog Mix 75/25

Generic Name
75% intermediate-acting lispro suspension and 25% rapid-acting lispro solution

Rx Only

Dosage Forms
Injection 100 units/mL (10 mL vial and 3 mL cartridge for pen use)

Pregnancy Category B

⊙ Insulin Glargine

Brand Names
Lantus, Lantus SoloStar

Generic Name
Insulin glargine (long-acting insulin)

Rx Only

Dosage Forms
Injection 100 units/mL (10 mL vial and 3 mL cartridge for pen use)

Pregnancy Category C

Dosing
- When changing to insulin glargine from once-daily NPH, the initial dose of insulin glargine should be the same. When changing to insulin glargine from

twice-daily NPH, the initial dose of insulin glargine should be reduced by 20% and adjusted according to patient response.

- Administer once daily
- Starting dose in a type 2 diabetic patient is 10 units at bedtime and then titrate according to patient response

◉ Insulin Detemir

Brand Names
Levemir, Levemir FlexPen

Generic Name
Insulin detemir (long-acting insulin)

Rx Only

Dosage Forms
Injection 100 units/mL (10 mL vial and 3 mL cartridge for pen use)

Pregnancy Category B

Dosing
- Indicated for once-daily or twice-daily dosing
- Once daily is dosed SUB-Q with the evening meal or at bedtime
- Twice daily is dosed every 12 hours

◉ Insulin Aspart

Brand Names
NovoLog, NovoLog FlexPen

Generic Name
Insulin aspart (rapid-acting insulin)

Rx Only

Dosage Forms
Injection 100 units/mL (10 mL vial and 3 mL cartridge for pen use)

Pregnancy Category B

Dosing
- Administer SUB-Q 15 minutes before or immediately after starting a meal
- May be administered by continuous subcutaneous infusion (insulin pump)

◉ 70% Intermediate-Acting Insulin Aspart Suspension and 30% Rapid-Acting Aspart Solution

Brand Name
NovoLog Mix 70/30

Generic Name
70% intermediate-acting insulin aspart suspension and 30% rapid-acting aspart solution

Rx Only

Dosage Forms
Injection 100 units/mL (10 mL vial and 3 mL cartridge for pen use)

Pregnancy Category B

Comparison of Insulin Products
Refer to **Table 2-1**.

TABLE 2-1 Comparison of Insulin Products				
Product	Onset (hours)	Peak (hours)	Duration (hours)	Appearance
Rapid-Acting Insulin				
Insulin aspart (NovoLog)	0.25	1–2	3–5	Clear
Insulin glulisine (Apidra)	0.25	1	3–4	Clear
Insulin lispro (Humalog)	0.25	0.5–1.5	3–4	Clear
Short-Acting Insulin				
Regular insulin (Humulin R, Novolin R)	0.5–1	2–3	3–6	Clear
Intermediate-Acting Insulin				
NPH insulin (Humulin N, Novolin N)	2–4	6–10	10–16	Cloudy
Long-Acting Insulin				
Insulin detemir (Levemir)	4	N/A	12–24	Clear
Insulin glargine (Lantus)	4	N/A	24	Clear

SULFONYLUREAS

Introduction

The sulfonylureas are used as adjunctive therapy to diet and exercise in patients with type 2 diabetes mellitus. Although periodically used as monotherapy, sulfonylureas are more commonly used in combination with other oral antidiabetic agents, sometimes in the same formulation, in patients who do not reach glycemic goals. General dosing guidelines are to start with a low dose and titrate upward according to patient response while monitoring for signs and symptoms of hypoglycemia, which is a common adverse effect of the drug class. Use cautiously in patients with renal or hepatic impairment. HbA1c reductions are between 1% and 2%.

Mechanism of Action for the Drug Class

Lowers blood glucose by stimulating insulin release from the beta cells of the pancreatic islets

Usage for the Drug Class
Type 2 diabetes mellitus*

Pregnancy Category C for the Drug Class
Except for glyburide (pregnancy category B)

Adverse Reactions for the Drug Class: Most Common
Hypoglycemia, GI distress, dizziness

Adverse Reactions for the Drug Class: Rare/Severe/Important
SIADH (most commonly with chlorpropamide); disulfiram-like reactions

Major Drug Interactions for the Drug Class
Drugs Affecting Sulfonylureas
- Anticoagulants, azole antifungals, gemfibrozil-enhanced hypoglycemic effects
- Beta blockers cause decreased hypoglycemic effects; also may mask signs and symptoms of hypoglycemia

Sulfonylureas' Effects on Other Drugs
Digoxin: Increased levels

Contraindications for the Drug Class
Diabetes complicated by ketoacidosis, with or without coma; Type 1 diabetes mellitus; diabetes complicated by pregnancy

Counseling Points for the Drug Class
Monitor glucose as directed and be aware of the signs and symptoms of hypoglycemia

Members of the Drug Class
In this section: Glimepiride, glipizide, glyburide
Others: Chlorpropamide, tolazamide, tolbutamide

⊙ Glimepiride
Brand Name
Amaryl

Generic Name
Glimepiride

Rx Only

Dosage Form
Tablet

Dosing
- Initial dose: 1–2 mg once daily at breakfast
- Maintenance dose: 1–8 mg once daily

⊙ Glipizide
Brand Names
Glucotrol, Glucotrol XL

Generic Names
Glipizide, glipizide extended-release

Rx Only

Dosage Forms
Tablet, extended-release tablet

Dosing
- Initial dose:
  - Glucotrol: 2.5–5 mg once daily 30 minutes before breakfast
  - Glucotrol XL: 5 mg extended-release once daily with breakfast
- Maintenance dose:
  - Glucotrol: 10–40 mg daily (> 15 mg/day should be divided)
  - Glucotrol XL: 5–20 mg extended-release once daily

⊙ Glyburide
Brand Names
DiaBeta, Micronase, Glynase PresTab

Generic Name
Glyburide

Rx Only

Dosage Form
Tablet

Dosing

DiaBeta and Micronase

- Initial dose: 1.25–5 mg once daily with breakfast
- Maintenance dose: 1.25–20 mg once daily; may give as single or divided doses

Glynase PresTab

- Initial dose: 1.5–3 mg once daily with breakfast
- Maintenance dose: 1.5–12 mg once daily; may give as single or divided doses

THIAZOLIDINEDIONES

Introduction

The thiazolidinediones decrease insulin resistance by enhancing insulin-receptor sensitivity. They are used as adjuncts to diet and exercise in patients with type 2 diabetes mellitus. Although periodically used as monotherapy, thiazolidinediones are more frequently used in combination with other oral antidiabetic agents in patients who do not reach glycemic goals. Recent clinical data suggest that patients taking thiazolidinediones may be at an increased risk of myocardial infarction and death; thus, they should be used with caution in patients with a history of previous cardiac disease. They are contraindicated in patients with NYHA class III or IV heart failure. A structurally similar thiazolidinedione, troglitazone, was removed from the market due to cases of liver failure and death. It is recommended to avoid use in patients with hepatic dysfunction. HbA1c reductions are between 1% and 1.5%.

Mechanism of Action for the Drug Class

Thiazolidinediones increase insulin sensitivity by affecting the peroxisome proliferator-activated receptor gamma (PPAR-γ). Acting as an agonist to this receptor, thiazolidinediones decrease insulin resistance in adipose tissue, skeletal muscle, and the liver.

Usage for the Drug Class

Type 2 diabetes mellitus*

Adverse Reactions for the Drug Class: Most Common

Weight gain, edema, hypoglycemia (when used with other oral antidiabetic drugs that may cause hypoglycemia)

Adverse Reactions for the Drug Class: Rare/Severe/Important

Hepatic failure, heart failure, anemia, ovulation in anovulatory premenopausal women, bone loss, bladder cancer, macular edema

Major Drug Interactions for the Drug Class

Drugs Affecting Thiazolidinediones

- Gemfibrozil: Increased levels
- Rifampin: Decreased levels

Thiazolidinediones' Effects on Other Drugs

Oral contraceptives: Decreased efficacy

Contraindications for the Drug Class

Patients with NYHA class III and IV heart failure; active liver disease (alanine aminotransferase [ALT] > 2.5 times the upper limit of normal)

Counseling Points for the Drug Class

Report signs and symptoms of liver dysfunction and/or shortness of breath immediately

Members of the Drug Class

In this section: Pioglitazone
Others: Rosiglitazone

◉ Pioglitazone

Brand Name

Actos

Generic Name

Pioglitazone

Rx Only

Dosage Form

Tablet

Pregnancy Category C

Dosing

- Initial dose:
  - 15–30 mg once daily without regard to meals
  - Limit initial dose to 15 mg once daily in patients with NYHA class I and II heart failure
- Maintenance dose:
  - 15–45 mg once daily
  - Maximum recommended dose is 15 mg once daily in patients taking strong CYP2C8 inhibitors (e.g., gemfibrozil)

REVIEW QUESTIONS

1. Which of the following is the drug of choice for initial treatment of a patient with newly diagnosed type 2 diabetes and no contraindications?

   a. Lantus
   b. Glucophage
   c. Actos
   d. Amaryl

2. Which of the following is *not* a brand name of metformin?

   a. Glumetza
   b. Fortamet
   c. DiaBeta
   d. Riomet

3. Which of the following is the correct initial starting dose for metformin?

   a. 500 mg PO BID
   b. 1,000 mg PO BID
   c. 1,500 mg PO BID
   d. 2,000 mg PO BID

4. Which of the following is the average HbA1c reduction with metformin?

   a. 0.7–1%
   b. 1–1.5%
   c. 1–2%
   d. 1.5–2%

5. Which of the following works primarily by decreasing hepatic glucose production?

   a. Micronase
   b. Januvia
   c. Glucophage
   d. Actos

6. Which of the following is the mechanism of action of sitagliptin?

   a. Decreases hepatic glucose production
   b. Inhibits di-peptidyl peptidase-4
   c. Stimulates peripheral glucose uptake
   d. Acts as a direct GLP-1 agonist

7. Which class of drugs may cause SIADH in rare instances?

   a. Biguanides
   b. Sulfonylureas
   c. Insulin
   d. DPP-4 inhibitors

8. Which of the following medications does *not* cause weight gain?

   a. Metformin
   b. Glyburide
   c. Insulin detemir
   d. Pioglitazone

9. Which of the following medications is indicated for the treatment of diabetic ketoacidosis?

   a. Glucophage
   b. Actos
   c. Insulin
   d. Januvia

10. Which insulin product comes in a highly concentrated 500 units/mL, 20 mL vial and should be used with caution?

    a. NPH
    b. Glargine
    c. Regular
    d. Detemir

11. Humulin 70/30 contains which of the following?

    a. 70% NPH and 30% regular insulin
    b. 30% NPH and 70% regular insulin
    c. 70% glargine and 30% regular insulin
    d. 30% glargine and 70% regular insulin

12. Which of the following should be discontinued immediately and a healthcare provider notified if unexplained myalgia, malaise, or hyperventilation occurs?

    a. Pioglitazone
    b. Glipizide
    c. Sitagliptin
    d. Metformin

13. Which of the following is *not* a member of the sulfonylurea drug class?

    a. Glipizide
    b. Sitagliptin
    c. Glyburide
    d. Glimepiride

14. Which of the following is an example of a biguanide?

    a. Amaryl
    b. Actos
    c. Glucophage
    d. Januvia

15. Insulin is released from which of the following?

    a. Beta cells of the liver
    b. Alpha cells of the pancreas
    c. Beta cells of the pancreas
    d. Alpha cells of the liver

16. Which of the following is the typical initial starting dose of insulin?

    a. 0.1–0.5 unit/kg per day
    b. 0.5–1 unit/kg per day
    c. 1–5 units/kg per day
    d. 5–10 units/kg per day

17. A patient's CrCl is 10–50 mL/min. What is the appropriate dosing of insulin for this patient?

    a. Administer 100% normal dose
    b. Administer 75% normal dose
    c. Administer 50% normal dose
    d. Administer 10% normal dose

18. When switching a patient from twice-daily insulin NPH to glargine, which of the following is the appropriate initial dose of glargine?

    a. Increase by 20% and adjusted accordingly
    b. Increase by 10% and adjusted accordingly
    c. Decrease by 20% and adjusted accordingly
    d. Decrease by 10% and adjusted accordingly

19. Humulin R insulin should be dosed:

    a. 15 minutes prior to a meal.
    b. 30 minutes prior to a meal.
    c. 30 minutes after a meal.
    d. at bedtime.

20. Which of the following is the maintenance dose of glyburide?

    a. 1–8 mg once daily
    b. 2.5–5 mg once daily
    c. 1.25–20 mg once daily
    d. 10–40 mg once daily

21. Which class of antidiabetic drugs works primarily by activation of adenosine monophosphate-activated protein kinase (AMPK)?

    a. Biguanides
    b. Sulfonylureas
    c. Thiazolidinediones
    d. Di-peptidyl peptidase-4 inhibitors

22. What is the average HbA1c reduction expected with sitagliptin?

    a. 0.7–1%
    b. 1–1.5%
    c. 1–2%
    d. 1.5–2%

23. When initiating insulin glargine in a patient with type 2 diabetes not well controlled on metformin therapy, the most common starting dose is:

    a. 5 units before each meal.
    b. 10 units before breakfast and 10 units before dinner.
    c. 10 units before each meal.
    d. 10 units at bedtime.

24. Which of the following is the maximum dose of Glipizide-XL?

    a. 5 mg once daily
    b. 10 mg once daily
    c. 20 mg once daily
    d. 40 mg once daily

25. Recent clinical data suggest patients taking which of the following classes of antidiabetic drugs are at an increased risk for myocardial infarction and death?

    a. Di-peptidyl peptidase inhibitors
    b. Biguanides
    c. Thiazolidinediones
    d. Insulin

26. Which of the following increases plasma concentrations of metformin and should not be used concomitantly with metformin?

    a. Cimetidine
    b. Ranitidine
    c. Omeprazole
    d. Lansoprazole

27. Which of the following insulin products cannot be administered by continuous subcutaneous infusion (insulin pump)?

    a. Regular
    b. Glulisine
    c. NPH
    d. Lispro

28. Pioglitazone can cause which of the following rare adverse reactions?

    a. Metallic taste
    b. Weight loss
    c. Bone loss
    d. Lactic acidosis

29. Which of the following antidiabetic drugs can be used for antipsychotic-induced weight gain?

    a. Glyburide
    b. Sitagliptin
    c. Insulin
    d. Metformin

30. The enzyme di-peptidyl peptidase is responsible for which of the following?

    a. Active absorption of glucose into the bloodstream
    b. Passive reabsorption of glucose from kidney
    c. Breakdown of active GLP-1 to inactive GLP-1
    d. Active absorption of carbohydrates from gastrointestinal tracts

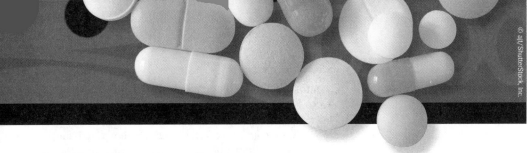

Anti-Infective Agents

Jason C. Gallagher, PharmD, BCPS
Carol Holtzman, PharmD, MSc

AMINOGLYCOSIDES

Introduction

Aminoglycosides are bactericidal, Gram-negative agents that are used to treat serious infections. They are notable for their toxicities, namely nephrotoxicity and ototoxicity. They often are used empirically and then the patient is transitioned to safer agents as culture results become available. Gentamicin and tobramycin are extremely similar drugs, with virtually identical pharmacokinetics and dosing. Only minor differences in spectra separate them. Neomycin is combined with polymyxin and used topically for superficial infections.

Mechanism of Action for the Drug Class

Aminoglycosides irreversibly bind to the 30S ribosomal subunit, disrupting bacterial protein synthesis and resulting in cell death.

Members of the Drug Class

In this section: Gentamicin, tobramycin, neomycin-polymyxin B
Others: Amikacin, streptomycin

◉ Gentamicin

Brand Name
Garamycin

Generic Name
Gentamicin

Rx Only

Dosage Form
Injection

Usage

Systemic aerobic Gram-negative infections of the bloodstream, lung, skin and soft tissue, bone, CNS, abdomen, heart, including those caused by *Pseudomonas aeruginosa*;* systemic infections (in particular those of the bloodstream and/or heart) caused by staphylococci, streptococci, or enterococci (treatment must be in combination with a cell-wall active agent for Gram-positive infections)

Pregnancy Category D

Dosing

- Initial dose:
  - Conventional dosing: 1.5–2 mg/kg per dose every 8 hours based on ideal or adjusted body weight
  - Extended-interval dosing: 5–7 mg/kg per day based on ideal or adjusted body weight
- Renal dosage adjustment: Dosing must be individualized based on CrCl and therapeutic drug monitoring

Pharmacokinetic Monitoring

Peaks associated with efficacy range from 5–10 µg/mL, with higher concentrations for more severe or resistant infections. Troughs associated with decreased nephrotoxicity range from < 1–2 µg/mL. Extended-interval dosing is monitored via nomograms with concentrations measured 6-14 hours from the time of administration. Do not use traditional peak and trough concentrations to monitor aminoglycosides dosed this way.

Adverse Reactions: Most Common

Electrolyte wasting (particularly potassium and magnesium); nephrotoxicity, manifesting usually as increased serum creatinine before changes in urine output are seen

---

* Throughout the text, an asterisk (*) is used to indicate the most common uses of a drug.

Adverse Reactions: Rare/Severe/Important

Ototoxicity; neuromuscular blockade

Major Drug Interactions

Drugs Affecting Gentamicin

Concomitant oto- or nephrotoxic agents: Additive oto- or nephrotoxicity

Gentamicin's Effect on Other Drugs

Neuromuscular blocking agents: Potentiated neuromuscular blockade

Essential Monitoring Parameters

Peaks and troughs should be monitored, particularly during extended therapy. If extended-interval dosing is used, gentamicin concentrations should be monitored and measured by a nomogram.

Counseling Point

Report any changes in hearing function or decline in urination to a healthcare practitioner immediately

Key Points

- Monitor serum peak and trough levels to ensure nontoxic levels. Nephrotoxicity is associated with elevated trough concentrations.
- Ototoxicity is irreversible. Patients receiving extended courses of aminoglycosides must have hearing monitored. Aminoglycosides should be discontinued at the first sign of hearing or balance problems.
- Extended-interval dosing may be more effective and less nephrotoxic than traditional dosing. However, it is not ideal for patients with changing renal function.
- Dosage should be based on ideal or adjusted body weight, not total body weight

◉ Tobramycin

Brand Names

Tobrex, Tobi (inhalation)

Generic Name

Tobramycin

Rx Only

Usage

- IV: Same as gentamicin
- Inhalation: Given to improve pulmonary function in cystic fibrosis by decreasing bacterial colony counts

Pregnancy Category D

Dosing

- IV: Same as gentamicin
- Inhalation: 300 mg every 12 hours

Essential Monitoring Parameters

Peaks and troughs should be monitored, particularly during extended therapy. If extended-interval dosing is used, tobramycin concentrations should be monitored and measured by a nomogram.

Key Points

- All of the preceding points for gentamicin apply to tobramycin. Tobramycin has slightly better activity against *Pseudomonas aeruginosa* than gentamicin, and gentamicin has slightly better Gram-positive activity than tobramycin, but they are otherwise very similar.
- Inhalation therapy with tobramycin is used to prevent exacerbations in cystic fibrosis patients. It should not be used as monotherapy to treat pneumonia.

◉ Neomycin-Polymyxin B

Brand Name

Neosporin

Generic Name

Neomycin-polymyxin B

OTC

Dosage Forms

Topical ointment or cream

Usage

Minor skin infections

Pregnancy Category C

Dosing

Apply to affected area three to four times daily

Adverse Reactions: Most Common

Local irritation

Counseling Points

- Do not use for deep wounds, puncture wounds, animal or human bites, or serious burns
- Do not apply to the eyes
- Cover treated area with a gauze or bandage
- See a healthcare provider if the wound does not begin to heal in a few days

Key Points

- Neomycin is an aminoglycoside antibiotic. It is often coupled with polymyxin B in a topical formulation with the brand name Neosporin. Note that not all products that contain the Neosporin name contain the neomycin/polymyxin B combination.
- Topical antibiotics are not effective in the treatment of skin infections that are any more severe than superficial

ANTIMYCOBACTERIAL AGENTS

Introduction

Mycobacteria such as *Mycobacterium tuberculosis* have cell walls that have a very different anatomy than other bacteria. Many antibiotics are not active against mycobacteria. Isoniazid and rifampin are both highly active against *M. tuberculosis* and are the two most important drugs in the treatment of tuberculosis. They are often used in combination in the treatment of tuberculosis, usually with other agents as well.

Mechanism of Action for the Drug Class

Isoniazid inhibits the synthesis of mycolic acids, an essential component of the mycobacterial cell wall. Rifampin inhibits the synthesis of RNA by preventing the action of RNA polymerase. Its activity is not specific to mycobacteria.

Members of the Drug Class

In this section: isoniazid, rifampin
Others: ethambutol, pyrazinamide, rifabutin, rifapentine

◉ Isoniazid

Brand Names
Laniazid, Nydrazid

Generic Name
Isoniazid

Rx Only

Dosage Forms
Tablet, solution, injection

Usage
Treatment of active and latent tuberculosis

Pregnancy Category C

Dosing
- Active tuberculosis: 5 mg/kg daily (maximum of 300 mg/dose) or 15 mg/kg two to three times weekly (maximum of 900 mg/dose)
- Latent tuberculosis: 5 mg/kg daily (maximum of 300 mg/dose)
- Hepatic impairment: In patients with moderate to severe hepatic dysfunction, consider reducing the dose or extending the dosing interval

Adverse Reactions: Most Common
Peripheral neuropathy, elevated liver function tests, abdominal pain

Adverse Reactions: Rare/Severe/Important
Hepatitis, hypersensitivity, anemia, thrombocytopenia, systemic lupus erythematosus

Major Drug Interactions

Drugs Affecting Isoniazid
- Cycloserine, ethionamide: Potentiated nervous system toxicity
- Ethanol: Increased hepatotoxicity

Isoniazid's Effect on Other Drugs
- Carbamazepine: Increased levels
- Phenytoin: Increased levels
- Serotonergic agents: Potential serotonin syndrome secondary to the weak MAO-inhibiting effect of isoniazid

Counseling Points
- Avoid alcohol intake while on isoniazid to prevent liver damage
- Report persistent abdominal pain (≥ 3 days), dark urine, fever, or fatigue because these may be signs of liver problems

Key Points
- For treatment of active tuberculosis, must be part of a multidrug regimen
- Administer with pyridoxine (vitamin B_6) to prevent peripheral neuropathy
- Common abbreviation is INH

◉ Rifampin

Brand Names
Rifadin, Rimactane

Generic Name
Rifampin

Rx Only

Dosage Forms
Capsule, injection

Usage
Active and latent tuberculosis, treatment of asymptomatic carriers of *Neisseria meningitides*, synergistic therapy for various infections (such as endocarditis) with other antibiotics

Pregnancy Category C

Dosing
- 600 mg IV or PO every 24 hours
- Hepatic impairment: In patients with moderate to severe hepatic dysfunction, consider reducing the dose or extending the dosing interval

Adverse Reactions: Most Common
Nausea, vomiting, cramps, rash, fever, drowsiness, elevated liver function tests

Adverse Reactions: Rare/Severe/Important

Hypersensitivity, hyperbilirubinemia, thrombocytopenia

Major Drug Interactions

Drugs Affecting Rifampin

- Antacids: May reduce absorption of rifampin
- Cotrimoxazole: May increase the levels of rifampin
- Isoniazid or halothane: Potentiate hepatotoxicity

Rifampin's Effect on Other Drugs

- Rifampin is a potent inducer of many hepatic enzymes, particularly those of the cytochrome P450 system. Careful monitoring of patients on concomitant drugs that are metabolized via the liver is recommended.
- Examples of drugs that are known to be cleared more rapidly by rifampin include phenytoin, disopyramide, quinidine, warfarin, azole antifungals, diltiazem, nifedipine, barbiturates, beta blockers, chloramphenicol, clarithromycin, digoxin, oral contraceptives, doxycycline, oral hypoglycemic agents, levothyroxine, methadone, narcotic analgesics, tricyclic antidepressants, tacrolimus, cyclosporine, and theophylline. Decreased therapeutic effects of these drugs are common with coadministration.

Counseling Point

Rifampin will turn bodily fluids orange/red. This includes tears, urine, and sweat. Contact lenses may be stained by this red color and should not be worn during rifampin therapy.

Key Points

- Always screen patients for drug interactions when rifampin therapy is started. If interactions cannot be avoided, careful monitoring is required.
- Rifabutin is a related drug with somewhat less potent enzyme induction that may be used in place of rifampin for some indications
- In the treatment of active tuberculosis, combination therapy is always needed. Rifampin cannot be used alone.
- Unlike most other antimycobacterial drugs, rifampin's activity is not limited to mycobacteria. It is sometimes used in combination with other antibacterial drugs for the treatment of resistant or difficult-to-treat bacterial infections.

PENICILLINS

Introduction

Penicillins were the second class of antibiotics to be developed. They comprise a very large class of antibiotics and range from agents with broad antimicrobial spectra to those with more narrow spectra. Some agents in this class can be given orally.

Mechanism of Action for the Drug Class

Penicillins limit bacterial cell growth in susceptible bacteria by inhibiting transpeptidase enzymes (also known as penicillin-binding proteins). This prevents cross-linking of peptidoglycan strands, thereby inhibiting synthesis of the bacterial cell wall.

Adverse Reactions for the Drug Class: Most Common

Nausea, vomiting, diarrhea, rash

Adverse Reactions for the Drug Class: Rare/Severe/Important

Hypersensitivity, anaphylaxis, seizures, pseudomembranous colitis

Major Drug Interactions for the Drug Class

Drugs Affecting Penicillins

- Probenecid: Decreases the renal tubular secretion of penicillins, resulting in increased and prolonged serum concentrations
- Chloramphenicol, macrolides, sulfonamides, and tetracyclines interfere with the bactericidal effects of penicillins

Counseling Points for the Drug Class

Complete the entire prescription. Do not stop taking the medication when you feel better.

Key Points for the Drug Class

Use with caution in patients who are allergic to other beta-lactam antibiotics

Members of the Drug Class

In this section: Amoxicillin, amoxicillin/clavulanate, penicillin

Others: Ampicillin, cloxacillin, dicloxacillin, nafcillin, oxacillin, piperacillin, piperacillin/tazobactam, ticarcillin/clavulanate

◉ Amoxicillin

Brand Names

Amoxil, Trimox

Generic Name

Amoxicillin

Rx Only

Dosage Forms

Capsule, tablet, suspension

Usage

Upper respiratory tract infections,* urinary tract infections, skin and skin structure infections, *Helicobacter pylori* infection*

Dosing

- Adults:
  - Mild to moderate infections: 250 mg three times daily or 500 mg twice daily
  - Moderate to severe infections: 500 mg three times daily or 875 mg twice daily
- Children: 20–40 mg/kg three times daily or 25–45 mg/kg twice daily
- Renal dosage adjustment: Adjust with a CrCl of < 30 mL/min

Pregnancy Category B

Key Points

- Amoxicillin and ampicillin have nearly identical antimicrobial spectra, but amoxicillin has much better oral absorption
- Resistance to amoxicillin among *Escherichia coli* is high, so it is not an ideal choice for urinary tract infections

⊙ Amoxicillin/Clavulanate

Brand Name

Augmentin

Generic Name

Amoxicillin/clavulanate

Rx Only

Dosage Forms

Tablet, suspension

Usage

Upper and lower respiratory tract infections,* skin and skin structure infections,* urinary tract infections, mixed aerobic and anaerobic infections

Pregnancy Category B

Dosing

- Dosing is based on the amoxicillin component
- Adults:
  - Mild to moderate infections: 250 mg three times daily or 500 mg twice daily
  - Moderate to severe infections: 500 mg three times daily or 875 mg twice daily

- Children:
  - Otitis media: 45 mg/kg per day in two divided doses or 40 mg/kg per day in three divided doses
  - Less severe infections: 25 mg/kg/day in two divided doses or 20 mg/kg/day in three divided doses
- Renal dosage adjustment: Adjust with a CrCl < 30 mL/min

Counseling Point

To minimize adverse gastrointestinal events, take at the start of a meal

Key Points

- Twice-daily dosing is associated with significantly less diarrhea
- The 250 and 500 mg tablets contain the same quantity of clavulanic acid; therefore, do not substitute two 250 mg tablets for one 500 mg tablet
- Amoxicillin/clavulanate has a significantly broader antimicrobial spectrum than amoxicillin alone. This is advantageous in treating some potentially drug-resistant infections but is not needed in those likely to be drug susceptible.

⊙ Penicillin

Brand Names

Beepen-VK, Pen-VK, Veetids

Generic Name

Penicillin

Rx Only

Dosage Forms

Tablet, oral solution

Usage

Streptococcal infections, uncomplicated anthrax, necrotizing ulcerative gingivitis, prophylaxis of pneumococcal infections, prophylaxis of recurrent rheumatic fever

Pregnancy Category B

Dosing

- 250–500 mg two to three times daily
- Renal dosage adjustment: If CrCl < 10 or dialysis, then administer twice daily

CEPHALOSPORINS

Introduction

Cephalosporins are beta-lactam antibiotics and one of the largest classes of antibiotics. They are more resistant to beta-lactamase enzymes (enzymes produced by bacteria to destroy beta-lactams) than penicillins, although beta-lactamases that destroy cephalosporins have since evolved. They have more broad-spectrum antimicrobial activity than penicillins; activity that broadens in spectrum, moving "down" the generations from first- to fourth-generation agents. The cephalosporins listed here are among the most frequently used and are representative of the much larger category of drugs.

Mechanism of Action for the Drug Class

Inhibit bacterial cell growth in susceptible bacteria by inhibiting transpeptidase enzymes (also known as penicillin-binding proteins). This prevents the cross-linking of peptidoglycan strands, thereby inhibiting the synthesis of the bacterial cell wall.

Adverse Reactions for the Drug Class: Most Common

Hypersensitivity, rash, diarrhea

Adverse Reactions for the Drug Class: Rare/Severe/Important

Anaphylaxis, bone marrow suppression, *Clostridium difficile*–associated diarrhea

Counseling Points for the Drug Class

- Complete the entire prescription
- Report any signs of an allergic reaction, such as a rash or hives, to your healthcare provider immediately

Key Point for the Drug Class

Use with caution in patients who are allergic to penicillin derivatives. Cross-reactivity between the two types of beta-lactams seems to be lower than initially suggested, but is still possible.

Members of the Drug Class

In this section: Cefprozil, cefdinir, ceftriaxone, cefuroxime, cephalexin

Others: Cefaclor, cefadroxil, cefamandole, cefazolin, cefixime, cefonicid, cefoperazone, cefonicid, cefotaxime, cefotetan, cefoxitin, cefprozil, ceftazidime, ceftibuten, ceftizoxime, cephalexin, cephalothin, cephapirin, loracarbef, moxalactam

◉ Cefprozil

Brand Name
Cefzil

Generic Name
Cefprozil

Dosage Forms
Tablet, suspension

Usage
Upper and lower respiratory tract infections,* uncomplicated skin and skin structure infections,* tonsillitis

Dosing
- Adults: 250–500 mg twice daily
- Children: 7.5 mg/kg twice daily or 20 mg/kg daily, depending on the indication
- Renal dosage adjustment: Reduce dose 50% with a creatinine clearance of < 30 mL/min

Adverse Reactions: Most Common
Nausea, vomiting

Major Drug Interactions
Drugs Affecting Cefprozil
Probenecid: Increases concentrations of cefprozil through impaired excretion

Key Points
- The oral suspension contains phenylalanine and should be avoided in patients with phenylketonuria
- This is a second-generation cephalosporin

◉ Cefdinir

Brand Name
Omnicef

Generic Name
Cefdinir

Rx Only

Dosage Forms
Capsule, suspension

Usage
Upper and lower respiratory infections,* uncomplicated skin and skin structure infections

Pregnancy Category B

Dosing
- Most indications: 300 mg twice daily or 600 mg once daily
- Renal dosage adjustment: If CrCl < 30 mL/min, then 300 mg once daily

Key Points
Cefdinir is a third-generation cephalosporin

⊙ Ceftriaxone

Brand Name

Rocephin

Generic Name

Ceftriaxone

Rx Only

Dosage Forms

Injection (IV and IM)

Usage

Upper and lower respiratory tract infections,* skin and skin structure infections, urinary tract infections,* gonorrhea,* pelvic inflammatory disease, bacteremia, endocarditis, bone and joint infections, intra-abdominal infections, meningitis,* surgical prophylaxis, Lyme disease

Pregnancy Category B

Dosing

- Adults:
  - 1–2 g given once or twice daily; maximum daily dose not to exceed 4 g
  - Meningitis: 2 g IV every 12 hours
  - Gonorrhea: 250 mg IM given once
- Pediatrics:
  - 50–75 mg/kg given daily (in one or two divided doses); maximum daily dose should not exceed 2 g
  - Meningitis: 100 mg/ kg daily (in one to two divided doses); maximum daily dose should not exceed 4 g

Adverse Reactions: Most Common

Injection site irritation; biliary sludging in neonates

Key Points

- In patients receiving long-term therapy, ceftriaxone-calcium may deposit in the gallbladder. This has been associated with symptoms of gallbladder disease. This salt deposition and subsequent symptoms are reversible upon discontinuation of ceftriaxone therapy.
- In neonates, calcium and ceftriaxone can form complexes that deposit in lung and kidney tissue and may be fatal. Alternative cephalosporins should be used.
- Biliary sludging may lead to jaundice in neonates. Alternative cephalosporins should be used in neonates.
- This is a third-generation cephalosporin
- Patients being treated for gonorrhea should receive concomitant therapy for chlamydia

⊙ Cefuroxime

Brand Name

Ceftin

Generic Name

Cefuroxime

Rx Only

Dosage Forms

Tablet, suspension, injection

Usage

Upper and lower respiratory tract infections,* uncomplicated skin and skin structure infections, urinary tract infections,* gonorrhea,* tonsillitis, early Lyme disease

Pregnancy Category B

Dosing

- Adults: 250–500 mg twice daily
- Pediatrics (younger than 12 years): 20–30 mg/kg per day divided into two doses (maximum daily dose: 1 g)
- Gonorrhea (adults): 1 g given once
- Renal dosage adjustment: Dose every 24 hours with a CrCl of < 10 mL/min

Key Points

- Available both intravenously and orally, unlike many beta-lactam antibiotics
- This is a second-generation cephalosporin and has a similar antimicrobial spectrum to cefprozil
- Patients being treated for gonorrhea should receive concomitant therapy for chlamydia

⊙ Cephalexin

Brand Names

Keflex, Keftab

Generic Name

Cephalexin

Rx Only

Dosage Forms

Capsule, suspension

Usage

Upper respiratory tract infections,* uncomplicated skin and soft tissue infections,* urinary tract infections

Pregnancy Category B

Dosing

- Adults: 1–4 g daily in divided doses; most commonly 250 mg four times daily
- Pediatrics: 25–50 mg/kg per day in two to four divided doses; in the treatment of acute otitis media, 75–100 mg/kg per day in four divided doses should be given
- Renal dosage adjustment: Interval should be increased with a CrCl < 40 mL/min

Key Points

- Most commonly used for skin infections, but it is ineffective against methicillin-resistant *Staphylococcus aureus* (MRSA). As MRSA increases, the usefulness of cephalexin decreases for skin infections caused by *S. aureus*. Cephalexin remains highly active against streptococci that cause skin infections.
- This is a first-generation cephalosporin

FLUOROQUINOLONES

Introduction

Fluoroquinolones are among the most frequently used antibiotics. Their utility is driven by their relatively broad antimicrobial spectra and their once- or twice-daily dosing strata. All are available both intravenously and orally, making transitional therapy easy in the inpatient setting. Unfortunately, frequent utilization of fluoroquinolones has led to inevitable increases in antimicrobial resistance, particularly in *P. aeruginosa* and *E. coli*.

Mechanism of Action for the Drug Class

Fluoroquinolones inhibit DNA gyrase (topoisomerase II) and topoisomerase IV, which results in an inability for bacterial DNA to supercoil; this results in a bactericidal effect

Pregnancy Category C for the Drug Class

Adverse Reactions for the Drug Class: Most Common

Headache, dizziness, confusion, photosensitivity, nausea, diarrhea

Adverse Reactions for the Drug Class: Rare/Severe/Important

QTc prolongation, hypotension, tremor, seizures, skin reactions, hepatitis, acute interstitial nephritis, arthropathy, tendon rupture (Achilles tendon), hypoglycemia, pseudomembranous colitis

Major Drug Interactions for the Drug Class

Drugs Affecting Fluoroquinolones

Di- and trivalent cations: Greatly decrease oral fluoroquinolone absorption

Fluoroquinolones' Effects on Other Drugs

QTc-prolonging drugs: Potentiated QTc prolongation, possibly leading to polymorphic ventricular tachycardia

Counseling Points for the Drug Class

- Complete the full prescribed course of therapy
- Separate administration from di- and trivalent cations by at least 2 hours
- Avoid excessive exposure to sunlight; use sunscreen if exposure is unavoidable

Key Points for the Drug Class

- The safety and efficacy of fluoroquinolones in children < 18 years of age (except for the use of ciprofloxacin following exposure to inhalational anthrax and in children with cystic fibrosis), pregnant women, and lactating women has not been established. They are generally avoided in these populations for that reason.

Members of the Drug Class

In this section: Ciprofloxacin, levofloxacin, moxifloxacin
Others: Gemifloxacin, ofloxacin

◉ Ciprofloxacin

Brand Names

Cipro, Cipro XR

Generic Name

Ciprofloxacin

Rx Only

Dosage Forms

Tablet, extended-release tablet, suspension, injection, ophthalmic solution and ointment, otic suspension

Usage

Upper and lower respiratory tract infections,* urinary tract infections,* intra-abdominal infections,* skin and soft tissue infections, osteomyelitis, infectious diarrhea, gonorrhea, anthrax

Dosing

- Oral: 250–750 mg twice daily dependent on the location and severity of infection
- Oral extended-release: 500–1,000 mg daily for urinary tract infections
- IV: 200–400 mg twice or three times daily dependent on the location and severity of infection
- Renal dosage adjustment: Required with CrCl of < 30–50 mL/min

Major Drug Interactions

Drugs Affecting Ciprofloxacin

NSAIDs: May increase the risk of CNS stimulation and/or seizures

Ciprofloxacin's Effect on Other Drugs

- Theophylline: Concentrations increase by 33% on average, but may be much higher
- Phenytoin: Both increased and decreased levels have been reported; close monitoring is recommended
- Warfarin: Enhanced anticoagulant effect

Key Points

- Ciprofloxacin has less Gram-positive activity than other fluoroquinolones, and treatment failures have been reported in streptococcal pneumonia. It is better used in hospital-acquired pneumonia than community-acquired pneumonia.

- Ciprofloxacin is one of two fluoroquinolones with clinically useful activity against *P. aeruginosa*, although resistance to it is high in many hospitals
- Resistance in *Neisseria gonorrhea* to fluoroquinolones has risen to the point that they are no longer preferred agents in the treatment of gonorrhea

◉ Levofloxacin

Brand Name
Levaquin

Generic Name
Levofloxacin

Rx Only

Dosage Forms
Tablet, injection

Usage
Upper and lower respiratory tract infections,* urinary tract infections,* skin and soft tissue infections*

Dosing
- 250–750 mg once daily, depending on indication
- Renal dosage adjustment: See **Table 3-1**

Major Drug Interactions
Drugs Affecting Levofloxacin
NSAIDs: May increase the risk of CNS stimulation and/or seizures

Levofloxacin's Effect on Other Drugs
Antidiabetic agents: May result in enhanced hypoglycemic effect

Key Points
- Levofloxacin has strong Gram-negative and Gram-positive activity, and it is useful in both hospital- and community-acquired infections such as pneumonia
- Levofloxacin is one of two fluoroquinolones with clinically useful activity against *P. aeruginosa*, although resistance to it is high in many hospitals

- Some indications for levofloxacin use higher dosing to shorten the course of therapy (e.g., community-acquired pneumonia)
- Levofloxacin has excellent absorption and is given in equivalent doses orally and intravenously

◉ Moxifloxacin

Brand Name
Avelox

Generic Name
Moxifloxacin

Rx Only

Dosage Forms
Tablet, injection

Usage
Upper and lower respiratory tract infections,* skin and soft tissue infections,* intra-abdominal infections

Dosing
- 400 mg once daily
- No renal dose adjustment is necessary

Key Points
- Unlike most other fluoroquinolones (including the two listed here), moxifloxacin is not eliminated by the kidney but is instead excreted via the biliary tract. For this reason, it is not used in the treatment of urinary tract infections.
- Moxifloxacin has potent activity against many Gram-positive organisms and has more activity against anaerobic bacteria than other fluoroquinolones. This increases its utility in intra-abdominal infections.
- Moxifloxacin lacks activity against *P. aeruginosa* and is more suitable for therapy of community-acquired pneumonia than hospital-acquired pneumonia

3

Anti-Infective Agents

TABLE 3–1 Renal Dosage Adjustment for Levofloxacin

Dose with Normal Renal Function	CrCl 20–49 mL/min	CrCl 10–19 mL/min
750 mg daily	750 mg every 48 hours	750 mg × 1, then 500 mg every 48 hours
500 mg daily	500 mg × 1, then 250 mg every 24 hours	500 mg × 1, then 250 mg every 48 hours
250 mg daily	250 mg daily	250 mg every 48 hours

GLYCOPEPTIDES

Introduction

The glycopeptides are cell-wall synthesis inhibitors of Gram-positive organisms. The rise of antimicrobial resistance among *S. aureus* has led to vancomycin becoming one of the most commonly used antibiotics in hospitals. The poor bioavailability of vancomycin necessitates IV therapy for systemic infections, although it is given orally for *Clostridium difficile* infections of the colon.

Mechanism of Action for the Drug Class

Glycopeptides bind to D-alanyl-D-alanine in the growing bacterial cell wall, preventing the elongation of peptidoglycan strands and halting cell wall synthesis. They are only effective against Gram-positive organisms.

Members of the Drug Class

In this section: Vancomycin
Others: Teicoplanin (outside the United States), telavancin (a lipoglycopeptide)

⊙ Vancomycin

Brand Name

Vancocin

Generic Name

Vancomycin

Rx Only

Dosage Forms

Injection, capsule

Usage

- Injection: Treatment of systemic infections caused by Gram-positive organisms, including those of the respiratory tract,* bloodstream,* skin and skin structure,* gastrointestinal system, and genitourinary tract
- Oral: Treatment of *C. difficile* infection*

Pregnancy Category B (Oral) and C (Injection)

Dosing

- Oral: 125–500 mg every 6 hours
- Injection:
  - Adults: 15–20 mg/kg twice daily
  - Children: 10 mg/kg per dose given every 6 hours
  - Infants: Loading dose of 15 mg/kg followed by 10 mg/kg every 12 hours (first week of life) or every 8 hours (> 1 week of life up to 1 month of life)
  - Doses are individualized by patient characteristics, infection severity, and renal function
- Renal dosage adjustment: Dose of the intravenous formulation needs to be reduced based on creatinine clearance. Most clinicians reduce doses of vancomycin at a CrCl of 50–60 mL/min.

Pharmacokinetic Monitoring

- Therapeutic troughs are generally considered to be from 10 to 20 mg/L, depending on characteristics of the infecting organism and the type of infection. Troughs of > 15–20 mg/L are associated with nephrotoxicity.
- Peaks are no longer routinely monitored
- Evidence correlating vancomycin concentrations with efficacy is lacking

Adverse Reactions: Most Common

Infusion related: "red man's syndrome" (rash, flushing, tachycardia, hypotension), phlebitis, nephrotoxicity (higher doses)

Adverse Reactions: Rare/Severe/Important

Bone marrow suppression (rare), hypersensitivity (rare)

Major Drug Interactions

Drugs Affecting Vancomycin

Nephrotoxic or ototoxic agents: Enhanced toxicity

Vancomycin's Effect on Other Drugs

Anesthesia: May result in enhanced histamine release and rash

Counseling Point

Nurses: Administer vancomycin at a rate of 1 g/hour to prevent infusion-related toxicity

Key Points

- Vancomycin is a drug of choice for infections caused by MRSA
- Closely monitor patients on concomitant nephrotoxic or ototoxic agents
- Oral therapy is ineffective for the treatment of systemic infection
- Systemic therapy is ineffective for the treatment of enterocolitis or pseudomembranous colitis

LINCOSAMIDES

Introduction

Clindamycin is the only commonly used lincosamide. Clindamycin has good activity against staphylococci, streptococci, and anaerobic organisms. It is being used more frequently for the treatment of skin infections due to the increase in MRSA infections seen in the community.

Mechanism of Action for the Drug Class

Clindamycin binds to the 50S subunit of bacterial ribosomes, suppressing protein synthesis.

Members of the Drug Class

In this section: Clindamycin
Other: Lincomycin

⦿ Clindamycin

Brand Name

Cleocin

Generic Name

Clindamycin

Rx Only

Dosage Forms

Capsule, injection

Usage

Skin and skin structure infections,* aspiration pneumonia, intra-abdominal infections*

Pregnancy Category B

Dosing

- Adults:
  - Oral: 150–450 mg every 6–8 hours
  - IV: 300–900 mg every 6–8 hours
- Pediatrics: 8–20 mg/kg per day oral or IV in three to four divided doses
- Hepatic dosage adjustment: In patients with moderate to severe hepatic dysfunction, consider reducing the dose or extending the dosing interval

Adverse Reactions: Most Common

Abdominal pain, diarrhea, nausea, vomiting, rash, pruritus

Adverse Reactions: Rare/Severe/Important

Pseudomembranous colitis, hypersensitivity, jaundice, severe skin eruption

Major Drug Interactions

Clindamycin's Effect on Other Drugs

Neuromuscular blocking agents: Enhanced neuromuscular blockade

Counseling Point

To avoid esophageal irritation, take clindamycin capsules with a full glass of water

Key Points

- *C. difficile*-associated disease, including pseudomembranous colitis, has been associated with all classes of antibiotics, but clindamycin is perhaps most closely associated with it in the minds of many clinicians. It is a popular exam question.
- Many, but not all, strains of MRSA are susceptible to clindamycin. Community-associated strains are much more likely to be susceptible than hospital-acquired strains. Unlike trimethoprim-sulfamethoxazole, clindamycin is active against both strains of MRSA and most streptococci that cause skin infections.
- In addition to the *C. difficile*-associated disease risk that it causes, like many antibiotics clindamycin commonly causes diarrhea that is not related to *C. difficile*

MACROLIDES

Introduction

Macrolides are antibiotics commonly used for respiratory tract infections. Although they are generally well tolerated, clarithromycin and erythromycin are strong inhibitors of the cytochrome P450 enzyme system, and clinicians must be wary of drug interactions with them.

Mechanism of Action for the Drug Class

Macrolides inhibit bacterial protein synthesis by binding to the 50S ribosomal subunit, generally resulting in a bacteriostatic effect

Adverse Reactions for the Drug Class: Most Common

Nausea, diarrhea, abdominal pain, pain at injection site (IV), rash, elevated liver function tests

Adverse Reactions for the Drug Class: Rare/Severe/Important

Allergic reaction, QTc prolongation

Members of the Drug Class

In this section: Azithromycin, clarithromycin, erythromycin
Others: Dirithromycin, troleandomycin

⊙ Azithromycin

Brand Names
Zithromax, Z-pak, Zmax

Generic Name
Azithromycin

Rx Only

Dosage Forms
Capsule, tablet, suspension, injection

Usage
Community-acquired upper and lower respiratory tract infections,* chlamydia, treatment and prophylaxis of *Mycobacteria avium intracellulare* complex (MAI or MAC),* skin and skin structure infections, syphilis

Pregnancy Category B

Dosing
- Adults:
  - Most indications: 500 or 250 mg once daily
  - Z-pak is 500 mg on day 1, followed by 250 mg on days 2–5
  - Zmax is a single 2 g dose
  - Prevention of MAC: 1,200 mg once weekly
  - Treatment of disseminated MAC: 600 mg daily
- Pediatrics:
  - Most indications: 5–12 mg/kg once daily
  - Otitis media can be 30 mg/kg once

Adverse Reactions: Most Common
Pain at injection site (IV)

Major Drug Interactions
In drug interaction studies, azithromycin has not been reported to result in metabolic interactions associated with other macrolides. However, monitoring is suggested in patients receiving digoxin, theophylline, ergotamine derivatives, triazolam, warfarin, and other agents known to be metabolized via the cytochrome P450 enzyme system.

Counseling Points
- Capsules and suspension (bottle) should not be administered with food (at least 1 hour before or 2 hours after a meal)
- Suspension powder packet and tablet may be administered without regard to meals
- Parenteral product should not be given as a bolus injection or intramuscularly
- Patients who vomit immediately after taking azithromycin may need to be redosed, but they should not do this without consulting their healthcare provider

Key Points
- Rising resistance rates to macrolides in *Streptococcus pneumoniae* have led to decreased efficacy for azithromycin. It should not be used as monotherapy in severely ill patients with pneumonia.

- Azithromycin has a very long terminal half-life, which allows for short-course therapy for many indications
- In 2012, the FDA published a warning that azithromycin therapy was associated with a small but increased risk of cardiovascular death compared to some other antibiotics. This prompted a warning to clinicians about the concern, but no specific recommendation was offered except to be aware of possible QTc prolongation and arrhythmias with antibiotic use.

⊙ Clarithromycin

Brand Names
Biaxin, Biaxin-XL

Generic Name
Clarithromycin

Rx Only

Dosage Forms
Tablet, extended-release tablet, suspension

Usage
Community-acquired upper and lower respiratory tract infections,* skin and skin structure infections, treatment of MAI or MAC,* treatment of *H. pylori* infection (in combination with amoxicillin and omeprazole or lansoprazole)

Pregnancy Category C

Dosing
- Adults:
  - Most indications: 250–500 mg every 12 hours
  - Extended-release: 1,000 mg every 24 hours
- Pediatrics: 7.5 mg/kg every 12 hours
- Renal dosage adjustment: Dose adjusted with a CrCl < 60 mL/min

Adverse Reactions: Most Common
Altered taste

Adverse Reactions: Rare/Severe/Important
Prolonged QTc interval (especially when administered with concomitant drugs that prolong the QTc interval); severe hepatic dysfunction

Major Drug Interactions
Drugs Affecting Clarithromycin
Ritonavir will increase the concentration of clarithromycin by 77% and its metabolite by 100%

Clarithromycin's Effect on Other Drugs
- Theophylline concentrations: Increase by 20% on average
- Carbamazepine levels will increase
- Warfarin: Enhanced anticoagulant effect
- Digoxin levels: Increase significantly

- Ergot derivatives: May result in acute ergot toxicity; combination is contraindicated
- QTc-prolonging drugs: Potentiated QTc prolongation, possibly leading to polymorphic ventricular tachycardia

Contraindications

Concomitant administration with cisapride, pimozide, or terfenadine

Counseling Points

- Take tablets and suspension without regard to meals
- Take extended-release tablets with food

Key Points

- Drug interactions reported with erythromycin are likely to occur with clarithromycin
- Patients receiving drugs that are metabolized by the cytochrome P450 enzyme system should be closely monitored

◉ Erythromycin

Brand Names

Ery-Tab, E-Mycin, EES, EryPed, Ilosone

Generic Name

Erythromycin

Rx Only

Dosage Forms

Ophthalmic ointment; topical ointment, gel, and solution; multiple oral formulations; injection

Usage

Community-acquired upper and lower respiratory tract infections,* skin and skin structure infections, chlamydia, conjunctivitis,* preoperative bowl preparation*

Pregnancy Category B

Dosing

- Adults:
  - Mild to moderate infection: 250–500 mg four times daily
  - Severe infection: 500–1,000 mg every 6 hours

- Pediatrics:
  - Mild to moderate infection: 7.5–12.5 mg (base)/kg four times daily
  - Severe infection: 15–25 mg/kg (base) four times daily

Adverse Reactions: Most Common

Infusion site pain (IV), phlebitis, prolonged QTc interval, diarrhea

Adverse Reactions: Rare/Severe/Important

Hepatotoxicity (estolate form), ototoxicity (high dose)

Major Drug Interactions

Erythromycin's Effect on Other Drugs

- Carbamazepine, valproic acid: Increased levels
- Cyclosporine: Increased levels
- Ergot derivatives: Increased levels (contraindicated)
- Many HmG-CoA reductase inhibitors: Increased risk of rhabdomyolysis
- Midazolam, triazolam: Decreased clearance, prolonged sedative effect
- Theophylline: Increased concentrations
- Warfarin: Potentiated anticoagulant effect
- QTc-prolonging drugs: Potentiated QTc prolongation, possibly leading to polymorphic ventricular tachycardia

Counseling Points

- Take with a full glass of water
- Report persistent abdominal pain (> 3 days duration)
- Report any changes in hearing function

Key Points

- Dosing varies based on the specific salt used
- Erythromycin is commonly used off-label as a pro-motility agent because it directly stimulates motilin receptors in the gut. This effect also causes more diarrhea with erythromycin than with other macrolides.
- Patients receiving drugs that are metabolized by the cytochrome P450 enzyme system should be monitored closely

NITROIMIDAZOLE

Introduction

Metronidazole is the only commonly used nitroimidazole. It is unique in that it only has clinically useful activity against anaerobic organisms and is thus frequently used in anaerobic infections. It is also a drug of choice for treating *C. difficile* infections.

Mechanism of Action for the Drug Class

In susceptible organisms, metronidazole is reduced to unidentified polar products, which result in cytotoxic antimicrobial effects.

Members of the Drug Class

In this section: Metronidazole
Other: Tinidazole

⊙ Metronidazole

Brand Name

Flagyl

Generic Name

Metronidazole

Rx Only

Dosage Forms

Tablet, extended-release tablet, capsule, injection, topical gel

Usage

Treatment of anaerobic bacterial infections,* C. difficile infection,* trichomoniasis, amebiasis, giardiasis, bacterial vaginosis, pelvic inflammatory disease,* rosacea, Helicobacter pylori infection (in combination with other drugs), prophylaxis in gastrointestinal surgery

Pregnancy Category B

Dosing

- Adults:
  - Most indications: 250–500 mg oral or IV two to four times daily
  - Trichomoniasis: Can be treated with 2,000 mg orally once
- Pediatrics: 15–50 mg/kg per day in three divided doses
- Hepatic dosage adjustment: In patients with moderate to severe hepatic dysfunction, consider reducing the dose or extending the dosing interval

Adverse Reactions: Most Common

Nausea, metallic taste, peripheral neuropathy

Adverse Reactions: Rare/Severe/Important

Pancreatitis, hypersensitivity, stomatitis, confusion, dizziness, seizures

Major Drug Interactions

Drugs Affecting Metronidazole

- Alcohol: May result in a mild disulfiram reaction
- Phenobarbital: Decreased half-life of metronidazole

Metronidazole's Effect on Other Drugs

- Warfarin: Potentiated anticoagulant effect, possibly leading to bleeding events
- Disulfiram: Acute psychosis and confusion
- Lithium: Increased levels

Counseling Points

- Be aware of possible metallic taste
- Minimize alcohol intake due to potential mild disulfiram reaction

Key Points

- Metronidazole is inferior to oral vancomycin for the treatment of severe C. difficile infection but equivalent for mild to moderate infection. It is generally used as a first-line agent in mild to moderate cases due to its significantly lower cost. Unlike vancomycin, it can be given intravenously for C. difficile infection and is an option in patients with a bowel obstruction.
- Metronidazole has excellent bioavailability and is given in similar oral and intravenous doses
- Metronidazole also is given intravaginally to treat bacterial vaginosis

FOLIC ACID SYNTHESIS INHIBITORS

Introduction

The folic acid synthesis inhibitors, trimethoprim and the sulfonamides, work synergistically to prevent bacterial growth and replication. The sulfonamides were the first antibiotics made available and introduced the antibiotic era. They are still used today, most commonly in trimethoprim/sulfamethoxazole, where the two active ingredients work together in susceptible bacteria.

Mechanism of Action for the Drug Class

Trimethoprim inhibits folate utilization by inhibiting dihydrofolate reductase in bacteria. Sulfamethoxazole and other sulfonamides compete with para-aminobenzoic acid (PABA) in an earlier step in folate synthesis that only exists in bacteria. The two types of drugs have synergistic activity in many bacteria.

Members of the Drug Class

In this section: Trimethoprim/sulfamethoxazole
Others: Sulfadiazine, sulfisoxazole; topical formulations

⊙ Trimethoprim/Sulfamethoxazole

Brand Names

Bactrim, Septra

Generic Name

Trimethoprim/sulfamethoxazole

Rx Only

Dosage Forms

Tablet, suspension, injection

Usage

Urinary tract infections,* upper and lower respiratory tract infections, skin and skin structure infections,* treatment and prophylaxis of *Pneumocystis jiroveci* pneumonia,* prophylaxis of toxoplasmosis, traveler's diarrhea

Pregnancy Category C

Contraindicated in late pregnancy (see Key Points)

Dosing

- Adults:
  - Most indications: 1 DS tablet or equivalent (800 mg sulfamethoxazole/160 mg trimethoprim) twice daily
  - Urinary tract infections: 1 DS tablet twice daily
  - *Pneumocystis* prophylaxis: 1 DS tablet daily or three times a week; 1 SS (400 mg sulfamethoxazole/80 mg trimethoprim) daily
  - Toxoplasmosis prophylaxis: 1 DS tablet daily
  - *P. jiroveci* pneumonia: 15–20 mg/kg per/day of trimethoprim component divided in three to four doses
- Children:
  - Most indications: 8–10 mg/kg per day of trimethoprim component divided in three to four doses
  - *P. jiroveci* pneumonia: Same as adult dosing
- Renal dosage adjustment:
  - CrCl of 15–30 mL/min: 50% of the usual dose
  - Listed as contraindicated with CrCl < 15 mL/min but is sometimes still given in lower doses

Adverse Reactions: Most Common

Nausea, vomiting, anorexia, rash, urticaria, hyperkalemia, arthralgia, myalgia, hepatitis

Adverse Reactions: Rare/Severe/Important

Toxic epidermal necrolysis, fulminant hepatic necrosis, agranulocytosis, bone marrow suppression, crystalluria, renal failure, anaphylaxis

Major Drug Interactions

Trimethoprim/Sulfamethoxazole's Effect on Other Drugs

- Thiazides: Concomitant use has been associated with thrombocytopenia with purpura in elderly patients
- Phenytoin: Increased half-life by 39%
- Methotrexate: Increased free concentrations
- Oral hypoglycemic agents: Potentiated hypoglycemia
- Digoxin: Serum levels may increase

Counseling Points

- Take oral product with a full glass of water
- Monitor for signs of hypersensitivity

Key Points

- Dosing is based on the trimethoprim component
- The combination is commonly abbreviated as *TMP/SMX, TMP/SMZ,* or *co-trimoxazole*
- The 5:1 ratio of sulfamethoxazole to trimethoprim is consistent among all dosage forms
- Trimethoprim competes with creatinine for renal secretion. Serum creatinine values may increase during therapy but not reflect true renal dysfunction. However, trimethoprim/sulfamethoxazole can lead to renal dysfunction through crystallization or acute interstitial nephritis.
- Trimethoprim/sulfamethoxazole is pregnancy category C, but it is contraindicated during late-stage pregnancy because sulfonamides can lead to kernicterus in the newborn. For some patients, the benefits of therapy may outweigh this risk because infection in the mother can have dire consequences for the fetus.

TETRACYCLINES

Introduction

Tetracyclines are broad-spectrum antibiotics that have lost much of their utility due to increases in bacterial resistance. They are still useful for many indications, however, and they are drugs of choice in several tickborne diseases.

Mechanism of Action for the Drug Class

Tetracyclines inhibit bacterial protein synthesis by reversibly binding to the 30S ribosomal subunit, resulting in a bacteriostatic effect.

Pregnancy Category D for the Drug Class

Adverse Reactions for the Drug Class: Most Common

Nausea, vomiting, diarrhea, gastrointestinal pain, rash, photosensitivity reactions, dizziness

Adverse Reactions for the Drug Class: Rare/Severe/Important

Hypersensitivity, tooth discoloration with prolonged use

Major Drug Interactions for the Drug Class

Drugs Affecting Tetracyclines

Di- and trivalent cations: Greatly decrease absorption of tetracyclines

Tetracyclines' Effects on Other Drugs

- Concurrent use of tetracyclines and methoxyflurane has been reported to result in fatal renal toxicity
- Enhance the activity of warfarin
- Diminish effect of cell-wall active bactericidal antibiotics when used concomitantly (e.g., beta-lactams)
- May render oral contraceptives less effective

Counseling Points for the Drug Class

- Administration to children is likely to result in discoloration of the teeth, particularly with prolonged use. Use in children 8 years of age and younger only when the benefit outweighs the risk.
- Dispose of all unused medication; use of outdated tetracycline products may result in Fanconi syndrome, a disorder characterized by kidney damage
- Separate from multivalent cation–containing compounds (including milk) by at least 2 hours

Members of the Drug Class

In this section: Doxycycline, minocycline
Others: Demeclocycline, tetracycline, tigecycline (a glycylcycline)

◉ Doxycycline

Brand Name

Vibramycin

Generic Name

Doxycycline

Rx Only

Dosage Forms

Capsule, suspension, injection

Usage

Community-acquired upper and lower respiratory tract infections,* chlamydia,* Rocky Mountain spotted fever, typhus fever, Q fever, rickettsialpox, tick fevers caused by rickettsiae, Lyme disease, plague, tularemia

Dosing

- Adults: 100 mg twice daily
- Children < 100 lb: 2 mg/lb divided into two doses on the first day, then 1 mg/lb daily thereafter

◉ Minocycline

Brand Names

Minocin, Solodyn (extended-release formulation)

Generic Name

Minocycline

Rx Only

Dosage Forms

Capsule, tablet, suspension, injection

Usage

Community-acquired upper and lower respiratory tract infections,* acne,* skin and soft tissue infections,* Rocky Mountain spotted fever, typhus fever, Q fever, rickettsialpox, Lyme disease, plague, tularemia

Dosing

- Normal-release formulation
  - Adults: 200 mg once, then 100 mg twice daily
  - Children (> 8 years of age): 4 mg/kg once, then 2 mg/kg twice daily
- Extended-release formulation: 45–135 mg once daily, based on weight
- Renal dosage adjustment: Use not recommended in renal failure

Key Point

Extended-release minocycline is only approved for the treatment of acne. The normal-release formulation of minocycline is used for this indication as well.

NITROFURANS

Introduction

Nitrofurantoin is the only available nitrofuran. It has one use, the treatment of acute uncomplicated cystitis (a urinary tract infection). Therapeutic concentrations of nitrofurantoin are not reached anywhere in the body but the urinary tract. It has become more useful over time as resistance to fluoroquinolones, trimethoprim/sulfamethoxazole, and other first-line drugs has increased, particularly in *E. coli*.

Mechanism of Action for the Drug Class

The mechanism of nitrofurantoin is not exactly known, but it is known to inhibit several bacterial enzyme systems, including acetyl coenzyme A, thus interfering with metabolism and possibly cell-wall synthesis

◉ Nitrofurantoin

Brand Names

Macrodantin, Macrobid

Generic Names

Nitrofurantoin, nitrofurantoin macrocrystals (Macrobid)

Rx Only

Dosage Form

Capsule

Usage

Urinary tract infections (acute uncomplicated cystitis)

Pregnancy Category B

Contraindicated at term (see Key Points)

Dosing

- Macrobid: 100 mg twice daily
- Macrodantin: 50–100 mg four times daily
- Renal dosage adjustment: Contraindicated in patients with a CrCl < 60 mL/min

Adverse Reactions: Most Common

Nausea, headache, diarrhea, rash, dizziness

Adverse Reactions: Rare/Severe/Important

Chronic, subacute, or acute pulmonary hypersensitivity; hepatic toxicity; lupus-like syndrome; exfoliative dermatitis; peripheral neuropathy (may be irreversible); cholestatic jaundice

Major Drug Interactions

Drugs Affecting Nitrofurantoin

- Antacids containing magnesium trisilicate: Decreased absorption of nitrofurantoin
- Probenecid: Increased nitrofurantoin levels

Counseling Point

Take with food to enhance tolerability and absorption

Key Points

- Nitrofurantoin therapy will produce a false-positive urine glucose test
- Not for use for any infection other than uncomplicated cystitis
- Unlike fluoroquinolones and trimethoprim/sulfamethoxazole, nitrofurantoin is pregnancy category B and often is used in pregnant women. However, it can cause hemolytic anemia in newborns and should be avoided in pregnant women who are at term.

CYCLIC LIPOPEPTIDES

Introduction

Daptomycin is the only currently available cyclic lipopeptide. It is an IV-only agent with potent bactericidal therapy against many Gram-positive bacteria, including strains of methicillin-resistant *Staphylococcus aureus* and vancomycin-resistant enterococci. Resistance to daptomycin is currently rare, but has been reported in staphylococci and enterococci.

Mechanism of Action for the Drug Class

Daptomycin inserts itself into the cell membrane of Gram-positive bacteria through a calcium-dependent process, leading to holes in the membrane that leak essential intracellular cations and cell death.

Members of the Drug Class

In this section: Daptomycin

◉ Daptomycin

Brand Name

Cubicin

Generic Name

Daptomycin

Rx Only

Dosage Form

Injection

Usage

Skin and skin structure infections,* bacteremia,* endocarditis, urinary tract infections

Pregnancy Category B

Dosing

- Skin and skin structure infections: 4 mg/kg daily
- Bacteremia and endocarditis: 6 mg/kg daily
- Renal dosage adjustment: If CrCl < 30 mL/min, administer every other day

Adverse Reactions: Most Common

Myopathy, CPK elevation

Adverse Reactions: Rare/Severe/Important

Eosinophilic pneumonia, rhabdomyolysis

Major Drug Interactions

Drugs Affecting Daptomycin

HMG-CoA reductase inhibitors: Increased risk of CPK elevations, myopathy

Counseling Points
- Report any muscle pain or changes in urine color immediately
- If you are administering this drug yourself at home, do not double-up doses if a day of drug is missed. This can increase the risk of muscle toxicity.

Key Points
- Daptomycin is useful in that it is active against both methicillin-resistant *S. aureus* and vancomycin-resistant enterococci, but resistance to it does occur rarely. Verify susceptibility through testing.
- Daptomycin distributes to the lungs, but it is inactivated by pulmonary surfactant and cannot be used for the treatment of respiratory infections such as pneumonia
- Daptomycin can be given both by IV infusion and IV push, which can be convenient for outpatient infusion centers

ANTIFUNGALS, POLYENES

Introduction
Polyenes are one of the oldest classes of antifungals. Two agents are available: amphotericin B, which is given systemically, and nystatin, which is given as topical therapy only. Neither drug can be given orally for systemic fungal infections. Adverse reactions with IV amphotericin B are considerable.

Mechanism of Action for the Drug Class
Polyenes bind to ergosterol in the fungal cell wall, causing cell-wall instability and leakage of cytoplasmic contents

Members of the Drug Class
In this section: Amphotericin B, nystatin

◉ Amphotericin B
Brand Names
Amphocin, Fungizone

Generic Name
Amphotericin B deoxycholate

Rx Only

Dosage Form
Injection

Usage
Systemic fungal infections caused by yeasts, molds, and dimorphic fungi;* empiric antifungal therapy in febrile neutropenia;* leishmaniasis

Pregnancy Category B

Dosing
- 0.3–1.5 mg/kg per day
- Note: Lipid formulations of amphotericin B are available and are given in much higher doses. Fatal overdoses have occurred when the incorrect formulation has been given at the incorrect dose.

Adverse Reactions: Most Common
Nephrotoxicity, electrolyte wasting (primarily potassium and magnesium), infusion reactions (fever, chills, nausea, flushing, tachycardia, hypotension)

Adverse Reactions: Rare/Severe/Important
Bronchospasm, hypoxia, arrhythmias, anemia, hypersensitivity

Major Drug Interactions
Drugs Affecting Amphotericin B
- Concomitant nephrotoxic agents potentiate nephrotoxicity (including, but not limited to, cyclosporine, pentamidine, aminoglycosides, colistin, cisplatin, vancomycin)
- Corticosteroids: May potentiate the potassium-wasting effect

Key Points
- Premedicate with diphenhydramine and/or acetaminophen to minimize infusion reactions
- Ensure adequate hydration by providing boluses of saline before and after the infusion to reduce the incidence of nephrotoxicity
- Infuse over at least 2 hours to decrease infusion-related reactions
- Lipid formulations of amphotericin B are commercially available. These agents tend to have a better adverse-event profile. Recommended dosing and administration is quite different for these products.

◉ Nystatin
Brand Name
Mycostatin

Generic Name
Nystatin

Rx Only

Dosage Forms
Suspension, powder, oral and vaginal tablets, cream, ointment

Usage

Treatment and prophylaxis of cutaneous, mucocutaneous, and superficial candidal infections

Pregnancy Category C (Oral and Topical) and A (Vaginal)

Dosing

- Tablet: 500,000–1 million units three times daily
- Suspension: 400,000–600,000 units four times daily. Patient should swish in the mouth before swallowing when treating oral candidiasis.

- Topical: Apply two to three times a daily to affected area
- Vaginal: 1 vaginal tablet at bedtime daily

Adverse Reactions: Most Common

Mild nausea, vomiting (tablet)

Counseling Points

- Do not apply in large quantity to open wound
- Cover medicated area with a gauze or bandage

Key Point

Not effective for systemic fungal infections

ANTIFUNGALS, TRIAZOLES

Introduction

The introduction of the azole antifungals changed the way systemic fungal infections were treated. The excellent bioavailability of some of these drugs allows for oral therapy of systemic infections.

Mechanism of Action of the Drug Class

Azole antifungals inhibit the production of ergosterol, a component of the fungal cell membrane, by inhibiting fungal cytochromes P450

Adverse Reactions for the Drug Class: Most Common

Vomiting, abdominal pain, nausea, diarrhea, rash

Adverse Reactions for the Drug Class: Rare/Severe/Important

Elevated liver function tests (rare severe hepatic toxicity), hypersensitivity

Major Drug Interactions for the Drug Class

All agents inhibit the cytochrome P450 system and increase concentrations of drugs metabolized via this pathway

Members of the Drug Class

In this section: Fluconazole, itraconazole, voriconazole
Others: Ketoconazole, numerous topical agents, posaconazole

◉ Fluconazole

Brand Name

Diflucan

Generic Name

Fluconazole

Rx Only

Dosage Forms

Tablet, suspension, injection

Usage

Candida infections of the vagina, oropharyngeal cavity, esophagus, bloodstream, and visceral organs;* cryptococcal meningitis*

Pregnancy Category D

However, pregnancy category C for one-time doses for vaginal infections

Dosing

- Adults:
  - Most indications: 200–800 mg once daily
    - Patients with serious infections such as candidemia should first receive a loading dose of twice the maintenance, then the maintenance dose 24 hours later
  - Vaginal candidiasis: 150 mg once
- Pediatrics: 3–12 mg/kg once daily
- Renal dosage adjustment: Decrease dose 50% with CrCl < 50 mL/min

Major Drug Interactions

Drugs Affecting Fluconazole

- Hydrochlorothiazide: Increases fluconazole concentrations
- Rifampin: Decreases fluconazole concentrations

Fluconazole's Effect on Other Drugs

- Drugs metabolized via CYP450: Increased concentrations. Notable examples: Phenytoin, cyclosporine, tacrolimus, HmG-CoA reductase inhibitors, theophylline.
- Warfarin: Potentiated anticoagulant effect

Counseling Point

Women being treated with fluconazole for vaginal yeast infections should be told that symptoms (such as itching and irritation) are unlikely to subside on day 1 of therapy, even though the infection is successfully treated

Key Points

- Fluconazole has high bioavailability, and oral and intravenous doses are equivalent
- Patients prescribed fluconazole should always be screened for drug interactions
- Unlike other azoles, fluconazole has appreciable renal elimination and needs to be adjusted in renal dysfunction

◉ Itraconazole

Brand Name
Sporanox

Generic Name
Itraconazole

Rx Only

Dosage Forms
Capsule, oral solution

Usage
Candidiasis, mold infections, dimorphic fungal infections, onychomycosis*

Pregnancy Category C

Dosing
100–400 mg daily; doses > 200 mg/day should be divided twice daily

Adverse Reactions: Most Common
Hypokalemia, rash

Adverse Reactions: Rare/Severe/Important
Negative inotropic effect, especially in patients with underlying congestive heart failure

Major Drug Interactions

Drugs Affecting Itraconazole

- Inducers of CYP450: Decrease itraconazole concentrations
- Inhibitors of CYP450: Increase itraconazole concentrations
- Antacids, H2-receptor antagonists, proton pump inhibitors: Decrease itraconazole absorption

Itraconazole's Effect on Other Drugs

- Drugs metabolized by CYP450: Increased concentrations
- Cisapride, quinidine, dofetilide: QTc prolongation via inhibition of metabolism

Contraindications
Coadministration with cisapride, pimozide, quinidine, or dofetilide; heart failure

Counseling Points

- Oral solution and capsules are not interchangeable
- Take capsules with food; can add a cola beverage to enhance bioavailability

Key Points

- Oral solution has significantly better bioavailability than oral capsules (area under the curve [AUC] increased by 149%)
- Patients prescribed itraconazole should always be screened for drug interactions
- Oral solution does not have to be taken with food; the capsules should be administered with food. In addition, acid-suppressing agents have less of an effect on the bioavailability of the oral solution.

◉ Voriconazole

Brand Name
Vfend

Generic Name
Voriconazole

Rx Only

Dosage Forms
Tablet, suspension, injection

Usage
Primary therapy of invasive aspergillosis,* invasive candidiasis, esophageal candidiasis, mold infections*

Pregnancy Category D

Dosing

- IV: 6 mg/kg every 12 hours twice, then 3–4 mg/kg every 12 hours
- Oral: Either same as IV dosage or 400 mg every 12 hours twice, then 200 mg every 12 hours (100 mg every 12 hours for patients < 40 kg)
- Renal dosage adjustment: Injection is not recommended for patients with a CrCl < 50 mL/min due to accumulation
- Hepatic dosage adjustment:
  - Mild to moderate dysfunction (Child-Pugh class A or B): Reduce maintenance dose 50%
  - Not recommended in severe hepatic dysfunction

Adverse Reactions: Most Common
Rash, visual events, hepatic enzyme elevations

Adverse Reactions: Rare/Severe/Important
Hepatic failure, visual hallucinations, gastrointestinal disturbances

Major Drug Interactions

Drugs Affecting Voriconazole

- Inducers of CYP450: Decrease voriconazole concentrations
- Inhibitors of CYP450: Increase voriconazole concentrations

Voriconazole's Effect on Other Drugs

Drugs metabolized by CYP450: Increased concentrations

Contraindications

Coadministration with sirolimus, rifampin, rifabutin, efavirenz, ritonavir, long-acting barbiturates, terfenadine, astemizole, cisapride, pimozide, quinidine, ergot alkaloids, carbamazepine

Counseling Points

- Visual effects are common and dose related. They usually go away after the first few doses.
- Although the IV form is relatively contraindicated with a CrCl < 50 mL/min, it may be used when the benefits of therapy outweigh the risks of cyclodextrin accumulation

Key Points

- Injection contains the solubilizer beta-cyclodextrin, which can accumulate in renal dysfunction
- Patients prescribed voriconazole should always be screened for drug interactions
- Patients on voriconazole should have their liver function tests monitored closely

---

ANTIVIRALS, ANTIHERPES AGENTS

Introduction

Acyclovir is a commonly used antiviral agent for many types of herpesvirus infections. Due to the low bioavailability of the oral form and the need for frequent administration, the prodrug valacyclovir was developed. The only other differences between the two drugs are pharmacokinetic.

Mechanism of Action of the Drug Class

Acyclovir is a competitive inhibitor of viral DNA synthesis. Valacyclovir is a prodrug that is rapidly converted to acyclovir in vivo.

Adverse Reactions for the Drug Class: Most Common

Nausea, vomiting, diarrhea

Adverse Reactions for the Drug Class: Rare/Severe/Important

Thrombotic thrombocytopenic purpura (immunocompromised host), anaphylaxis, rash, renal failure, dizziness, agitation, crystalluria

Major Drug Interactions for the Drug Class

Drugs Affecting Acyclovir/Valacyclovir

Probenecid: Increase in the mean half-life and AUC of acyclovir

Counseling Points for the Drug Class

- Initiate therapy as soon as possible; for genital herpes, ideally during the prodromal period; other diseases, at the onset of rash
- Take oral products with a full glass of water to decrease potential for crystallization in the kidney

Members of the Drug Class

In this section: Acyclovir, valacyclovir
Other: Famciclovir

⊙ Acyclovir

Brand Name

Zovirax

Generic Name

Acyclovir

Rx Only

Dosage Forms

- Oral: Capsule (200 mg); suspension (200 mg/5 mL); tablet (400 mg, 800 mg)
- Parenteral: Concentrate (25 mg/mL; 50 mg/mL); infusion (500 mg, 1 g)

Usage

Mucosal, cutaneous, ocular, and systemic herpes simplex infection, including genital herpes;* varicella-zoster virus infection, including chicken pox and herpes zoster (shingles);* herpes encephalitis (IV)

Pregnancy Category B

Dosing

- Genital herpes:
  - Initial episode: 200 mg five times daily *or* 400 mg three times daily for 7–10 days
  - Initial episode (prostatitis): 400 mg five times daily for 10 days *or* 800 mg three times daily for 7–10 days
  - Severe initial episode: 5–10 mg/kg IV every 8 hours for 2–7 days or until clinical improvement is observed, followed by oral antiviral therapy to complete a total course of at least 10 days of therapy
  - Recurrent episodes: 200 mg five times daily *or* 400 mg three times daily *or* 800 mg twice daily for 5 days
  - Chronic suppressive therapy: 400 mg twice daily *or* 200 mg 3–5 times daily for up to 1 year

- Varicella (chicken pox): Initiate therapy within 24–48 hours of the appearance of rash
    - Immunocompetent children 2 years of age and older < 40 kg: 20 mg/kg four times daily for 5 days
    - Immunocompetent patient > 40 kg: 800 mg per dose four times daily for 5 days
    - Herpes zoster (shingles): Initiate therapy within 24–48 hours of the appearance of rash
    - Immunocompetent adults and children ≥ 12 years of age: 800 mg five times daily for 7–10 days
    - HIV-infected patient with dermatomal zoster: 800 mg five times daily for 7–10 days
    - Immunocompromised patients ≥ 12 years of age: 10 mg/kg IV every 8 hours for 7 days
    - Immunocompromised patients ≤ 12 years of age: 20 mg/kg IV every 8 hours for 7 days
- Herpes simplex virus infection:
    - Mucosal or cutaneous infection:
        - Adults: 400 mg five times daily for 7–14 days
        - Children: 10 mg/kg/dose three times daily for 7–14 days
    - Parenteral:
        - Adults: 5 mg/kg IV every 8 hours for 7 days
        - Children: 10 mg/kg IV every 8 hours for 7 days
    - Encephalitis:
        - Adults ≥ 12 years of age: 10 mg/kg IV every 8 hours for at least 10 days
        - Children ≥ 12 years of age: 20 mg/kg IV every 8 hours for at least 10 days

- Renal dosage adjustment:
    - Oral therapy: Dose adjust with CrCl < 10–25 mL/min
    - IV therapy: Dose adjust with CrCl < 50 mL/min

◉ Valacyclovir

Brand Name
Valtrex

Generic Name
Valacyclovir

Dosage Forms
Caplet

Usage
Herpes zoster infection,* genital herpes (initial, recurrent, or suppressive therapy)*

Dosing
- Treatment: 500–1,000 mg every 8–12 hours
- Suppression: 500–1,000 mg daily
- Renal dose adjustment: Decrease dose with a CrCl < 30–49 mL/min

---

ANTIVIRALS, ANTI-INFLUENZA AGENTS

Introduction
Influenza is a common, easily spread infection that is seasonal. Because it evolves so frequently, designing effective vaccines and drugs that always work is nearly impossible. Oseltamivir is an oral drug for the treatment of influenza that can shorten the duration of illness, particularly when it is started quickly after influenza symptoms begin. Like all anti-influenza agents, its effectiveness is dependent on the susceptibility of the dominant influenza strains of the season.

Mechanism of Action of the Drug Class
Oseltamivir is a neuraminidase inhibitor. It prevents the influenza viral neuraminidase enzyme from releasing new virions (viruses) from infected host cells, preventing further replication.

Members of the Drug Class
In this section: Oseltamivir
Others: Zanamivir, amantadine, rimantadine

◉ Oseltamivir

Generic Name
Oseltamivir

Brand Name
Tamiflu

Rx Only

Dosage Form
Capsule

Usage
Treatment of influenza,* prophylaxis of influenza in unvaccinated persons

Pregnancy Category C

Dosing
- Adults and children > 12 years
    - Treatment of influenza: 75 mg twice daily for 5 days (may be extended in severe infections)
    - Prophylaxis of influenza infection: 75 mg daily

- Children 1–12 years: All doses are twice daily for treatment, once daily for prophylaxis
  - < 16 kg: 30 mg
  - 16–23 kg: 45 mg
  - 24–40 kg: 60 mg
  - > 40 kg: Adult dosing
- Renal dosage adjustment:
  - Treatment with CrCl 10–30 mL/min: 75 mg once daily
  - Prophylaxis with CrCl 10–30 mL/min: 75 mg every other day or 30 mg daily

Adverse Reactions: Most Common

Headache, vomiting

Adverse Reactions: Rare/Severe/Important

Neuropsychiatric effects (particularly in children), hypersensitivity including Stevens-Johnson syndrome

Major Drug Interactions

Oseltamivir's Effect on Other Drugs

Oseltamivir may diminish the immunologic effect of the live, attenuated influenza vaccine (nasal vaccine)

Counseling Points

- Oseltamivir is not a substitute for the seasonal influenza vaccine. It should only be used for prophylaxis of influenza in patients who cannot be vaccinated, such as those with severe egg allergy.
- The sooner oseltamivir is started, the more effective it is likely to be. It may not help patients who are already recovering from influenza.
- Patients who do not receive the vaccine and contract influenza need to be vaccinated for influenza after they have recovered

Key Points

- Oseltamivir is most effective when started early. Although the package insert says it must be started within 48 hours of symptoms beginning, clinicians often start it later, particularly for severely ill or hospitalized patients.
- Oseltamivir is active against both influenza A and B strains, but dominant strains in the community may be resistant in any given year

ANTIRETROVIRALS, NUCLEOSIDE/NUCLEOTIDE REVERSE TRANSCRIPTASE INHIBITORS

Introduction

Nucleoside/nucleotide reverse transcriptase inhibitors (NRTIs) are antiretrovirals for the treatment of HIV. Currently, it is recommended that antiretroviral regimens contain at least two NRTIs in combination with another class of antiretrovirals, such as a non-nucleoside reverse transcriptase inhibitor, a protease inhibitor, an integrase inhibitor, or a CCR5 antagonist in treatment-naive patients. All NRTIs except abacavir are renally eliminated and require renal dosage adjustments. They also have minimal drug–drug interactions. Mitochondrial toxicities causing lactic acidosis, hepatic steatosis, peripheral neuropathy, pancreatitis, and lipoatrophy are less commonly associated with the NRTIs lamivudine, emtricitabine, abacavir, and tenofovir. These NRTIs are now the most commonly used agents.

Mechanism of Action for the Drug Class

NRTIs competitively inhibit the essential viral enzyme reverse transcriptase, preventing viral replication

Members of the Drug Class

In this section: Lamivudine, emtricitabine, tenofovir, abacavir
Others: Didanosine, stavudine, zidovudine

◉ Lamivudine

Brand Names

Epivir, Epivir-HBV, Epzicom (coformulated with abacavir), Combivir (coformulated with zidovudine), Trizivir (coformulated with abacavir and zidovudine)

Generic Name

Lamivudine

Rx Only

Dosage Forms

Tablet, oral solution

Usage

HIV infection,* chronic hepatitis B

Pregnancy Category C

Dosing

- 300 mg daily or 150 mg twice daily for HIV; 100 mg daily for hepatitis B
- Renal dosage adjustment:
  - CrCl 30–49 mL/min: 150 mg daily
  - CrCl 15–29 mL/min: 150 mg × 1, then 100 mg daily
  - CrCl 5–14 mL/min: 150 mg × 1, then 50 mg daily
  - CrCl < 5 mL/min: 50 mg × 1, then 25 mg daily

Adverse Reactions: Most Common

No common reactions

Adverse Reactions: Rare/Severe/Important

Lactic acidosis with hepatic steatosis; severe acute exacerbation of hepatitis may occur in HBV-coinfected patients who discontinue emtricitabine

Major Drug Interactions

Concomitant administration with emtricitabine should be avoided because they are chemically related

Contraindication

Concomitant administration with emtricitabine is contraindicated

Key Points

- Lamivudine or emtricitabine is almost always part of combination antiretroviral therapy
- Although well tolerated with minimal toxicity, lamivudine has a low genetic barrier to resistance
- Due to minimal toxicity, renal dosage adjustments for patients with severe renal impairment (CrCl < 10 mL/min) often do not decrease to less than 150 mg daily
- Commonly abbreviated as 3TC

◉ Emtricitabine

Brand Names

Emtriva, Truvada (coformulated with tenofovir)

Generic Name

Emtricitabine

Rx Only

Dosage Forms

Capsule, oral solution

Usage

HIV infection,* chronic hepatitis B

Pregnancy Category B

Dosing

- 200 mg capsule daily or 240 mg (24 mL) oral solution daily
- Renal dosage adjustment:
  - CrCl 30–49 mL/min: 200 mg every 2 days (capsule), 120 mg daily (solution)
  - CrCl 15–29 mL/min: 200 mg every 3 days (capsule), 80 mg daily (solution)
  - CrCl < 15 mL/min (including hemodialysis): 200 mg every 4 days (capsule), 60 mg daily (solution), administered after dialysis

Adverse Reactions: Most Common

Hyperpigmentation/skin discoloration

Adverse Reactions: Rare/Severe/Important

Lactic acidosis with hepatic steatosis; severe acute exacerbation of hepatitis may occur in HBV-coinfected patients who discontinue emtricitabine

Major Drug Interactions

Concomitant administration with lamivudine should be avoided because they are chemically related

Contraindication

Concomitant administration with lamivudine is contraindicated

Key Points

- Lamivudine or emtricitabine are almost always part of combination antiretroviral therapy
- Although well tolerated with minimal toxicity, emtricitabine has a low genetic barrier to resistance
- Commonly abbreviated as FTC

◉ Tenofovir

Brand Names

Viread, Truvada (coformulated with emtricitabine), Atripla (coformulated with emtricitabine and efavirenz), Complera (coformulated with emtricitabine and rilpivirine), Stribild (coformulated with emtricitabine, cobicistat, and elvitegravir)

Generic Name

Tenofovir

Rx Only

Dosage Forms

Tablet, powder

Usage

HIV infection,* chronic hepatitis B

Pregnancy Category B

Dosing

- Usual dose: 300 mg daily
- Renal dosage adjustment:
  - CrCl 30–49 mL/min: 300 mg every 2 days
  - CrCl 10–29 mL/min: 300 mg every 3 to 4 days
  - Hemodialysis: 300 mg daily for 7 days after dialysis

Adverse Reactions: Most Common

Asthenia, headache, nausea, vomiting, diarrhea, flatulence

Adverse Reactions: Rare/Severe/Important

Nephrotoxicity, decreased bone mineral density, lactic acidosis with hepatic steatosis

Major Drug Interactions

Drug Affecting Tenofovir

Adefovir: Increased nephrotoxicity

Tenofovir's Effect on Other Drugs

Atazanavir: Decreased concentrations. When given together, ritonavir must be given as well.

Essential Monitoring Parameters

Renal function (urinalysis every 6 months and serum creatinine every 3 months)

Counseling Point

Adverse effects such as asthenia, headache, nausea, vomiting, diarrhea, and flatulence should subside in 4 weeks

Key Points

- Tenofovir and emtricitabine are the two NRTIs most commonly used in combination antiretroviral therapy
- Avoid the use of tenofovir in patients with baseline renal impairment
- Do not coadminister with adefovir for hepatitis B infection
- Commonly abbreviated as TDF

⊙ Abacavir

Brand Names

Ziagen, Epzicom (coformulated with lamivudine)

Generic Name

Abacavir

Rx Only

Dosage Forms

Tablet, oral solution

Usage

HIV infection

Pregnancy Category C

Dosing

- Usual dose: 600 mg once daily or 300 mg twice daily
- Hepatic dosage adjustment:
  - Child-Pugh score 5–6: 200 mg twice daily
  - Child-Pugh score > 6: contraindicated

Adverse Reactions: Most Common

No common reactions

Adverse Reactions: Rare/Severe/Important

Hypersensitivity reaction (symptoms may include fever, rash, nausea, vomiting, malaise or fatigue, or respiratory symptoms such as sore throat, cough, or shortness of breath; increased risk if HLA-B5701 positive), lactic acidosis with hepatic steatosis

Major Drug Interactions

Abacavir's Effect on Other Drugs

- Methadone: Increased clearance, possibly leading to withdrawal
- Ribavirin: Increased risk of lactic acidosis

Essential Monitoring Parameters

Hypersensitivity reaction (fever, rash, nausea, vomiting, malaise or fatigue, or respiratory symptoms such as sore throat, cough, or shortness of breath)

Contraindications

Any manifestation of a hypersensitivity reaction; patients who test positive for HLA-B5701 (relative contraindication). Rechallenging with abacavir after an initial reaction can be fatal.

Counseling Point

Report the following signs/symptoms because they may be associated with a hypersensitivity reaction: fever, rash, nausea, vomiting, malaise or fatigue, or respiratory symptoms, such as sore throat, cough, or shortness of breath

Key Points

- Patients should undergo genetic testing for the presence of the HLA-B5701 allele before starting; if positive, do not give because it is predictive of hypersensitivity
- Avoid in patients at high risk of cardiovascular disease; studies have shown an association between abacavir and an increased risk for myocardial infarction
- Commonly abbreviated as ABC

ANTIRETROVIRALS, NON-NUCLEOSIDE REVERSE TRANSCRIPTASE INHIBITORS

Introduction

Non-nucleoside reverse transcriptase inhibitors (NNRTIs) are antiretrovirals used in the treatment of HIV. They are often used in combination with nucleoside/nucleotide reverse transcriptase inhibitors (NRTIs). They tend to have a low genetic barrier to resistance, except for second-generation NNRTIs, such as etravirine and rilpivirine. Etravirine and rilpivirine tend to have fewer adverse effects compared to efavirenz and nevirapine, but currently are not preferred agents in treatment-naive patients. Drug interactions are common because agents in this class are substrates, as well as inducers and inhibitors, of the CYP450 enzyme system.

Mechanism of Action for the Drug Class

NNRTIs inhibit the essential viral enzyme reverse transcriptase in a noncompetitive manner, preventing viral replication

Members of the Drug Class

In this section: Efavirenz
Others: Nevirapine, etravirine, rilpivirine

⊙ Efavirenz

Brand Names

Sustiva, Atripla (coformulated with tenofovir and emtricitabine)

Generic Name

Efavirenz

Rx Only

Dosage Forms

Capsule, tablet

Usage

HIV infection

Pregnancy Category D

Dosing

- 600 mg daily on an empty stomach
- Hepatic dosage adjustment:
  - Child-Pugh score < 7: No dosage adjustment recommended; use with caution
  - Child-Pugh score ≥ 7: Use not recommended

Adverse Reactions: Most Common

Dizziness, somnolence, insomnia, abnormal dreams, confusion, abnormal thinking, impaired concentration, hallucinations, elevated transaminases, hyperlipidemia, rash

Adverse Reactions: Rare/Severe/Important

Grade 3 or 4 rash (has rarely progressed to Stevens-Johnson syndrome)

Major Drug Interactions

CYP 3A4 substrate, inhibitor, and inducer

Medications That Should Not Be Administered with Efavirenz
Other NNRTIs, oral midazolam, triazolam, cisapride, pimozide, ergot alkaloids, and voriconazole (at standard doses)

Drug Interactions with Efavirenz That May Require Dosage Adjustments or Monitoring
Itraconazole, ketoconazole, posaconazole, voriconazole, carbamazepine, phenobarbital, phenytoin, clarithromycin, rifabutin, rifampin, calcium channel blockers, St. John's wort, HMG-CoA reductase inhibitors, ethinyl estradiol, methadone, and warfarin

Essential Monitoring Parameters

Liver function tests every 3 months, lipid panel yearly (if normal)

Contraindications

Concomitant administration with other NNRTIs, oral midazolam, triazolam, cisapride, pimozide, ergot alkaloids, and voriconazole (at standard doses)

Counseling Points

- Take on an empty stomach at bedtime
- Adherence is essential for successful treatment of HIV. Medications are not a cure.

Key Points

- Avoid in women of childbearing potential because efavirenz should not be used in the first trimester of pregnancy
- Avoid in patients with unstable psychiatric disease due to adverse CNS effects
- Commonly abbreviated as EFV

ANTIRETROVIRALS, PROTEASE INHIBITORS

Introduction

The protease inhibitors (PIs) are antiretrovirals used in the treatment of HIV. They are often used in combination with nucleoside/nucleotide reverse transcriptase inhibitors. Most PIs have low oral bioavailability due to hepatic first-pass metabolism. As a result, almost all PIs should be given with ritonavir to pharmacokinetically "boost" levels of the primary PI. Drugs in this class have a high genetic barrier to resistance. Most are substrates and inhibitors of the CYP450 enzyme system and can cause clinically significant drug–drug interactions. The PIs are often associated with adverse effects such as gastrointestinal intolerance, lipodystrophy, glucose intolerance, and dyslipidemia.

Mechanism of Action for the Drug Class

Inhibit the essential viral enzyme protease, preventing viral maturation

Members of the Drug Class

In this section: Ritonavir, lopinavir/ritonavir, atazanavir, darunavir
Others: Fosamprenavir, indinavir, nelfinavir, saquinavir, tipranavir

⊙ Ritonavir

Brand Names
Norvir, Kaletra (coformulated with lopinavir)

Generic Name
Ritonavir

Rx Only

Dosage Forms
Capsule, tablet, oral solution

Usage
Used as a pharmacokinetic "booster" for other protease inhibitors

Pregnancy Category B

Dosing
Usual dose (as a pharmacokinetic "booster"): 100–400 mg daily in one to two divided doses

Adverse Reactions: Most Common
Nausea, vomiting, diarrhea, abdominal pain

Major Drug Interactions
Medications That Should Not Be Administered Concomitantly with Ritonavir

Simvastatin, lovastatin, cisapride, pimozide, oral midazolam, triazolam, ergot alkaloids, amiodarone, flecainide, propafenone, quinidine, rifampin, St. John's wort, fluticasone

Drug Interactions with Ritonavir That May Require Dosage Adjustment or Monitoring

Itraconazole, ketoconazole, posaconazole, voriconazole, carbamazepine, lamotrigine, phenobarbital, phenytoin, valproic acid, clarithromycin, rifabutin, alprazolam, diazepam, HMG-CoA reductase inhibitors, methadone, phosphodiesterase type 5 inhibitors, bosentan, digoxin, calcium channel blockers, hormonal contraceptives, and psychiatric medications

Counseling Points
- Gastrointestinal discomfort is likely during the initiation of therapy but should subside within 4 weeks
- Keep ritonavir capsules in the refrigerator
- Take with food to decrease gastrointestinal side effects

Key Points
- Ritonavir is no longer used as a primary PI due to low tolerance at effective doses but is frequently used as a pharmacokinetic "booster" for other PIs via inhibition of the CYP450 system
- Commonly abbreviated as RTV, or "/r" in combination regimens

⊙ Lopinavir/Ritonavir

Brand Name
Kaletra

Generic Name
Lopinavir/ritonavir

Rx Only

Dosage Forms
Tablet, oral solution

Usage
HIV infection

Dosing
- Usual dose:
  - Lopinavir 400 mg + ritonavir 100 mg (2 tablets) twice daily
  - Lopinavir 800 mg + ritonavir 200 mg (4 tablets) once daily in patients with fewer than three lopinavir resistance-associated substitutions and who are not pregnant or receiving efavirenz, nevirapine, fosamprenavir, nelfinavir, carbamazepine, phenobarbital, or phenytoin
- Concomitant administration with efavirenz, nevirapine, fosamprenavir, or nelfinavir:
  - Lopinavir 500 mg + ritonavir 125 mg twice daily (combination of different formulations)
  - Lopinavir 533 mg + ritonavir 133 mg (6.7 mL oral solution) twice daily with food
- Hepatic dosage adjustments: Use with caution in patients with hepatic impairment

Adverse Reactions: Most Common
Asthenia, gastrointestinal disturbance, dyslipidemia, elevated transaminases

Adverse Reactions: Rare/Severe/Important
PR interval prolongation, QT interval prolongation with possible polymorphic ventricular tachycardia

Major Drug Interactions
Medications That Should Not Be Administered with Lopinavir/Ritonavir

Amiodarone, flecainide, propafenone, quinidine, pimozide, cisapride, oral midazolam, triazolam, rifampin, voriconazole, lovastatin, simvastatin, fluticasone, ergot alkaloids, fluticasone, St. John's wort

Drug Interactions with Lopinavir/Ritonavir That May Require Dosage Adjustment or Monitoring

Itraconazole, ketoconazole, posaconazole, carbamazepine, lamotrigine, phenobarbital, phenytoin, valproic acid, clarithromycin, rifabutin, alprazolam, diazepam, HMG-CoA reductase inhibitors, methadone, phosphodiesterase type 5 inhibitors, bosentan, digoxin, calcium channel blockers, hormonal contraceptives, and psychiatric medications

3

Anti-Infective Agents

Essential Monitoring Parameters

Liver function tests every 3 months, lipid panel yearly (if normal)

Counseling Points

- Gastrointestinal discomfort is likely during the initiation of therapy but should subside within 4 weeks
- Take with food to decrease gastrointestinal side effects

Key Points

- Lopinavir is pharmacokinetically limited as monotherapy and should always be administered in concert with ritonavir
- Once-daily formulation should only be administered to treatment-naive patients without concurrent CYP450 inducers or pregnancy
- Commonly abbreviated as LPV/r or LPV/RTV

⊙ Atazanavir

Brand Name

Reyataz

Generic Name

Atazanavir

Rx Only

Dosage Form

Capsule

Usage

HIV infection

Pregnancy Category B

Dosing

- Boosted or treatment-experienced patients or with tenofovir: Atazanavir 300 mg + ritonavir 100 mg once daily
- Unboosted and PI-naive patients: Atazanavir 400 mg once daily
- Concomitant administration with efavirenz and treatment-naive patients: Atazanavir 400 mg + ritonavir 100 mg once daily
- Hepatic dosage adjustment:
  - Child-Pugh score 7–9: Atazanavir 300 mg daily
  - Child-Pugh score > 9: Not recommended

Adverse Reactions: Most Common

Indirect hyperbilirubinemia, gastrointestinal disturbance, elevated transaminases, rash

Adverse Reactions: Rare/Severe/Important

Nephrolithiasis, PR interval prolongation

Major Drug Interactions

Medications That Should Not Be Administered with Atazanavir

Etravirine, nevirapine, indinavir, nevirapine, simvastatin, lovastatin, rifampin, cisapride, pimozide, quinidine, oral midazolam, triazolam, ergot alkaloids, irinotecan, St. John's wort, proton pump inhibitors (if unboosted)

Drug Interactions with Atazanavir That May Require Dosage Adjustment or Monitoring

- Itraconazole, ketoconazole, posaconazole, carbamazepine, lamotrigine, phenobarbital, phenytoin, valproic acid, clarithromycin, rifabutin, alprazolam, diazepam, HMG-CoA reductase inhibitors, methadone, phosphodiesterase type 5 inhibitors, bosentan, digoxin, calcium channel blockers, hormonal contraceptives, and psychiatric medications
- Acid-reducing agents: Drug-regimen modification is required due to the need for gastric acidity to absorb atazanavir. Specific recommendations are available and differ between acid-reducing agents and the level of treatment experience of the patient.

Essential Monitoring Parameters

Liver function tests and total bilirubin every 3 months, lipid panel yearly (if normal)

Counseling Points

- Gastrointestinal discomfort is likely during the initiation of therapy but should subside within 4 weeks
- Take with food and drink plenty of water
- Do not take antacids without first talking to your physician
- You may notice that the color of your skin turns yellow; talk to your physician

Key Points

- Use with caution in patients taking acid-reducing agents. Many of these agents are overused, and it may be possible to discontinue them.
- Commonly abbreviated as ATV

⊙ Darunavir

Brand Name

Prezista

Generic Name

Darunavir

Rx Only

Dosage Form

Tablet

Usage

HIV infection

Pregnancy Category C

Dosing

- Treatment-naive or treatment-experienced patients with no darunavir resistance–associated mutations: Darunavir 800 mg + ritonavir 100 mg daily with food
- Treatment-experienced patients with at least one darunavir resistance–associated mutation: Darunavir 600 mg + ritonavir 100 mg twice daily with food
- Hepatic dosage adjustments: If Child-Pugh score > 9, use is not recommended

Adverse Reactions: Most Common

Gastrointestinal disturbance, dyslipidemia, elevated transaminases, rash

Adverse Reactions: Rare/Severe/Important

Hypersensitivity

Major Drug Interactions

Medications That Should Not Be Administered with Darunavir

Simvastatin, lovastatin, rifampin, cisapride, pimozide, oral midazolam, triazolam, ergot alkaloids, carbamazepine, phenobarbital, phenytoin, amiodarone, lidocaine, quinidine, fluticasone

Drug Interactions with Darunavir That May Require Dosage Adjustment or Monitoring

Acid-reducing agents, itraconazole, ketoconazole, posaconazole, carbamazepine, lamotrigine, phenobarbital, phenytoin, valproic acid, clarithromycin, rifabutin, alprazolam, diazepam, HMG-CoA reductase inhibitors, methadone, phosphodiesterase type 5 inhibitors, bosentan, digoxin, calcium channel blockers, hormonal contraceptives, and psychiatric medications

Essential Monitoring Parameters

Liver function tests every 3 months, lipid panel yearly (if normal)

Counseling Points

- Gastrointestinal discomfort is likely during the initiation of therapy but should subside within 4 weeks
- Take with food to decrease gastrointestinal side effects and for increased absorption of the drug

Key Points

- Use caution in patients with sulfa allergies due to sulfa moiety in darunavir
- Do not give without ritonavir
- Commonly abbreviated as DRV

INTEGRASE INHIBITORS (ANTIRETROVIRALS)

Introduction

Integrase inhibitors are antiretrovirals used in the treatment of HIV. They are often used in combination with NRTIs. Compared to the PIs and NNRTIs, integrase inhibitors are extremely well tolerated and have limited adverse effects.

Mechanism of Action for the Drug Class

Integrase inhibitors inhibit the essential viral enzyme integrase, preventing integration of the proviral gene into human DNA

Members of the Drug Class

In this section: Raltegravir
Others: Elvitegravir

⊚ Raltegravir

Brand Name
Isentress

Generic Name
Raltegravir

Rx Only

Dosage Form
Tablet

Usage
HIV infection

Pregnancy Category C

Dosing
- 400 mg twice daily
- Concomitant administration with rifampin: 800 mg twice daily
- Hepatic dosing adjustment: Use with caution in cases of severe hepatic impairment

Adverse Reactions: Most Common

No common reactions

Adverse Reactions: Rare/Severe/Important

Creatine phosphokinase elevation

Major Drug Interactions

Drugs Affecting Raltegravir

Rifampin: Decreases raltegravir concentrations, necessitating dose increases of raltegravir

Counseling Point

Adherence is essential for successful treatment of HIV. Medications are not a cure.

Key Point

Although well tolerated with minimal drug interactions, raltegravir has a low genetic barrier to resistance

REVIEW QUESTIONS

1. Concomitant use of lamivudine is contraindicated with which of the following antiretrovirals?
   a. Tenofovir
   b. Abacavir
   c. Emtricitabine
   d. Zidovudine

2. Which of the following antiretrovirals can be used for the treatment of chronic hepatitis B?
   a. Darunavir
   b. Atazanavir
   c. Abacavir
   d. Tenofovir

3. Which of the following antiretrovirals causes renal toxicity?
   a. Abacavir
   b. Raltegravir
   c. Efavirenz
   d. Tenofovir

4. Which of the following antiretrovirals requires genetic testing for HLA-B*5701 in order to test for risk of hypersensitivity reaction?
   a. Atazanavir
   b. Zidovudine
   c. Abacavir
   d. Lopinavir

5. Which of the following antiretrovirals is in pregnancy category D?
   a. Tenofovir
   b. Efavirenz
   c. Raltegravir
   d. Darunavir

6. Which of the following antiretrovirals is used to pharmacokinetically "boost" the levels of other protease inhibitors?
   a. Atazanavir
   b. Darunavir
   c. Ritonavir
   d. Lopinavir

7. Which of the following antiretrovirals already comes coformulated with ritonavir?
   a. Darunavir
   b. Atazanavir
   c. Lopinavir
   d. Abacavir

8. Which of the following is *not* an adverse effect of atazanavir?
   a. Hyperbilirubinemia
   b. Renal toxicity
   c. Rash
   d. Elevated transaminases

9. Which of the following drugs is contraindicated with darunavir and ritonavir?
   a. Lisinopril
   b. Metformin
   c. Simvastatin
   d. Warfarin

10. The dose of raltegravir needs to be increased from 400 mg twice daily to 800 mg twice daily when coadministered with which of the following?
    a. Phenytoin
    b. Rifampin
    c. St. John's Wort
    d. Carbamazepine

11. Which class of antiretrovirals generally needs to be dose adjusted for renal impairment?
    a. Nucleoside/nucleotide reverse transcriptase inhibitors
    b. Non-nucleoside reverse transcriptase inhibitors
    c. Protease inhibitors
    d. Integrase inhibitors

12. Which of the following is an adverse effect of efavirenz?
    a. Lipoatrophy
    b. Vivid dreams
    c. Mitochondrial toxicity
    d. PR interval prolongation

13. Which of the following antiretrovirals causes minimal drug–drug interactions?
    a. Atazanavir
    b. Efavirenz
    c. Ritonavir
    d. Raltegravir

14. Which of the following antiretrovirals has a sulfa moiety?
    a. Zidovudine
    b. Efavirenz
    c. Darunavir
    d. Atazanavir

15. Which of the following classes of antiretrovirals generally causes gastrointestinal upset?

    a. Nucleoside/nucleotide reverse transcriptase inhibitors
    b. Non-nucleoside reverse transcriptase inhibitors
    c. Protease inhibitors
    d. Integrase inhibitors

16. Which of the following drugs is used for the treatment of latent tuberculosis?

    a. Abacavir
    b. Isoniazid
    c. Gentamicin
    d. Vancomycin

17. Which of the following drugs is active against *Pseudomonas aeruginosa*?

    a. Amoxicillin
    b. Omnicef
    c. Tobramycin
    d. Vancomycin

18. Which of the following drugs inhibits the activity of bacterial topoisomerases?

    a. Gentamicin
    b. Levaquin
    c. Azithromycin
    d. Metronidazole

19. Which of the following drugs is *only* useful for treating infections caused by anaerobic bacteria?

    a. Tetracycline
    b. Bactrim
    c. Metronidazole
    d. Cubicin

20. Which of the following drugs commonly causes fevers and chills during the infusion?

    a. Amphotericin B
    b. Fluconazole
    c. Itraconazole
    d. Voriconazole

21. Which of the following drugs is contraindicated in patients with heart failure?

    a. Valtrex
    b. Sporanox
    c. Diflucan
    d. Cefdinir

22. Which of the following antiviral drugs is effective in the treatment of influenza?

    a. Epivir
    b. Tamiflu
    c. Valtrex
    d. Zovirax

23. Which of the following drugs treats skin infections caused by methicillin-resistant *Staphylococcus aureus*?

    a. Cubicin
    b. Macrobid
    c. Flagyl
    d. Tobramycin

24. Which of the following drugs is known to cause eosinophilic pneumonia?

    a. Amoxicillin
    b. Daptomycin
    c. Septra
    d. Vancomycin

25. Which of the following drugs is available as a single-dose formulation?

    a. Amoxicillin
    b. Azithromycin
    c. Levofloxacin
    d. Avelox

26. Which of the following indications is oral Vancocin used for?

    a. Skin infections caused by methicillin-resistant *Staphylococcus aureus*
    b. Urinary tract infections
    c. *Clostridium difficile* infections
    d. Pneumonia

27. Which of the following drugs causes bodily fluids such as urine to appear orange-red?

    a. Biaxin
    b. Diflucan
    c. Rifampin
    d. Vancocin

28. Which of the following drugs can cause jaundice in neonates?

    a. Cefdinir
    b. Ceftriaxone
    c. Cefuroxime
    d. Cephalexin

29. Which of the following drugs should *not* be used for community-acquired pneumonia?

    a. Cipro
    b. Levaquin
    c. Avelox
    d. Azithromycin

30. Which of the following drugs is a potent inducer of the cytochrome P450 system?

    a. Biaxin
    b. Erythromycin
    c. Rifadin
    d. Isoniazid

Anti-Infective Agents

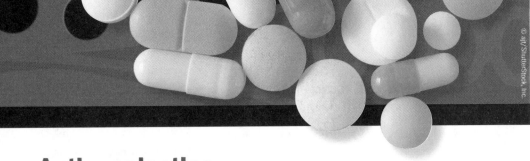

Antineoplastics

Rachel Clark-Vetri, PharmD, BCOP

ALKYLATING AGENTS

Introduction

Alkylating agents are a large drug class of chemotherapeutic agents composed of drugs used in adults and children to treat a number of malignant and nonmalignant diseases. The most notable side effects include bone marrow suppression, nausea and vomiting, and mucositis, as well as long-term complications, such as sterility and secondary malignancies. These drugs have a wide dosing range based on the indication and route of administration.

Mechanism of Action for the Drug Class

Alkylating agents form strong covalent bonds with DNA, inhibiting replication and causing bond breaks and cell death. These agents are directly toxic to DNA and are considered cell-cycle nonspecific, meaning that they can cause cell death regardless of the phase of cell division.

Members of the Drug Class

In this section: Cyclophosphamide, temozolomide
Others: Bendamustine, busulfan, carmustine, chlorambucil, dacarbazine, ifosfamide, lomustine, mechlorethamine, melphalan, procarbazine, thiotepa

⊚ Cyclophosphamide

Brand Name
Cytoxan

Generic Name
Cyclophosphamide

Rx Only

Dosage Forms
Injection, tablet

Usage

- Oncologic: Hodgkin and non-Hodgkin lymphoma,* chronic lymphocytic leukemia (CLL),* acute myelogenous leukemia (AML),* acute lymphocytic leukemia (ALL),* multiple myeloma, neuroblastoma, breast cancer,* testicular cancer, ovarian cancer, lung cancer, stem cell immobilization, Ewing sarcoma, rhabdomyosarcoma, mycosis fungoides, Wilms' tumor
- Nononcologic: Severe rheumatoid disorders, Wegener's granulomatosis, myasthenia gravis, multiple sclerosis, systemic lupus erythematosus, lupus nephritis, autoimmune hemolytic anemia, idiopathic thrombocytic purpura (ITP), antibody-induced pure red cell aplasia, nephrotic syndrome in children

Pregnancy Category D

Dosing

- Individual protocols specify dosing for specific indications and institutions
- Usual doses:
  - Oral: 50–100 mg/m² per day up to 14 days continuous therapy
  - IV: Single dose of 400–1,800 mg/m², which may be repeated at 2- to 4-week intervals
- Juvenile rheumatoid arthritis: 10 mg/kg IV every 2 weeks
- High dose: 1.8 g/m² IV daily for 4 days (total of 7.2 g/m²) or 50 mg/kg daily for 4 days
- Renal dosage adjustment:
  - CrCl < 10 mL/min: Administer 75% of normal dose
  - Hemodialysis: Administer 50% of dose post hemodialysis
- Hepatic dosage adjustment:
  - Bilirubin 3.1–5 mg/dL: Administer 75% of dose
  - Bilirubin > 5 mg/dL: Avoid use

---

* Throughout the text, an asterisk (*) is used to indicate the most common uses of a drug.

Adverse Reactions: Most Common

Leukopenia, nausea and vomiting, alopecia, diarrhea, mucositis, amenorrhea

Adverse Reactions: Rare/Severe/Important

Hemorrhagic cystitis, sterility, secondary malignancies, SIADH, cardiac necrosis, renal tubular necrosis, skin rash

Major Drug Interactions

Drugs Affecting Cyclophosphamide

Antineoplastics: Enhance bone marrow suppression

Cyclophosphamide's Effect on Other Drugs

- Succinylcholine: Decreases metabolism
- Vaccines: Diminishes therapeutic effect of vaccines via immunosuppression
- Warfarin: Increases bleeding risk

Contraindications

Severely depressed bone marrow function

Counseling Points

- Drink plenty of fluids (3–4 L daily) for at least 24 hours after an IV dose
- Report any painful urination or discolored or bloody urine
- Take oral doses early in the day

Key Points

- Doses > 1 g/m² are likely to require uroprotection with Mesna to prevent hemorrhagic cystitis
- Monitor patients for signs of leukopenia and infection
- Give patient antiemetics to prevent nausea and vomiting

◉ Temozolomide

Brand Name

Temodar

Generic Name

Temozolomide

Rx Only

Dosage Forms

Capsule, injection

Usage

Malignant glioblastoma,* refractory anaplastic astrocytoma*

Pregnancy Category D

Dosing

- Anaplastic astrocytoma (refractory): Oral, IV:
  - Initial dose: 150 mg/m² daily for 5 days; repeat every 28 days
  - Subsequent doses: 100–200 mg/m² daily for 5 days per treatment cycle
- Glioblastoma multiforme (newly diagnosed, high-grade glioma): Oral, IV:
  - Concomitant phase: 75 mg/m² daily for 42 days with focal radiotherapy
  - Maintenance phase: Begin 4 weeks after concomitant phase completion. Cycle 1: 150 mg/m²/day for 5 days; repeat every 28 days. Cycles 2–6: May increase to 200 mg/m²/day for 5 days every 28 days.
- Renal dosage adjustment: If CrCl < 36 mL/min/m², use with caution

Adverse Reactions: Most Common

Leukopenia, anemia, alopecia, nausea

Adverse Reactions: Rare/Severe/Important

Pancytopenia, Stevens-Johnson syndrome, severe life-threatening opportunistic infections, pneumonitis

Major Drug Interactions

Drugs Affecting Temozolomide

- Clozapine: Increases risk of agranulocytosis
- Valproic acid: Increases toxicity

Temozolomide's Effects on Other Drugs

Vaccines: Efficacy may be diminished

Contraindications

Hypersensitivity to temozolomide or dacarbazine, severely depressed bone marrow function

Counseling Points

- Swallow capsules whole with a glass of water. Do not chew or open the capsules.
- The incidence of nausea and vomiting is decreased when taken on an empty stomach and/or at bedtime
- Take capsules consistently either with food or without food (absorption is affected by food)

Key Points

- *Pneumocystis carinii* pneumonia (PCP) prophylaxis should be given concurrently with radiation
- No live virus vaccines should be given during therapy
- Antiemetics should be given to prevent nausea and vomiting
- Increased MGMT (O-6-methylguanine-DNA methyltransferase) activity/levels within tumor tissue is associated with temozolomide resistance

Introduction

Anthracyclines are a group of antineoplastic drugs used to treat a variety of malignant diseases, including both hematologic and solid tumors. Given only as an IV treatment, they are most notable for their risk of causing cardiotoxicity. They are vesicants that can cause severe skin necrosis if extravasation occurs.

Mechanism of Action for the Drug Class

Inhibition of DNA and RNA synthesis by intercalation of DNA base pairs and inhibition of DNA repair by topoisomerase

Members of the Drug Class

In this section: Doxorubicin
Others: Daunorubicin, epirubicin, idarubicin, mitoxantrone

◉ Doxorubicin

Brand Name
Adriamycin

Generic Name
Doxorubicin

Rx Only

Dosage Form
Injection

Usage

Acute lymphoblastic leukemia (ALL), acute myeloid leukemia (AML), Hodgkin disease, malignant lymphoma,* soft tissue and bone sarcomas, thyroid cancer, small cell lung cancer, breast cancer,* gastric cancer, ovarian cancer, bladder cancer, neuroblastoma, Wilms' tumor, multiple myeloma

Pregnancy Category D

Dosing

- Individual protocols specify dosing for specific indications and institutions
- Children:
  - 30–75 mg/m^2 per dose every 3–4 weeks *or*
  - 20–30 mg/m^2 per dose once weekly *or*
  - 60–90 mg/m^2 given as a continuous infusion over 96 hours every 3–4 weeks
- Adults:
  - 60–75 mg/m^2 per dose every 3–4 weeks *or*
  - 20–30 mg/m^2 daily for 3 days every 4 weeks *or*
  - 60 mg/m^2 per dose every 2 weeks (dose dense)
- Hepatic dosage adjustment:
  - Transaminases two to three times the upper limit of normal: Administer 75% of dose
  - Bilirubin 1.2–3 mg/dL or transaminases more than three times the upper limit of normal: Administer 50% of dose
  - Bilirubin 3.1–5 mg/dL: Administer 25% of dose
  - Bilirubin > 5 mg/dL: Do not administer

Adverse Reactions: Most Common

Leukopenia, anemia, thrombocytopenia, nausea and vomiting, alopecia, diarrhea, mucositis, amenorrhea

Adverse Reactions: Rare/Severe/Important

Acute and delayed cardiotoxicity, sterility, secondary malignancy

Major Drug Interactions

Drugs Affecting Doxorubicin
- Cyclosporine: May increase doxorubicin levels
- Paclitaxel: Reduces the clearance of doxorubicin
- Trastuzumab: May increase cardiotoxicity of doxorubicin

Doxorubicin's Effect on Other Drugs
- Digoxin: Levels may be decreased
- Phenytoin: Levels may be decreased
- Radiation: Severe skin reactions are possible

Contraindications

Recent myocardial infarction, severe myocardial insufficiency, severe arrhythmia; previous therapy with high cumulative doses of doxorubicin, daunorubicin, idarubicin, or other anthracycline and anthracenediones; baseline neutrophil count < 1,500/mm^3; severe hepatic impairment

Counseling Points

- This drug may darken your urine for 24–48 hours
- Watch for fever, malaise, sore mouth or throat, pain or swelling at injection site

Key Points

- Dose adjustments may be needed for patients with inadequate marrow reserve
- No live virus vaccines should be given during therapy
- Doxorubicin is a vesicant. Extravasation should be treated with topical dimethylsulfoxide and cold compresses or dexrazoxane.
- Patients should have ejection fraction measured before starting therapy
- Monitor patients for signs of infection and mucositis
- Premedicate with antiemetics to prevent nausea and vomiting
- A liposomal formulation of doxorubicin (Doxil) is available. However, note that the two formulations have different indications and dosing regimens and cannot be substituted for each other.

4

Antineoplastics

ANTIESTROGENS

Introduction

The available antiestrogens are selective estrogen receptor modulators (SERMs) commonly used for the treatment of breast cancer. Tamoxifen and raloxifene are also approved to prevent breast cancer in patients who are at high risk of the disease.

Mechanism of Action for the Drug Class

Compete with estrogen for binding sites in target tissues such as the breast, decreasing the effects of estrogen in those tissues.

Members of the Drug Class

In this section: Tamoxifen
Others: Toremifene, raloxifene

◉ Tamoxifen

Brand Name
Nolvadex

Generic Name
Tamoxifen

Rx Only

Dosage Form
Tablet

Usage
Breast cancer; reduction in breast cancer incidence in high-risk women;* treatment of ductal carcinoma in situ

Pregnancy Category X

Dosing
- Treatment of metastatic breast cancer: 20–40 mg daily
- Adjuvant treatment for breast cancer, ductal carcinoma in situ, and reduction of breast cancer risk: 20 mg daily for 5 years

Adverse Reactions: Most Common

Hot flashes, mood changes, vaginal discharge or bleeding, menstrual irregularities, weight gain

Adverse Reactions: Rare/Severe/Important

Blood clots, hair loss, bone pain, endometrial hyperplasia, cataracts

Major Drug Interactions

Drugs Affecting Tamoxifen
- Strong inhibitors or inducers of CYP2C9, CYP2D6, and CYP3A4: Increase or decrease efficacy (may increase risk of breast cancer)
- SSRIs: Decrease effectiveness

Tamoxifen's Effect on Other Drugs
Warfarin: Increases anticoagulant effects

Contraindications

Women who require concomitant anticoagulant therapy, women with a history of deep vein thrombosis or pulmonary embolus, pregnancy

Counseling Points

- Take steps to avoid pregnancy when taking tamoxifen and during the 2 months after discontinuation
- Annual PAP smear and pelvic exam are recommended while on therapy
- Annual eye exams are recommended while on therapy

Key Points

- The benefits of tamoxifen as a treatment for breast cancer are firmly established and far outweigh the potential risks for most women
- Tamoxifen may help decrease bone loss in postmenopausal women
- Patients require annual screening for endometrial cancer while on therapy

ANTIMETABOLITES

Introduction

This large class of antineoplastic drugs is similar in structure to naturally occurring compounds. All the agents in this class cause GI side effects to varying degrees, depending on the agent, dose, and route of administration. Each agent also is associated with unique side effects.

Mechanism of Action for the Drug Class

These compounds kill tumor cells by inhibiting DNA synthesis by a specific mechanism or they incorporate themselves into DNA, causing apoptosis. They generally have greater toxicity in rapidly growing cancer cells than normal cells of the host, but many of their toxicities arise from host cell effects.

Members of the Drug Class

In this section: Capecitabine, cytarabine, 5-fluorouracil, gemcitabine, mercaptopurine, methotrexate, pemetrexed
Others: Cladribine, fludarabine, floxuridine, hydroxyurea, nelarabine, thioguanine

◉ Capecitabine

Brand Name
Xeloda

Generic Name
Capecitabine

Rx Only

Dosage Form
Tablet

Usage
Metastatic colorectal cancer,* adjuvant therapy of colon cancer,* metastatic breast cancer,* gastric cancer,* pancreatic cancer,* esophageal cancer, ovarian cancer, metastatic renal cell cancer, neuroendocrine tumors, metastatic CNS lesions

Pregnancy Category D

Dosing
- Individual protocols specify dosing for specific indications and institutions
- Usual dose: 1,000–1,250 mg/m^2 PO twice daily
- Renal dosage adjustment:
  - CrCl 30–50 mL/min: Administer 75% of dose
  - CrCl < 30 mL/min: Contraindicated
- Hepatic dosage adjustment: Avoid in severe impairment

Adverse Reactions: Most Common
Leukopenia, anemia, thrombocytopenia, nausea and vomiting, diarrhea, mucositis, skin discoloration, palmar-plantar erythrodysesthesias, eye irritation

Adverse Reactions: Rare/Severe/Important
Chest pain, venous thrombosis

Major Drug Interactions
Drugs Affecting Capecitabine
Leucovorin: Enhances toxic effect

Capecitabine's Effect on Other Drugs
Phenytoin: Increases serum concentration

Contraindications
Known deficiency of dihydropyrimidine dehydrogenase (DPD), severe renal impairment (CrCl < 30 mL/min)

Counseling Points
- Report any fever, mouth sores, rashes, or diarrhea
- Avoid sunlight exposure and use sunscreen when exposure cannot be avoided
- Take with food
- Avoid use of antacids within 2 hours of taking medicine
- Do not crush, chew, or dissolve tablets

Key Points
- No live virus vaccines should be given during therapy
- Food reduces the rate and extent of absorption of capecitabine
- May cause a painful rash on the hands and feet

◉ Cytarabine

Brand Name
ARA-C

Generic Name
Cytarabine

Rx Only

Dosage Form
Injection

Usage
Treatment of acute myelogenous leukemia (AML),* acute lymphocytic leukemia (ALL),* chronic myelogenous leukemia (blast phase),* and lymphomas; prophylaxis and treatment of meningeal leukemia

Pregnancy Category D

Dosing
- Individual protocols specify dosing for specific indications and institutions
- Usual IV doses:
  - Children: 75–200 mg/m^2 for 5- to 10-day therapy
  - Adults:
    - 100–200 mg/m^2 daily for 5–10 days *or*
    - 100 mg/m^2 daily for 7 days *or*
    - 100 mg/m^2 per dose every 12 hours for 7 days *or*
    - High dose: 1–3 g/m^2 every 12 hours for up to 12 doses
- Usual intrathecal doses:
  - Adults: 5–75 mg/m^2 per dose every 2–7 days
  - Children:
    - 30 mg/m^2 per dose
    - Children < 3 years of age: Dose based on age
- Renal dosage adjustment:
  - No adjustment needed for 100–200 mg/m^2
  - High dose, CrCl 46–60 mL/min: Administer 60% of dose
  - High dose, CrCl 31–45 mL/min: Administer 50% of dose
  - High dose, CrCl < 30 mL/min: Avoid use
- Hepatic dosage adjustment: Reduce dose in severe dysfunction

Adverse Reactions: Most Common

Mucositis, diarrhea, nausea and vomiting, leucopenia, anemia, thrombocytopenia, conjunctivitis, alopecia

Adverse Reactions: Rare/Severe/Important

Chest pain, tumor lysis syndrome, neurotoxicity, coma, rash, skin desquamation, ocular toxicity

Counseling Points

- No live virus vaccines should be given during therapy
- Watch for fever, mouth sores, and diarrhea
- Stay well hydrated by drinking lots of fluids during therapy
- Report any changes in mental status
- May cause nausea and vomiting
- Increased risk of infection

Key Points

- Monitor for mental status changes during therapy
- Patients require aggressive hydration and antiemetic therapy
- May require prophylaxis for tumor lysis syndrome
- Myelosuppression can be severe and prolonged
- Patients require steroid eye drops to prevent ocular toxicities

⊙ 5-Fluorouracil

Brand Names

5-FU, Efudex

Generic Name

5-Fluorouracil

Rx Only

Dosage Forms

Injection, topical cream, topical solution

Usage

Treatment of carcinomas of the breast,* colon,* rectum,* pancreas,* stomach; head and neck cancer; anal cancer; cervical cancer; topically for the management of actinic or solar keratoses and superficial basal cell carcinomas*

Pregnancy Category D

Dosing

- Individual protocols specify dosing for specific indications and institutions
- IV bolus:
  - 500–600 mg/m^2 per day weekly *or*
  - 425 mg/m^2 daily on days 1–5 every 4 weeks
- Continuous IV infusion:
  - 1,000 mg/m^2 daily for 4–5 days every 3–4 weeks *or*
  - 300–400 mg/m^2 daily *or*
  - 225 mg/m^2 daily for 5–8 weeks (with radiation therapy)
- Topical: Apply to lesions twice daily for 2–4 weeks

- Renal dosage adjustment: After dialysis, administer 50% of dose
- Hepatic dosage adjustment: If bilirubin ≥ 5 mg/dL, avoid use

Adverse Reactions: Most Common

Leukopenia, anemia, thrombocytopenia, nausea and vomiting, diarrhea, mucositis, skin discoloration, palmar-plantar erythrodysesthesias, eye irritation; skin irritation with topical

Adverse Reactions: Rare/Severe/Important

Chest pain

Major Drug Interactions

Drugs Affecting 5-Fluorouracil

Leucovorin: Increases both toxic effects and efficacy

5-Fluorouracil's Effect on Other Drugs

- Carvedilol: Increases serum concentrations
- Natalizumab: Increases toxicities
- Phenytoin: Increases serum concentration
- Warfarin: Increases bleeding risk

Counseling Points

- No live virus vaccines should be given during therapy
- Watch for fever, mouth sores, and diarrhea
- Avoid sunlight exposure and use sunscreen when exposure cannot be avoided
- Wash hands after using topical formulation
- Avoid drinking alcohol while taking this medication

Key Points

- Patients with a genetic deficiency of dihydropyrimidine dehydrogenase have increased systemic toxicities
- May be an irritant if it extravasates from the vein
- May cause severe diarrhea and mucositis

⊙ Gemcitabine

Brand Name

Gemzar

Generic Name

Gemcitabine

Rx Only

Dosage Form

Injection

Usage

Metastatic breast cancer;* locally advanced or metastatic non-small cell lung cancer (NSCLC) or pancreatic cancer;* advanced, relapsed ovarian cancer, bladder cancer, cervical cancer, Hodgkin disease, non-Hodgkin lymphomas, small cell lung cancer,* hepatobiliary cancers*

Pregnancy Category D

Dosing

- Individual protocols specify dosing for specific indications and institutions
- 1,000 mg/m² per day IV weekly up to 7 weeks followed by 1 week rest
- Renal dosage adjustment: Caution with severe impairment; no specific recommendations on dose reductions are available

Adverse Reactions: Most Common

Leukopenia, thrombocytopenia, anemia, diarrhea, skin rash, nausea, flulike symptoms, peripheral edema, proteinuria

Adverse Reactions: Rare/Severe/Important

Hematuria, hepatotoxicity

Major Drug Interactions

Gemcitabine's Effect on Other Drugs

- Bleomycin: Increases risk of pulmonary toxicity
- Fluorouracil: Increases serum concentration
- Warfarin: Increases bleeding risk

Counseling Points

- Watch for fever, bleeding, and bruising
- Flu symptoms can be severe; analgesics may be used to decrease these effects

Key Points

- No live virus vaccines should be given during therapy
- Rash is usually self-limiting
- Thrombocytopenia is common
- Flulike symptoms may require the use of acetaminophen or NSAIDs
- Gemcitabine is a radiosensitizer and will increase the toxicity of radiation therapy if used concurrently

⦿ Mercaptopurine

Brand Name
Purinethol

Generic Name
Mercaptopurine

Rx Only

Dosage Form
Tablet

Usage
Treatment (maintenance and induction) of acute lymphoblastic leukemia (ALL);* steroid-sparing agent for corticosteroid-dependent Crohn's disease (CD) and ulcerative colitis (UC); maintenance of remission in CD; fistulizing CD

Pregnancy Category D

Dosing

- Individual protocols specify dosing for specific indications and institutions
- Oncologic indications:
  - Induction: 2.5–5 mg/kg daily
  - Maintenance: 1.5–2.5 mg/kg daily or 80–100 mg/m² daily given once daily
- Reduction of steroid use in CD or UC, maintenance of remission in CD or fistulizing disease (unlabeled uses):
  - Initial: 50 mg PO daily
  - May increase by 25 mg daily every 1–2 weeks as tolerated to target dose of 1–1.5 mg/kg daily
- Renal dosage adjustment:
  - CrCl < 50 mL/min: Administer every 48 hours
  - Hemodialysis: Administer every 48 hours
- Hepatic dosage adjustment: Reduced dosage may be required

Adverse Reactions: Most Common

Leukopenia, thrombocytopenia, anemia, hepatotoxicity, drug fever, hyperpigmentation and rash

Adverse Reactions: Rare/Severe/Important

Encephalopathy, ascites

Major Drug Interactions

Drugs Affecting Mercaptopurine
Allopurinol: Increases mercaptopurine levels

Mercaptopurine's Effect on Other Drugs
Warfarin: Effects may be inhibited

Counseling Points

- Watch for fever, malaise, bleeding, and bruising
- Take on an empty stomach

Key Points

- No live virus vaccines should be given during therapy
- Administration in the evening (versus morning administration) may lower the risk of relapse
- Dosage adjustment with concurrent allopurinol: Reduce mercaptopurine dosage by a quarter to a third of the usual dose
- TPMT genotyping may identify individuals at risk for toxicity
- Do not use the terms *6-mercaptopurine* or *6-MP* when writing prescriptions. The use of these terms has been associated with sixfold overdosage.

⦿ Methotrexate

Brand Name
Rheumatrex

Generic Name
Methotrexate

Rx Only

Dosage Forms

Injection, tablet

Usage

- Nononcologic: Treatment of psoriasis (severe, recalcitrant, disabling) and severe rheumatoid arthritis (RA),* including polyarticular-course juvenile rheumatoid arthritis (JRA); ectopic pregnancy;* Crohn's disease (CD)
- Oncologic: Treatment of trophoblastic neoplasms (gestational choriocarcinoma, chorioadenoma destruens, and hydatidiform mole),* acute lymphoblastic leukemia (ALL),* meningeal leukemia,* breast cancer, head and neck cancer (epidermoid), cutaneous T-cell lymphoma (advanced mycosis fungoides), lung cancer (squamous cell and small cell), advanced non-Hodgkin lymphomas, osteosarcoma

Pregnancy Category X

Dosing

- Adult:
  - Individual protocols specify dosing for specific indications and institutions
  - Antineoplastic dosage range: Range is wide, from 30–40 mg/m^2 per week IV to 100–12,000 mg/m^2 with leucovorin rescue
  - RA: 7.5 mg PO once weekly or 2.5 mg PO every 12 hours for three doses per week, not to exceed 20 mg per week
  - Psoriasis:
    - 2.5–5 mg/dose PO every 12 hours for three doses given weekly *or*
    - 10–25 mg/dose PO or IM given once weekly
  - Ectopic pregnancy and abortion: 50 mg/m^2 IM once
  - Note that doses for oncologic indications are frequently much higher than for other uses
- Children:
  - JRA: 10 mg/m^2 PO or IM once weekly, then 5–15 mg/m^2 per week as a single dose or as three divided doses given 12 hours apart
  - Antineoplastic dosage range:
    - Oral, IM: 7.5–30 mg/m^2 per week or every 2 weeks
    - IV: Range: 10 mg/m^2 bolus dosing to 18,000 mg/m^2. Continuous infusion over 6–42 hours: Doses over 150 mg/m^2 will require leucovorin rescue.
    - Pediatric solid tumors:
      - < 12 years: 12 g/m^2 (dosage range: 12–18 g)
      - ≥ 12 years: 8 g/m^2 (maximum dose: 18 g)
    - Acute lymphoblastic leukemias
      - High-dose IV: Loading dose: 200 mg/m^2 followed by a 24-hour infusion of 1200 mg/m^2/day

- Oral: Induction of remission in acute lymphoblastic leukemias: 3.3 mg/m^2/day for 4–6 weeks
      - Oral, IM: Remission maintenance: 20–30 mg/m^2 two times/week
    - Meningeal leukemia: 6–12 mg/dose intrathecal based on age, up to a maximum of 12 mg/dose
- Renal dosage adjustment:
  - CrCl 61–80 mL/min: Administer 75% of dose
  - CrCl 51–60 mL/min: Administer 70% of dose
  - CrCl 10–50 mL/min: Administer 30–50% of dose
  - CrCl < 10 mL/min: Avoid use
  - Hemodialysis: Not dialyzable (0–5%); supplemental dose is not necessary
  - Peritoneal dialysis effects: Supplemental dose is not necessary
- Hepatic dosage adjustment:
  - Bilirubin 3.1–5 mg/dL or transaminases more than three times the upper limit of normal: Administer 75% dose
  - Bilirubin > 5 mg/dL: Do not administer

Adverse Reactions: Most Common

- Dependent on dose and route of administration
- Intrathecal 12 mg/m^2: Headache, myelosuppression, nausea
- Low oral dose (< 50 mg/week): Hepatotoxicity
- Moderate IV dose (50–100 mg/m^2): Leukopenia, nausea, vomiting, thrombocytopenia, anemia, diarrhea, mucositis
- High IV dose (> 100 mg/m^2): Severe nausea and vomiting, alopecia, hepatotoxicity, renal toxicity, life-threatening myelosuppression and mucositis (must give with leucovorin rescue)

Adverse Reactions: Rare/Severe/Important

Renal failure, arachnoiditis, encephalopathy (intrathecal administration), demyelinating encephalopathy, hepatotoxicity, sterility

Major Drug Interactions

Drugs Affecting Methotrexate

- Ciprofloxacin: May increase the serum concentration of methotrexate
- Cyclosporine: May increase the serum concentration of methotrexate
- NSAIDs: May reduce the excretion of methotrexate
- Penicillin: May decrease the excretion of methotrexate
- Proton pump inhibitors: May reduce the excretion of methotrexate
- Salicylates: Reduce methotrexate renal clearance and may displace methotrexate from binding sites
- Sulfonamides: Reduce methotrexate renal clearance and may displace methotrexate from binding sites

Methotrexate's Effect on Other Drugs

Cyclosporine: Levels may be increased

Contraindications

Pregnancy, breast-feeding, alcoholism, alcoholic liver disease or other chronic liver disease

Counseling Points

- Watch for fever, malaise, bleeding, bruising, sore mouth and throat, and flank pain
- Avoid prolonged exposure to sunlight

Key Points

- No live virus vaccines should be given during therapy
- Cannot be administered with radiation therapy
- Use preservative-free solution when preparing methotrexate for intrathecal administration
- Doses between 1 and 500 mg/m^2 may require leucovorin rescue, and doses > 500 mg/m^2 require leucovorin rescue:
  - IV, IM, Oral: Leucovorin 10–15 mg/m^2 every 6 hours for 8 or 10 doses, starting 24 hours after the start of methotrexate infusion. Continue until the methotrexate level is ≤ 0.1 micromolar (10^{-7} M).
  - Leucovorin calcium must be given when using high doses of methotrexate to avoid severe life-threatening myelosuppression and mucositis.
- Avoid use in patients with third spacing such as ascites and effusions because of the reservoir effect
- Note that there is a wide spectrum of doses for methotrexate depending on the indication. The antineoplastic doses are much higher than those for other inflammatory conditions, and logic should be used when the dose is assessed. Antineoplastic doses to a patient with rheumatoid arthritis can be fatal.

◉ Pemetrexed

Brand Name

Alimta

Generic Name

Pemetrexed

Rx Only

Dosage Form

Injection

Usage

Mesothelioma,* non-small cell lung cancer*

Pregnancy Category D

Dosing

- IV: 500 mg/m^2 dose given once every 21 days
- Renal dosage adjustment: Use not recommended with a CrCl < 45 mL/min
- Hepatic dosage adjustment: If Grade 3 (5.1–20 times the upper limit of normal) *or* 4 (> 20 times upper limit of normal) transaminase elevation during treatment, then reduce pemetrexed dose to 75% of previous dose

Adverse Reactions: Most Common

Leukopenia, anemia, nausea, rash, stomatitis, fatigue, diarrhea

Adverse Reactions: Rare/Severe/Important

Interstitial pneumonia, severe cutaneous reactions, severe infections, hepatotoxicity

Major Drug Interactions

Drugs Affecting Pemetrexed

Ibuprofen: Increases concentration of pemetrexed

Pemetrexed's Effects on Other Drugs

Vaccines: Diminishes effect

Counseling Points

- Avoid use of NSAIDS several days before and after pemetrexed dosing
- Report any sign of infection, rash, or allergic reaction
- Take vitamin supplement as prescribed

Key Points

- Oral folic acid and injectable B$_{12}$ must be given while on pemetrexed therapy to reduce neutropenia
- Oral steroid therapy is required before and after pemetrexed to prevent rash

---

AROMATASE INHIBITORS

Introduction

Aromatase inhibitors are used in the adjuvant treatment of breast cancer as well as metastatic disease in postmenopausal females with hormone-positive tumors.

Mechanism of Action of the Drug Class

These drugs competitively inhibit aromatase, an enzyme that converts androgens to estrogens. Some breast cancers are stimulated by estrogen and progesterone, and this reduces the available hormones in postmenopausal women.

Members of the Drug Class

In this section: Letrozole
Others: Anastrozole, exemestane

◉ Letrozole

Brand Name
Femara

Generic Name
Letrozole

Rx Only

Dosage Form
Tablet

Usage
Adjuvant and metastatic treatment of breast cancer,* ovarian cancer

Pregnancy Category X

Dosing
- Advanced breast cancer in postmenopausal women: 2.5 mg daily
- Adjuvant treatment for breast cancer in postmenopausal women: 2.5 mg daily for 5 years
- Ovarian cancer in postmenopausal women: 2.5 mg daily
- Hepatic dosage adjustment: In cases of severe hepatic dysfunction, reduce dose by 50% (2.5 mg every other day)

Adverse Reactions: Most Common
Musculoskeletal pain, nausea, hot flashes, headache, night sweats, weight gain, edema

Adverse Reactions: Rare/Severe/Important
Hypercholesterolemia, bone loss

Major Drug Interactions
Drugs Affecting Letrozole
Tamoxifen: May decrease the concentration of letrozole

Letrozole's Effects on Other Drugs
CYP2A6 substrates: Letrozole may increase the effects of

Contraindications
Pregnancy

Counseling Points
- May cause nausea, hot flashes, musculoskeletal pain, and headache
- Can increase the risk of bone fractures and the development of osteoporosis

Key Points
- Aromatase inhibitors should only be used in postmenopausal women
- Aromatase inhibitors have been studied in the adjuvant treatment of breast cancer
- Aromatase inhibitors are well tolerated
- Bone loss is one of the most common concerns

MONOCLONAL ANTIBODIES

Introduction

Monoclonal antibodies comprise a group of targeted therapies that kill tumors by targeting oncogenes (i.e., genetic abnormalities of tumor cells). All of them have the risk of infusion reactions and skin rashes. Monoclonal antibodies are available for many other nononcologic diseases; only those used in the treatment of cancer are discussed here.

Mechanism of Action for the Drug Class

These drugs are engineered antibodies that are human, murine, or chimeric combinations that target abnormal antigen and oncogenes on tumor cells. By binding to these receptors on tumor cells extracellularly, internal signaling pathways to grow and spread are inhibited, or "turned off," leading to cell death. Cetuximab and trastuzumab target epidermal growth factor receptors (EGFRs), whereas bevacizumab targets vascular endothelial growth factor (VEGF). Rituximab targets the antigen CD20 found on B-cell lymphocytes.

Members of the Drug Class

In this section: Bevacizumab, cetuximab, rituximab, trastuzumab
Others: Alemtuzumab, panitumumab

◉ Bevacizumab

Brand Name
Avastin

Generic Name
Bevacizumab

Rx Only

Dosage Form

Injection

Usage

Metastatic colorectal cancer;* nonsquamous, non-small cell lung cancer;* renal cell carcinoma;* malignant glioblastoma;* metastatic breast cancer

Pregnancy Category C

Dosing

- 5 or 10 mg/kg IV every 2 weeks *or*
- 15 mg/kg IV every 3 weeks

Adverse Reactions: Most Common

Hypertension, proteinuria, rash, hypersensitivity reactions

Adverse Reactions: Rare/Severe/Important

Arterial thrombosis, bleeding, poor wound healing, nephrotic syndrome, bowel perforation, reversible leuko-encephalopathy

Major Drug Interactions

Drugs Affecting Bevacizumab

Sunitinib: May increase toxicity

Bevacizumab's Effects on Other Drugs

- Irinotecan: Increases toxicity
- Sunitinib: Increases hypertensive effects
- Sorafenib: Increases toxicity
- Anthracyclines: Increases cardiotoxicity

Contraindications

Use within 4 weeks of surgery, uncontrolled hypertension

Counseling Points

- Report any signs of bleeding or thrombosis
- Hypersensitivity reactions and rash may occur

Key Points

- Monitor blood pressure with treatment visits, and treat hypertension if needed
- Monitor for proteinuria
- Monitor for signs of bleeding

◉ Cetuximab

Brand Name

Erbitux

Generic Name

Cetuximab

Rx Only

Dosage Form

Injection

Usage

Metastatic K-RAS negative colorectal cancer,* head and neck cancer,* EGFR+ non-small cell lung cancer

Pregnancy Category C

Dosing

- Initial loading dose: 400 mg/m² IV
- Maintenance dose: 250 mg/m² IV weekly

Adverse Reactions: Most Common

Hypersensitivity, acneiform rash, diarrhea, hypomagnesemia

Adverse Reactions: Rare/Severe/Important

Sepsis, severe infusion reactions

Counseling Points

- Report any rashes
- Acne rash is an expected reaction. It may require treatment with topical or oral antibiotics.
- Avoid direct sunlight for 2 months after therapy is completed

Key Points

- Magnesium, potassium, and calcium levels should be monitored
- Acneiform rash may require treatment with antibiotics if severe
- Premedication with corticosteroid and diphenhydramine is recommended to prevent hypersensitivity reactions

◉ Rituximab

Brand Name

Rituxan

Generic Name

Rituximab

Rx Only

Dosage Form

Injection

Usage

B-cell non-Hodgkin lymphoma,* chronic lymphocytic leukemia (CLL),* rheumatoid arthritis (RA),* Burkitt's lymphoma, CNS lymphoma, Hodgkin lymphoma (lymphocyte predominant); MALT lymphoma (gastric and nongastric), splenic marginal zone lymphoma, small lymphocytic lymphoma (SLL), Waldenström's macroglobulinemia, autoimmune hemolytic anemia in children, chronic idiopathic thrombocytopenic purpura, refractory pemphigus vulgaris, systemic autoimmune diseases (other than RA), steroid-refractory chronic graft-versus-host disease

Pregnancy Category C

Dosing

- Usual dosing: 375 mg/m^2 IV weekly
- RA: 1,000 mg on days 1 and 15 in combination with methotrexate
- Infusion notes:
  - Initial infusion: Start rate of 50 mg/hour; if there is no reaction, increase the rate 50 mg/hour every 30 minutes, to a maximum of 400 mg/hour
  - Subsequent infusions: If patient did not tolerate initial infusion well, follow initial infusion guidelines. If patient tolerated initial infusion, start at 100 mg/hour; if there is no reaction, increase the rate by 100 mg/hour every 30 minutes, to a maximum of 400 mg/hour.
  - If a reaction occurs, slow or stop the infusion. If the reaction abates, restart the infusion at 50% of the previous rate.

Adverse Reactions: Most Common

Infusion reaction, tumor lysis syndrome, lymphopenia, rash, nausea, myalgias, arthralgias

Adverse Reactions: Rare/Severe/Important

Severe and sometimes fatal mucocutaneous reactions (lichenoid dermatitis, paraneoplastic pemphigus, Stevens-Johnson syndrome, toxic epidermal necrolysis, and vesiculobullous dermatitis); anaphylaxis; progressive multifocal leukoencephalopathy; bowel obstruction and perforation

Major Drug Interactions

Rituximab's Effect on Other Drugs

Antihypertensives: Hypotension may be increased

Counseling Points

- Immediately report any shortness of breath or chest tightness or fever and chills during treatments
- The risk of infection is increased while on treatment

Key Points

- No live virus vaccines during therapy
- Infusion-related reactions are common. Monitor the patient during the infusion.

- Pretreatment with acetaminophen and diphenhydramine is recommended
- Reactivation of hepatitis B and other serious viral infections (possibly new or reactivated) have been reported

◉ Trastuzumab

Brand Name

Herceptin

Generic Name

Trastuzumab

Rx Only

Dosage Form

Injection

Usage

Early stage and metastatic breast cancer*

Pregnancy Category D

Dosing

IV 4 mg/kg loading dose, then 2 mg/kg weekly or 6 mg/kg every 3 weeks

Adverse Reactions: Most Common

Infusion-related reactions, rash, nausea, diarrhea

Adverse Reactions: Rare/Severe/Important

Cardiotoxicity, pulmonary toxicity

Major Drug Interactions

Trastuzumab's Effect on Other Drugs

- Anthracyclines: Increase cardiotoxicity
- Myelosuppressive chemotherapy: Increases infection risk

Counseling Point

Report immediately any shortness of breath or chest tightness or fever and chills during treatments

Key Point

Patients should have ejection fraction measured before starting therapy

PLATINUM COMPOUNDS

Introduction

Similar to alkylating agents, platinum compounds are cell cycle–nonspecific agents that are directly toxic to DNA by causing strand breaks to form. They are used in the treatment of a variety of malignant diseases. All of them cause some degree of neurotoxicity but also possess unique toxicities.

Mechanism of Action for the Drug Class

Form strong covalent bonds with DNA, inhibiting replication and causing cell death

Members of the Drug Class

Carboplatin, cisplatin, oxaliplatin

⊙ Carboplatin

Brand Name

Paraplatin-AQ

Generic Name

Carboplatin

Rx Only

Dosage Form

Injection

Usage

Treatment of ovarian cancer,* lung cancer,* head and neck cancer,* endometrial cancer, esophageal cancer, bladder cancer,* breast cancer, cervical cancer, CNS tumors, germ cell tumors, osteogenic sarcoma, and high-dose therapy with stem cell/bone marrow support

Pregnancy Category D

Dosing

- Individual protocols specify dosing for specific indications and institutions
- Children:
  - Solid tumor: 300–600 mg/m² once every 4 weeks
  - Brain tumor: 175 mg/m² weekly for 4 weeks every 6 weeks, with a 2-week recovery period between courses
- Adults:
  - 300–360 mg/m² IV every 3–4 weeks or target area under the curve (AUC) of 5–7 mg given every 3 weeks dosed by the Calvert equation
    - Calvert equation: Dose = AUC (glomerular filtration rate [GFR] + 25)
  - Autologous bone marrow transplant: 1,600 mg/m² (total dose) IV divided over 4 days
- Renal dosage adjustment:
  - Renal dosing based on the Calvert equation: Dose = AUC (GFR + 25)
  - CrCl 41–59 mL/min: Initiate at 250 mg/m²
  - CrCl 16–40 mL/min: initiate at 200 mg/m²

Adverse Reactions: Most Common

Leucopenia, anemia, thrombocytopenia, nausea and vomiting, peripheral neuropathies, alopecia

Adverse Reactions: Rare/Severe/Important

Ototoxicity, hypersensitivity

Major Drug Interactions

Drugs Affecting Carboplatin

Aminoglycosides: Increase risk of ototoxicity

Carboplatin's Effect on Other Drugs

Taxanes: Increase bone marrow suppression

Contraindications

Severe allergic reaction to carboplatin, cisplatin, other platinum-containing formulations, mannitol, or any component of the formulation; should not be used in patients with severe bone marrow depression or significant bleeding

Counseling Points

- This drug may cause severe fetal defects; avoid pregnancy and breast-feeding during therapy
- Drink plenty of fluids after chemotherapy
- Severe nausea and vomiting could occur for several days after chemotherapy
- Contact your healthcare provider if you are unable to keep food or fluids down
- Contact your healthcare provider if there is any hearing loss

Key Points

- No live virus vaccines during therapy
- May be an irritant if it extravasates from the vein
- Hypersensitivity risk increases with more than six treatments

⊙ Cisplatin

Brand Names

Platinol, Platinol-AQ

Generic Names

Cisplatin, CDDP

Rx Only

Dosage Form

Injection

Usage

Bladder cancer,* testicular cancer,* ovarian cancer,* head and neck cancer,* breast cancer,* gastric cancer, esophageal cancer, cervical cancer,* prostate cancer, non-small cell lung carcinoma (NSCLC),* small cell lung cancer,* Hodgkin and non-Hodgkin lymphoma, neuroblastoma, sarcoma, myeloma, melanoma, mesothelioma, osteosarcoma

Pregnancy Category D

Dosing

- Individual protocols specify dosing for specific indications and institutions
- Children:
  - 37–100 mg/m² every 21–28 days *or*
  - 15–20 mg/m² daily for 5 days every 3–4 weeks
- Adults:
  - 10–20 mg/m² daily for 5 days every 3–4 weeks *or*
  - 50–120 mg/m² every 3–4 weeks
  - Maximum dose: 120 mg/m² per cycle
  - High-dose bone marrow transplant: 55 mg/m² daily for 3 days, 165 mg/m² total

- Renal dosage adjustment:
  - CrCl 46–60 mL/min: Administer 75% of dose
  - CrCl 31–45 mL/min: Administer 50% of dose
  - CrCl < 30 mL/min: Consider use of alternative drug
  - Hemodialysis: Administer 50% of normal dose postdialysis

Adverse Reactions: Most Common

Nausea and vomiting, peripheral neuropathies, anemia, alopecia, nephrotoxicity, electrolyte imbalances

Adverse Reactions: Rare/Severe/Important

Ototoxicity

Major Drug Interactions

Drugs Affecting Cisplatin

- Aminoglycosides: Increase nephrotoxicity
- Amifostine: Can reduce nephrotoxicity
- Taxanes: Increase bone marrow suppression

Cisplatin's Effect on Other Drugs

- Topotecan: Reduces clearance
- Vinorelbine: Increases risk of neutropenia

Contraindications

Hypersensitivity to cisplatin, other platinum-containing compounds, or any component of the formulation (anaphylactic-like reactions have been reported); pre-existing renal impairment; myelosuppression; hearing impairment

Counseling Points

- This drug may cause severe fetal defects; avoid pregnancy and breast-feeding during therapy
- Drink plenty of fluids after chemotherapy
- Severe nausea and vomiting could occur for several days after chemotherapy
- Contact your healthcare provider if you are unable to keep food or fluids down
- Contact your healthcare provider if there is any hearing loss

Key Points

- Verify any dose > 100 mg/m²
- Assess renal function prior to administration
- Assess electrolytes, particularly potassium and magnesium, and replace as needed
- IV hydration should be given before and after cisplatin therapy
- Mannitol or furosemide can be given to reduce nephrotoxicity
- Highly emetogenic; premedicate to prevent nausea and vomiting
- Patients should also receive antiemetics after chemotherapy to prevent delayed emesis
- Ototoxicity is more pronounced in children

◉ Oxaliplatin

Brand Name

Eloxatin

Generic Name

Oxaliplatin

Rx Only

Dosage Form

Injection

Usage

Colorectal cancer,* head and neck cancers,* gastric cancer, pancreatic cancer

Pregnancy Category D

Dosing

- Individual protocols specify dosing for specific indications and institutions
- Typically dosed 85 mg/m² IV every 2 weeks with 5-fluorouracil regimens
- Renal dosage adjustment: If CrCl < 30 mL/min, reduce dose from 85 mg/m² to 65 mg/m²

Adverse Reactions: Most Common

Leucopenia, anemia, thrombocytopenia, nausea and vomiting, peripheral neuropathies, thermal dysesthesias, alopecia

Adverse Reactions: Rare/Severe/Important

Hypersensitivity reactions, peripheral neuropathies, pulmonary fibrosis, hepatotoxicity, reversible posterior leukoencephalopathy

Major Drug Interactions

Oxaliplatin's Effects on Other Drugs

- Taxanes: Increase bone marrow suppression
- Vaccines: May have diminished effect

Contraindications

Severe allergic reaction to carboplatin, cisplatin, other platinum-containing formulations, mannitol, or any component of the formulation; should not be used in patients with severe bone marrow depression or significant bleeding

Counseling Points

- Allergic reaction can occur during the infusion
- Report any sign of infection, bleeding, or bruising
- Report any numbness or tingling in hands and feet
- Do not eat or drink anything cold 3 to 4 days after chemotherapy; everything must be warm or room temperature
- Wear gloves in cold weather
- Breathing cold air may cause throat pain

TAXANES

Introduction

This class of antineoplastics is used to treat a wide range of malignancies. Taxanes can be used alone as monotherapy or in combination with other antineoplastics. From a toxicity standpoint, they are most notable for causing bone marrow suppression and peripheral neuropathies.

Mechanism of Action for the Drug Class

Taxanes stabilize the microtubule bundles by promoting assembly and preventing depolymerization, thereby inhibiting cell replication

Members of the Drug Class

In this section: Docetaxel, paclitaxel
Others: Cabazitaxel

⊙ Docetaxel

Brand Name

Taxotere

Generic Name

Docetaxel

Rx Only

Dosage Form

Injection

Usage

Breast cancer,* locally advanced or metastatic non-small cell lung cancer,* hormone-refractory metastatic prostate cancer,* advanced gastric adenocarcinoma, locally advanced squamous cell head and neck cancer, bladder cancer, ovarian cancer, small cell lung cancer, soft tissue sarcoma

Pregnancy Category D

Dosing

- Individual protocols specify dosing for specific indications and institutions
- Dosage range: 60–100 mg/m^2/dose every 3–4 weeks *or* 35 mg/m^2 weekly
- Hepatic dosage adjustment: Avoid if either of the following are present: Total bilirubin > than the upper limit of normal or aspartate aminotransferase/alanine aminotransferase > 1.5 times the upper limit of normal concomitant with alkaline phosphatase > 2.5 times the upper limit of normal

Adverse Reactions: Most Common

Fluid retention syndrome, leukopenia, anemia, thrombocytopenia, alopecia, peripheral neuropathies, myalgias, arthralgias, diarrhea, stomatitis, mild nausea

Adverse Reactions: Rare/Severe/Important

Skin desquamation, hypersensitivity, oncolysis

Major Drug Interactions

Drugs Affecting Docetaxel

- Azole antifungals: Decrease metabolism of docetaxel, raising concentrations
- Carboplatin, cisplatin: Increase myelosuppression

Contraindications

Severe hypersensitivity to other medications containing polysorbate 80; neutrophil count < 1,500/mm^3

Counseling Points

- No live virus vaccines during therapy
- Watch for fever, malaise
- Risk of infection is increased; report any fever or infection

Key Points

- Extravasation can cause tissue necrosis
- Must premedicate with a corticosteroid to reduce fluid retention
- Administer taxane derivatives before platinum derivative when given as sequential infusions to limit toxicity

⊙ Paclitaxel

Brand Name

Taxol

Generic Name

Paclitaxel

Rx Only

4

Antineoplastics

Dosage Form

Injection

Usage

Breast cancer,* non-small cell lung cancer,* locally advanced squamous cell head and neck cancer,* bladder cancer, ovarian cancer,* small cell lung cancer, adenocarcinomas of unknown primary and AIDS-related Kaposi sarcoma

Pregnancy Category D

Dosing

- Individual protocols specify dosing for specific indications and institutions
- Dosage range: 135–200 mg/m² per dose every 3–4 weeks *or* 80–100 mg/m² weekly
- Hepatic dosage adjustment: (3-hour infusion):
  - Transaminase levels < 10 times the upper limit of normal and bilirubin level 1.26–2 times the upper limit of normal: 135 mg/m²
  - Transaminase levels < 10 times the upper limit of normal and bilirubin level 2.01–5 times the upper limit of normal: 90 mg/m²
  - Transaminase levels ≥ 10 times the upper limit of normal and bilirubin level > 5 times the upper limit of normal: Avoid use

Adverse Reactions: Most Common

Bradycardia, flushing, leukopenia, anemia, thrombocytopenia, alopecia, peripheral neuropathies, myalgias, arthralgias, diarrhea, stomatitis, mild nausea

Adverse Reactions: Rare/Severe/Important

Hypersensitivity, skin rashes

Major Drug Interactions

Drugs Affecting Paclitaxel

- Azole antifungals: Decrease the metabolism of paclitaxel, increasing concentrations
- Carboplatin, cisplatin: Increase myelosuppression
- Trastuzumab: Enhances neutropenia

Paclitaxel's Effect on Other Drugs

Anthracyclines: Increase cardiotoxicity

Contraindications

Hypersensitivity to paclitaxel, Cremophor EL (polyoxyethylated castor oil), or any component of the formulation

Counseling Points

- No live virus vaccines during therapy
- Peripheral neuropathies can occur with continued use
- Risk of infection is increased; report any fever or infection

Key Points

- Severe bone marrow suppression is possible and may require dose reduction
- Monitor blood pressure regularly while drug is infusing
- Extravasation can cause tissue necrosis
- Must premedicate with a corticosteroid, diphenhydramine, and histamine-2 blocker to prevent hypersensitivity
- Paclitaxel is a radiosensitizer and will increase the effect and toxicity of radiation therapy
- Administer a taxane derivative before a platinum derivative when given as sequential infusions to limit toxicity

TOPOISOMERASE INHIBITORS

Introduction

Members of this class of antineoplastics, also known as podophyllotoxins, are extracted from the mandrake plant, with recorded use dating back to colonial America as a cathartic agent. Today, etoposide is the most commonly used agent in the class and has important utility in the treatment of a variety of tumors, including pediatric leukemias, lymphomas, lung cancer, and testicular cancer.

Mechanism of Action for the Drug Class

Antineoplastics in this class are cell cycle–specific and arrest cell division in the premitotic phase by inhibiting topoisomerase enzymes that are required for normal DNA repair. Etoposide inhibits TOPO-II enzymes, whereas topotecan and irinotecan inhibit TOPO I enzymes. Both topotecan and irinotecan are frequently used agents for multiple solid tumors such as ovarian, lung, and colorectal cancers.

Members of the Drug Class

In this section: Etoposide, irinotecan, topotecan
Others: Teniposide

◉ Etoposide

Brand Name

VePesid

Generic Name

Etoposide

Rx Only

Dosage Forms

Capsule, injection

Usage

Ovarian cancer (oral),* small cell lung cancer,* testicular cancer*

Pregnancy Category D

Dosing

- Individual protocols specify dosing for specific indications and institutions
- Oral: 30–50 mg/m² on days 1–21 every 28 days
- IV:
  - 80–120 mg/m² on days 1–3 every 21 days *or*
  - 100 mg/m² on days 1–5 every 21 days
- Nonseminoma, metastatic (high-dose regimens): 750 mg/m² per day IV administered 5, 4, and 3 days before peripheral blood stem cell infusion
- Renal dosage adjustment:
  - CrCl 15–50 mL/min: Administer 75% of dose
  - CrCl < 15 mL/min: Data not available; consider further dose reductions

Adverse Reactions: Most Common

Leukopenia, anemia, thrombocytopenia, alopecia, nausea, vomiting

Adverse Reactions: Rare/Severe/Important

Severe skin reactions, hypotension, extravasation. Note that the following may occur with higher doses used in stem cell transplantation: Alopecia, ethanol intoxication, hepatitis, hypotension (infusion related), metabolic acidosis, mucositis, nausea and vomiting (severe), secondary malignancy, skin lesions (resembling Stevens-Johnson syndrome).

Major Drug Interactions

Drugs Affecting Etoposide

- Atovaquone: May increase levels
- CYP3A4 inducers or major substrates: May diminish effect
- CYP3A4 inhibitors: May increase effect or toxicity
- Phenytoin: May decrease blood levels
- St. John's wort: May decrease levels

Etoposide's Effect on Other Drugs

- Other substrates of CYP3A4: May decrease effect
- Vaccines: May have a diminished effect
- Warfarin: Effects may be enhanced

Counseling Points

- Watch for fever, malaise, sore mouth or throat, pain or swelling at injection site
- No live virus vaccines during therapy
- Risk of infection is increased; report any fever or infection

Key Points

- IV administration commonly given in a regimen with additional chemotherapy agents
- Oral etoposide has poor bioavailability but is used as single agent in advanced ovarian cancer
- Leukopenia and alopecia are the most common adverse effects seen with typical dosing. High doses used pre-stem cell transplant have more significant adverse effects.

◉ Irinotecan

Brand Name

Camptosar

Generic Name

Irinotecan

Rx Only

Dosage Form

Injection

Usage

Metastatic colorectal cancer,* non-small cell lung cancer, ovarian cancer, gastric cancer, small cell lung cancer, pancreatic cancer, central nervous system cancer, cervical cancer

Pregnancy Category D

Dosing

- Individual protocols specify dosing for specific indications and institutions
- Metastatic colorectal cancer:
  - 125 mg/m² weekly for 4 weeks on and 2 weeks off of a 6-week cycle *or*
  - 350 mg/m² IV once every 3 weeks
- Hepatic dosage adjustment:
  - Bilirubin > the upper limit of normal to ≤ 2 mg/dL: Consider reducing initial dose by one dose level
  - Bilirubin > 2 mg/dL: Use is not recommended

Adverse Reactions: Most Common

Leukopenia, anemia, thrombocytopenia, diarrhea, cramping, nausea, vomiting, dehydration

Adverse Reactions: Rare/Severe/Important

Dehydration, diarrhea, colitis, intestinal perforation

Major Drug Interactions

Drugs Affecting Irinotecan

- Bevacizumab: May enhance the adverse/toxic effect
- Carbamazepine: May decrease the serum concentration
- CYP3A4 inducers or major substrates: May diminish effect
- CYP3A4 inhibitors: May increase effect or toxicity
- Phenytoin: May decrease blood levels
- St. John's wort: May decrease levels

4

Antineoplastics

Irinotecan's Effect on Other Drugs
- Other substrates of CYP3A4: May decrease effects
- Vaccines: May have a diminished effect
- Warfarin: Effects may be enhanced

Counseling Points
- No live virus vaccines during therapy
- Loperamide should be used at the first sign of diarrhea
- Report any signs of infection, bleeding, or bruising
- Report any diarrhea or cramping and vomiting

Key Points
- Patients should be given loperamide as needed for delayed diarrhea
- Acute diarrhea and cramping during the infusion is a cholinergic reaction and should be treated with atropine

◉ Topotecan

Brand Name
Hycamtin

Generic Name
Topotecan

Rx Only

Dosage Forms
Capsule, injection

Usage
Ovarian cancer,* small cell lung cancer,* cervical cancer

Pregnancy Category D

Dosing
- Individual protocols specify dosing for specific indications and institutions
- IV: 1.5 mg/m^2 per day for 5 days every 21 days
- Oral: 2.3 mg/m^2 daily for 5 days every 21 days
- Renal dosage adjustment:
  - CrCl 20–39 mL/min: Reduce dose to 0.75 mg/m^2
  - CrCl < 20 mL/min: Insufficient data available for dosing recommendation

Adverse Reactions: Most Common
Leukopenia, anemia, thrombocytopenia, diarrhea

Adverse Reactions: Rare/Severe/Important
Interstitial lung disease, neutropenic colitis, neutropenic fevers

Major Drug Interactions
Drugs Affecting Topotecan
- Cisplatin: May increase toxicity
- Clozapine: May increase the risk of agranulocytosis

Topotecan's Effect on Other Drugs
Vaccines: May have a diminished effect

Contraindications
Neutropenia

Counseling Points
- No live virus vaccines during therapy
- Report any signs of infection, bleeding, or bruising
- Risk of infection is increased; report any fevers
- Report any unresolved diarrhea, nausea, or vomiting
- Capsules must be swallowed whole with or without food

Key Points
- Use of prophylactic G-CSF can reduce the incidence of neutropenic fevers
- Do not administer chemotherapy if ANC < 1,500/mm^3 or platelets < 100,000/mm^3

TYROSINE KINASE INHIBITORS

Introduction
Tyrosine kinase inhibitors are a large class of oral targeted agents available to treat cancers. Each inhibits the protein tyrosine kinase and has an effect on specific growth factor receptors that stimulate tumor growth.

Mechanism of Action for the Drug Class
Tyrosine kinase inhibitors are a new class of agents that specifically target genetic abnormalities in cancers that push the cell to divide, grow, and spread. These agents inhibit the oncogene proteins intracellularly, blocking the signaling pathway and ultimately slowing or stopping tumor cell proliferation. Erlotinib targets the tyrosine kinase of EGFR (epidermal growth factor), whereas imatinib targets the Philadelphia chromosome.

Members of the Drug Class
In this section: Erlotinib, imatinib
Others: Axitinib, dasatinib, lapatinib, nilotinib, sorafenib, sunitinib

⊙ Erlotinib

Brand Name
Tarceva

Generic Name
Erlotinib

Rx Only

Dosage Form
Tablet

Usage
Non-small cell lung cancer,* pancreatic cancer*

Pregnancy Category D

Dosing
- 100 or 150 mg oral daily
- Smokers: A dose increase to a maximum of 300 mg (with careful monitoring) may be required in patients who continue to smoke
- Hepatic dosage adjustment: If total bilirubin > 3 times the upper limit of normal and/or transaminases are > 5 times the upper limit of normal, then interrupt or discontinue treatment

Adverse Reactions: Most Common
Diarrhea, nausea, edema

Adverse Reactions: Rare/Severe/Important
Severe skin reactions, GI perforation, interstitial pneumonitis, hepatoxicity

Major Drug Interactions
Drugs Affecting Erlotinib
- Antacids: May decrease absorption
- CYP3A4 inhibitors: May increase toxicity
- CYP3A4 inducers: May decrease efficacy
- Grapefruit: May increase serum concentration
- Proton pump inhibitors: May reduce serum concentrations

Erlotinib's Effect on Other Drugs
Warfarin: Effects may be enhanced

Counseling Points
- Take on an empty stomach
- Avoid grapefruit or grapefruit juice around dosing time
- Maintain adequate hydration
- Report any rashes, swelling, or respiratory symptoms
- Notify your healthcare provider right away if your smoking status changes

Key Points
- Food will increase bioavailability
- Verify smoking status; smokers require higher dosing
- Dose adjustments needed if used with CYP3A4 inhibitors or inducers or major substrates

⊙ Imatinib

Brand Name
Gleevec

Generic Name
Imatinib

Rx Only

Dosage Form
Tablet

Usage
Gastric stromal cell tumor,* chronic myelogenous leukemia,* Ph-positive acute lymphoblastic leukemia, dermatofibrosarcoma protuberans, hypereosinophilic syndrome, myelodysplastic disease, desmoid tumors

Pregnancy Category D

Dosing
- Adults: 400 mg daily; up to 800 mg daily in divided doses
- Children: 260–340 mg/m² daily; maximum of 600 mg daily
- Renal dosage adjustment:
  - Mild impairment: No adjustment
  - Moderate impairment of CrCl 20–39 mL/min: Administer 50% of dose
  - Severe impairment of CrCl < 20 mL/min: Use not recommended
- Hepatic dosage adjustment:
  - Mild to moderate impairment: No adjustment
  - Severe impairment: Reduce dose by 25%

Adverse Reactions: Most Common
Fluid retention, nausea, diarrhea, rash, leukopenia, thrombocytopenia, anemia, myalgias, arthralgias, muscle cramps

Adverse Reactions: Rare/Severe/Important
Hepatotoxicity, heart failure, severe bullous dermatologic reactions, hemorrhage

Major Drug Interactions
Drugs Affecting Imatinib
- Azole antifungals: Increase serum concentration
- Lansoprazole: Enhances the dermatologic adverse effects of imatinib; monitoring is necessary

Imatinib's Effect on Other Drugs
- Carbamazepine: Inhibits carbamazepine metabolism, increasing carbamazepine concentrations and toxicity
- Digoxin: Decreases absorption
- Codeine: Diminishes therapeutic effect due to inhibition of codeine conversion to active metabolite

- Colchicine, cyclosporine, fentanyl: Serum levels may increase
- Fludarabine: Therapeutic effects may be diminished
- Simvastatin: Metabolism may be reduced
- Tamoxifen: Therapeutic effects may be diminished
- Tramadol: Therapeutic effects may be diminished
- Warfarin: Bleeding effects may be increased

Counseling Points
- Take with food and/or large glass of water
- Report any fevers, bleeding, bruising, or flank pain
- Report any shortness of breath

Key Points
- Edema can progress to pulmonary edema
- Edema is worse in the elderly
- Food may reduce GI irritation

VINCA ALKALOIDS

Introduction
Vinca alkaloids are derived from natural plant sources and are used to treat hematologic and solid tumors. They are usually part of a combination regimen, frequently in pediatric malignancies. The class is known for its neurotoxicity, with vincristine having the highest incidence and grade, limiting the possible dosing.

Mechanism of Action for the Drug Class
Vinca alkaloids prevent microtubule assembly, thereby preventing cell mitosis and ultimately causing cell death

Members of the Drug Class
In this section: Vincristine
Others: Vinblastine, vinorelbine

◉ Vincristine

Brand Name
Oncovin

Generic Name
Vincristine

Rx Only

Dosage Form
Injection

Usage
Acute lymphocytic leukemia,* Hodgkin lymphoma, non-Hodgkin lymphoma,* Wilms' tumor,* neuroblastoma, rhabdomyosarcoma

Pregnancy Category D

Dosing
- Adult IV: 2 mg max per dose
- Children:
  - ≤ 10 kg: 0.05 mg/kg once weekly
  - > 10 kg: 1.5–2 mg/m²; frequency may vary based on protocol

- Hepatic dosage adjustment:
  - Total bilirubin greater than the upper limit of normal: Avoid use
  - Aspartate aminotransferase/alanine aminotransferase > 1.5 times the upper limit of normal concomitant with alkaline phosphatase > 2.5 times the upper limit of normal: Avoid use

Adverse Reactions: Most Common
Peripheral neuropathies, constipation, jaw pain, depression, confusion

Adverse Reactions: Rare/Severe/Important
Ileus, uric acid nephropathy

Major Drug Interactions
Drugs Affecting Vincristine
- CYP3A4 inhibitors: May increase toxicity
- CYP3A4 inducers: May decrease efficacy

Contraindications
Patients with demyelinating form of Charcot-Marie-Tooth syndrome

Counseling Points
- Constipation may occur, requiring laxative therapy
- Report any numbness and tingling in hands and feet
- Report any change in mental status
- Report any jaw pain

Key Points
- Extravasation can cause tissue necrosis
- IV use only: Vincristine should be clearly labeled NOT FOR INTRATHECAL USE
- Dosing is usually capped at 2 mg per dose due to its neurotoxicity; any dose exceeding this should be questioned
- If given on its own, it does not require antiemetics
- If given alone, it does not cause bone marrow suppression
- Jaw pain is more common with the first dose
- Use of laxatives can prevent constipation and possible ileus
- Avoid eye contamination

Introduction

The agents in this class have unique mechanisms and play a role in treating multiple myeloma. Lenalidomide has become an important oral agent in the treatment of multiple myeloma, whereas bortezomib is an injectable agent.

Mechanism of Action for the Drug Class

Lenalidomide acts as an immunomodulator and also has antiangiogenic properties. Its mechanism is not completely understood. Bortezomib is the first of a new class of proteasome inhibitors that inhibit proteasomes, enzyme complexes that regulate protein homeostasis within the cell, ultimately leading to cell-cycle arrest and cell death.

Members of the Drug Class

In this section: Bortezomib, lenalidomide
Others: Thalidomide

◉ Bortezomib

Brand Name
Velcade

Generic Name
Bortezomib

Rx Only

Dosage Form
Injection

Usage
Multiple myeloma,* mantle cell lymphoma

Pregnancy Category D

Dosing
IV, SUB-Q: 1.3 mg/m^2 days 1, 4, 8, 11, 22, 25, 29, and 32 of a 42-day treatment cycle

Adverse Reactions: Most Common
Leukopenia, anemia, thrombocytopenia, nausea, herpes reactivation, peripheral neuropathies, hypotension

Adverse Reactions: Rare/Severe/Important
Hepatotoxicity, reversible posterior leukoencephalopathy, tumor lysis syndrome, pneumonitis

Major Drug Interactions
Drugs Affecting Bortezomib
- Ascorbic acid: May diminish therapeutic effect
- Moderate CYP2C19 inhibitors: May decrease metabolism
- Strong CYP3A4 inducers: May increase metabolism
- Moderate CYP3A4 inhibitors: May decrease metabolism

- Grapefruit juice: May increase levels
- Green tea: May reduce effect
- St Johns wort: May decrease serum concentration

Bortezomib's Effect on Other Drugs
Clopidogrel: Decreases serum concentrations of the active metabolite(s) and decreases effect

Contraindications
Allergy to boron or mannitol

Counseling Points
- Reports any signs of infection, bleeding, or bruising
- Numbness and tingling in hands and feet can occur with continued therapy
- Avoid use of ascorbic acid, green tea, and grapefruit juice on treatment days
- No live virus vaccines during therapy

Key Points
- Consider prophylaxis of herpes simplex infections with antivirals
- Peripheral neuropathies can be severe
- Caution with using SSRIs while on therapy
- Not for intrathecal use; fatalities reported

◉ Lenalidomide

Brand Name
Revlimid

Generic Name
Lenalidomide

Rx Only

Dosage Form
Capsule

Usage
Myelodysplastic syndrome (MDS), multiple myeloma*

Pregnancy Category X

Dosing
- Multiple myeloma: 25 mg PO once daily for 21 days of a 28-day treatment cycle
- Myelodysplastic syndrome (MDS) with deletion 5q: 10 mg PO once daily

Adverse Reactions: Most Common
Leukopenia, anemia, thrombocytopenia, thromboembolism, pruritus, rash

Adverse Reactions: Rare/Severe/Important
Severe skin rashes, including Stevens-Johnson syndrome; hepatotoxicity; secondary malignancies

4

Antineoplastics

Major Drug Interactions

Drugs Affecting Lenalidomide

- Dexamethasone: Increases thrombosis risk
- Immunosuppressants: Increase immunosuppressive effect

Lenalidomide's Effect on Other Drugs

Vaccines: Diminished effect

Contraindication

Pregnancy

Counseling Points

- No live vaccines during therapy
- Report any fevers, bleeding, or bruising
- Report any sign of a clot, shortness of breath, or swelling in an extremity
- Woman of childbearing years must use birth control to avoid pregnancy
- Stop therapy if you become pregnant

Key Points

- May cause birth defects; do not use during pregnancy (contraindication). Patients must avoid pregnancy while taking lenalidomide.
- Women of childbearing potential: Pregnancy test 10–14 days *and* 24 hours prior to initiating therapy, weekly during the first 4 weeks of treatment, then every 2–4 weeks through 4 weeks after therapy discontinued
- Distribution is restricted; physicians, pharmacists, and patients must be registered with the RevAssist program
- Thrombosis prophylaxis is recommended if using with dexamethasone

REVIEW QUESTIONS

1. Cyclophosphamide, an alkylating agent commonly used for breast cancer, can cause which of the following side effects?

   a. Constipation
   b. Hemorrhagic cystitis
   c. Infusion reactions
   d. Peripheral neuropathies

2. Temozolomide is classified in which of the following drug classes?

   a. Vinca alkaloids
   b. Antimetabolites
   c. Alkylators
   d. Aromatase inhibitors

3. Which of the following would be a likely indication for using oral Temodar?

   a. Breast cancer
   b. Colon cancer
   c. Malignant glioblastoma
   d. Acute myelogenous leukemia

4. Which of the following requires baseline assessment of cardiac output prior to starting treatment?

   a. Doxorubicin
   b. Vincristine
   c. Cyclophosphamide
   d. Pemetrexed

5. Which of the following should be dose adjusted for hepatic impairment?

   a. Topotecan
   b. Etoposide
   c. Cisplatin
   d. Doxorubicin

6. Which of the following has a category X pregnancy rating?

   a. Lenalidomide
   b. Doxorubicin
   c. Cisplatin
   d. Irinotecan

7. Use of paroxetine, a SSRI, should be avoided in patients receiving tamoxifen because paroxetine

   a. increases the risk of thrombosis.
   b. may decrease the efficacy of tamoxifen.
   c. may increase the risk of serotonin syndrome.
   d. may increase tamoxifen levels.

8. Which of the following is true regarding capecitabine?

   a. It is given intravenously.
   b. It is dosed once daily.
   c. It can cause palmar-plantar erythrodysethesias.
   d. It is a topoisomerase inhibitor.

9. Corticosteroid ophthalmic should be used to prevent severe chemical conjunctivitis for which of the following agents?

   a. Cytarabine
   b. Mercaptopurine
   c. Temozolomide
   d. Cisplatin

10. Flulike symptoms are common with which of the following agents?

    a. Capecitabine
    b. Topotecan
    c. Gemcitabine
    d. Vincristine

11. Leucovorin is given as a rescue to prevent life-threatening bone marrow suppression from high doses of which of the following chemotherapies?

    a. 5-Fluorouracil
    b. Pemetrexed
    c. Cytarabine
    d. Methotrexate

12. Which vitamin supplements should be given with pemetrexed to avoid increased toxicities?

    a. Folic acid and vitamin B_6
    b. Folic acid and vitamin B_{12}
    c. Folic acid and vitamin C
    d. Thiamine and vitamin B_{12}

13. Pemetrexed is approved for use in which of the following cancers?

    a. Mesothelioma and non-small cell lung cancer
    b. Non-small cell lung cancer and breast cancer
    c. Colon cancer
    d. Prostate cancer

14. Which of the following is a major concern of long-time use of letrozole?

    a. Bone loss
    b. Bone marrow suppression
    c. Endometrial cancer
    d. Osteonecrosis of the jaw

15. Which of the following monoclonal antibodies targets vascular endothelial growth factor?

    a. Cetuximab
    b. Rituximab
    c. Trastuzumab
    d. Bevacizumab

16. Which of the following is a major concern when giving monoclonal antibodies?

    a. Renal toxicity
    b. Bone marrow suppression
    c. Nausea and vomiting
    d. Hypersensitivity reactions

17. When administering bevacizumab, it is important to monitor which of the following with each treatment visit?

    a. Blood pressure
    b. Potassium
    c. Serum creatinine
    d. Liver function tests

18. Which of the following rashes is commonly seen with cetuximab?

    a. Butterfly
    b. Stevens-Johnson
    c. Acneiform
    d. Contact dermatitis

19. When used to treat lymphoma, rituximab has a high incidence of which of the following?

    a. Infusion reactions
    b. Nausea and vomiting
    c. Hepatotoxicity
    d. Mucositis

20. Trastuzumab, which is frequently given sequentially after doxorubicin therapy for breast cancer, is associated with an increased risk of which of the following?

    a. Pulmonary toxicity
    b. Cardiac toxicity
    c. Bone marrow suppression
    d. Secondary malignancies

21. Dosing of carboplatin is commonly done using the Calvert equation, which estimates the dose needed to attain a desired area under the curve (AUC). This is estimated using which of the following?

    a. Renal function
    b. Hepatic function
    c. Platelet count
    d. Body surface area

22. Which of the following daily doses is too high for cisplatin?

    a. 75 mg/m²
    b. 150 mg/m²
    c. 60 mg/m²
    d. 25 mg/m²

23. Which of the following chemotherapy doses is *incorrect*?

    a. Oxaliplatin IV 85 mg/m²
    b. Vincristine IV 4 mg
    c. Methotrexate IV 40 mg/m²
    d. Docetaxel IV 60 mg/m²

24. Patients receiving oxaliplatin should avoid cold food and drinks for multiple days after chemotherapy because of which of the following side effects?

    a. Peripheral neuropathies
    b. Nausea and vomiting
    c. Thermal dysesthesias
    d. Skin rashes

25. Which of the following agents should be avoided in patients with significant hepatic impairment?

    a. Docetaxel
    b. Cisplatin
    c. Topotecan
    d. Trastuzumab

26. Which of the following agents requires premedication with diphenhydramine to prevent a hypersensitivity reaction?

    a. Vincristine
    b. Etoposide
    c. Paclitaxel
    d. Imatinib

27. Irinotecan causes cell death by inhibiting which of the following?

    a. Topoisomerase II
    b. Topoisomerase I
    c. Asparaginase
    d. Tyrosine kinase

28. Etoposide is given orally to treat which of the following cancers?

    a. Testicular cancer
    b. Small cell lung cancer
    c. Ovarian cancer
    d. Colon cancer

29. Which of following adverse effects of irinotecan is of most concern?

    a. Alopecia
    b. Nausea
    c. Diarrhea
    d. Renal toxicity

30. Which statement regarding topotecan is true?

    a. It is only available as an injection.
    b. It has a low risk of neutropenia.
    c. The use of G-CSF is recommended.
    d. The dose should be reduced in cases of hepatic impairment.

Cardiovascular Agents

Anna M. Wodlinger Jackson, PharmD, BCPS

ALPHA-1 ADRENERGIC BLOCKERS

Introduction

Alpha-1 adrenergic blockers are used in the treatment of hypertension. Drugs in this class are usually not the first-line agent of choice because more effective agents are available. They are more commonly used in the treatment of benign prostatic hyperplasia (BPH).

Mechanism of Action for the Drug Class

Alpha-1 adrenergic blockers cause vasodilation by selectively blocking postsynaptic alpha-1 adrenergic receptors, resulting in dilation of both peripheral arterioles and veins. They also relax smooth muscles in the prostate and bladder neck. Tamsulosin is selective for alpha-receptors in the prostate and does not have a therapeutic effect on blood pressure, although orthostatic hypotension is still possible, as with other members of this class.

Rx Only for the Drug Class

Usage for the Drug Class

Treatment of hypertension (not first-line choice) and BPH,* symptomatic treatment of bladder outlet obstruction or dysfunction (tamsulosin), facilitation of expulsion of ureteral stones (tamsulosin)

Adverse Reactions for the Drug Class: Most Common

Dizziness, headache, orthostatic hypotension, syncope, flushing (tamsulosin)

Adverse Reactions for the Drug Class: Rare/Severe/Important

Intraoperative floppy iris syndrome (in patients undergoing cataract surgery), priapism, symptoms of angina

Major Drug Interactions for the Drug Class

Drugs Affecting Alpha-1 Adrenergic Blockers

Concomitant antihypertensive agents and phosphodiesterase-5 inhibitors: Additive hypotension

Alpha-1 Adrenergic Blockers' Effects on Other Drugs

Antihypertensive agents: Additive hypotension

Counseling Points for the Drug Class

- These drugs may cause dizziness or drowsiness (take at night to avoid)
- Use caution when getting up from a sitting or lying down position
- May require 1–2 weeks of therapy before improvement of BPH symptoms

Members of the Drug Class

In this section: Doxazosin, tamsulosin, terazosin
Others: Alfuzosin, phenoxybenzamine, phentolamine, prazosin, silodosin

⊚ Doxazosin

Brand Names
Cardura, Cardura XL

Generic Name
Doxazosin

Dosage Forms
Tablet, extended-release tablet

Pregnancy Category C

---

* Throughout the text, an asterisk (*) is used to indicate the most common uses of a drug.

Dosing

- Initial dose: 1 mg daily
- Dosage adjustment: Up to 16 mg daily (maximum for BPH is usually 8 mg)

Counseling Point

Do not crush, split, or chew the XL formulation

Key Points

- Although indicated for the treatment of hypertension, doxazosin is not often used as a first-line agent. It is more commonly used for the treatment of BPH.
- The extended-release formula is a nondeformable matrix that is expelled in the stool. Be cautious when using for patients with known stricture/narrowing of the GI tract.

◉ Tamsulosin

Brand Name

Flomax

Generic Name

Tamsulosin

Dosage Form

Capsule

Pregnancy Category B

Dosing

- Initial dose: 0.4 mg daily
- Dosage adjustment: Can increase in 2–4 weeks to maximum of 0.8 mg daily

Counseling Point

Do not crush, chew, or open capsule

Key Points

- Because it is a selective alpha-agonist, it has minimal effects on blood pressure and is used only for the treatment of BPH
- Avoid concomitant use of phosphodiesterase-5 inhibitors (sildenafil, tadalafil, vardenafil)

◉ Terazosin

Brand Name

Hytrin

Generic Name

Terazosin

Dosage Form

Capsule

Pregnancy Category C

Dosing

- Initial dose: 1 mg daily
- Dosing adjustment: Up to 20 mg daily

Key Point

Although indicated for the treatment of hypertension, terazosin is not often used as a first-line agent. It is more commonly used for the treatment of BPH. Watch for orthostatic hypotension and signs of dizziness.

ALPHA-2 ADRENERGIC AGONISTS

Introduction

The alpha-2 adrenergic agonists are used for the treatment of hypertension, although usually not as a first-line agent of choice. They also have many unlabeled uses.

Mechanism of Action for the Drug Class

The stimulation of alpha-2 adrenergic receptors in the brain stem by these agents results in reduced sympathetic outflow from the CNS and a decrease in peripheral resistance, renal vascular resistance, heart rate, and blood pressure

Members of the Drug Class

In this section: Clonidine
Others: Dexmedetomidine, guanabenz, guanfacine, methyldopa

◉ Clonidine

Brand Names

Catapres, Catapres-TTS-1, Catapres-TTS-2, Catapres-TTS-3, Duraclon, Kapvay

Generic Name

Clonidine

Rx Only

Dosage Forms

Tablet, transdermal patch, injection (epidural solution)

Usage

Hypertension,* alcohol withdrawal, attention deficit hyperactivity disorder,* cancer pain (intraspinal administration), diabetes-associated diarrhea, dysmenorrhea, glaucoma, opioid or nicotine withdrawal, impulse control disorder, menopausal flushing (hot sweats), migraine prophylaxis, severe pain, tic disorder, restless leg syndrome

Pregnancy Category C

Dosing

- Initial dose for hypertension:
  - Tablet: 0.1 mg twice daily
  - Transdermal: Start with Catapres-*TTS-1* applied once every 7 days
  - May need to overlap oral therapy for 1–2 days when initiating transdermal
- Dosing adjustments:
  - Tablet: Can increase in weekly intervals by 0.1 mg to a maximum dose of 2.4 mg daily. Can give in 2–4 daily doses.
  - Transdermal: Increase in 1- to 2-week intervals

Adverse Reactions: Most Common

CNS depression, constipation, dry mouth, dizziness, drowsiness, orthostatic hypotension

Adverse Reactions: Rare/Severe/Important

AV block, bradycardia, contact dermatitis (transdermal)

Major Drug Interactions

Drugs Affecting Clonidine

- Concomitant antihypertensive agents: Additive hypotension
- Tricyclic antidepressants: Decrease hypotensive effects
- Beta blockers: Additive bradycardia. Discontinuation of clonidine during concurrent use of a beta blocker may increase the risk of clonidine-withdrawal hypertensive crisis. It is preferred to discontinue the beta blocker several days prior to clonidine discontinuation.
- CNS depressants: Additive CNS effects

Clonidine's Effect on Other Drugs

Cyclosporine: Increases levels

Counseling Points

- Do not stop clonidine abruptly because it may cause rebound hypertension and other withdrawal symptoms (agitation, headache, tremor)
- Apply transdermal patch weekly to clean hairless area of upper outer arm or chest and rotate site weekly
- Oral therapy and transdermal therapy may overlap for 1–2 days until the full effect of transdermal therapy occurs
- The transdermal patch may contain metal; must remove before an MRI

Key Points

- Clonidine is a very effective blood pressure–lowering agent. It is often added to other antihypertensive therapies in patients with resistant hypertension. The risk of rebound hypertension is high if the patient discontinues clonidine abruptly.
- The transdermal route takes 2–3 days for full therapeutic effect
- Clonidine is commonly used for a variety of indications other than the treatment of hypertension

---

ADRENERGIC AGONISTS

Introduction

The adrenergic agonist class of drugs includes agents that stimulate alpha-1 and/or beta-1 receptors. Some agents work on either receptor, whereas some work on both, resulting in vasoconstriction, increased cardiac contractility, or both. These agents are only used in hospital settings for critically ill patients with severe hypotension or cardiogenic shock who require close monitoring.

Members of the Drug Class

In this section: Dobutamine, dopamine, epinephrine, norepinephrine, phenylephrine

◉ Dobutamine

Brand Name

Dobutrex

Generic Name

Dobutamine

Rx Only

Mechanism of Action

A synthetic catecholamine that stimulates beta-1 receptors, resulting in increased contractility (positive inotrope) and heart rate. Hemodynamic effects include increased cardiac output and stroke volume, with minimal lowering of blood pressure.

Dosage Forms

IV (injection and premixed infusion)

Usage

Cardiogenic shock/severe decompensated heart failure,* stress echocardiography

Pregnancy Category B

Dosing

- Initial dose: 2.5 µg/kg/min
- Dosage adjustment: Up to 15–20 µg/kg/min; doses of up to 40 µg/kg/min may be required, although benefit beyond 20 µg/kg/min not likely

Adverse Reactions: Most Common

Increased heart rate/tachyarrhythmia

Adverse Reactions: Rare/Severe/Important

Ventricular arrhythmias

Major Drug Interactions

Drugs Affecting Dobutamine

- Negative inotropes (beta blockers, verapamil/diltiazem): Decrease efficacy
- IV drugs: Check for compatibility when infusing through same line

Essential Monitoring Parameters

Blood pressure, heart rate, cardiac output/cardiac index, ECG

Key Points

- Only indicated for use in patients with severely decompensated heart failure and reduced cardiac output. Its use in stable heart failure patients is associated with increased mortality.
- Close hemodynamic monitoring is necessary

◉ Dopamine

Brand Name

None

Generic Name

Dopamine

Rx Only

Mechanism of Action

Effects are dose-related and dependent upon patient clinical status. Low doses (0.5–2 µg/kg/min) stimulate dopaminergic receptors, resulting in vasodilation of renal, mesenteric, coronary, and intracerebral vasculature. Intermediate doses (2–10 µg/kg/min) stimulate beta-1 receptors, causing increased myocardial contractility and cardiac output (positive inotrope). High rates of infusion (10–20 µg/kg/min) stimulate alpha-receptors, causing vasoconstriction and increased blood pressure.

Dosage Form

IV (injection and premixed infusion)

Usage

Adjunct treatment of shock (cardiac decompensation, septic),* symptomatic bradycardia or heart block

Pregnancy Category C

Dosing

- Low dose: 0.5–2 µg/kg/min
- Intermediate dose: 2–10 µg/kg/min
- High dose: 10–20 µg/kg/min
- Very high dose: 20–50 µg/kg/min

Adverse Reaction: Most Common

Increased heart rate/tachyarrhythmia

Adverse Reactions: Rare/Severe/Important

Ventricular arrhythmias, limb necrosis (with higher rates of infusion)

Major Drug Interactions

Drugs Affecting Dopamine

- Negative inotropes (beta blockers, verapamil/diltiazem): Decrease efficacy
- Vasodilators: Decrease efficacy
- IV drugs: Check for compatibility when infusing through same line

Essential Monitoring Parameters

Blood pressure, heart rate, cardiac output/cardiac index, ECG

Key Points

- Dopamine is primarily used as adjunctive therapy in patients with hemodynamic compromise/shock. Doses used depend on the goal of therapy, and patient response varies depending on the clinical situation.
- Close hemodynamic monitoring and dose adjustment is necessary

◉ Epinephrine

Brand Name

Adrenalin, EpiPen, Twinject

Generic Name

Epinephrine

Rx Only

Mechanism of Action

Epinephrine is a sympathomimetic catecholamine with numerous uses based on various mechanisms of action. Epinephrine is a very potent activator of alpha-receptors, resulting in vasoconstriction and decreased vascular permeability. It also stimulates beta-receptors, resulting in relaxation of bronchial smooth muscle and stimulation of heart rate and cardiac contractility.

Dosage Forms

Injection (vials and prefilled autoinjectors), solution for inhalation

Usage

Advanced cardiovascular life support (*ACLS*; ventricular fibrillation/pulseless ventricular tachycardia, pulseless electrical activity, asystole),* anaphylactic reactions,* bradycardia, bronchospasms/asthma/wheezing, shock/hypotension

Pregnancy Category C

Dosing

- ACLS:
  - IV: 1 mg every 3–5 minutes until return of spontaneous circulation
  - Endotracheal administration: 2–2.5 mg
- Anaphylaxis:
  - SUB-Q or IM (IM preferred): 0.2–0.5 mg (prefilled autoinjectors contain 0.3 mg)
  - IV: 0.1 mg
- Shock/hypotension:
  - Continuous infusion: 2–10 µg/min (up to 35 µg/min)

Adverse Reactions: Most Common

Increased heart rate/tachyarrhythmia, headache, hyperglycemia, tremor

Adverse Reactions: Rare/Severe/Important

Ventricular arrhythmias, limb necrosis (with higher rates of infusion), worsening coronary artery disease or cerebrovascular disease

Major Drug Interactions

Drugs Affecting Epinephrine

- Negative inotropes (beta blockers, verapamil/diltiazem): Decrease efficacy
- Vasodilators: Decrease efficacy
- IV drugs: Check for compatibility when infusing through same line

Essential Monitoring Parameters

Blood pressure, heart rate, cardiac output/cardiac index, ECG

Counseling Points

- Autoinjectors should be administered into the anterolateral aspect of the middle third of the thigh and can be administered through clothing if necessary
- A second dose should always be available and can be administered if response to first dose is inadequate. More than 2 doses should only be administered under medical care.

Key Points

- Epinephrine is used for a variety of acute indications, often in situations requiring immediate treatment. Its actions on alpha- and beta-receptors result in

effective treatment of anaphylaxis, wheezing, and arrhythmias/circulatory shock.
- Close hemodynamic monitoring and dose adjustment is necessary when administering as continuous infusion

⊙ Norepinephrine

Brand Name

Levophed

Generic Name

Norepinephrine

Rx Only

Mechanism of action

Stimulates alpha-receptors, resulting in vasoconstriction, and beta-receptors, resulting in increased heart rate and cardiac contractility

Dosage Form

Injection

Usage

Treatment of shock/hypotension*

Pregnancy Category C

Dosing

- Initial dose: 2–4 µg/min
- Dosage adjustment: Up to 20 µg/min
- Weight-based dosing: 0.01–3 µg/kg/min

Adverse Reactions: Most Common

Increased heart rate/tachyarrhythmia, headache, anxiety

Adverse Reactions: Rare/Severe/Important

Ventricular arrhythmias, limb/skin necrosis

Major Drug Interactions

Drugs Affecting Norepinephrine

- Negative inotropes (beta blockers, verapamil/diltiazem): Decrease efficacy
- Vasodilators: Decrease efficacy
- IV drugs: Check for compatibility when infusing through same line

Essential Monitoring Parameters

Blood pressure, heart rate, cardiac output/cardiac index, ECG

Key Points

- Norepinephrine is used primarily to increase blood pressure in patients with hypotension and shock
- Close hemodynamic monitoring and dosage adjustment is necessary

Phenylephrine

Brand Names

Numerous OTC combination products, including Pedia-Care, Sudafed PE, Neo-Synephrine

Generic Name

Phenylephrine

Rx (IV) and OTC (Oral, Opthalmic, Nasal Spray)

Mechanism of Action

Phenylephrine is a sympathomimetic agent with only alpha-receptor activity. Stimulation of alpha-receptors results in systemic arterial vasoconstriction, resulting in increased blood pressure. Vasoconstriction results in reflex bradycardia and decreased cardiac output in patients with heart failure.

Dosage Forms

Injection, liquid solution, tablet, nasal spray

Usage

Hypotension/shock* (IV only), decongestant* (oral, nasal spray, ophthalmic drops), vasoconstrictor in regional anesthesia

Pregnancy Category C

Dosing

- IV: 100–180 µg/min up to 300 µg/min
- Weight-based dosing: 0.5–9 µg/kg/min
- Oral: 10 mg every 4 hours as needed

Adverse Reactions: Most Common

Increased heart rate/tachyarrhythmia, headache, hyperglycemia, tremor

Adverse Reactions: Rare/Severe/Important

Limb necrosis (with higher rates of infusion), worsening coronary artery disease or cerebrovascular disease

Major Drug Interactions

Drugs Affecting Phenylephrine

- Vasodilators: Decrease efficacy
- IV drugs: Check for compatibility when infusing through same line

Contraindications

Oral: Cardiovascular disease, hypertension, narrow-angle glaucoma

Essential Monitoring Parameters

Blood pressure, heart rate, cardiac output/cardiac index

Counseling Point

Do not take for more than 7 days. If symptoms do not resolve, seek medical care.

Key Points

- Phenylephrine is a potent vasoconstrictor used intravenously in the treatment of hypotension and shock. Oral formulations, often in combination with other ingredients, exist for treatment of congestion.
- Close hemodynamic monitoring and dosage adjustment are necessary when administering as continuous infusion
- The properties of phenylephrine administered intravenously compared to administration via other routes are so different that they resemble different drugs. The oral and nasal spray formulations of phenylephrine do have some systemic absorption, although their systemic effects are minimal compared to the IV form.

ANGIOTENSIN-CONVERTING ENZYME INHIBITORS

Introduction

The angiotensin-converting enzyme (ACE) inhibitors are widely used for various cardiovascular diseases. They are effective for the treatment of hypertension and are the foundation of therapy for heart failure and left ventricular dysfunction. In addition, they are used for the prevention and treatment of diabetic nephropathy.

Mechanism of Action for the Drug Class

These agents act primarily through suppression of the renin–angiotensin–aldosterone system. They inhibit ACE, thereby inhibiting the conversion of angiotensin I to angiotensin II, a potent vasoconstrictor.

Rx Only for the Drug Class

Usage for the Drug Class

Diabetic nephropathy,* heart failure,* hypertension,* left ventricular dysfunction after myocardial infarction, acute myocardial infarction

Pregnancy Category D for the Drug Class

Adverse Reactions for the Drug Class: Most Common

Hypotension, hyperkalemia, cough, taste disorder (captopril)

Adverse Reactions for the Drug Class: Rare/Severe/Important

Angioedema (contraindication for use), azotemia, and renal failure in susceptible patients (e.g., volume depleted); neutropenia/agranulocytosis (captopril); avoid use in patients with bilateral renal artery stenosis, hepatic syndrome

Major Drug Interactions for the Drug Class

Drugs Affecting ACE Inhibitors

- Concomitant antihypertensive agents: Additive hypotension
- Angiotensin II receptor blockers, potassium-sparing diuretics, trimethoprim/sulfamethoxazole: Increase risk of hyperkalemia
- Angiotensin receptor blockers and aldosterone antagonists: Use in combination with ACE inhibitors should be avoided due to increased risk of hyperkalemia
- Diuretics: May potentiate renal insufficiency in volume-depleted patients
- NSAIDs: Reduce hypotensive effect of ACE inhibitors

ACE Inhibitors' Effects on Other Drugs

- Antihypertensive agents: Additive hypotension
- Cyclosporine: Increase nephrotoxicity
- Lithium: Increase serum levels
- Potassium-sparing diuretics, potassium supplements: May cause elevated potassium levels

Contraindication for the Drug Class

Angioedema with previous ACE inhibitor use

Essential Monitoring Parameters for the Drug Class

Renal function (serum creatinine), potassium, blood pressure

Counseling Points for the Drug Class

- Laboratory work will be needed periodically to monitor therapy (potassium, serum creatinine)
- Seek help immediately if swelling in face, lips, tongue, or throat occurs
- Avoid salt substitutes containing potassium
- Women: Notify your physician if pregnancy is suspected

Key Point for the Drug Class

ACE inhibitors are widely used for the treatment of hypertension, heart failure, and other cardiovascular diseases. Some potentially fatal adverse effects are associated with their use, so appropriate monitoring and patient counseling are necessary.

Members of the Drug Class

In this section: Benazepril, captopril, enalapril/enalaprilat, fosinopril, lisinopril, quinapril, ramipril
Others: Moexipril, perindopril, trandolapril

◉ Benazepril

Brand Name
Lotensin

Generic Name
Benazepril

Dosage Form
Tablet

Dosing

- Initial dose: 10 mg daily
- Dosage adjustment:
  - Up to 40 mg daily in 1–2 divided doses
  - Doses up to 80 mg daily may be tried, although increased efficacy using doses beyond 40 mg is limited
- Renal dosage adjustment: If CrCl < 30 mL/min, consider starting at lower doses (5 mg daily)

◉ Captopril

Brand Name
Capoten

Generic Name
Captopril

Dosage Form
Tablet

Dosing

- Initial dose: 6.25–25 mg two to three times daily
- Dosage adjustment: Up to 450 mg daily in 3 divided doses
- Renal dosage adjustment: Consider starting at lower doses

Key Point

The use of captopril is often limited to the inpatient setting because it is administered three times a day. Other ACE inhibitors with more convenient dosing regimens (once or twice daily) are available.

◉ Enalapril

Brand Name
Vasotec

Generic Name
Enalapril

Dosage Forms
Tablet, injection (as enalaprilat)

Dosing

- Initial dose:
  - Oral: 2.5 mg two times daily (can be given daily for hypertension)
  - IV: 1.25 mg every 6 hours (doses as low as 0.625 mg recommended in some patients)
- Dosage adjustment:
  - Oral: Up to 40 mg per day in 2 divided doses
  - IV: Up to 5 mg every 6 hours
- Renal dosage adjustment: Consider starting at lower doses
- IV to oral conversion:
  - 0.625 mg IV every 6 hours to 2.5 mg PO daily
  - 1.25 mg IV every 6 hours to 5 mg PO daily

Key Points

Enalaprilat is a more potent activated form of enalapril with an extended half-life that is administered via IV. It should be used cautiously because it can decrease blood pressure precipitously for prolonged periods of time.

◉ Fosinopril

Brand Name
Monopril

Generic Name
Fosinopril

Dosage Form
Tablet

Dosing

- Initial dose: 10 mg daily
- Dosage adjustment: Up to 40 mg daily in 1–2 doses

◉ Lisinopril

Brand Names
Prinivil, Zestril

Generic Name
Lisinopril

Dosage Form
Tablet

Dosing

- Initial dose: 5–10 mg daily
- Dosage adjustment: Up to 40 mg daily (up to 80 mg daily in hypertension)
- Renal dosage adjustment: Consider starting at lower doses (2.5 mg)

◉ Quinapril

Brand Name
Accupril

Generic Name
Quinapril

Dosage Form
Tablet

Dosing

- Initial dose: 10–20 mg daily (in 1–2 doses)
- Dosage adjustment: Up to 40 mg daily in 2 divided doses (up to 80 mg daily in hypertension)
- Renal dosage adjustment: Consider starting at lower doses

◉ Ramipril

Brand Name
Altace

Generic Name
Ramipril

Dosage Forms
Capsule, tablet

Dosing

- Initial dose: 2.5 mg daily
- Dosage adjustment: Up to 20 mg daily in 1–2 divided doses
- Renal dosage adjustment: Consider starting at lower doses

Key Point

Ramipril is also indicated to reduce the risk of myocardial infarction, stroke, and death from cardiovascular causes in patients who are at increased risk of these events

ANGIOTENSIN II RECEPTOR BLOCKERS

Introduction

Angiotensin II receptor blockers (ARBs) are widely used for the treatment of cardiovascular diseases. They are primarily used for the treatment of hypertension and as an alternative to ACE inhibitors for the treatment of heart failure and diabetic nephropathy. Although they also work along the renin–angiotensin–aldosterone system, they have an advantage over ACE inhibitors in that they do not cause cough as ACE inhibitors do. Although the agents in this class are largely similar, there are differences in their pharmacokinetics and their approved indications, depending on the disease states in which they have been studied.

Mechanism of Action for the Drug Class

These agents suppress the renin–angiotensin–aldosterone system. They block the binding of angiotensin II to the AT1 receptor, thereby inhibiting the effects of angiotensin II, which is a potent vasoconstrictor.

Rx Only for the Drug Class

Usage for the Drug Class

Hypertension,* diabetic nephropathy,* heart failure* (select ARBs), myocardial infarction

Pregnancy Category D for the Drug Class

Adverse Reactions for the Drug Class: Most Common

Hyperkalemia, hypotension

Adverse Reactions for the Drug Class: Rare/Severe/Important

Increased serum creatinine, angioedema

Major Drug Interactions for the Drug Class

Drugs Affecting ARBs

- Concomitant antihypertensive agents: Additive hypotension
- Potassium supplements and potassium-sparing diuretics: Potential additive increases in potassium
- ACE inhibitors, potassium-sparing diuretics, trimethoprim/sulfamethoxazole: Increase risk of hyperkalemia
- ACE inhibitor and aldosterone antagonists: Use in combination with ARBs should be avoided due to increased risk of hyperkalemia

ARBs' Effects on Other Drugs

Lithium: May reduce elimination

Essential Monitoring Parameters for the Drug Class

Renal function (serum creatinine), potassium, blood pressure

Counseling Points for the Drug Class

- Laboratory work will be needed periodically to monitor therapy (potassium, serum creatinine)
- Women: Notify your physician if pregnancy is suspected

Key Point for the Drug Class

ARBs are used widely for the treatment of cardiovascular diseases. They are often used in patients intolerant of ACE inhibitors who have heart failure (candesartan, losartan, valsartan only).

Members of the Drug Class

In this section: Irbesartan, losartan, olmesartan, valsartan
Others: Azilsartan, candesartan, eprosartan, telmisartan

◉ Irbesartan

Brand Name
Avapro

Generic Name
Irbesartan

Dosage Form
Tablet

Dosing
- Initial dose: 75–150 mg daily
- Dosage adjustment: Up to 300 mg daily

Key Point
Not recommended for heart failure

◉ Losartan

Brand Name
Cozaar

Generic Name
Losartan

Dosage Form
Tablet

Dosing
- Initial dose: 25–50 mg daily
- Dosage adjustment: Up to 100 mg daily in 1–2 divided doses

Key Point
Additional indication includes reducing the risk of stroke in patients with hypertension and left ventricular hypertrophy

◉ Olmesartan Medoxomil

Brand Name
Benicar

Generic Name
Olmesartan medoxomil

Dosage Form
Tablet

Dosing
- Initial dose: 20 mg once daily
- Dosage adjustment: Up to 40 mg daily

Valsartan

Brand Name
Diovan

Generic Name
Valsartan

Dosage Form
Tablet

Dosing
- Initial dose: 40–160 mg daily
- Dosage adjustment: Up to 320 mg daily in 1–2 divided doses

Key Point
Preferred ARB in patients with heart failure

ANTIANGINALS, RANOLAZINE

Introduction

Ranolazine is a unique agent whose exact mechanism of action is unknown. It does not rely on decreased heart rate or myocardial workload for its antianginal effects. It is used in patients with continued angina symptoms despite maximum therapy with other antianginals or who cannot tolerate additional antianginal therapy due to low heart rate or blood pressure.

Mechanism of Action for the Drug Class

The exact mechanism of ranolazine is unknown. One possible mechanism is inhibition of the inward sodium channel in the ischemic myocardium, resulting in decreased calcium influx and decreased ventricular tension and oxygen consumption. Another postulated mechanism is that ranolazine inhibition of fatty acid oxygenation results in increased glucose oxidation and generation of more ATP per molecule of oxygen.

Ranolazine

Brand Name
Ranexa

Generic Name
Ranolazine

Rx Only

Dosage Form
Extended-release tablet

Usage
Treatment of chronic angina*

Pregnancy Category C

Dosing
- Initial dose: 500 mg twice daily
- Dosage adjustment: Up to 1,000 mg twice daily
- Renal dosage adjustment: No specific recommendations; however, levels increased by 50% in patients with renal dysfunction

Adverse Reactions: Most Common
Dizziness, QTc prolongation

Adverse Reactions: Rare/Severe/Important
Torsade de pointes

Major Drug Interactions
Drugs Affecting Ranolazine
- Diltiazem, erythromycin, verapamil, and other moderate CYP3A inhibitors: Ranolazine dose should not exceed 500 mg twice daily
- Strong CYP3A inhibitors: Increased risk of QTc prolongation, avoid use
- QTc-prolonging drugs: Increased risk of QTc prolongation

Ranolazine's Effect on Other Drugs
- Simvastatin: Dose should not exceed 20 mg daily
- Substrates of P-glycoprotein: Increases risk of toxicity

Contraindications
Use with caution in patients with QTc prolongation; contradicted for patients with any degree of hepatic cirrhosis

Essential Monitoring Parameter
EKG (QTc interval)

Counseling Points
- Do not crush, break, or chew tablet
- Ranolazine should not be used to treat an acute angina episode

Key Points
- Ranolazine is used for the treatment of chronic angina symptoms. Because it does not affect heart rate or blood pressure, it is used when patients cannot tolerate other antianginal agents.
- EKG must be monitored closely because the QTc interval can be prolonged

ANTIARRHYTHMICS, AMIODARONE

Introduction

Amiodarone is the most commonly used antiarrhythmic agent. It is used for rate and rhythm control of atrial fibrillation and to treat and prevent ventricular arrhythmias. It has a very long terminal half-life of approximately 2 months and a large volume of distribution and thus requires large loading doses administered over several weeks.

Mechanism of Action for the Drug Class

Amiodarone is considered a class III antiarrhythmic medication; however, it exhibits characteristics of all four Vaughan-Williams antiarrhythmic medication classes. Amiodarone slows intraventricular conduction by blocking sodium channels, slows the heart rate, and impedes AV node conduction by blocking beta-adrenergic receptors and calcium channels and prolongs atrial and ventricular repolarization by inhibiting potassium channels.

◉ Amiodarone

Brand Names
Cordarone, Pacerone

Generic Name
Amiodarone

Dosage Forms
Tablet, injection

Rx Only

Usage
Atrial arrhythmias,* life-threatening ventricular arrhythmias,* prevention of postoperative atrial fibrillation in cardiothoracic surgery,* prevention of ventricular arrhythmias in patients with internal cardioverter-defibrillators*

Pregnancy Category D

Dosing
- Oral:
  - Loading dose of 800–1,600 mg per day in divided doses for 1–3 weeks until adequate arrhythmia control is achieved (usually up to 10 g total)
  - Maintenance dose: 200–400 mg per day
- IV: Loading dose of 150–300 mg in 20–30 mL NS followed by 1 mg/min for 6 hours, then 0.5 mg/minute for 18 hours. Infusion can be continued for up to 4 weeks. Should switch to oral as soon as possible.

Adverse Reactions: Most Common
Bradycardia, corneal microdeposits, hypotension (more common with IV), hypothyroidism, nausea, vomiting (especially with higher doses), phlebitis (IV form), photosensitivity, prolonged QTc interval

Adverse Reactions: Rare/Severe/Important
Blue/gray skin discoloration, hyperthyroidism, liver toxicity, pulmonary toxicity

Major Drug Interactions
Drugs Affecting Amiodarone
- Drugs that prolong the QTc interval: May increase the QTc-prolonging effect of amiodarone
- Beta blockers, diltiazem, digoxin, and verapamil: May cause excessive atrioventricular block
- Cimetidine: Decreases metabolism
- Fluconazole, ketoconazole, voriconazole, itraconazole, posaconazole, azithromycin: Increase QT prolongation
- Darunavir, boceprevir, delavirdine, telaprevir, saquinavir, indinavir, nelfinavir, ritonavir, tipranavir, lopinavir, atazanavir, amprenavir, fosamprenavir: Increase risk of amiodarone cardiotoxicity

Amiodarone's Effect on Other Drugs
- Cyclosporine, tacrolimus, sirolimus: Increases levels
- Lovastatin, simvastatin: Increases risk of myopathy
- Digoxin: Increases levels
- Warfarin: Increases effects

Contraindications
Severe bradycardia, second- or third-degree AV block, cardiogenic shock

Counseling Points
- Take with food to decrease adverse GI effects
- Use sunscreen or stay out of sun to prevent burns
- Schedule regular blood work for thyroid and liver function

Key Points
- Although amiodarone is the most commonly used antiarrhythmic agent for atrial and ventricular arrhythmias, it should be reserved for patients with life-threatening arrhythmias due to its substantial toxicity. Patients should be hospitalized for initiation of therapy and need to be monitored and counseled appropriately to limit toxicity.
- IV admixtures must be made in glass or non-PVC containers (for all infusions expected to run more than 1 hour)

Introduction

Digoxin is the only available digitalis glycoside and is one of the oldest medications used for the treatment of heart failure. Although it is still frequently utilized in heart failure, it is no longer a first-line choice because other agents (ACE inhibitors, beta blockers) have been proven more effective at reducing morbidity and mortality. Digoxin also has a role as a rate-control agent in the treatment of atrial fibrillation.

Mechanism of Action for the Drug Class

Inhibits sodium-potassium ATPase, leading to an increase in the intracellular concentration of sodium, thus stimulating sodium–calcium exchange. This increases the intracellular concentration of calcium, leading to increased contractility. Enhances vagal tone to directly suppress the atrioventricular node, which increases effective refractory period and decreases conduction velocity resulting in decreased ventricular rate.

◉ Digoxin

Brand Names

Lanoxin, Digitek, Lanoxicaps

Generic Name

Digoxin

Rx Only

Dosage Forms

Tablet, capsule, solution, injection

Usage

Heart failure (stage C),* supraventricular arrhythmias*

Pregnancy Category C

Dosing

- Loading dose:
  - 8–12 µg/kg ideal body weight (adjust for renal function). Average loading dose is 0.75–1 mg.
  - Administration recommendations: Roughly half of the total loading dose administered as the first dose, with the remaining portion divided and administered every 6–8 hours initially
- Maintenance dose: 0.125–0.5 mg daily
- Renal dosage adjustment (both loading and maintenance doses should be adjusted):
  - CrCl 10–50 mL/min: Administer 25–75% of dose or full dose every 36 hours
  - CrCl < 10 mL/min: Administer 10–25% of dose or full dose every 48 hours
  - End-stage renal disease: Reduce dose by 50%

Pharmacokinetic Monitoring

- Monitor levels after at least 6 hours following administration (usually prior to next dose)
- Obtain levels within 12–24 hours of initiating therapy if a loading dose is given or within 3–5 days following initiation if no loading dose is given
- Usual range 0.5–0.8 ng/dL for heart failure, 0.8–2 ng/dL for arrhythmias

Adverse Reactions: Most Common

Anorexia, diarrhea, dizziness, headache, nausea

Adverse Reactions: Rare/Severe/Important

Atrial tachycardia, AV dissociation, blurred or yellow vision, hallucinations, heart block, ventricular fibrillation/tachycardia

Major Drug Interactions

Drugs Affecting Digoxin

- Amiodarone (reduce digoxin dose by 50%), boceprevir, clarithromycin, conivaptan, cyclosporine, diltiazem, dronedarone (reduce dose by 50%), erythromycin, fluconazole, itraconazole, quinidine, quinine, ritonavir, saquinavir, telaprevir, tetracyclines, verapamil: Increase digoxin serum levels
- Cholestyramine, colestipol, kaolin-pectin, sucralfate: Decrease digoxin therapeutic effects
- Diuretic-induced electrolyte decreases (potassium, magnesium) may predispose patients to digitalis-induced arrhythmias

Digoxin's Effect on Other Drugs

Although beta blockers or calcium channel blockers and digoxin may be useful in combination to control atrial fibrillation, their additive effects on AV node conduction may result in advanced or complete heart block

Essential Monitoring Parameters

Digoxin levels (to check for toxicity or compliance), renal function (serum creatinine), heart rate/ECG periodically

Counseling Points

- Take digoxin at the same time every day
- Notify your healthcare provider if any signs of toxicity occur (e.g., nausea, vomiting, blurry vision)

Key Points

- Although digoxin is not a first-line choice, it is often used in the treatment of symptomatic heart failure and atrial fibrillation
- Digoxin has a narrow therapeutic index, and dosing must be adjusted for renal function, weight, and heart failure status. Appropriate monitoring of renal function is necessary to avoid toxicity.
- Loading doses are typically not necessary for patients with heart failure

ANTIARRHYTHMICS, SOTALOL

Introduction

Sotalol has activity as both a beta blocker and as a class III antiarrhythmic. It is used for rate and rhythm control in patients with atrial fibrillation.

Mechanism of Action for the Drug Class

Sotalol has both nonselective beta-adrenergic blockade and class III antiarrhythmic actions that prolong cardiac action potential duration by inhibiting potassium channels

◉ Sotalol

Brand Names

Betapace, Betapace AF, Sorine

Generic Name

Sotalol

Rx Only

Dosage Forms

Tablet, IV solution

Usage

Atrial fibrillation,* life-threatening ventricular arrhythmias

Pregnancy Category B

Dosing

- Initial dose:
  - Initiate treatment in a setting where continuous ECG monitoring is possible
  - Initial dose is based on CrCl:
    - ◆ CrCl > 60 mL/min: 80 mg twice daily
    - ◆ CrCl 40–60 mL/min: 80 mg daily
    - ◆ CrCl < 40 mL/min: Contraindicated
- Maintenance dose: Up to 160 mg twice daily
- Renal dosage adjustment (of maintenance dose):
  - CrCl 30–60 mL/min: Administer daily
  - CrCl < 40 mL/min: Contraindicated (atrial fibrillation)
  - CrCl 10–30 mL/min: Consider increasing dosing interval to every 36 to 48 hours (ventricular arrhythmias)

Adverse Reactions: Most Common

Bradycardia, dizziness, dyspnea, fatigue, QT interval prolongation (avoid if baseline QTc > 450 msec; discontinue or decrease dose if QTc ≥ 500 msec during therapy)

Adverse Reactions: Rare/Severe/Important

Bronchospasm, heart block, torsades de pointes

Major Drug Interactions

Drugs Affecting Sotalol

- Calcium channel blockers: Increase bradycardia
- Digoxin: Increases proarrhythmic risk
- Drugs that prolong the QTc interval: Increase the QTc-prolonging effect of sotalol
- Fluconazole, itraconazole, ketoconazole, voriconazole: Increase risk of cardiotoxicity
- Antacids containing aluminum oxide or magnesium hydroxide: Reduce absorption

Sotalol's Effect on Other Drugs

Although calcium channel blockers and digoxin may be useful in combination with sotalol to control atrial fibrillation, their additive effects on AV node conduction may result in advanced or complete heart block

Contraindications

Baseline QTc interval > 450 msec, long QT syndrome, heart failure (cardiogenic shock, uncontrolled heart failure), CrCl < 40 mL/min, hypokalemia, bradycardia, second- or third-degree AV block

Essential Monitoring Parameters

EKG (QTc interval), serum creatinine, heart rate

Counseling Point

Routine blood tests are required to monitor renal function

Key Points

- Initiation of therapy and dosage adjustments should occur in a hospital setting with continuous monitoring
- Betapace and Betapace AF should not be substituted for each other
- Renal function and QTc interval must be monitored closely and dosing adjustments made accordingly
- Electrolyte abnormalities (hypokalemia, hypomagnesemia) should be corrected prior to initiation
- Avoid use in patients with heart failure

Introduction

Atropine is an anticholinergic agent used primarily intravenously for bradycardia during *advanced cardiovascular life support* (*ACLS*). It is also available in ophthalmic form to produce mydriasis. Many other anticholinergic medications exist that are used for noncardiac indications, ranging from pulmonary diseases to incontinence. These are discussed elsewhere.

Mechanism of Action for the Drug Class

Atropine competitively blocks the action of acetylcholine on all muscarinic receptors. Anticholinergic activity in smooth muscle, secretory glands, and CNS results in tachycardia, dried secretions, and bronchodilation.

◉ Atropine

Brand Names

AtroPen, Atropine Care, Isopto Atropine

Generic Name

Atropine

Rx Only

Dosage Forms

Injection, ophthalmic ointment and solution

Usage

Antidote for mushroom poisoning, bradycardia/heart block,* cycloplegic refraction, mydriasis induction, organophosphate poisoning, poisoning by parasympathomimetic drug, premedication for anesthetic procedure, uveitis

Pregnancy Category C

Dosing

- Bradycardia: 0.5 mg IV, repeat every 3–5 minutes up to 3 mg
- Poisoning: Dosing depends on poison
- Preanesthesia: 0.4–0.6 mg IV, IM, or SUB-Q; repeat every 4–6 hours as needed to inhibit salivation/secretions

Adverse Reactions: Most Common

Flushing, tachycardia

Adverse Reactions: Rare/Severe/Important

Acute organic brain syndrome (confusion, delirium, restlessness, somnolence, psychosis), anhidrosis, arrhythmias, paralytic ileus, urinary retention

Major Drug Interactions

None

Contraindications

Narrow-angle glaucoma (ophthalmic), pyloric stenosis

Essential Monitoring Parameters

Blood pressure, heart rate, mental status

Key Point

Atropine is a potent anticholinergic agent used primarily in the management of bradycardia/heart block. Ophthalmic formulations are also commonly used to produce mydriasis.

ANTIDIURETIC HORMONE

Introduction

Vasopressin has multiple mechanisms and is primarily used to increase blood pressure in patients with hypotension/septic shock. It can replace other pressor agents in some patients.

Mechanism of Action for the Drug Class

Vasopressin acts on vasopressin receptors V_1 and V_2. Stimulation of the V_2 receptor is greater than V_1 and causes increased water permeability in the renal tubule, resulting in decreased urine volume. In addition, vasopressin is a direct vasoconstrictor and increases blood vessel response to catecholamines and acts on portal blood pressure to restrict blood flow to esophageal varices.

◉ Vasopressin

Brand Name

Pitressin

Generic Name

Vasopressin

Rx Only

Dosage Form

Injection

Usage

Advanced cardiovascular life support (*ACLS*; pulseless arrest),* diabetes insipidus, esophageal varices, GI hemorrhage, shock/hypotension*

Pregnancy Category C

Dosing

- Diabetes insipidus: 5–10 units IM/SUB-Q two to four times daily as needed
- Variceal hemorrhage: 0.2–0.4 units/min continuous infusion (doses up to 0.8 units/min have been used)
- ACLS: 40 units IV/IO
- Shock/hypotension: 0.01–0.04 units/min

Adverse Reactions: Most Common

Headache, abdominal cramps, nausea, vomiting, tremor

Adverse Reactions: Rare/Severe/Important

Heart failure, decreased cardiac output, limb/skin necrosis, myocardial infarction

Major Drug Interactions

Drugs Affecting Vasopressin

- Vasodilators: Decrease efficacy
- IV drugs: Check for compatibility when infusing through same line

Essential Monitoring Parameters

Blood pressure, heart rate, cardiac output/cardiac index, ECG

Key Points

- Vasopressin is used primarily in pulseless arrest during ACLS and to increase blood pressure in patients with hypotension and shock
- Close hemodynamic monitoring and titration of dose is necessary

BETA BLOCKERS

Introduction

Beta-adrenergic antagonists, commonly called beta blockers, are one of the most widely used cardiovascular medications. They have multiple clinical effects and are very effective at preventing morbidity and mortality for several disease states, although they can be sedating to patients.

Mechanism of Action for the Drug Class

Beta blockers competitively block response to beta-adrenergic stimulation at the receptor level, which results in decreases in heart rate, myocardial contractility, blood pressure, and myocardial oxygen demand. Beta-1 selective agents selectively block beta-1 receptors with little to no effect on beta-2 receptors, whereas nonselective agents antagonize both types.

Members of the Drug Class

In this section: Atenolol, carvedilol, labetalol, metoprolol, nebivolol, propranolol
Others: Betaxolol, bisoprolol, esmolol, nadolol, timolol

Rx Only for the Drug Class

Usage for the Drug Class

- Cardiovascular uses: Angina,* arrhythmias,* heart failure (bisoprolol, carvedilol, and metoprolol XL only),* hypertension,* myocardial infarction,* premature ventricular contractions, adjunctive management of pheochromocytoma, prevention of postoperative cardiac complications in noncardiovascular surgery
- Noncardiovascular uses: Essential tremors, migraine prophylaxis, adjunctive therapy in the treatment of Parkinson disease, alcohol withdrawal syndrome, aggressive behavior, treatment of antipsychotic-induced akathisia, prevention of esophageal varices rebleeding, treatment of anxiety, adjunctive treatment in schizophrenia and acute panic, prevention of gastric bleeding in portal hypertension, and treatment of thyrotoxicosis symptoms

Pregnancy Category D for the Drug Class

Adverse Reactions for the Drug Class: Most Common

Bradycardia, decreased sexual ability, dizziness, hypotension, fatigue, lethargy

Adverse Reactions for the Drug Class: Rare/Severe/Important

Heart block, worsening heart failure symptoms, bronchoconstriction (nonselective or selective at higher doses), exacerbations of Raynaud's disease, depression

Major Drug Interactions for the Drug Class

Drugs Affecting Beta Blockers

Amiodarone, clonidine, digoxin, diltiazem, dronedarone, verapamil: Enhance AV nodal inhibition

Beta Blockers' Effects on Other Drugs

Oral antidiabetic agents, insulin: May mask the symptoms of hypoglycemia

Contraindications for the Drug Class

Sinus bradycardia, cardiogenic shock, second- or third-degree heart block

Essential Monitoring Parameters for the Drug Class

Heart rate, blood pressure

Counseling Points for the Drug Class

- Do not abruptly stop taking medication. Beta blockers should be gradually tapered when stopping to avoid tachycardia, hypertension, and/or ischemia.
- These medications may increase blood glucose. They may also mask the symptoms of hypoglycemia.
- May decrease heart rate and blood pressure. Tell your healthcare provider if you experience any dizziness or lightheadedness.

Key Points for the Drug Class

- Beta blockers are one of the most widely used cardiovascular agents because they are very effective for the treatment of many cardiovascular diseases. They are also used for some off-label uses not associated directly with cardiovascular disease.
- Nonselective beta blockers should not be used in patients with asthma because they can lead to asthma exacerbations. Selective agents should be used cautiously.

⊙ Atenolol (beta-1 selective)

Brand Name

Tenormin

Generic Name

Atenolol (beta-1 selective)

Dosage Form

Tablet

Dosing

- 25–100 mg daily
- Use lower doses or increase the dosing interval in elderly and patients with renal dysfunction due to significantly increased half-life
- Renal dosage adjustment:
  - CrCl 15–35 mL/min: Maximum dose of 50 mg once daily
  - CrCl < 15 mL/min: Maximum dose 50 mg every other day

⊙ Carvedilol (nonselective with alpha-1 blockade)

Brand Names

Coreg, Coreg CR

Generic Name

Carvedilol (nonselective with alpha-1 blockade)

Dosage Forms

Tablet, extended-release capsule

Dosing

- Nonextended release: 3.125–50 mg twice daily
- Extended release: 10–80 mg daily

Key Points

- Recommended for heart failure
- Conversion from immediate-release to extended-release is not 1:1
- Inhibits alpha-1 receptors as well, unlike most other beta blockers

⊙ Labetalol (nonselective with alpha-1 blockade)

Brand Names

Trandate, Normodyne

Generic Name

Labetalol (nonselective with alpha-1 blockade)

Dosage Forms

Tablet, injection

Dosing

- Oral: 100 mg twice daily, can be given up to 2,400 mg daily in divided doses
- IV:
  - Repeat boluses: 20–80 mg slow IV push every 10 minutes up to total 300 mg until response
  - Continuous infusion: 0.5–2 mg/min up to total 300 mg. In rare instances when clinically necessary (i.e., BP lowering in aortic dissection), continuous infusions up to 8 mg/min can be utilized. Close monitoring of blood pressure and heart rate is necessary.

Key Points

- Often used for hypertension and hypertensive emergencies, in part due to the availability of an IV form
- Inhibits alpha-1 receptors as well, unlike most other beta blockers

⊙ Metoprolol Tartrate

Brand Names

Lopressor, Toprol XL

Generic Names

Metoprolol tartrate, metoprolol succinate (beta-1 selective)

Dosage Forms

Tablet, injection

Dosing

- Initial dose:
  - Oral: 25–50 mg twice daily (once daily if XL formulation)
  - IV: 1.25–5 mg every 6–12 hours

- Dosage adjustments:
  - Oral: Up to 450 mg in divided daily doses (once daily if XL formulation)
  - IV: Up to 15 mg every 3–6 hours

Key Point

Only the extended-release formulation (metoprolol succinate) is recommended for use in heart failure patients

⊙ Nebivolol (beta-1 selective)

Brand Name

Bystolic

Generic Name

Nebivolol (beta-1 selective)

Dosage Form

Tablet

Dosing

- Initial dose:
  - Hypertension: 5 mg daily
  - Heart failure in adults age > 70 years: 1.25 mg daily
- Dosing adjustments: Up to 40 mg daily

Key Point

Limited data suggest that nebivolol may be effective for heart failure in elderly patients (age > 70 years)

⊙ Propranolol (nonselective)

Brand Names

Inderal, Inderal LA, InnoPran XL

Generic Name

Propranolol (nonselective)

Dosage Forms

Tablet, sustained-release capsule, oral solution, injection

Dosing

- Initial dose:
  - Oral: 40 mg twice daily (once daily if long-acting formulation)
  - IV: 1–3 mg every 2 minutes up to 10 mg
- Dosage adjustments: Up to 320 mg PO in 2–4 divided daily doses (once daily if long-acting formulation)

Key Points

- Propranolol is the beta blocker of choice for treatment of thyroid storm
- Propranolol is also used for the treatment of performance anxiety, although other beta blockers also are used

CALCIUM CHANNEL BLOCKERS, BENZOTHIAZEPINES

Introduction

Diltiazem is the only member of the benzothiazepine class of calcium channel blockers. It is commonly used for the treatment of hypertension and heart rate control in patients with atrial fibrillation due to its effects on both blood pressure and cardiac conduction.

Mechanism of Action for the Drug Class

These drugs inhibit the movement of calcium ions across the cell membranes. The effects on the cardiovascular system include relaxation of coronary vascular smooth muscle and coronary vasodilation. They also increase myocardial oxygen delivery and depress both impulse formation and conduction velocity in the atrioventricular node.

⊙ Diltiazem

Brand Names

Cardizem, Cardizem CD, Cardizem LA, Cartia XT, Dilacor XR, Dilt-CD, Dilt-XR, Diltia XT, Diltzac, Matzim LA, Taztia XT, Tiazac

Generic Name

Diltiazem

Rx Only

Dosage Forms

Tablet, extended-release tablet, extended-release capsule, injection

Usage

Atrial arrhythmias,* chronic stable angina, diabetic nephropathy, hypertension,* paroxysmal supraventricular tachycardias, pulmonary hypertension, variant angina

Pregnancy Category C

Dosing

- PO: 120–540 mg per day (in one to four divided doses, depending on the drug formulation)
- IV:
  - Bolus: 10–25 mg (0.25 mg/kg actual body weight) given over 2 minutes
  - Continuous infusion: 5–15 mg/hour
  - IV to PO conversion: Oral dose = [rate (mg/hr) × 3 + 3] × 10

Adverse Reactions: Most Common

Bradycardia, dizziness, lightheadedness, flushing, headache, hypotension, peripheral edema

Adverse Reactions: Rare/Severe/Important

Third-degree AV block, decreased heart contractility (worsening symptoms of heart failure), dermatologic reactions, gingival hyperplasia

Major Drug Interactions

Drugs Affecting Diltiazem

- CYP3A4 inhibitors: Increase effects
- Azole antifungal agents: Increase hypotensive effect
- Carbamazepine: Decreases hypotensive effect
- Clarithromycin, erythromycin: Decrease metabolism
- Rifampin: Decreases hypotensive effect
- Sildenafil: Increases hypotensive effect

Diltiazem's Effect on Other Drugs

- Antihypertensive medications: Additive hypotensive effects
- Amiodarone, beta blockers, and digoxin: Enhanced decrease in AV node conduction, increased risk of bradycardia
- Increased concentration of drugs metabolized by CYP3A4 (cyclosporine, HMG-CoA reductase inhibitors, tacrolimus)
- Phenytoin: Decreases metabolism

Contraindications

Atrial fibrillation/flutter with an accessory bypass tract, cardiogenic shock/heart failure, second- or third-degree heart block

Counseling Points

- Take on an empty stomach if possible
- Do not crush long-acting formulations
- Capsules may be opened and the contents sprinkled on applesauce, which can be swallowed without chewing

Key Points

- Diltiazem is used for the treatment of hypertension, angina, and atrial fibrillation. It should be avoided in patients with myocardial infarction and/or heart failure because it is a negative inotrope.
- Extended-release formulations are either daily or twice-daily dosing. Check with specific manufacturer recommendations.

CALCIUM CHANNEL BLOCKERS, DIHYDROPYRIDINES

Introduction

The dihydropyridine calcium channel blockers are widely used for the treatment of hypertension. They do not affect heart rate or contractility to the same extent as diltiazem and verapamil.

Mechanism of Action for the Drug Class

These drugs inhibit movement of calcium ions across the cell membranes. The effects on the cardiovascular system include relaxation of coronary vascular smooth muscle and coronary vasodilation. They also increase myocardial oxygen supply.

Rx Only for the Drug Class

Usage for the Drug Class

Chronic stable angina,* diabetic nephropathy, hypertension,* prevention/treatment of altitude sickness, pulmonary hypertension, Raynaud's disease, vasospastic angina*

Pregnancy Category C for the Drug Class

Adverse Reactions for the Drug Class: Most Common

Dizziness/lightheadedness, flushing, headache, hypotension, peripheral edema

Adverse Reactions for the Drug Class: Rare/Severe/Important

Orthostasis

Major Drug Interactions for the Drug Class

Drugs Affecting Dihydropyridines

- CYP3A4 inhibitors: Increase effects
- Carbamazepine: Decreases hypotensive effect
- Sildenafil: Increases hypotensive effect
- Azole antifungal agents: Increase hypotensive effects
- Rifampin: Decreases hypotensive effect

Dihydropyridines' Effects on Other Drugs

- Antihypertensive agents: Additive hypotension
- Simvastatin, tacrolimus: Increases effects/toxicity

Counseling Points for the Drug Class

- These medications can be taken without regard to meals
- Do not stop therapy abruptly

Key Points for the Drug Class

- The dihydropyridine calcium channel blockers are used primarily for the treatment of hypertension. They also have a role in the treatment of chronic stable angina.

- Immediate-release formulations of nifedipine are no longer recommended due to increased mortality compared to extended-release formulations, although both forms are still available.

Members of the Drug Class

In this section: Amlodipine, felodipine, nifedipine
Others: Clevidipine, isradipine, nicardipine, nimodipine, nisoldipine

◉ Amlodipine

Brand Name
Norvasc

Generic Name
Amlodipine

Dosage Form
Tablet

Dosing
2.5–10 mg daily

Key Point
Amlodipine has a long half-life and therefore can be dosed once daily. It is not an extended-release formulation and therefore can be crushed.

◉ Felodipine

Brand Name
Plendil

Generic Name
Felodipine

Dosage Form
Extended-release tablet

Dosing
2.5–20 mg daily

◉ Nifedipine

Brand Names
Adalat CC, Afeditab CR, Nifediac CC, Nifedical XL, Procardia, Procardia XL

Generic Name
Nifedipine

Dosage Forms
Capsule, extended-release tablet

Dosing
30–180 mg per day (in 3 doses or once daily, depending on the formulation)

Key Points
- Immediate-release formulation is not recommended for use
- Extended-release formulation contains nondeformable matrix, which is expelled in stool. Caution using in patients with a known stricture/narrowing of the GI tract.
- Nifedipine has negative inotropic effects and may worsen heart failure symptoms

CALCIUM CHANNEL BLOCKERS, PHENYLALKYLAMINES

Introduction

Verapamil is the only available member of the phenylalkylamine class of calcium channel blockers. It is used for the treatment of hypertension and heart rate control in patients with atrial fibrillation.

Mechanism of Action for the Drug Class

Verapamil inhibits the movement of calcium ions across the cell membranes. The effects on the cardiovascular system include relaxation of coronary vascular smooth muscle, coronary vasodilation, and decreased myocardial contractility. It also increases myocardial oxygen delivery and depresses both impulse formation and conduction velocity in the atrioventricular node.

◉ Verapamil

Brand Names
Calan, Calan SR, Covera-HS, Isoptin SR, Verelan, Verelan PM

Generic Name
Verapamil

Rx Only

Dosage Forms
Tablet, extended-release tablet, sustained-release tablet, capsule, injection

Usage

- Cardiovascular uses: Atrial fibrillation and flutter,* chronic stable angina, hypertension,* unstable angina, variant angina
- Noncardiovascular uses: Manic manifestations of bipolar disorder, migraine prophylaxis

Pregnancy Category C

Dosing

- Oral: 120–480 mg per day (given daily or in divided doses, depending on the formulation)
- IV: 2.5–5 mg over 2 minutes. May repeat every 15–30 minutes up to maximum of 30 mg.
- Renal dosage adjustment: If CrCl < 10 mL/min, administer 50–75% of normal dose

Adverse Reactions: Most Common

Bradycardia, constipation (up to 42%), dizziness/lightheadedness, gingival hyperplasia, headache, hypotension, peripheral edema

Adverse Reactions: Rare/Severe/Important

Worsening of heart failure, increased hepatic enzymes

Major Drug Interactions

Drugs Affecting Verapamil

- Amiodarone, beta blockers: Increase risk of bradycardia
- Carbamazepine: Decreases hypotensive effect
- Clarithromycin, erythromycin: Increase levels
- Fluconazole, itraconazole: Increase effects

Verapamil's Effect on Other Drugs

- Digoxin: Increases levels
- Dofetilide: Increases levels, leading to ventricular arrhythmias (contraindicated)
- Cyclosporine, tacrolimus: Increase levels
- Phenytoin: Decreases metabolism
- Theophylline: Increased levels
- Lovastatin, simvastatin, atorvastatin: Increase levels/toxicity

Contraindications

Severe left ventricular dysfunction/cardiogenic shock/heart failure, second- or third-degree AV block, atrial fibrillation/flutter with an accessory bypass tract

Essential Monitoring Parameters

Blood pressure, heart rate, constipation

Counseling Points

- Take sustained-release product with food or milk; other formulations may be taken without regard to food
- Sprinkling contents of capsules onto food does not affect absorption
- Do not crush or chew extended- or sustained-release products

Key Points

- Verapamil is used for the treatment of hypertension and atrial fibrillation. It should be avoided in patients with acute myocardial infarction and/or heart failure because it is a negative inotrope. Patients must be counseled on the side effects, particularly constipation.
- Dosing intervals vary based on the product

LOOP DIURETICS

Introduction

The loop diuretics are very effective at reducing edema in patients who are volume overloaded. They are used to treat symptoms of congestion in patients with heart failure and other diseases that cause fluid retention/overload. They have been supplanted by more effective agents in the treatment of hypertension.

Mechanism of Action for the Drug Class

Loop diuretics are named as such because they primarily inhibit the reabsorption of sodium and chloride at the thick ascending limb of the loop of Henle, increasing the excretion of sodium, water, chloride, calcium, and magnesium.

Members of the Drug Class

In this section: Furosemide
Others: Bumetanide, ethacrynic acid, torsemide

◉ Furosemide

Brand Name
Lasix

Generic Name
Furosemide

Rx Only

Dosage Forms
Tablet, oral solution, injection

Usage
Edema,* hypertension

Pregnancy Category C

Dosing
- Oral:
  - Initial dose: 20–40 mg once or twice daily
  - Dosage adjustment: Up to 600 mg per day in 2–4 divided doses
- IV:
  - IV bolus: Doses of 10–200 mg administered every 6–12 hours or as needed
  - Continuous infusion: 10–40 mg/hour
  - Oral bioavailability is poor; therefore equivalent IV dose is 50% of PO dose

Adverse Reactions: Most Common
Dehydration, electrolyte depletion, hyperuricemia, hypochloremic alkalosis, hypotension, orthostasis

Adverse Reactions: Rare/Severe/Important
Renal function impairment, ototoxicity (increased risk with higher doses and rapid IV administration), skin rash

Major Drug Interactions
Drugs Affecting Furosemide
NSAIDs: Decrease diuresis

Furosemide's Effects on Other Drugs
- Aminoglycosides: Increase ototoxicity
- Lithium: Increases levels
- Digoxin: Increases risk of toxicity due to furosemide-induced hypokalemia

Essential Monitoring Parameters
Blood pressure, renal function (serum creatinine, urine output), electrolytes (K, Mg)

Counseling Points
- Avoid taking before bedtime
- Take with food or milk to reduce GI irritation
- With the possibility of hypokalemia, there may be a need for additional potassium in the diet or supplements; do not change your diet without first checking with your healthcare provider
- Use caution when getting up suddenly from a lying or sitting position
- Be cautious in using alcohol, while standing for long periods or exercising, and during hot weather because of enhanced orthostatic hypotensive effects
- Regular monitoring of laboratory tests (potassium, serum creatinine) and blood pressure is necessary to ensure safe use of the drug and avoid adverse effects

Key Points
- Furosemide is commonly used to treat edema. It must be monitored closely to make sure electrolyte disturbances and hypotension do not occur.
- Furosemide is more commonly used than bumetanide, but sometimes formulary or other concerns necessitate use of one drug in place of the other. A 40 mg dose of oral furosemide is roughly equivalent to a 1 mg dose of oral bumetanide. For IV administration, the ratio is 20:1 furosemide to bumetanide.

NITRATES

Introduction
The nitrates are used for the treatment of angina, both unstable and chronic stable types. They are available in several formulations and dosage forms that differ in their onset and duration of action.

Mechanism of Action for the Drug Class
Nitrates relax vascular smooth muscle by stimulating intracellular cyclic guanosine monophosphate production. They cause predominantly venous dilation with some dose-dependent arterial effects.

Members of the Drug Class
In this section: Isosorbide mononitrate, nitroglycerin (sublingual)
Others: Isosorbide dinitrate, nitroglycerin (capsules, injection, topical ointment, transdermal patch, translingual spray)

Rx Only for the Drug Class

Usage for the Drug Class
- Cardiovascular uses: Angina,* heart failure, hypertension, pulmonary hypertension
- Noncardiovascular uses: Esophageal spastic disorders, anal fissure (topical)

Pregnancy Category C for the Drug Class

Adverse Reactions for the Drug Class: Most Common

Bradycardia, headache, hypotension, lightheadedness, syncope, weakness

Major Drug Interactions for the Drug Class

Drugs Affecting Nitrates

- Alcohol: Can cause severe hypotension and syncope
- Calcium channel blockers: May increase orthostatic hypotension
- Sildenafil, tadalafil, vardenafil: Increase hypotensive effects (avoid use within 24 hours of each other)

Nitrates' Effects on Other Drugs

- Antihypertensive agents: Additive hypotension
- Ergot derivatives: Increase effects

Contraindications for the Drug Class

Systolic BP < 90 mm Hg, heart rate < 50 bpm, acute right ventricular infarction

Essential Monitoring Parameters for the Drug Class

Blood pressure, heart rate, headache

Counseling Points for the Drug Class

- Extended-release tablets and capsules: Do not crush or chew. Administer doses so that a "nitrate-free interval" of 10–12 hours occurs.
- Sublingual tablets: Place under tongue or between cheek and gum. Rest during administration, preferably seated. Do not swallow tablets. Should feel a slight burning sensation under the tongue, which means the drug is working. Do not remove tablets from original glass container.
- Transdermal patch: Apply once daily to skin site free of hair and not subject to excessive movement. Avoid areas with cuts or irritations. Do not apply to distal parts of the extremities. Use caution when discarding so as to keep out of the reach of children or pets. Remove at night for a 12-hour "nitrate-free interval." May contain metal; remove prior to MRI.
- Headaches may occur and are a sign that the medication is working. Do not alter dosage schedule; aspirin or acetaminophen may be used to relieve pain.

Key Point for the Drug Class

Nitrates are the drug of choice for quick relief of angina symptoms. They are also used for long-term prevention of angina symptoms. However, they not recommended as first-line treatment in patients with recent myocardial infarction (beta blockers are preferred).

◉ Isosorbide Mononitrate

Brand Names

Imdur, Ismo, Monoket

Generic Name

Isosorbide mononitrate

Dosage Forms

Tablet, extended-release tablet

Dosing

20–240 mg daily (divided doses if not the extended-release formulation)

Key Point

Used for long-term treatment of chronic angina

◉ Nitroglycerin (sublingual)

Brand Name

Nitrostat

Generic Name

Nitroglycerin (sublingual)

Dosage Form

Sublingual tablet

Dosing

0.3–0.6 mg repeated at 5-minute intervals up to 3 doses as needed for relief of anginal attack. If pain continues after one tablet, notify physician immediately. May use prophylactically 5–10 minutes before activities that precipitate an attack.

Key Points

- Sublingual tablets are used for the relief of angina attacks only. They are not used for long-term treatment of angina.
- Sublingual tablets must be stored in original containers away from humidity and moisture.
- Patients should not crush sublingual tablets; they should just place under tongue and allow to dissolve.

PHOSPHODIESTERASE ENZYME INHIBITORS

Introduction

The phosphodiesterase inhibitor milrinone is a positive inotrope used in the treatment of decompensated heart failure. In addition to being a positive inotrope, it results in significant decreases in blood pressure.

Mechanism of Action for the Drug Class

Inhibition of the enzyme cAMP phosphodiesterase results in increased cAMP in cardiac and vascular muscle. Increased cAMP increases intracellular calcium, thereby increasing contractility in cardiac muscle (positive inotrope) and relaxation in vasculature (vasodilation).

Rx Only for the Drug Class

Members of the Drug Class

In this section: Milrinone
Other: Amrinone (not available in the United States)

◉ Milrinone

Brand Name
Primacor

Generic Name
Milrinone

Dosage Forms
IV (injection and premixed infusion)

Usage
Acute decompensated heart failure,* palliation of symptoms in end-stage heart failure*

Pregnancy Category C

Dosing
- Initial dose: 0.1 μg/kg/min
- Maximum dose: Up to 0.75 μg/kg/min (doses up to 1 μg/kg/min can be used but are unlikely to result in significant improvement)

- Renal dosage adjustments: Half-life is increased, consider starting at lower end of dosing range and titrating more slowly

Adverse Reactions: Most Common
Arrhythmias, hypotension

Adverse Reactions: Rare/Severe/Important
Ventricular arrhythmias

Major Drug Interactions
Drugs Affecting Milrinone
Negative inotropes: Decrease efficacy

Contraindication
Significant hypotension (use with caution)

Essential Monitoring Parameters
Cardiac output/cardiac index, blood pressure, EKG

Key Points
- Milrinone is commonly used for the treatment of acute decompensated and end-stage heart failure. It increases cardiac output and is a potent vasodilator. Blood pressure must be monitored closely.
- Use is associated with increased risk of arrhythmias/mortality; therefore, the benefit must outweigh risk

POTASSIUM-SPARING DIURETICS, ALDOSTERONE ANTAGONISTS

Introduction

The aldosterone antagonists can be used as diuretics; however, they are more commonly used as adjunctive therapy to prevent morbidity and mortality in patients with stage C or D heart failure

Mechanism of Action for the Drug Class

Aldosterone antagonists competitively inhibit aldosterone, which binds to aldosterone receptors of the distal tubules in the kidney. This action increases the excretion of sodium chloride and water, but not potassium and hydrogen ions. Spironolactone may also block the effect of aldosterone on arteriolar smooth muscle.

Rx Only for the Drug Class

Members of the Drug Class

In this section: Spironolactone
Other: Eplerenone

◉ Spironolactone

Brand Name
Aldactone

Generic Name
Spironolactone

Dosage Form
Tablet

Usage
Edema or ascites in patients with cirrhosis of the liver,* heart failure,* hyperaldosteronism, hypertension, hypokalemia, acne in women, hirsutism

Pregnancy Category C

Dosing
- Heart failure, hypertension: 12.5–25 mg daily
- Edema: 25–200 mg per day in 1–2 divided doses
- Renal dosage adjustment:
  - CrCl 10–50 mL/min: Administer lower initial doses
  - CrCl < 10 mL/min: Avoid use

Adverse Reactions: Most Common

Hyperkalemia, cramping, diarrhea

Adverse Reactions: Rare/Severe/Important

Gynecomastia, renal dysfunction

Major Drug Interactions

Drugs Affecting Spironolactone

Potassium supplements: Increase risk of hyperkalemia

Spironolactone's Effects on Other Drugs

ACE inhibitors, ARBs, trimethoprim: Increase risk of hyperkalemia

Contraindications

- In heart failure: Serum creatinine > 2 mg/dL in women or > 2.5 mg/dL in men
- Potassium > 5 mEq/L

Essential Monitoring Parameters

Renal function (serum creatinine, urine output), potassium, blood pressure

Counseling Point

Avoid ingestion of foods high in potassium or use of salt substitutes or other potassium supplements without the advice of your healthcare provider

Key Points

- Spironolactone is used as a diuretic in patients with cirrhosis of the liver. Use in these patients requires much higher dosing (up to 200 mg daily) than what is recommended in patients with heart failure (maximum 50 mg daily). The main role of spironolactone in patients with heart failure is to reduce morbidity and mortality.
- Patients must be monitored closely for hyperkalemia and renal dysfunction because these could result in potentially fatal adverse effects (hyperkalemia-induced arrhythmias)

THIAZIDE DIURETICS

Introduction

The thiazide diuretics are recommended for first-line therapy in the treatment of hypertension. They can also be used in patients with edema, often in combination with a loop diuretic for synergistic effects.

Mechanism of Action for the Drug Class

Inhibit reabsorption of sodium and chloride in the distal tubules, resulting in increased urinary excretion of sodium and chloride

Members of the Drug Class

In this section: Hydrochlorothiazide
Others: Bendroflumethiazide, chlorothiazide, chlorthalidone, methyclothiazide

◉ Hydrochlorothiazide

Brand Name

Microzide

Generic Name

Hydrochlorothiazide

Rx Only

Dosage Forms

Tablet, capsule

Usage

- Cardiovascular uses: Hypertension,* edema
- Noncardiovascular use: Treatment of lithium-induced diabetes insipidus

Pregnancy Category B

Dosing

- 12.5–50 mg daily
- Renal dosage adjustment: Ineffective if CrCl < 30 mL/min (except in combination with loop diuretics)

Adverse Reactions: Most Common

Hypokalemia, orthostatic hypotension, stomach upset

Adverse Reactions: Rare/Severe/Important

Gout, hypercalcemia, hypochloremic alkalosis, photosensitivity

Major Drug Interactions

Drugs Affecting Hydrochlorothiazide

- Loop diuretics: Enhance diuresis
- NSAIDs: May decrease efficacy of thiazides

Hydrochlorothiazide's Effect on Other Drugs

- Digoxin: Thiazide-induced hypokalemia may precipitate digitalis-induced arrhythmias
- Dofetilide: Increases levels, leading to ventricular arrhythmias (contraindicated)
- Lithium: Increases levels

Counseling Points

- Take in the morning to avoid increased urination at night
- Antihypertensive effects may take several days

Key Points

- The thiazide diuretics can be used in the treatment of mild hypertension. They can also be used for edema; however, they often only work for mild edema, and a loop diuretic is often required for more severe edema associated with heart failure.
- The 50 mg dose of hydrochlorothiazide has increased adverse effects without added efficacy and should generally be avoided

---

VASODILATORS, HYDRALAZINE

Introduction

Hydralazine is used for the treatment of refractory hypertension and heart failure. It is often not used as first-line treatment because of its inconvenient dosing schedule. It is sometimes used in heart failure in combination with nitrates in patients who do not respond to or are intolerant of ACE inhibitors or ARBs.

Mechanism of Action for the Drug Class

Hydralazine directly relaxes vascular smooth muscle, resulting in peripheral vasodilation

◉ Hydralazine

Brand Name

Apresoline

Generic Name

Hydralazine

Rx Only

Dosage Forms

Tablet, injection

Usage

Hypertension,* heart failure* (in combination with nitrate therapy)

Pregnancy Category C

Dosing

- Initial dose:
  - Oral: 10 mg four times daily
  - IV: 10–20 mg every 4–6 hours

- Dosage adjustments: Up to 300 mg daily in 3–4 divided doses
- Renal dosage adjustment: If CrCl 10–50 mL/min, then administer every 8–12 hours

Adverse Reactions: Most Common

Angina, headache, nausea/vomiting, tachycardia

Adverse Reactions: Rare/Severe/Important

Drug-induced lupus-like syndrome (with higher doses)

Major Drug Interactions

None

Essential Monitoring Parameters

Blood pressure, heart rate

Counseling Points

- Hydralazine must be taken three to four times daily
- Let your healthcare provider know if any lupus-like symptoms develop (fever, arthralgia, myalgia, malaise, pleuritic chest pain, edema, maculopapular facial rash)

Key Points

- Hydralazine is effective in the treatment of hypertension. It is also used for the treatment of heart failure in combination with nitrate therapy.
- Patient compliance may be an issue because it must be taken multiple times a day
- Hydralazine is a classic example of a drug that causes lupus-like syndrome. This adverse effect abates with discontinuation.

VASODILATORS, NITROPRUSSIDE

Introduction

Nitroprusside is a short-acting, potent vasodilator used in hypertensive crisis and following cardiac surgery. High doses and prolonged infusions are associated with increased toxicity, and close monitoring is necessary for safe use.

Mechanism of Action for the Drug Class

Nitroprusside acts on venous and arterial smooth muscle to decrease peripheral resistance and cause vasodilation

⊙ Nitroprusside

Brand Name
Nitropress

Generic Name
Nitroprusside

Rx Only

Dosage Form
Injection

Usage
Hypertensive crisis,* heart failure, controlled hypotension during surgery

Pregnancy Category C

Dosing
- Initial dose: 0.3 µg/kg/min
- Dosage adjustments: Up to 10 µg/kg/min (doses > 3 µg/kg/min and renal/hepatic impairment increase risk of toxicity)
- May coinfuse with sodium thiosulfate to decrease risk of toxicity

Adverse Reactions: Most Common
Flushing, headache, nausea and vomiting

Adverse Reactions: Rare/Severe/Important
Cyanide and thiocyanate toxicity, increased intracranial pressure, methemoglobinemia, metabolic acidosis

Major Drug Interactions
IV drugs: Check for compatibility when infusing through same line

Contraindications
Use cautiously in patients with renal and/or hepatic impairment

Essential Monitoring Parameters
Blood pressure, heart rate, cyanide toxicity (increased risk with hepatic impairment), thiocyanate toxicity (increased risk with renal impairment)

Key Points
- Nitroprusside is a very effective antihypertensive medication. Its fast onset and short half-life allows for immediate effects and close titration of dose.
- Severe toxicities are associated with increased dose and prolonged use. Therefore, transition to oral therapy should occur as soon as possible (avoid infusions > 72 hours).

COMBINATION DRUG THERAPIES

Introduction

The use of antihypertensive agents in combination is common. To decrease the pill burden and improve compliance, combination antihypertensive therapies combine two active drugs into one pill. These formulations should not be used as initial therapy because they are not easy to titrate and should therefore only be used once it is known what doses of medication a patient requires. Most combinations include a thiazide diuretic. Available combination products are summarized in **Table 5-1**.

Other Combination Products
Amlodipine/olmesartan, amlodipine/telmisartan, amlodipine/valsartan, clonidine/chlorthalidone

Multiple Combination Products
Amlodipine/olmesartan/hydrochlorothiazide, amlodipine/valsartan/hydrochlorothiazide

TABLE 5-1 Combination Antihypertensive Agents

Drug Class	Brand Name(s)	Generic Names	Other Similar Drugs
ACE inhibitor in combination with HCTZ	Zestoric, Prinzide	Lisinopril/HCTZ	Benazepril/HCTZ, captopril/HCTZ, enalapril/HCTZ, fosinopril/HCTZ, moexipril/HCTZ, quinapril/HCTZ, ramipril/HCTZ
ARB in combination with thiazide diuretic	Hyzaar	Losartan/HCTZ	Azilsartan/chlorthalidone, Candesartan/HCTZ, eprosartan/HCTZ, irbesartan/HCTZ, olmesartan/HCTZ, telmisartan/HCTZ, valsartan/HCTZ
Dihydropyridine calcium channel blocker in combination with ACE inhibitor	Lotrel	Amlodipine/benazepril	None
Beta blockers in combination with thiazide diuretic	Ziac	Bisoprolol/HCTZ	Atenolol/chlorthalidone, nadolol/bendroflumethiazide, metoprolol/HCTZ, propranolol/HCTZ
Thiazide diuretic in combination with potassium-sparing diuretic	Dyazide, Maxzide, Maxzide-25	Triamterene/HCTZ	Hydrochlorothiazide/spironolactone

REVIEW QUESTIONS

1. Which of the following has the least effect on blood pressure?

   a. Doxazosin
   b. Prazosin
   c. Tamsulosin
   d. Terazosin

2. Which of the following is the primary indication for alpha-1 adrenergic blockers?

   a. Acute myocardial infarction
   b. Benign prostatic hypertrophy
   c. Deep venous thrombosis
   d. Venous stasis

3. Which of the following statements regarding clonidine is incorrect?

   a. Clonidine patches should be changed daily.
   b. Abrupt discontinuation of clonidine may result in rebound hypertension.
   c. Overlapping of oral and transdermal clonidine may be necessary when initiating transdermal therapy.
   d. Clonidine may cause bradycardia.

4. Which of the following is *not* a side effect of clonidine?

   a. Constipation
   b. Drowsiness
   c. Dry mouth
   d. Renal dysfunction

5. Which of the following agents is a pure alpha-receptor agonist?

   a. Dobutamine
   b. Dopamine
   c. Milrinone
   d. Phenylephrine

6. Which of the following is a side effect of dobutamine?

   a. Hypersensitivity to sun
   b. Limb necrosis
   c. Ventricular arrhythmias
   d. Both B and C

7. Epinephrine can be used for all of the following, *except*:

   a. anaphylaxis.
   b. bradycardia.
   c. hypertensive emergency.
   d. ventricular fibrillation (ACLS).

8. Which of the following is *not* a side effect of ACE inhibitors?

   a. Angioedema
   b. Bradycardia
   c. Cough
   d. Hyperkalemia

9. Which of the following dosing regimens is *incorrect*?

   a. Captopril 25 mg PO daily
   b. Enalapril 20 mg PO twice daily
   c. Lisinopril 40 mg PO daily
   d. Ramipril 5 mg PO twice daily

10. Which of the following is an essential monitoring parameter for angiotensin receptor blockers (ARBs)?

    a. Blood pressure
    b. Potassium
    c. Serum creatinine (renal function)
    d. All of the above

11. Which of the following is the preferred ARB for patients with heart failure?

    a. Bosentan
    b. Irbesartan
    c. Telmisartan
    d. Valsartan

12. Which of the following is the most significant adverse effect associated with ranolazine?

    a. Diarrhea
    b. Hypotension
    c. Torsade de pointes
    d. Valvular insufficiency

13. Ranolazine is used for the treatment of which of the following?

    a. Atrial fibrillation
    b. Chronic stable angina
    c. Hypertension
    d. Peripheral vascular disease

14. Which of the following regarding amiodarone dosing is true?

    a. Amiodarone loading dose should be administered over several days to weeks.
    b. Amiodarone loading dose must be infused immediately over 1 hour to be effective.
    c. Amiodarone loading doses must be administered IV.
    d. Amiodarone does not require a loading dose.

15. Patients taking amiodarone should be counseled on all of the following, *except*:

    a. avoid foods containing vitamin K.
    b. schedule regular blood work for thyroid and liver function.
    c. take with food to decrease adverse GI effects.
    d. use sunscreen or stay out of sun to prevent burns.

16. Which of the following statements regarding digoxin is *false*?

    a. Digoxin levels should be drawn at least 6 hours following administration once the patient is at steady-state.
    b. Digoxin has minimal effects on hemodynamics and therefore is a first-line agent for the treatment of atrial fibrillation.
    c. Dosing should be adjusted for congestive heart failure status, renal function, and weight.
    d. Signs of toxicity include nausea, vomiting, and vision changes.

17. Which of the following is the appropriate dose of sotalol in patients on hemodialysis?

    a. 80 mg twice daily
    b. 80 mg daily
    c. 160 mg twice daily
    d. Sotalol is contraindicated in patients on hemodialysis.

18. Drug interactions with sotalol include each of the following, *except*:

    a. digoxin.
    b. fluconazole.
    c. ipratropium.
    d. QT-prolonging drugs.

19. Which of the following best describes the mechanism of action of atropine?

    a. Alpha-agonist
    b. Anticholinergic
    c. Beta-agonist
    d. Cholinergic

20. Vasopressin can be used for all of the following indications, *except*:

    a. ACLS (pulseless arrest).
    b. GI hemorrhage.
    c. peripheral vascular disease.
    d. shock/hypotension.

21. Which of the following is an appropriate starting dose for vasopressin in the treatment of shock/hypotension?

    a. 0.01 units/min
    b. 0.2 units/min
    c. 40 units/min
    d. None of the above, vasopressin should not be used for shock/hypotension.

22. Which of the following beta blocker and selectivity pairings is *incorrect*?

    a. Atenolol: beta-1 selective
    b. Carvedilol: beta-1 selective
    c. Metoprolol: beta-1 selective
    d. Propranolol: nonselective

23. Which of the following beta blockers is *not* recommended for patients with heart failure?

    a. Atenolol
    b. Bisoprolol
    c. Carvedilol
    d. Metoprolol XL

24. Which of the following beta blockers requires dosing adjustment in patients with renal dysfunction?

    a. Atenolol
    b. Carvedilol
    c. Metoprolol
    d. Propranolol

25. Which of the following is not available in an IV formulation?

    a. Enalapril
    b. Labetalol
    c. Losartan
    d. Metoprolol

26. Which of the following does *not* interact with diltiazem?

    a. Clarithromycin
    b. CYP3A4 inhibitors
    c. Fluconazole
    d. Gentamicin

27. Which of the following is the typical dosing range for oral diltiazem?

    a. 10–40 µg daily
    b. 120–540 µg daily
    c. 10–40 mg day
    d. 120–540 mg daily

28. Amlodipine belongs to which class of calcium channel blockers?

    a. Benzothiazepines
    b. Dihydropyridines
    c. Phenylalkylamines
    d. Amlodipine is not a calcium channel blocker.

29. Which calcium channel blocker should not be administered in the immediate-release formulation due to increased risk of mortality?

    a. Diltiazem
    b. Felodipine
    c. Nifedipine
    d. Verapamil

30. Which of the following is *not* a side effect of verapamil?

    a. Bradycardia
    b. Constipation
    c. Hepatotoxicity
    d. Worsening heart failure

Central Nervous System Agents

Donna Leverone, PharmD
Susan Kent, PharmD, CGP
Neela Bhajandas, PharmD

5-HT RECEPTOR ANTAGONISTS

Introduction

Eletriptan, rizatriptan, and sumatriptan are selective agonists of vascular serotonin type 1–like receptors for the acute management of migraine headache with or without aura. Injectable sumatriptan is also indicated for the acute treatment of cluster headache. They are highly effective in many patients but must be avoided in those with concurrent cardiovascular disease. These agents should not be used for prophylaxis of migraine or cluster headache.

Mechanism of Action for the Drug Class

$5\text{-}HT_{1B/1D}$ receptor agonist at extracerebral and intracranial blood vessels, likely resulting in vasoconstriction and decreased trigeminal nerve transmission

Members of the Drug Class

In this section: Eletriptan, rizatriptan, sumatriptan
Others: Almotriptan, frovatriptan, naratriptan, zolmitriptan

◉ Eletriptan

Brand Name
Relpax

Generic Name
Eletriptan

Rx Only

Dosage Form
Tablet

Usage
Acute treatment of migraine in adults, with or without aura*

Pregnancy Category C

Dosing

- Initial dose: 20–40 mg; may repeat after 2 hours if headache returns
- Maximum single dose: 40 mg
- Maximum daily dose: 80 mg
- Renal dosage adjustment: No dosing adjustment needed; monitor for increased blood pressure
- Hepatic dosage adjustment:
  - Mild to moderate impairment: No adjustment needed
  - Severe impairment: Use is contraindicated

Adverse Reactions: Most Common

Nausea, asthenia, somnolence

Adverse Reactions: Rare/Severe/Important

Chest pain, coronary artery spasm, myocardial infarction, peripheral ischemia, transient myocardial ischemia, cerebrovascular accident, seizure

Major Drug Interactions

Drugs Affecting Eletriptan

- CYP3A4 inhibitors (fluconazole, ketoconazole, itraconazole, nefazodone, clarithromycin, ritonavir, nelfinavir): May increase peak plasma concentrations of eletriptan. Avoid administration of eletriptan within 72 hours of drugs with documented potent CYP3A4 inhibition.
- Ergot alkaloids (ergot,*ne, dihydroergotamine, methysergide) and other $5\text{-}HT_1$ receptor agonists: Additive vasospastic effects. Use within 24 hours is contraindicated.
- Selective serotonin-reuptake inhibitors (SSRIs) and selective serotonin and norepinephrine reuptake inhibitors (SNRIs): Risk for serotonin syndrome
- Propranolol: Potential pharmacokinetic interaction (increases the maximum plasma concentrations of eletriptan); no dosage adjustment required

---

* Throughout the text, an asterisk (*) is used to indicate the most common uses of a drug.

Contraindications

Known or suspected ischemic heart disease, coronary vasospasm (Prinzmetal variant angina), other serious underlying cardiovascular disease (uncontrolled hypertension), cerebrovascular syndromes, or peripheral vascular ischemia (ischemic bowel disease). Concomitant use with another 5-HT$_1$ receptor agonist within 24 hours. Concomitant use with an ergot alkaloid within 24 hours. Basilar or hemiplegic migraine. Severe hepatic impairment (Child-Pugh grade C).

Counseling Points

- Take at first sign of migraine. This drug only treats migraine and will not prevent migraine headaches from occurring. Take exactly as directed; do not redose if no response is achieved.
- Take a second dose 2 or more hours after the first. Do not take more than 80 mg per day.
- Report signs/symptoms of ischemic cardiac syndrome (angina, myocardial infarction, stroke, or transient ischemic attack) or ischemic bowel disease (sudden severe abdominal pain, bloody diarrhea)
- Report any shortness of breath, tightness, pain, pressure, or heaviness in chest, throat, jaw, or neck after taking eletriptan and do not take eletriptan again until evaluated by a healthcare provider
- Report signs/symptoms of serotonin syndrome (agitation, hallucinations, tachycardia, hyperthermia, labile blood pressure, hyperreflexia, incoordination, diarrhea, nausea, and vomiting)
- Do not take eletriptan within 24 hours of using an ergot alkaloid or another 5-HT$_1$ agonist
- Do not take eletriptan within 72 hours of using CYP3A4 inhibitors
- Female patients: Inform healthcare provider of plans to become pregnant or breast-feed

Key Points

- A complete history and physical and medication history are imperative prior to initiating eletriptan
- Eletriptan should be used only in patients with a clear diagnosis of migraine
- Take exactly as directed; do not redose if no response is achieved
- Be aware of important drug–drug interactions and serious cardiac effects

◉ Rizatriptan

Brand Names
Maxalt, Maxalt MLT

Generic Name
Rizatriptan

Rx Only

Dosage Forms
Tablets, film-coated and orally disintegrating (MLT)

Usage

Acute treatment of migraine, with or without aura, in adults and children 6–17 years of age;* tension-type headache in adults

Pregnancy Category C

Dosing

- Adults:
  - 5 or 10 mg, may repeat after 2 hours
  - Maximum dose: 30 mg/24 hour
- Children:
  - Safety and efficacy not established in pediatric patients < 6 years of age
  - 6–17 years, < 40 kg:
    - 5 mg
    - Maximum dose: 1 dose/24 hours
  - 6–17 years, ≥ 40 kg:
    - 10 mg
    - Maximum dose: 1 dose/24 hours
- Dosage adjustment with *concomitant propranolol*:
  - Adults: 5 mg; maximum is 3 doses in 24-hour period
  - Children ages 6–17 years, < 40 kg: Do not use
  - Children ages 6–17 years, ≥ 40 kg: 5 mg; maximum 1 dose/24 hours

Adverse Reactions: Most Common

Nausea, asthenia, dizziness, somnolence, fatigue

Adverse Reactions: Rare/Severe/Important

Chest pain, coronary artery spasm, hypertension, myocardial infarction, peripheral ischemia, ventricular arrhythmia, ischemic colitis, anaphylaxis, angioedema, analgesic overuse headache, cerebrovascular accident, serotonin syndrome

Major Drug Interactions

Drugs Affecting Rizatriptan

- Ergot alkaloids (ergotamine, dihydroergotamine, methysergide) and other 5-HT$_1$ receptor agonists: Additive vasospastic effects. Use within 24 hours is contraindicated.
- Monoamine oxidase inhibitors (MAOIs; phenelzine, selegiline, tranylcypromine): Potential pharmacokinetic interaction (increased systemic exposure to rizatriptan and active metabolite). Use of rizatriptan within 2 weeks of MAOI therapy is contraindicated.
- Propranolol: Potential pharmacokinetic interaction (increased plasma concentrations of rizatriptan). Maximum rizatriptan dosage of 5 mg per single dose and 3 doses per 24-hour period recommended.
- SSRIs and SNRIs: Risk for life-threatening serotonin syndrome. Observe patients carefully during treatment initiation, with dosage increases, or when another serotonergic agent is started.

Contraindications

Known or suspected ischemic heart disease, coronary vasospasm (Prinzmetal variant angina), other serious underlying cardiovascular disease (uncontrolled hypertension), cerebrovascular syndromes, or peripheral vascular ischemia (ischemic bowel disease). Concomitant use with another 5-HT$_1$ receptor agonist within 24 hours. Concomitant use with an ergot alkaloid within 24 hours. Concurrent or recent (within 2 weeks) treatment with an MAOI. Basilar or hemiplegic migraine.

Counseling Points

- Take at first sign of migraine. This drug only treats migraine and will not prevent migraine headaches from occurring. Take exactly as directed; do not redose if no response is achieved.
- Separate doses by at least 2 hours. Maximum of 30 mg per 24-hour period. Maximum of 1 dose in a 24-hour period for children (6–17 years of age).
- The rizatriptan orally disintegrating tablet is packaged in a blister in an aluminum pouch. Peel open blister pack right before dosing with dry hands. Place the tablet on the tongue, allow it to disintegrate, and then swallow. Administration with liquid is not needed.
- Overuse of migraine drugs may cause a worsening of headache or an increase in the frequency of headache
- Report signs/symptoms of ischemic cardiac syndrome (angina, myocardial infarction, stroke, or TIA) or ischemic bowel disease (sudden severe abdominal pain, bloody diarrhea)
- Report any shortness of breath, tightness, pain, pressure, or heaviness in chest, throat, jaw, or neck after taking rizatriptan and do not take rizatriptan again until evaluated by a healthcare provider
- Report signs/symptoms of serotonin syndrome (agitation, hallucinations, tachycardia, hyperthermia, labile BP, hyperreflexia, incoordination, diarrhea, nausea, and vomiting)
- Do not take rizatriptan within 24 hours of using an ergot alkaloid or another 5-HT$_1$ agonist
- Do not take rizatriptan within 2 weeks of using an MAOI
- Female patients: Inform healthcare provider of plans to become pregnant or breast-feed

Key Points

- A complete history and physical and medication history are imperative prior to initiating rizatriptan
- Rizatriptan should be used only in patients with a clear diagnosis of migraine
- Be familiar with dosage adjustments for patients taking concomitant propranolol
- Be aware of important drug–drug interactions and serious cardiac effects

◉ Sumatriptan

Brand Names

Imitrex, Sumavel DosePro, Alsuma

Generic Names

Sumatriptan, sumatriptan succinate

Rx Only

Dosage Forms

- Sumatriptan succinate: Film-coated tablet, injection (SUB-Q use only)
- Sumatriptan: Nasal solution

Usage

Acute treatment of migraine in adults with or without aura,* acute treatment of cluster headache episodes (SUB-Q injection)

Pregnancy Category C

Dosing

- Oral:
  - Initial dose: 25–100 mg, repeat after 2 hours if needed
  - Maximum dose: 200 mg/24 hours
- Injectable:
  - 6 mg SUB-Q, repeat in 1 hour if needed
  - Maximum dose: 6 mg/dose and 12 mg/24 hours
- Nasal spray:
  - 5–20 mg (10 mg given as one 5 mg spray in each nostril)
  - If headache returns, may repeat dose once after 2 hours
  - Maximum dose: 40 mg/24 hours
- Renal dosage adjustment: No formal recommendations. Use caution in hemodialysis patients.
- Hepatic dosage adjustment:
  - Bioavailability of oral sumatriptan is increased with liver disease. If treatment is needed, do not exceed single doses of 50 mg.
  - Use of all dosage forms is contraindicated with severe hepatic impairment
- Concomitantly with MAOIs: Decreased doses should be considered in injectable form and contraindicated in oral form. Sumatriptan autoinjector should not be used because it is only available as a 6 mg fixed dose.

Adverse Reactions: Most Common

Paresthesias, hot/cold skin sensations, chest discomfort, flushing, fatigue, somnolence, nausea, vomiting, unpleasant taste in mouth, dry mouth, headache, photosensitivity, vertigo, injection site reactions (with injectable)

Adverse Reactions: Rare/Severe/Important

Chest, jaw, neck tightness, coronary vasospasm, myocardial infarction, arrhythmia, ischemic colitis, blindness and/or vision impairment, seizure, serotonin syndrome

Major Drug Interactions

Drugs Affecting Sumatriptan

Sibutramine, monoamine oxidase inhibitors (MAOIs), ergotamines: Increase risk of serotonin syndrome

Essential Monitoring Parameters

Reduction in migraine headache severity indicates efficacy. ECG during initial dosing in patients with risk factors for coronary artery disease and among patients who develop signs or symptoms of angina with administration of sumatriptan. Cardiovascular function and risk factors should be monitored at baseline and periodically thereafter.

Contraindications

Ischemic heart disease (angina, myocardial infarction, cerebrovascular accident, transient ischemic attack), peripheral vascular syndromes, uncontrolled hypertension, ischemic bowel disease, severe hepatic impairment (Child-Pugh C), hemiplegic or basilar migraine, hypersensitivity, use of an ergotamine derivative (dihydroergotamine, methysergide) within 24 hours, use of another 5-HT$_1$ agonist within 24 hours, use of an MAOI within 2 weeks of sumatriptan therapy

Counseling Points

- Take at first sign of migraine. This drug only treats migraine and will not prevent migraine headaches from occurring. Take exactly as directed; do not redose if no response is achieved.
- Follow exact instructions for use. Do not redose if no response is achieved.
- Do not take sumatriptan within 24 hours of using an ergot medication or another serotonin agonist. Do not take sumatriptan with recent use of an MAOI (2 weeks).
- Wear sunscreen and proper clothing when in the sun
- Report any risk factors for heart disease or any unusual side effects immediately (chest tightness or pain, acute abdominal pain, excessive drowsiness)

Key Points

- A complete history and physical and medication history are imperative prior to initiating sumatriptan
- Sumatriptan should only be used in patients with a clear diagnosis of migraine
- Demonstrate proper SUB-Q injection technique and syringe/needle disposal
- Be aware of important drug–drug interactions and cardiac effects

ANOREXIANTS

Introduction

Obesity is increasing in prevalence worldwide. To be successful in weight loss, it has been suggested that a goal weight should be predefined and a weight loss program should be developed that includes diet, exercise, behavior modification, and possibly a pharmacologic agent. Debate continues on the appropriateness of weight loss medications due to the controversy surrounding the deaths and medical complications caused by the combination product Fen-Phen (fenfluramine and phentermine). Phentermine is still available.

Mechanism of Action for the Drug Class

Phentermine is a sympathomimetic amine that stimulates the CNS. It is structurally related to the amphetamines. Phentermine stimulates the CNS and elevates blood pressure. The mechanism of action in treating obesity is unknown.

Members of the Drug Class

In this section: Phentermine
Others: Benzphetamine, phendimetrazine

⊙ Phentermine

Brand Names
Adipex-P, Ionamin, Suprenza

Generic Name
Phentermine

Rx Only
Class IV controlled substance

Dosage Forms
Tablet, capsule, orally disintegrating tablet (ODT)

Usage
Obesity* (short-term use)

Pregnancy Category X

Dosing
- Tablet/capsule: 15–37.5 mg daily (given in 1–2 divided doses)
- ODT formulation: 15–30 mg daily in the morning

Adverse Reactions: Most Common

Increased blood pressure, palpitations, arrhythmias, GI discomfort, insomnia, nervousness, and dry mouth

Adverse Reactions: Rare/Severe/Important

Primary pulmonary hypertension, valvular heart disease, psychiatric reactions

Major Drug Interactions

Drugs Affecting Phentermine

Monoamine oxidase inhibitors (MAOIs): Contraindicated due to the risk of severe, possibly fatal adverse reactions

Contraindications

History of cardiovascular disease (e.g., congestive heart failure, arrhythmias, coronary artery disease, uncontrolled hypertension, stroke); hyperthyroidism; glaucoma; history of drug abuse; agitated psychological states; concurrent use or within 14 days following MAOI therapy; pregnancy; breastfeeding

Counseling Points

- Tablet/capsule: Take at breakfast or 1–2 hours after breakfast and avoid late night dosing
- ODT: Dissolve on the tongue and take before breakfast

Key Points

- Use for patients with a BMI $\geq$ 30 kg/m^2 or with patients with a BMI $\geq$ 27 kg/m^2 in the presence of other risk factors (controlled hypertension, diabetes mellitus, dyslipidemia)
- Should be used in conjunction with a weight management program
- Discontinue if weight loss has not occurred within the first 4 weeks of use
- Use with caution in diabetic patients. Glucose requirements may change.
- Contraindicated in patients with a history of drug abuse, cardiovascular disease, moderate to severe hypertension, pulmonary hypertension, hyperthyroidism, and glaucoma

BENZODIAZEPINES

Introduction

Benzodiazepines are utilized in a broad spectrum of CNS disorders, though primarily as antianxiety, anticonvulsant, or hypnotic agents. Benzodiazepines are Schedule IV medications and can be habit forming. As with use in other indications, if patients have used the benzodiazepine long term, they should be counseled not to discontinue the drug abruptly. A gradual taper is required to avoid rebound, relapse, and withdrawal symptoms. The agents within the class have many similarities, and the differences between them are mostly pharmacokinetic.

Mechanism of Action for the Drug Class

Benzodiazepines facilitate the activity of the inhibitory neurotransmitter GABA (gamma-aminobutyric acid) and other inhibitory transmitters by binding to specific benzodiazepine receptors

Adverse Reactions for the Drug Class: Most Common

Sedation, somnolence, memory impairment, coordination problems, dizziness, and dysarthria

Adverse Reactions for the Drug Class: Rare/Severe/Important

Withdrawal syndrome and respiratory depression (particularly with other CNS depressants)

Counseling Points for the Drug Class

- Avoid alcohol because it can lead to possibly fatal respiratory depression
- Avoid activities that require mental alertness (e.g., driving) until the effects of the medication are known and comfortable and whenever the dose is increased
- Avoid abrupt discontinuation

Key Points for the Drug Class

- The benzodiazepines are Schedule IV medications that may be habit forming. Be cautious using benzodiazepines in patients with a history of substance abuse.
- Patients who receive chronic benzodiazepines will need to be gradually tapered off of the medication
- Abrupt discontinuation should be avoided to prevent withdrawal symptoms, especially in patients with seizure disorders to prevent precipitating seizures
- Contraindicated in narrow-angle glaucoma and pregnancy

Members of the Drug Class

In this section: Alprazolam, clonazepam, diazepam, lorazepam
Others: Chlordiazepoxide, clorazepate, midazolam, oxazepam, estazolam, quazepam, triazolam

⊚ Alprazolam

Brand Names

Xanax, Xanax XR, Alprazolam Intensol, Niravam

Generic Name

Alprazolam

Rx Only

Class IV controlled substance

Dosage Forms

Tablet, extended-release tablet, orally disintegrating tablet (ODT), solution

Usage

Anxiety disorders,* panic disorders

Pregnancy Category D

Dosing

- Initial dose:
  - Anxiety: 0.25–0.5 mg three times daily
  - Panic disorders: 0.5 mg three times daily
- Hepatic dosage adjustment: Reduce dosing by 50% or avoid use in cases of hepatic impairment

Major Drug Interactions

Drugs Affecting Alprazolam

- CNS depressants and alcohol: Increase CNS depression
- Cimetidine, oral contraceptives, fluoxetine, valproic acid, azole antifungals: Increase serum concentrations (contraindicated with ketoconazole and itraconazole)

Contraindications

Narrow-angle glaucoma, concurrent use with itraconazole or ketoconazole, pregnancy

Counseling Points

- Do not chew, crush, or break extended-release tablets. Swallow whole.
- Do not push ODTs through the blister pack foil. Peel back foil, remove tablet with dry finger, and place the tablet on tongue. Medication does not require water.

Key Points

- Abuse potential may be higher with this agent compared to other benzodiazepines due to its rapid action
- Withdrawal symptoms are more likely with a short-acting benzodiazepine, such as alprazolam. Discontinue medication slowly (e.g., reduce daily dose by 0.5 mg every 3 days) especially when used for > 4 months or in patients receiving > 4 mg daily.

◉ Temazepam

Brand Name
Restoril

Generic Name
Temazepam

Rx Only
Class IV controlled substance

Dosage Form
Capsule

Pregnancy Category X

Usage

Short-term treatment of insomnia,* anxiety

Dosing

- Insomnia: 7.5–30 mg at bedtime
- Renal dosage adjustment: Use with caution in patients with renal impairment
- Hepatic dosage adjustment: Use with caution in patients with hepatic impairment

Adverse Reactions: Most Common

Sedation, somnolence, memory impairment, coordination problems, dizziness, emergence of complex behavior ("sleep driving")

Adverse Reactions: Rare/Severe/Important

Withdrawal syndromes and respiratory depression (especially additive with other CNS depressants or alcohol), anaphylaxis reactions (angioedema, dyspnea, throat closing, nausea, vomiting)

Major Drug Interactions

Temazepam's Effect on Other Drugs
CNS depressants: Additive CNS depression

Contraindications

Narrow-angle glaucoma, pregnancy

Counseling Points

- Ingesting alcoholic beverages during benzodiazepine therapy is very dangerous and must be avoided
- Take just before going to sleep and only when able to get a full night's sleep (i.e., 7–8 hours)
- Take only when needed and should be used for a short term (7–10 days) to prevent habit-forming use

Key Points

- As a drug class, all benzodiazepines are contraindicated in narrow-angle glaucoma and pregnancy
- Elderly patients are the most susceptible to adverse effects and should be started with the 7.5 mg dose

◉ Clonazepam

Brand Names
Klonopin, Klonopin Wafers

Generic Name
Clonazepam

Rx Only
Class IV controlled substance

Dosage Forms
Tablet, orally disintegrating tablet (ODT)

Usage

Panic disorder,* seizures (Lennox-Gastaut, akinetic, myoclonic, absence),* restless leg syndrome, social phobia, acute mania associated with bipolar, multifocal tic disorders

Pregnancy Category D

Dosing

- Seizure disorders:
  - Initial: 0.25–0.5 mg three times daily
  - Maintenance dose: 0.05–0.2 mg/kg
  - Maximum dose: 20 mg daily
- Panic disorders:
  - 0.25–0.5 mg twice or three times daily
  - Maximum dose: 4 mg daily
- Hepatic dosage adjustment: Contraindicated in severe hepatic disease

Major Drug Interactions

Drugs Affecting Clonazepam

- Phenytoin, carbamazepine, and phenobarbital: Decrease serum concentrations
- Azole antifungals: Increase serum concentrations
- CNS depressants and alcohol: Increase CNS depression

Contraindications

Narrow-angle glaucoma, severe hepatic impairment, pregnancy

Counseling Point

Do not push ODTs through the blister pack foil. Peel back foil, remove tablet with dry finger, and place the tablet on tongue. Medication does not require water.

Key Points

- Some clinicians use once-daily bedtime dosing due to the drug's long half-life
- Abrupt discontinuation should be avoided to prevent withdrawal symptoms, especially in patients with seizure disorders to prevent precipitating seizures
- During withdrawal of clonazepam in patients with seizure disorders another anticonvulsant may be indicated for simultaneous substitution

⊙ Diazepam

Brand Names

Valium, Diastat, Diazepam Intensol, Diastat AcuDial

Generic Name

Diazepam

Rx Only

Class IV controlled substance

Dosage Forms

Tablet, solution, injection, rectal gel

Usage

Anxiety disorders,* acute alcohol withdrawal, seizures (adjunctive therapy, status epilepticus),* skeletal muscle relaxant, preoperative and procedural sedation and amnesia

Pregnancy Category D

Dosing

- Anxiety disorders: Initial dose of 2–10 mg two to four times daily as needed
- Skeletal muscle relaxant (adjunct therapy): Initial dose of 2–10 mg PO three to four times daily
- Acute alcohol withdrawal: Initial dose of 5–10 mg three to four times daily as needed
- Status epilepticus:
  - Initial dose: 5–10 mg IV every 5–10 minutes
  - Maximum dose: 30 mg
- Hepatic dosage adjustment:
  - Mild hepatic insufficiency: Reduce dosing by 50% or avoid use
  - Severe hepatic disease: Contraindicated

Major Drug Interactions

Drugs Affecting Diazepam

- CNS depressants and alcohol: Increase CNS depression
- Cimetidine, oral contraceptives, fluoxetine, valproic acid, azole antifungals: Increase serum concentrations (contraindicated with ketoconazole and itraconazole)
- Ranitidine and antacids: Decrease serum concentrations

Contraindications

Myasthenia gravis, narrow-angle glaucoma, sleep apnea syndrome, severe respiratory insufficiency, severe hepatic insufficiency

Key Points

- Use with caution or not at all in the elderly due to its long half-life
- Risk of propylene glycol toxicity with the parenteral formulation; monitor closely when using higher doses or for prolonged periods of time
- Abrupt discontinuation should be avoided to prevent withdrawal symptoms, especially in patients with seizure disorders to prevent precipitating seizures

⊙ Lorazepam

Brand Names

Ativan, Lorazepam Intensol

Generic Name

Lorazepam

Rx Only

Class IV controlled substance

Dosage Forms

Tablet, solution, injection

Pregnancy Category D

Usage

Anxiety disorders,* seizures (status epilepticus),* insomnia, acute alcohol withdrawal,* sedation,* agitation,* antiemetic

Dosing

- Anxiety disorders: Initial dose of 1–10 mg daily in 2–3 divided doses
- Status epilepticus:
  - Initial dose: 4 mg IV can repeat in 10–15 minutes
  - Maximum dose: 8 mg
- Acute alcohol withdrawal: Initial dose of 1–2 mg four times daily
- Agitation: Initial dose of 1–2 mg
- IV sedation in ICU setting:
  - Intermittent: Initial dose of 0.02–0.06 mg/kg
  - Continuous infusion: Initial dose of 0.01–0.1 mg/kg per hour

Major Drug Interactions

Drugs Affecting Lorazepam

- CNS depressants and alcohol: Increase CNS depression
- Valproic acid and probenecid: Increase serum levels (reduce lorazepam dose by 50%)

Contraindications

Narrow-angle glaucoma, sleep apnea (with parenteral formulation), severe respiratory insufficiency (except with mechanical ventilation)

Key Points

- Risk of propylene glycol toxicity with the parenteral formulation; monitor closely when using higher doses or for prolonged periods of time (e.g., continuous infusion of ≥ 6 mg/hour for 48 hours)
- Although specific dose recommendations are not available, use with caution in patients with renal or hepatic impairment
- Abrupt discontinuation should be avoided to prevent withdrawal symptoms, especially in patients with seizure disorders to prevent precipitating seizures

NONBENZODIAZEPINE ANTIANXIETY AGENTS

Introduction

Buspirone is the only drug within this class. Although used for anxiety disorders, it is not a benzodiazepine and is chemically unrelated to other CNS agents. Unlike benzodiazepines, it lacks anticonvulsant and sedative properties and therefore has less overall clinical utility. However, buspirone lacks issues that can be problematic with benzodiazepine use. Buspirone is less sedating, has fewer CNS side effects, and has a higher threshold of interaction with other CNS depressants and alcohol. Physical dependency and withdrawal symptoms have not been seen with buspirone. Buspirone can be a good maintenance agent to use in patients who are unable to tolerate benzodiazepines due to undesirable side effects and interactions, patients with a history of drug or alcohol abuse, and the elderly.

Mechanism of Action for the Drug Class

Buspirone's mechanism of action is primarily unknown. The drug has a high affinity for serotonin receptors and a moderate affinity for dopamine type-2 receptors.

Members of the Drug Class

In this section: Buspirone

◉ Buspirone

Brand Name

BuSpar

Generic Name

Buspirone

Rx Only

Dosage Form

Tablet

Usage

Anxiety disorders,* aggression, depression, premenstrual syndrome, nicotine dependence

Pregnancy Category B

Dosing

- Initial dose: 15 mg daily in 2 divided doses.
- Dosage adjustments: Titrate by 5 mg daily every 2–3 days to a maximum dose of 60 mg daily (target for most patients is 20–30 mg daily divided)
- Renal dosage adjustment: Use is not recommended in patients with severe renal dysfunction
- Hepatic dosage adjustment: Use is not recommended in patients with severe hepatic dysfunction

Adverse Reactions: Most Common

Dizziness, lightheadedness, headache, nausea, nervousness, excitement

Adverse Reactions: Rare/Severe/Important

Extrapyramidal symptoms, restless leg syndrome

Major Drug Interactions

Major substrate of CYP3A4

Drugs Affecting Buspirone

- Erythromycin, cimetidine, ketoconazole, itraconazole, clarithromycin, diltiazem, verapamil, other 3A4 inhibitors: Increase serum levels
- Rifampin, phenytoin, phenobarbital, carbamazepine, fluoxetine: Decrease serum levels

Buspirone's Effect on Other Drugs

- Monoamine oxidase inhibitors (MAOIs): Warning of concomitant use due to risk of hypertensive crisis
- Haloperidol: Increases serum levels

Counseling Points

- Antianxiety effects may not be seen for at least a week or more
- Buspirone should not be stopped abruptly
- Avoid large quantities of grapefruit juice

Key Points

- Abuse potential is low compared to benzodiazepines
- Buspirone will not treat benzodiazepine withdrawal symptoms
- Because of the delayed onset of action, buspirone cannot be used to treat acute anxiety

ANTICONVULSANTS

Introduction

Anticonvulsants are used for a broad spectrum of CNS on- and off-label indications, including seizure disorders, trigeminal and postherpetic neuralgias, bipolar disorders, neuropathic pain, migraine, mood disorders, and many others. The treatment goal in epilepsy is seizure-free control on as few antiepileptic drugs (AEDs) as possible with few to no side effects. However, achieving a balance between superior efficacy and side effects is not easily obtainable for many patients due to the many adverse reactions affiliated with these medications. In addition, the FDA has issued a special drug class warning of increased suicide behavior or ideation for all AEDs. Patients and family members should be made aware of the increased risk of suicidal thoughts and behavior. With any AED, patients should check with their physician before discontinuing medication. A gradual taper in dose may be required to prevent seizures and status epilepticus. Many AEDs are a substrate of or strongly inhibit/induce the CYP enzymatic system, resulting in multiple drug interactions. In addition, pregnant patients who remain on AEDs should be encouraged to enroll in the North American Antiepileptic Drug Pregnancy Registry.

Mechanism of Action for the Drug Class

Multiple mechanisms of action are used within this drug class and in many cases are unknown. Effective seizure control typically augments CNS inhibitory processes or opposes excitatory processes. Generally, when used for seizure disorders, control is achieved through alteration of sodium, calcium, and/or potassium ion channels and/or neurotransmitters, including potentiating inhibitory gamma-aminobutyric acid (GABA) and antagonizing excitatory glutamate. The mechanism may be through direct activation/inhibition of an ion channel, receptor site, or changes in enzyme production, metabolism, or function.

Members of the Drug Class

In this section: Carbamazepine, gabapentin, lamotrigine, levetiracetam, oxcarbazepine, phenobarbital, phenytoin, pregabalin, topiramate, valproic acid and derivatives
Others: Ethosuximide, ezogabine, felbamate, fosphenytoin, lacosamide, methsuximide, pentobarbital, primidone, rufinamide, tiagabine, vigabatrin, zonisamide

◉ Carbamazepine

Brand Names

Carbatrol, Epitol, Equetro, Tegretol, Tegretol XR

Generic Name

Carbamazepine

Rx Only

Dosage Forms

Tablet, extended-release tablet, chewable tablet, extended-release capsule, suspension

Usage

Seizures (partial, generalized tonic-clonic seizures, and mixed types);* trigeminal neuralgia; acute manic and mixed episodes associated with bipolar 1 disorder (Equetro only); psychiatric disorders (unipolar depression, schizoaffective disorder, resistant schizophrenia, posttraumatic stress disorder); withdrawal from alcohol, cocaine, or benzodiazepines; restless leg syndrome; neuropathic pain; glossopharyngeal neuralgia; many others

Pregnancy Category D

Dosing

- Seizure disorders in adults and children > 12 years of age:
  - Initial dose:
    - Tablet or capsule: 200 mg twice a day
    - Suspension: 400 mg four times a day
  - Dosage adjustment: Increase at weekly intervals by ≤ 200 mg daily in divided doses until optimal control is attained
  - Usual maintenance dose: 800–1,200 mg daily
- Trigeminal neuralgia:
  - Initial dose:
    - Tablet or capsule: 100 mg twice daily on the first day
    - Suspension: 50 mg four times a day
  - Dosage adjustment: Increase by up to 200 mg daily in divided dosing as needed
  - Maximum dose: Do not exceed 1,200 mg daily
- Acute mania and mixed episodes with bipolar 1 disorder (Equetro only):
  - Initial dose: 200 mg twice a day
  - Dosage adjustment: Increase daily dose in increments of 200 mg daily until optimal response is achieved
  - Maximum dose: 1,600 mg daily

Pharmacokinetic Monitoring

Target serum concentrations: 4–12 μg/ml

Adverse Reactions: Most Common

Dizziness, drowsiness, ataxia, nausea, vomiting, diplopia, headache

Adverse Reactions: Rare/Severe/Important

Hematologic reactions (aplastic anemia, leukopenia, agranulocytosis, eosinophilia, thrombocytopenia), hepatic or renal dysfunction, dermatologic reactions (toxic epidermal necrolysis, Stevens-Johnson syndrome), SIADH, cardiac conduction disturbances, hyponatremia

Major Drug Interactions

Drugs Affecting Carbamazepine

- Carbamazepine induces its own metabolism
- Cimetidine, erythromycin, clarithromycin, fluoxetine, valproic acid, protease inhibitors, azole antifungals, isoniazid, propoxyphene, diltiazem, verapamil, loratadine, zileuton, and others: Increase carbamazepine serum concentrations
- Phenobarbital, primidone, rifampin, theophylline, and phenytoin: Decrease serum concentrations of carbamazepine

Carbamazepine's Effect on Other Drugs

- Alprazolam, bupropion, caspofungin, felbamate, lamotrigine, 10-monohydroxy metabolite (active metabolite of oxcarbazepine), phenytoin, protease inhibitors, citalopram, itraconazole, clozapine, cyclosporine, diazepam, olanzapine, risperidone, tiagabine, topiramate, valproic acid, zonisamide, doxycycline, oral contraceptives, theophylline, warfarin, and many others: Induces metabolism of these drugs, leading to decreased serum concentrations and possible therapeutic failure
- MAOIs and nefazodone: Concomitant use is contraindicated

Essential Monitoring Parameters

Serum carbamazepine concentrations, CBC, platelets, serum sodium, liver function tests

Counseling Points

- Do not crush or chew extended-release tablets or capsules. Extended-release tablet coating is not absorbed and is excreted in the feces. Tablet coatings may be noticeable in the stool. Capsules may be opened and sprinkled over applesauce.
- Notify your healthcare provider if any of the following symptoms occur: Unusual bleeding, bruising, fever, sore throat, rash ulcer in the mouth, muscle cramping, jaundice, or suicide ideation
- If using oral contraceptives, consider an additional or alternative method of birth control
- May cause drowsiness, dizziness, or blurred vision. Observe caution when driving or performing tasks requiring alertness, coordination, or physical dexterity until the effects of the medication are familiar.
- Do not drink alcohol because it can exacerbate CNS depression, somnolence, and dizziness

Key Points

- Carbamazepine has a U.S. black box warning for development of serious dermatologic reactions, including toxic epidermal necrolysis (TEN) or Stevens-Johnson syndrome, with an increased incidence in patients of Asian descent with the HLA-B*1502 allele. These patients should be screened for the presence of the HLA-B*1502 allele. If positive, carbamazepine should not be started.
- Carbamazepine has a black box warning for the development of aplastic anemia and agranulocytosis
- Carbamazepine is contraindicated for use in patients with a history of bone marrow suppression
- Carbamazepine is metabolized through CYP450 3A4 to an active metabolite, 10,11-epoxide. The active metabolite is metabolized through epoxide hydrolase. Carbamazepine is a strong inducer of CYP450 enzymes. Be alert to any new medications added or discontinued from a patient's drug regimen because this could affect medication blood levels or the levels of the active metabolite.
- Because of autoinduction, the half-life of the drug and its serum levels may change over the first few weeks of therapy. Patients must be observed closely and dosing must be individualized.

⊙ Gabapentin

Brand Names
Neurontin, Gralise, Horizant

Generic Names
Gabapentin, Gabapentin enacarbil

Rx Only

Dosage Forms
Tablet, extended-release tablet, capsule, suspension

Usage
Seizures (adjunctive therapy in the treatment of partial seizures with and without secondary generalization),* postherpetic neuralgia, pain (neuropathic, chronic, and postoperative pain), diabetic peripheral neuropathy,* restless leg syndrome,* vasomotor symptoms associated with menopause, fibromyalgia, social phobia, and many others

Pregnancy Category C

Dosing
- Adjunctive therapy for partial seizures and diabetic peripheral neuropathy with immediate-release formulation (Neurontin):
  - Initial therapy: 300 mg three times daily
  - Dosage adjustment: Increase at weekly intervals to 1.8 g daily
  - Maximum dose: Up to 3.6 g daily
- Neuropathic pain: Immediate-release dosing is 300 mg once a day
- Postherpetic neuralgia:
  - Immediate-release initial dose: Initiate therapy with 300 mg on day 1, 300 mg twice a day on day 2, and 300 mg three times a day on day 3. Titrate dose as needed for pain relief up to a daily dose of 1.8 g.
  - Extended-release (Gralise) initial dose: Initiate therapy with 300 mg once a day on day 1, titrate up to 600 mg once a day on day 2, 900 mg once daily on days 3–6, 1,200 mg once daily on days 7–10, 1,500 mg once daily on days 11–14, and 1,800 mg once daily thereafter
- Restless leg syndrome:
  - Immediate-release:
    - Initial therapy: Initiate therapy with 300 mg once daily 2 hours prior to bedtime
    - Dosage adjustment: Dose may be titrated up every 2 weeks until symptom relief.
    - Maintenance therapy: Typically 300–1,800 mg daily; doses > 600 mg daily are given in divided doses
  - Extended-release (Horizant): Initiate therapy with 600 mg once daily (5 P.M.) and titrate up to 1,200 mg daily.

- Renal dosage adjustment:
  - Immediate-release:
    - CrCl ≥ 60 mL/min: 300–1,200 mg three times a day
    - CrCl > 30–59 mL/min: 200–700 mg twice a day
    - CrCl > 15–29 mL/min: 200–700 mg once daily
    - CrCl 15 mL/min: 100–300 mg once daily
    - CrCl < 15 mL/min: Reduce daily dose in proportion to CrCl of 15 mL/min
    - End-stage renal disease (ESRD) or hemodialysis (HD): Utilize dosing of CrCl < 15 mL/min plus give an additional supplemental dose of 125–350 mg post-HD
  - Extended-release:
    - CrCl ≥ 60 mL/min: 1,800 mg once daily
    - CrCl > 30–59 mL/min: 600–1,800 mg once daily
    - CrCl < 30 mL/min: Not recommended
    - ESRD or HD: Not recommended

Adverse Reactions: Most Common
Fatigue, somnolence, dizziness, peripheral edema, nystagmus, ataxia

Adverse Reactions: Rare/Severe/Important
Aggressive behavior in children

Major Drug Interactions
Drugs Affecting Gabapentin

Aluminum-containing antacids: Decrease bioavailability by 20%

Counseling Point
Do not drink alcohol because it can exacerbate CNS depression, somnolence, and dizziness

Key Point
Immediate-release (Neurontin) and extended-release (Gralise, Horizant) are not interchangeable products due to differences in formulation, indication, and pharmacokinetics

⊙ Lamotrigine

Brand Names
Lamictal, Lamictal XR, Lamictal CD, Lamictal ODT

Generic Name
Lamotrigine

Rx Only

Dosage Forms
Tablet, extended-release tablet, chewable dispersible tablet, orally disintegrating tablet (ODT). Starter kits are available for initial dosing titration when patients are already receiving valproic acid (blue kit) or carbamazepine, phenytoin, phenobarbital, primidone, or rifampin (green kit). The orange starter kit is used when titration is not affected by another concomitant medication.

Usage

Adjunctive therapy for seizures (generalized seizures of Lennox-Gastaut syndrome, partial seizures, and primary generalized tonic-clonic seizures);* seizures conversion to monotherapy (partial seizures in patients who are currently taking valproic acid, carbamazepine, phenobarbital, phenytoin, or primidone as the single AED),* maintenance treatment of bipolar 1 disorder

Pregnancy Category C

Dosing

- Seizure disorders (adjunctive therapy) and bipolar disorder:
  - Initial dosing and titration schedules depend on concomitant medications. Initiating at a higher dose or titrating at an accelerated rate increases the incidence of lamotrigine-associated rash.
    - Concurrent use with valproic acid: Initial dose is 25 mg every other day for 1–2 weeks
    - Concurrent use with carbamazepine, phenobarbital, phenytoin, primidone, or rifampin: Initial dose is 50 mg a day for 1–2 weeks
    - Concurrent use with any other AED: Initial dose is 25 mg daily for 1–2 weeks
  - Dosage adjustments: Follow specific dosing guidelines for titration beyond weeks 1–2
- Seizure disorders (conversion to monotherapy): Follow specific guidelines to appropriately titrate lower doses of valproic acid, carbamazepine, phenobarbital, phenytoin, and primidone while increasing doses of lamotrigine
- Hepatic dosage adjustment: Reduce dosing by 25–50% and titrate to clinical effectiveness in moderate to severe hepatic impairment

Adverse Reactions: Most Common

Headache, dizziness, rash, diplopia, nausea, somnolence, ataxia, rhinitis, blurred vision, somnolence

Adverse Reactions: Rare/Severe/Important

Life-threatening dermatologic reactions (toxic epidermal necrolysis, Stevens-Johnson syndrome), hypersensitivity reactions, multiorgan failure/dysfunction, blood dyscrasias, aseptic meningitis

Major Drug Interactions

Drugs Affecting Lamotrigine

- Valproic acid: Increases lamotrigine concentrations and effects
- Oral contraceptives, rifampin, carbamazepine, phenytoin, primidone, oxcarbazepine, and phenobarbital: May decrease lamotrigine concentrations

Counseling Points

- Women should alert their physician if they plan on starting or stopping oral contraceptives. Levels of lamotrigine can fluctuate greatly for weeks "on" the pill vs. weeks "off" the pill.

- It is very important to slowly increase daily dosage as directed. Use a calendar to assist in this process.
- Notify your healthcare provider immediately if you develop a rash

Key Points

- Lamotrigine has a black box warning for risk of life-threatening serious rashes, including toxic epidermal necrolysis or Stevens-Johnson syndrome and/or rash-related deaths. The risk of rash is increased in the pediatric population, with concomitant use with valproic acid, with doses greater than the recommended initial dose, and when upward dose titration occurs too quickly. Patients should always be monitored for rash when starting therapy with this agent.
- Do not rechallenge a patient with lamotrigine if a rash has occurred with prior use
- This medication has been confused with the antifungal medication Lamisil

◉ Levetiracetam

Brand Names

Keppra, Keppra XR

Generic Name

Levetiracetam

Rx Only

Dosage Forms

Tablet, extended-release tablet, solution, injection

Usage

Seizures (adjunctive therapy for partial, myoclonic, and primary generalized tonic-clonic),* manic bipolar 1 disorder, migraine prophylaxis

Pregnancy Category C

Dosing

- Immediate release:
  - Initial dosing: 500 mg twice a day
  - Dosage adjustment: Titrate every 2 weeks up to 1,500 mg twice a day
- Extended release:
  - Initial dosing: 100 mg daily
  - Dosage adjustment: Titrate every 2 weeks up to 3,000 mg once daily
- Renal dosage adjustment:
  - Immediate-release:
    - CrCl < 80 mL/min: 500–1,500 mg twice daily
    - CrCl 50–80 mL/min: 500–1,000 mg twice daily
    - CrCl 30–50 mL/min: 25–750 mg twice daily
    - CrCl < 30 mL/min: 250–500 mg twice daily
    - ESRD on HD: 500–100 mg daily with a supplemental dose of 250–500 mg after HD

- Extended-release:
  - CrCl 50–80 mL/min: 1,000–2,000 mg daily
  - CrCl 30–50 mL/min: 500–1,500 mg daily
  - CrCl < 30 mL/min: 500–1,000 mg daily
  - ESDR on HD: Use immediate-release formulation

Adverse Reactions: Most Common

Asthenia, somnolence, dizziness, infection, decreased appetite, vomiting

Adverse Reactions: Rare/Severe/Important

Coordination difficulties, behavior abnormalities (depression, nervousness, mood swings, irritability, agitation)

Counseling Point

May cause drowsiness, dizziness, or blurred vision. Use caution when driving or performing tasks requiring alertness, coordination, or physical dexterity.

◉ Oxcarbazepine

Brand Name
Trileptal

Generic Name
Oxcarbazepine

Rx Only

Dosage Forms
Tablet, suspension

Usage
Seizures (monotherapy and adjunctive therapy in partial seizures),* bipolar disorders, neuropathic pain

Pregnancy Category C

Dosing
- Initial dose: 300 mg twice a day
- Dosage adjustment: Titrate dose up by 600 mg daily once a week to recommended dose of 600 mg twice a day
- Renal dosage adjustment: If CrCl < 30 mL/min, initiate dose at 150 mg twice a day

Adverse Reactions: Most Common
Dizziness, somnolence, diplopia, fatigue, nausea, vomiting, ataxia, abnormal vision, abdominal pain, tremor, dyspepsia, abnormal gait

Adverse Reactions: Rare/Severe/Important
Hyponatremia (monitoring serum levels should be considered during maintenance treatment), anaphylactic reactions and angioedema, multiorgan hypersensitivity reactions, dermatological reactions (TEN and/ or Stevens-Johnson syndrome), psychomotor slowing, hematologic (agranulocytosis, aplastic anemia, pancytopenia)

Major Drug Interactions

Drugs Affecting Oxcarbazepine

Phenobarbital, carbamazepine, valproic acid, phenytoin, and verapamil: Decrease serum concentrations of MHD (active metabolite), compromising effectiveness

Oxcarbazepine's Effect on Other Drugs

- Oral contraceptives, felodipine, and lamotrigine: Decreases serum concentrations
- Phenytoin and phenobarbital: Increases serum concentrations

Counseling Points

- If using oral contraceptives, consider an additional or alternative method of birth control
- May cause drowsiness, dizziness, or blurred vision. Observe caution when driving or performing tasks requiring alertness, coordination, or physical dexterity.
- Do not drink alcohol because it can exacerbate CNS depression, somnolence, and dizziness

Key Points

- Oxcarbazepine has an active metabolite, 10-monohydroxy metabolite (MHD)
- Of patients with a history of a hypersensitivity reaction to carbamazepine, approximately 25–30% experience a hypersensitivity reaction to oxcarbazepine
- Unlike carbamazepine, oxcarbazepine has not been shown to cause autoinduction
- Due to oxcarbazepine's strong inducing influence on the CYP450 enzymatic system, be alert to any new medications added or discontinued from a patient's drug regimen because it could affect medication blood concentrations

◉ Phenobarbital

Generic Name
Phenobarbital

Rx Only
Class IV controlled substance

Dosage Forms
Tablet, capsule, elixir, injection

Usage
Sedative/hypnotic, seizure disorders* (partial and generalized tonic-clonic seizures, status epilepticus)

Pregnancy Category D

Dosing

- Seizure disorders:
  - Loading dose: 10–20 mg/kg
  - Initial dose: 1–3 mg/kg per day
- Sedation: Initial dose of 30–120 mg daily in divided doses
- Renal dosage adjustment: If CrCl < 10 mL/min, administer doses every 12–16 hours
- Hepatic dosage adjustment: Reduce dose in hepatic impairment

Pharmacokinetic Monitoring

Target serum concentration: 10–40 µg/ml

Adverse Reactions: Most Common

Fatigue, drowsiness, decreased cognitive function, hyperactivity in children

Adverse Reactions: Rare/Severe/Important

Respiratory depression (contraindication in severe respiratory disorders), hepatotoxicity (contraindicated in severe liver dysfunction), rash (including Stevens-Johnson syndrome), osteomalacia (chronic administration), acute intermittent porphyria (contraindicated in porphyria), hematologic disorders

Major Drug Interactions

Drugs Affecting Phenobarbital

Cimetidine, felbamate, valproic acid: Increase serum concentrations

Phenobarbital's Effect on Other Drugs

- Carbamazepine, lamotrigine, 10-monohydroxy metabolite of oxcarbazepine, doxycycline, theophylline, verapamil, valproic acid, warfarin, zonisamide: Decreases serum concentrations
- Oral contraceptives and metronidazole: Decreases efficacy

Essential Monitoring Parameters

Phenobarbital serum concentrations, liver function tests

Counseling Points

- Avoid use with other CNS depressants, including alcohol, to prevent excessive sedation
- May cause drowsiness. Use caution when driving or performing tasks requiring alertness, coordination, or physical dexterity.
- If using oral contraceptives, consider an additional or alternative method of birth control

Key Points

- Schedule IV medication. Addiction is rare in patients taking phenobarbital for epilepsy, but this drug is contraindicated in patients with previous addiction to sedative/hypnotics.
- Due to phenobarbital's strong inducing influence on the CYP450 enzymatic system, be alert to any new medications added or discontinued from a patient's drug regimen because it could affect medication concentrations
- The half-life of this drug is approximately 80 hours. Maintenance dosing can be given at bedtime to decrease daytime sedation.

⊙ Phenytoin

Brand Names

Dilantin, Dilantin-125, Phenytek

Generic Name

Phenytoin

Rx Only

Dosage Forms

Capsule, extended-release capsule, chewable tablet, suspension, injection

Usage

Seizures* (generalized tonic-clonic and complex partial seizures and prevention and treatment of seizures occurring during or following head trauma/neurosurgery, status epilepticus)

Pregnancy Category D

Dosing

- Status epilepticus: Loading dose 15–20 mg/kg, maximum rate 50 mg/minute
- Seizure disorders: Initial dose of 100 mg three times a day titrated to target serum concentrations. Titrate dose to a therapeutic serum concentration.
- Obesity dosage adjustment: Use an adjusted body weight with a correction factor of 1.33 to account for a doubling of volume of distribution in obese patients

Pharmacokinetic Monitoring

Target serum concentration of 10–20 µg/ml total phenytoin, or free phenytoin serum concentrations of 1–2 µg/mL. Free fraction of phenytoin increases in low albumin states and CrCl < 10 mL/min.

Adverse Reactions: Most Common

Lethargy, fatigue, dizziness, blurred vision, nystagmus (an initial symptom of toxicity), cognitive impairment, gingival hyperplasia, acne, hirsutism, coarsening of facial features

Adverse Reactions: Rare/Severe/Important

Rash (Stevens-Johnson syndrome and TEN), osteomalacia, folate deficiency, blood dyscrasias, hepatitis, lupuslike reactions, lymphadenopathy, porphyria, arrhythmias following rapid IV administration, seizures and coma at toxic levels, teratogenic (fetal hydantoin syndrome)

Major Drug Interactions

Drugs Affecting Phenytoin

- Antacids: Decrease bioavailability
- Carbamazepine, chronic alcohol ingestion, folic acid, and valproic acid: Decrease serum concentration
- Cimetidine, acute alcohol ingestion, fluconazole, isoniazid, and warfarin: Increase serum concentration

Phenytoin's Effect on Other Drugs

- Carbamazepine, felbamate, lamotrigine, 10 monohydroxy metabolite of oxcarbazepine, tiagabine, topiramate, valproic acid, zonisamide, folic acid, and vitamin D: Decreases serum concentrations
- Lithium: Increases toxicity
- Oral contraceptives: Decreases efficacy

Essential Monitoring Parameters

Serum phenytoin levels or free phenytoin levels, liver function tests, albumin

Counseling Points

- Avoid alcoholic beverages
- If using oral contraceptives, consider an additional or alternative method of birth control

Key Points

- Phenytoin has a black box warning on the IV formulation for hypotension. The maximum rate of IV administration is 50 mg/min.
- Due to phenytoin's strong inducing influence on the CYP450 and UGT enzymatic system, be alert to any new medications added or discontinued from a patient's drug regimen because it could affect medication blood levels
- Drug interactions are complicated. Phenytoin is highly protein bound; thus drugs that displace phenytoin from protein-binding sites increase free phenytoin levels. Monitoring serum concentrations or free phenytoin levels if displacement from protein-binding sites is suspected and clinical response is important.
- The suspension formulation of this drug interacts with tube feedings. If a patient requires tube feedings, separate dosing of the suspension formulation at least 1–2 hours before and 1–2 hours after tube feeding. Consider switching to the injection formulation if interruption of tube feeding is not feasible.
- This drug is metabolized by Michaelis-Menten pharmacokinetics. Saturation of metabolism can occur at doses used clinically, resulting in a disproportionally large increase in the serum concentration compared to a small dosage increase. When serum concentrations are subtherapeutic, increase doses cautiously.
- Serum concentration levels need to be corrected for significant renal dysfunction and/or hypoalbuminemia. Alternatively, obtain a free phenytoin level.

⊙ Pregabalin

Brand Name

Lyrica

Generic Name

Pregabalin

Rx Only

Class V controlled substance

Dosage Forms

Capsule, solution

Usage

Seizures (adjunctive therapy for partial onset), diabetic peripheral neuropathy,* postherpetic neuralgia, fibromyalgia,* general anxiety disorder, central pain

Pregnancy Category C

Dosing

- Initial dose:
  - 50 mg three times a day *or*
  - 75 mg two times a day
- Dosage adjustment: Dose can be increased to a maximum of 300 mg daily within 1 week
- Maximum dose: 600 mg daily, except for fibromyalgia, for which the maximum dose is 450 mg daily
- Renal dosage adjustment:
  - CrCl < 60 mL/min: 150–600 mg daily in 2–3 divided doses
  - CrCl 30–60 mL/min: 72–300 mg daily in 2–3 divided doses
  - CrCl 15–30 mL/min: 25–150 mg daily in 1–2 divided doses
  - CrCl < 15 mL/min: 25–75 mg daily

Adverse Reactions: Most Common

Peripheral edema, increased appetite, weight gain, constipation, dry mouth, ataxia, dizziness, somnolence, euphoria, difficulty with concentrating and attention, blurred vision, diplopia

Adverse Reactions: Rare/Severe/Important

Angioedema, hypersensitivity reaction, creatine kinase elevations, thrombocytopenia, P-R interval prolongation

Counseling Points

- Let your healthcare provider know about any muscle pain or tenderness, swelling of face or mouth, or swelling of hands, legs, or feet
- May cause drowsiness. Use caution when driving or performing tasks requiring alertness, coordination, or physical dexterity

Key Point

Use with caution in patients with Class III or IV heart failure or concomitant medications known to cause peripheral edema, due to the propensity of pregabalin to cause edema

⊙ Topiramate

Brand Name
Topamax

Generic Name
Topiramate

Rx Only

Dosage Forms
Tablet, capsule

Usage
Seizures (monotherapy or adjunctive therapy for partial onset seizures and primary generalized tonic-clonic seizures, adjunctive treatment of seizures associated with Lennox-Gastaut syndrome),* prophylaxis of migraine headache,* diabetic neuropathy, cluster headache, neuropathic pain, bipolar disorder, withdrawal from alcohol, weight loss

Pregnancy Category D

Dosing
- Seizure disorders: Initial dose of 25–50 mg daily and increased weekly by 25–50 mg until an effective dose of 200–400 mg/ day is reached in 2 divided doses
- Migraine prophylaxis: Initial dose of 25 mg daily and then increased weekly by 25 mg until an effective dose is reached at 50 mg twice a day
- Renal dosage adjustment: If CrCl < 70 mL/min, start at 50% the usual adult dose
- Hepatic dosage adjustment: Use with caution in patients with hepatic impairment

Adverse Reactions: Most Common
CNS (dizziness, ataxia, somnolence, psychomotor slowing, confusion, nervousness, memory impairment), loss of appetite, anorexia, taste alteration, abnormal vision, fatigue, paresthesia

Adverse Reactions: Rare/Severe/Important
Metabolic acidosis, precipitation of manic or hypomanic states in patients with bipolar disorder, oligohidrosis, hyperthermia, depression, kidney stones (concomitant use with carbonic anhydrase inhibitors should be avoided), hyperammonemia and encephalopathy, acute myopia and secondary angle closure glaucoma

Major Drug Interactions
Drugs Affecting Topiramate
Phenytoin, carbamazepine, valproic acid, and lamotrigine: Decrease serum concentrations

Topiramate's Effect on Other Drugs
- Phenytoin and lithium: Increases serum concentrations
- Oral contraceptives: Decreases efficacy

Counseling Points
- Drink lots of fluid to prevent the formation of kidney stones
- Use caution with other CNS medications and alcohol due to increased risk of CNS side effects
- If using oral contraceptives, consider an additional or alternative method of birth control

Key Point
Concomitant use with other carbonic anhydrase inhibitors may increase the risk or severity of metabolic acidosis or kidney stones

⊙ Valproate Sodium

Brand Names
Depakene, Depacon, Depakote, Depakote ER, Depakote Sprinkle, Stavzor

Generic Names
Valproate sodium, valproic acid, and divalproex sodium (divalproex is converted to the active moiety, valproic acid, in the GI tract)

Rx Only

Dosage Forms
Tablet (immediate-, delayed-, and extended-release), capsule (immediate- and delayed-release), syrup, injection

Usage
Seizures (monotherapy and adjunctive therapy for simple and complex absence seizures, and complex partial seizures, adjunctive therapy for multiple seizure types),* manic episodes associated with bipolar disorder,* prophylaxis for migraine headaches,* mood disorders, status epilepticus, diabetic neuropathy

Pregnancy Category D

Dosing
- Seizure disorders:
  - Initial dose: 10–15 mg/kg per day in divided doses
  - Dosage adjustment: Titrate dose by 5–10 mg/kg per day weekly until a therapeutic response is observed or intolerable side effects
  - Maximum dose: 60 mg/kg per day
  - Extended-release formulation: Can be given once daily
  - Conversion from a stable dose of valproic acid and its derivatives to the extended-release formulation requires an 8–20% increase in total daily dose to maintain the same serum concentration
- Status epilepticus: IV loading dose of 15–45 mg/kg
- Mania:
  - Stavzor:
    - Initial dose: 750 mg in divided doses
    - Dosage adjustment: Titrate dose as rapidly as tolerated to control symptoms
    - Maximum dose of 60 mg/kg daily

- Depakote ER:
  - Initial dose: 25 mg/kg daily once daily
  - Dosage adjustment: Titrate to maximum of 60 mg/kg daily
- Migraine prophylaxis:
  - Stavzor:
    - Initial dose: 250 mg twice a day
    - Dosage adjustment: Titrate up to 1,000 mg daily
  - Depakote ER:
    - Initial dose: 500 mg daily for 7 days
    - Dosage adjustment: Titrate up to 500–1,000 mg daily based on response
- Hepatic dosage adjustment: Consider dose reduction in hepatic impairment. Use is contraindicated in severe liver dysfunction.

Pharmacokinetic Monitoring

Epilepsy target serum concentration is 50–100 µg/mL, although some patients may be well controlled on higher or lower serum concentrations. Mania target serum concentrations is 85–125 µg/mL.

Adverse Reactions: Most Common

Abdominal pain, nausea, vomiting, anorexia initially, weight gain with chronic use, drowsiness, ataxia, alopecia, blurred vision, asthenia

Adverse Reactions: Rare/Severe/Important

Hepatotoxicity (can be fatal, usually occurs within the first 6 months of therapy), pancreatitis (can be fatal), teratogenic, hyperammonemia, thrombocytopenia, hypothermia, multiorgan hypersensitivity, contraindicated in patients with urea cycle disorder

Major Drug Interactions

Drugs Affecting Valproate/Divalproex

- Phenytoin, phenobarbital, primidone, carbamazepine, lamotrigine, rifampin, carbapenem antibiotics, and topiramate: Decrease serum concentration
- Cimetidine, aspirin, and felbamate: Increase serum concentration

Valproate/Divalproex's Effect on Other Drugs

Benzodiazepines, zidovudine, tricyclic antidepressants, phenobarbital, 10, 11-carbamazepine epoxide (an active metabolite): Increases serum concentrations

Essential Monitoring Parameters

Valproic acid serum levels, liver function tests, serum ammonia levels

Counseling Point

Contact healthcare provider if nausea, vomiting, anorexia, lethargy, or jaundice occur because these may be signs of liver problems

Key Points

- There are black box warnings for hepatotoxicity, pancreatitis, and teratogenicity
- GI side effects can be reduced by using the delayed-release formulation
- Due to their inhibitory influence on the CYP450 enzymatic system, be alert to any new medications added or discontinued from a patient's drug regimen because it could affect medication concentrations
- Consider an alternative AED in women of childbearing age due to teratogenic risk

ANTIDEPRESSANTS, MISCELLANEOUS

Introduction

This group of antidepressants encompasses some first-line agents, especially in the presence of compelling indications. These agents may have fewer sexual side effects than the more commonly used selective serotonin reuptake inhibitors (SSRIs).

Mechanism of Action for the Drug Class

These agents have multiple mechanisms of action, including blocking the presynaptic reuptake of serotonin and/or norepinephrine, thereby increasing concentrations of these CNS neurotransmitters in the synapse. Bupropion is also a weak inhibitor of dopamine reuptake. Mirtazapine has central presynaptic alpha-2 adrenergic antagonism, which leads to increased release of serotonin and norepinephrine.

Counseling Points for the Drug Class

- All antidepressants require several weeks of continuous use before symptoms improve. Patients should be cautioned that some side effects will probably occur before the therapeutic effect.
- The most important aspect of treating depression may be that therapy must continue for 6–9 months after improvement. Stopping the drug therapy too soon greatly increases the risk of depression returning.

Key Points for the Drug Class

- There is a black box warning for all antidepressants that these drugs increase the risk of suicidal thinking and behavior in children, adolescents, and young adults (18–24 years of age) with major depressive disorder (MDD) and other psychiatric disorders
- Monitoring parameters for all antidepressants should include suicide ideation (especially at the beginning

of therapy or when doses are changed), mental status for efficacy, and the most common side effects of the individual agent. Side-effect monitoring is especially important because side effects can occur before therapeutic effects and negatively impact adherence.
- All antidepressants are contraindicated with the concomitant use of monoamine oxidase inhibitors (MAOIs) or sibutramine and use within 14 days of MAOI therapy.

Members of the Drug Class
In this section: Bupropion, mirtazapine, nefazodone, trazodone

◉ Bupropion

Brand Names
Wellbutrin, Wellbutrin-SR, Wellbutrin XL, Zyban, Budeprion

Generic Name
Bupropion

Rx Only

Dosage Forms
Tablet, sustained-release tablet, extended-release tablet

Usage
Depression,* smoking cessation*

Pregnancy Category C

Dosing
- Depression:
  - Immediate-release: Start with 100 mg twice daily and increase to the 300 mg target dose by day 4
  - Sustained- or extended-release: Start with 150 mg once daily in the morning. Increase to the 300 mg target dose by day 4
- Smoking cessation: Start with 150 mg daily for 3 days, then increase to 150 mg twice daily
- Renal dosage adjustment: Start with reduced dosage or dosing frequency and monitor carefully
- Hepatic dosage adjustment: Start with reduced dosage or dosing frequency and monitor carefully

Adverse Reactions: Most Common
Headache, insomnia, xerostomia, weight loss

Adverse Reactions: Rare/Severe/Important
Seizures

Major Drug Interactions
Major substrate of CYP2B6, strong inhibitor of CYP2D6

Drugs Affecting Bupropion
- CYP2B6 inhibitors: Increase concentrations
- CYP2B6 inducers: Decrease concentrations

Bupropion's Effect on Other Drugs
- Alcohol: Increases seizure risk
- Herbs used for depression and anxiety (e.g., kava kava, St. John's wort): Increases CNS depression
- CYP2D6 substrates: Increases concentrations

Contraindications
Seizure disorder, history of anorexia/bulimia

Counseling Points
- Patients should be aware that bupropion is marketed under the brand names Wellbutrin and Zyban. These are the same medication; they should not be taken together.
- Avoid alcohol because it can increase the risk for seizures. Excessive use or abrupt discontinuation of alcohol or sedatives can also increase seizure risk.
- Dry mouth and insomnia are common and may improve over time. If insomnia occurs, recommend taking the first dose as early as possible. The patient may also take the second dose 8 hours after the first.

Key Points
- There is a black box warning for neuropsychiatric effects when used in smoking cessation
- Bupropion was removed from the market many years ago due to the risk of seizures at doses > 450 mg daily. At that time, the recommended daily doses were higher.
- Bupropion is particularly useful for patients suffering sexual side effects or excessive sedation from other agents
- Start elderly patients at half the usual initial doses

◉ Mirtazapine

Brand Names
Remeron, Remeron Sol Tabs

Generic Name
Mirtazapine

Rx Only

Dosage Forms
Tablet, orally disintegrating tablet (ODT)

Usage
Depression

Pregnancy Category C

Dosing
- Initial dose: 15 mg daily at bedtime, increased to 30–45 mg daily
- Maximum dose: 45 mg daily
- Renal dosage adjustment: No specific recommendations are given. Start with reduced dosage and monitor carefully.
- Hepatic dosage adjustment: No specific recommendations are given. Start with reduced dosage and monitor carefully.

Adverse Reactions: Most Common

Somnolence, xerostomia, increased appetite, weight gain, increase cholesterol, constipation

Major Drug Interactions

Major substrate of CYP1A2, 2D6, and 3A4

Counseling Points

- Because sleepiness is common with mirtazapine, it is best to take before bedtime
- Weight gain and changes in cholesterol can occur
- SolTab is formulated to dissolve on the tongue without water

Key Points

- Paradoxically, higher doses (30–45 mg) may be less sedating than the initial 15 mg dose
- Mirtazapine may cause fewer sexual side effects as compared with the SSRIs
- Start elderly patients at half the usual initial dose
- Due to its effects on sleep and weight, mirtazapine is a good choice for patients with depression characterized by insomnia and loss of appetite

◉ Nefazodone

Brand Name

Serzone (has been removed from market as a brand name)

Generic Name

Nefazodone

Dosage Form

Tablet

Usage

Depression

Pregnancy Category C

Dosing

- Initial dose: 100 mg twice daily, increased to target dose of 300–600 mg daily
- Elderly patients: Reduce dose by half

Adverse Reactions: Most Common

Sedation, headache, dizziness

Adverse Reactions: Rare/Severe/Important

Liver failure (drug has a black box warning for hepatotoxicity)

Major Drug Interactions

- Major substrate of CYP2D6 and 3A4
- Strong inhibitor of CYP3A4, inducer of P-glycoprotein

Drugs Affecting Nefazodone

- CYP2D6 and 3A4 inhibitors such as amiodarone, erythromycin, grapefruit juice, diltiazem, verapamil: Increase concentrations
- CYP2D6 and 3A4 inducers: Decrease concentrations

Nefazodone's Effect on Other Drugs

Triazolam and alprazolam (contraindicated drugs), other benzodiazepines, some antipsychotic agents, lovastatin, simvastatin, and many others: Increases concentrations

Contraindications

Active liver disease, increased liver function tests, use during acute recovery phase post myocardial infarction

Key Points

- Due to hepatotoxicity (black box warning) and the availability of safer antidepressants, this agent is used infrequently
- Nefazodone is chemically related to trazodone, which may cause priapism. Rare cases of priapism have been reported.
- Nefazodone can be fairly sedating. Give larger portion of daily dosage at bedtime, if possible.
- Nefazodone has a low incidence of sexual dysfunction
- Medication errors are possible because of the similar-sounding and similar available doses of Seroquel (an antipsychotic agent)

◉ Trazodone

Brand Names

Desyrel, Oleptro

Generic Name

Trazodone

Rx Only

Dosage Forms

Tablet, extended-release tablet

Usage

Depression, nighttime sedation/insomnia*

Pregnancy Category C

Dosing

- Depression:
  - Initial dose: 150 mg daily divided in 2–3 doses
  - Dosage adjustment: Increase to 300–500 mg daily as a target dose for depression
  - Maximum dose:
    - Tablets: 600 mg daily
    - Extended-release tablets: 375 mg daily
- At bedtime for nighttime sedation:
  - Initial dose: 25–50 mg
  - Usual dose: 100–150 mg
  - Maximum dose: 200 mg

Adverse Reactions: Most Common

Sedation, dizziness, headache

Adverse Reactions: Rare/Severe/Important

Priapism

Major Drug Interactions

Major substrate of CYP3A4

Drugs Affecting Trazodone

CYP3A4 inhibitors (e.g., sibutramine, venlafaxine, protease inhibitors, some SSRIs): Increase concentrations

Trazodone's Effect on Other Drugs

Alcohol and other CNS depressants: Increases effects

Counseling Points

- Report prolonged or inappropriate erections
- Immediate-release formulations should be taken after meals
- Extended-release tablets should be taken on an empty stomach. Do not crush or chew the tablet.

Key Points

- Trazodone is often used as a hypnotic due to its sedative properties. Many authorities frown on such usage, especially when used with antipsychotic or other antidepressant therapy. If such dual therapy is improperly employed, patients should be thoroughly educated on the signs and symptoms of serotonin syndrome and be seen immediately if such symptoms occur.
- Anticholinergic effects may be seen with high doses
- Start elderly patients at half the usual initial doses

ANTIDEPRESSANTS, SEROTONIN-NOREPINEPHRINE REUPTAKE INHIBITORS

Introduction

This small class of newer antidepressants has fewer sexual side effects compared to selective serotonin reuptake inhibitors (SSRIs) and a patient-friendly adverse effect profile. Like SSRIs, serotonin-norepinephrine reuptake inhibitors (SNRIs) are first-line treatments for depression and anxiety. Duloxetine is also used for the management of certain pain syndromes. Norepinephrine activity is required in order to treat neuropathic pain, which is why SNRIs and tricyclic antidepressants (TCAs) are used for this indication but SSRIs are not.

Mechanism of Action for the Drug Class

These medications work in depression by blocking the neuronal reuptake of serotonin and norepinephrine. It is their action on norepinephrine that is responsible for their efficacy in neuropathic pain syndromes, as well as their toxicity profile of GI upset and increased blood pressure.

Counseling Points for the Drug Class

- All antidepressants require several weeks of continuous use before symptoms improve. Patients should be cautioned that some side effects will probably occur before the therapeutic effect.
- The most important aspect of treating depression is that therapy must continue for 6–9 months after the patient has shown improvement. Stopping the drug therapy too soon greatly increases the risk of relapse.
- Patients should be counseled on the signs and symptoms of serotonin toxicity, especially if on more than one medication that increases serotonin concentrations due to the increased risk of serotonin syndrome. Such symptoms include agitation, restlessness, diaphoresis, tachycardia, hyperthermia, nausea, vomiting, and loss of coordination.
- Avoid alcohol and maintain adequate hydration unless otherwise restricted
- Counsel patients on the black box warning and to be seen immediately or go to their local ER if symptoms of suicide ideation occur. Also counsel patients to report any sudden changes in mental status.

Key Points for the Drug Class

- There is a black box warning for all antidepressants that they increase the risk of suicidal thinking and behavior in children, adolescents, and young adults (18–24 years of age) with major depressive disorder (MDD) and other psychiatric disorders
- Monitoring parameters for all antidepressants should include suicide ideation (especially at the beginning of therapy or when doses are changed), mental status for efficacy, and the most common side effects of the individual agent. Side-effect monitoring is especially important because side effects can occur before therapeutic effects and negatively impact adherence.
- For all SNRIs, blood pressure should be monitored at baseline and periodically thereafter, with extra caution in hypertensive patients. Liver and kidney function should also be monitored and doses adjusted accordingly.
- All antidepressants are contraindicated with the concomitant use of MAOIs or sibutramine and use within 14 days of MAOI therapy
- Concomitant use of multiple agents that increase serotonin, such as SSRIs, SNRIs, and TCAs, should be avoided due to the risk for serotonin syndrome, a serious and potentially life-threatening reaction

If this combination is utilized, patients should be educated on the signs and symptoms of serotonin toxicity (see previous discussion). Other medications that can increase the risk for serotonin syndrome when used with antidepressants include triptans, linezolid, dextromethorphan, meperidine, and OTC treatments for depression, such as 5-HTP, SAMe, and St. John's wort.

Members of the Drug Class
In this section: Duloxetine, venlafaxine
Others: Desvenlafaxine, milnacipran

◉ Duloxetine
Brand Name
Cymbalta

Generic Name
Duloxetine

Rx Only

Dosage Forms
Delayed-release capsule, enteric-coated pellet

Usage
Depression,* generalized anxiety disorder (GAD), and the pain syndromes* associated with diabetic neuropathy, fibromyalgia, and chronic musculoskeletal pain

Pregnancy Category C

Dosing
- Initial dose: 40–60 mg daily in 1 or 2 doses
- Maximum dose: 120 mg daily
- Note: Doses > 60 mg daily have not been shown to be more effective
- Renal dosage adjustment: Avoid in patients with CrCl < 30 mL/min
- Hepatic dosage adjustment: Avoid in patients with hepatic impairment

Adverse Reactions: Most Common
Nausea, headache, somnolence, dry mouth, insomnia, other GI complaints

Adverse Reactions: Rare/Severe/Important
Syndrome of inappropriate antidiuretic hormone

Major Drug Interactions
- Major substrate of CYP1A2 and 2D6
- Moderate inhibitor of CYP2D6

Drugs Affecting Duloxetine
CYP2D6 and 1A2 inhibitors (paroxetine, fluvoxamine): Increase effects

Duloxetine's Effect on Other Drugs
Alcohol and other CNS depressants, thioridazine, beta-agonists: Increases effects

Contraindication
Uncontrolled narrow-angle glaucoma

Counseling Points
- Swallow capsule whole. Do not crush or chew.
- Monitor glucose closely in diabetic patients

Key Points
- May take 2–3 weeks to be effective. Doses may need to be titrated upward.
- Drug should be tapered off over a 2-week period when discontinuing therapy
- May be confused with fluoxetine (Prozac)

◉ Venlafaxine
Brand Names
Effexor, Effexor XR

Generic Name
Venlafaxine

Rx Only

Dosage Forms
Tablet, extended-release tablet, extended-release capsule

Usage
Depression,* generalized anxiety disorder (GAD),* seasonal affective disorder (SAD), panic disorder, hot flashes, obsessive compulsive disorder (OCD), ADHD, neuropathic pain, migraine prophylaxis

Pregnancy Category C

Dosing
- Initial dose for most indications: 75 mg daily that should be increased to 150 mg by days 4–7
- Target dose range: 150–225 mg daily (can divide dose for immediate-release tablets)
- Maximum dose:
  - Immediate-release: 375 mg daily
  - Extended-release: 225 mg daily
- Renal dosage adjustment: Reduce by 25–50% in patients with CrCl 10–70 mL/min
- Hepatic dosage adjustment: Reduce by 50% in mild to moderate impairment

Adverse Reactions: Most Common
Headache, insomnia, nervousness, somnolence, GI complaints, increased diastolic blood pressure, dizziness, sexual dysfunction

Adverse Reactions: Rare/Severe/Important
SIADH

Major Drug Interactions
Major substrate of CYP3A4 and 2D6

Drugs Affecting Venlafaxine
CYP2D6 and 3A4 inhibitors: Increase effects

Venlafaxine's Effects on Other Drugs
CNS depressants, trazodone: Increases effects

Counseling Points
- Take with food to decrease GI upset
- Extended-release capsules should be swallowed whole; do not crush or chew. Alternatively, contents may be emptied onto a spoonful of applesauce and swallowed without chewing.

Key Points
- Drug should be tapered off over a 2-week period when discontinuing therapy
- Not FDA approved for use in children
- Start elderly patients at half the usual initial dose

ANTIDEPRESSANTS, SELECTIVE SEROTONIN REUPTAKE INHIBITORS

Introduction

When the selective serotonin reuptake inhibitors (SSRIs) came to the market in the late 1980s, this class of antidepressants replaced the tricyclic antidepressants (TCAs) as first-line treatment for depression. Compared to TCAs, SSRIs have a much safer and more favorable side-effect profile. These agents are among the most widely prescribed medications in the United States. They are used for major depressive disorder (MDD) and various anxiety disorders, and their use for nonpsychiatric disorders is increasing.

Mechanism of Action for the Drug Class

SSRIs block presynaptic reuptake of serotonin, thereby increasing the concentration of this CNS neurotransmitter in the synapse

Counseling Points for the Drug Class

- All antidepressants require several weeks of continuous use before symptoms improve. Patients should be cautioned that some side effects will probably occur before the therapeutic effect.
- The most important aspect of treating depression may be that therapy must continue for 6–9 months after improvement. Stopping drug therapy too soon greatly increases the risk of depression returning.
- All SSRIs may cause somnolence or insomnia. Each patient's response should determine if once-daily dosing is in the morning or afternoon.
- Patients should be counseled on the signs and symptoms of serotonin toxicity, especially if on more than one medication that increases serotonin concentrations, due to the increased risk of serotonin syndrome. Such symptoms include agitation, restlessness, diaphoresis, tachycardia, hyperthermia, nausea, vomiting, and loss of coordination.
- Avoid alcohol and maintain adequate hydration unless otherwise restricted
- Counsel patients on the black box warning and to be seen immediately or go to their local ER if symptoms of suicide ideation occur. Also counsel patients to report any sudden changes in mental status.

Key Points for the Drug Class

- There is a black box warning for all antidepressants that these drugs increase the risk of suicidal thinking and behavior in children, adolescents, and young adults (18–24 years of age) with major depressive disorder (MDD) and other psychiatric disorders
- Monitoring parameters for all antidepressants should include suicide ideation (especially at the beginning of therapy or when doses are changed), mental status for efficacy, and the most common side effects of the individual agent. Side-effect monitoring is especially important because side effects can occur before therapeutic effects and negatively impact adherence.
- All antidepressants are contraindicated with the concomitant use of *monoamine oxidase inhibitors* (MAOIs) or sibutramine and use within 14 days of MAOI therapy
- Concomitant use of multiple agents that increase serotonin, such as SSRIs, SNRIs, and TCAs, should be avoided due to the risk for serotonin syndrome, a serious and potentially life-threatening reaction. If this combination is utilized, patients should be educated on the signs and symptoms of serotonin toxicity (see earlier discussion). Other medications that can increase the risk for serotonin syndrome when used with antidepressants include triptans, linezolid, dextromethorphan, meperidine, and OTC treatments for depression, such as 5-HTP, SAMe, and St. John's wort.

Members of the Drug Class

In this section: Citalopram, escitalopram oxalate, fluoxetine, paroxetine, sertraline
Others: Fluvoxamine, vilazodone

◉ Citalopram

Brand Name
Celexa

Generic Name
Citalopram

136 CHAPTER 6 *Central Nervous System Agents*

Rx Only

Dosage Forms
Tablet, oral solution

Usage
Depression,* obsessive compulsive disorder (OCD)

Pregnancy Category C

Dosing
- Initial dose: 20 mg daily, increased in 1–2 weeks to 40 mg daily if little or no response
- Maximum dose:
  - Due to the risk for dose-related QT-interval prolongation, the new recommended maximum dose is 40 mg daily
  - In patients > 60 years of age, poor metabolizers of CYP2C19, or patients on concurrent moderate-to-strong CYP2C19 inhibitors such as cimetidine: 20 mg daily
- Renal dosage adjustment: Use with caution in patients with CrCl < 20 mL/min
- Hepatic dosage adjustment: Do not exceed 20 mg in patients with hepatic impairment

Adverse Effects: Most Common
Nausea, loss of appetite; somnolence or insomnia, sexual dysfunction, headache, xerostomia, diaphoresis

Adverse Effects: Rare/Severe/Important
Hyponatremia, SIADH

Major Drug Interactions
- Major substrate of CYP2C19 and 3A4
- Contraindicated with pimozide

Drugs Affecting Citalopram
- Strong CYP2D6, 2C19, 3A4 inhibitors, including quinidine, some protease inhibitors, ticlopidine: Increase levels
- Carbamazepine and other strong CYP inducers: Decrease levels

Citalopram's Effect on Other Drugs
CNS depressants, buspirone, clozapine: Increases effect

Contraindications
Previously, use in patients with conditions known to have a risk of QT prolongation was contraindicated; however, those who require treatment with citalopram (i.e., no other alternative) may derive benefit from a low dose such as 20 mg as long as diligent ECG monitoring is employed

Counseling Point
Start elderly patients at half the usual initial doses

Key Point
Drug should be tapered off over a 2-week period when discontinuing therapy

◉ Escitalopram Oxalate

Brand Name
Lexapro

Generic Name
Escitalopram oxalate

Rx Only

Dosage Forms
Tablet, oral solution

Usage
Depression,* generalized anxiety disorder (GAD)*

Pregnancy Category C

Dosing
- Initial dose: 10 mg daily, which may be increased to 20 mg after 1–2 weeks
- Maximum dose: 20 mg daily
- Hepatic dosage adjustment:
  - Mild to moderate hepatic impairment:
    - Initial dose: 5 mg
    - Maximum dose: 10 mg
  - Severe hepatic impairment: Has not been studied, no recommendations available (use with caution)

Adverse Reactions: Most Common
Nausea, loss of appetite, somnolence or insomnia, headache, sexual dysfunction

Adverse Reactions: Rare/Severe/Important
Hyponatremia, SIADH

Major Drug Interactions
- Major substrate of CYP2C19 and 3A4
- Contraindicated with pimozide

Drugs Affecting Escitalopram
- Strong CYP2D6, 2C19, 3A4 inhibitors including quinidine, some protease inhibitors, ticlopidine: Increase effects
- Serotonin agonists (e.g., "triptans"): May result in serotonin syndrome

Escitalopram's Effect on Other Drugs
CNS depressants, buspirone, clozapine: Increases effects

Counseling Point
Start elderly patients at half the usual initial doses

Key Points
- Drug should be tapered off over a 2-week period when discontinuing therapy
- This drug is simply the S-enantiomer of citalopram and may not have advantages over citalopram. The dosing ratio between the two is 1:2 (i.e., 10 mg of escitalopram is equal to 20 mg of citalopram).

Fluoxetine

Brand Names

Prozac, Prozac Weekly, Sarafem

Generic Name

Fluoxetine

Rx Only

Dosage Forms

Capsule, tablet, delayed-release capsule for weekly dosing, oral solution

Usage

Depression,* obsessive compulsive disorder (OCD), bulimia nervosa, premenstrual dysphoric disorder (PMDD),* panic disorder with or without agoraphobia, in combination with olanzapine for treatment-resistant or bipolar I depression

Pregnancy Category C

Dosing

- Initial dose: 10–20 mg daily
- Dosage adjustments: Adjustments may be made every 2 weeks to a maximum dose of 80 mg daily
- OCD and bulimia nervosa: Often require high end of the dosage range
- Once-weekly dosing with 90 mg delayed-release capsule: May replace 20 mg daily dosage (rarely used product)
- Renal dosage adjustment: Use lower doses and monitor closely in patients with severe renal disease
- Hepatic dosage adjustment: Use lower doses and monitor closely in patients with severe hepatic disease

Adverse Reactions: Most Common

Nausea, loss of appetite, xerostomia, insomnia, sexual dysfunction, headache, anxiety, nervousness (CNS stimulation)

Adverse Reactions: Rare/Severe/Important

Hyponatremia, SIADH

Major Drug Interactions

- Major substrate for CYP2C9 and 2D6
- Strong inhibitor of CYP2D6, moderate inhibitor of CYP2C19 and 1A2
- Contraindicated with thioridazine and ziprasidone. Do not start these medications until 5 weeks after the discontinuation of fluoxetine.

Drugs Affecting Fluoxetine

- Carbamazepine: Decreases levels
- CYP2C9 and 2D6 inhibitors: Increase levels

Fluoxetine's Effect on Other Drugs

Alcohol, phenytoin, clozapine, tramadol, and others metabolized by CYP2D6, 1A2, and 2C19: Increases levels

Counseling Points

- Fluoxetine should always be taken in the morning to avoid insomnia. It is the most stimulating of the SSRIs.
- Do not crush, chew, or break Prozac Weekly capsules

Key Points

- Appetite suppression is common, and the drug is sometimes used for obesity
- The parent molecule and active metabolite, norfluoxetine, have a very long half-life. Therefore, steady-state concentrations may not be reached for weeks, and the drug may remain in the body for weeks after discontinuation.
- Use cautiously and at reduced dosages in elderly patients (because of its long half-life), if at all
- This medication is approved for use in children 7 years and older

Paroxetine

Brand Names

Paxil, Paxil CR, Pexeva

Generic Name

Paroxetine

Rx Only

Dosage Forms

Tablet, controlled-release tablet, extended-release tablet, oral suspension

Usage

Depression,* obsessive compulsive disorder (OCD),* panic disorder with or without agoraphobia, seasonal affective disorder (SAD), generalized anxiety disorder (GAD),* posttraumatic stress disorder,* premenstrual dysphoric disorder (PMDD)

Pregnancy Category D

Dosing

- Initial dose: 10–20 mg daily
- Dosage adjustment: May increase by 10 mg every 1–2 weeks
- Maximum dose: 60 mg daily
- Paxil CR:
  - Initial dose: 25 mg daily
  - Maximum dose: 62.5 mg daily
- OCD and panic disorder: Higher doses may be necessary

- Renal dosage adjustment: If CrCl < 30 mL/min:
  - Immediate-release:
    - Initial dose: 10 mg daily
    - Maximum dose: 40 mg daily
  - Paxil CR:
    - Initial dose: 12.5 mg daily
    - Maximum dose: 50 mg daily
- Hepatic dosage adjustment: Severe hepatic impairment:
  - Immediate-release:
    - Initial dose: 10 mg daily
    - Maximum dose: 40 mg daily
  - Paxil CR:
    - Initial dose: 12.5 mg daily
    - Maximum dose: 50 mg daily

Adverse Reactions: Most Common

Nausea, loss of appetite, somnolence or insomnia, headache, sexual dysfunction

Adverse Reactions: Rare/Severe/Important

Hyponatremia, SIADH

Major Drug Interactions

- Major substrate of CYP2D6
- Strong inhibitor of CYP2D6, moderate inhibitor of CYP2B6
- Contraindicated with tamoxifen and thioridazine

Drugs Affecting Paroxetine
- Buspirone, cimetidine, tramadol: Increase levels
- Carbamazepine: Decreases levels

Paroxetine's Effect on Other Drugs
- Strong inhibitor of CYP2D6 and moderate inhibitor of CYP2B6
- CNS depressants, beta blockers, carbamazepine, buspirone: Increases levels

Counseling Points

- Take in the morning to avoid insomnia
- Do not crush, chew, or break the controlled-release formulation

Key Points

- This medication should be tapered over several weeks for discontinuation
- Paroxetine causes more sexual dysfunction and anticholinergic side effects than other SSRIs
- Paroxetine has the most drug interactions of all of the SSRIs
- Use this agent cautiously and at reduced dosages in elderly patients
- There is no real advantage to the patented controlled-release formulation

◉ Sertraline

Brand Name

Zoloft

Generic Name

Sertraline

Rx Only

Dosage Forms

Tablet, solution

Usage

Depression,* obsessive compulsive disorder (OCD),* panic disorder,* posttraumatic stress disorder (PTSD),* seasonal affective disorder (SAD), generalized anxiety disorder (GAD), eating disorders

Pregnancy Category C

Dosing

- Initial dose: 25–50 mg daily, which is usually increased to an effective range of 100–200 mg daily
- Hepatic dosage adjustment: Use cautiously in patients with hepatic impairment due to extensive hepatic metabolism of this agent

Adverse Reactions: Most Common

Nausea, diarrhea, loss of appetite, somnolence or insomnia, headache, sexual dysfunction, dizziness, fatigue, xerostomia, tremors, diaphoresis

Adverse Reactions: Rare/Severe/Important

Hyponatremia, SIADH

Major Drug Interactions

- Major substrate of CYP2D6 and a minor substrate of many others
- Moderate inhibitor of CYP2B6, 2C19, 2D6, and 3A4
- Contraindicated with thioridazine, pimozide, and disulfiram

Drugs Affecting Sertraline
Strong CYP2D6 inhibitors: Increase effects

Sertraline's Effect on Other Drugs
Carbamazepine, phenytoin, CNS depressants, clozapine, risperidone: May increase effects

Key Points

- There are fewer clinically significant drug interactions with this agent compared to other SSRIs when used at lower doses, although these doses are often subtherapeutic (50–100 mg daily)
- On average, initial doses must be increased for full therapeutic effect, probably more so than with other SSRIs
- Start elderly patients at half the usual initial doses

Introduction

The tricyclic antidepressants (TCAs) are one of the oldest groups of antidepressant agents. Because of their many adverse effects, especially their anticholinergic and sedative properties, as well as the introduction of safer, more favorable agents such as the SSRIs, these medications are not frequently used for depression, nor are they considered first-line therapy. The possibility of death upon overdose is another drawback with these agents. These drugs are more commonly used for the treatment of chronic nerve pain conditions at lower doses than to treat depression. They still have a role in treatment-resistant depression (i.e., after therapeutic failure with several first-line agents).

Mechanism of Action for the Drug Class

TCAs block presynaptic reuptake of serotonin and norepinephrine, thereby increasing concentrations of these CNS neurotransmitters in the synapse. It is their action on norepinephrine that is responsible for their efficacy in neuropathic pain conditions.

Counseling Points for the Drug Class

- All antidepressants require several weeks of continuous use before symptoms improve. Patients should be cautioned that some side effects will probably occur before the therapeutic effect.
- The most important aspect of treating depression may be that therapy must continue for 6–9 months after improvement. Stopping drug therapy too soon greatly increases the risk of depression returning.
- Patients should be counseled on the signs and symptoms of serotonin toxicity, especially if on more than one medication that increases serotonin concentrations due to the increased risk of serotonin syndrome. Such symptoms include agitation, restlessness, diaphoresis, tachycardia, hyperthermia, nausea, vomiting, and loss of coordination.
- Orthostatic hypotension is possible with these agents. Advise patients to take a full minute at the side of the bed before getting up in the morning.
- Sedation decreases with continued treatment
- Recommend sugarless drinks, candies, and gum for dry mouth. More water is the easiest and most convenient "therapy" for dry mouth and to prevent constipation.
- Avoid alcohol and maintain adequate hydration unless otherwise restricted
- Counsel patients on the black box warning and to be seen immediately or go to their local ER if symptoms of suicide ideation occur. Also counsel patients to report any sudden changes in mental status.

Key Points for the Drug Class

- There is a black box warning for all antidepressants that these drugs increase the risk of suicidal thinking and behavior in children, adolescents, and young adults (18–24 years of age) with MDD and other psychiatric disorders
- Monitoring parameters for all antidepressants should include suicide ideation (especially at the beginning of therapy or when doses are changed), mental status for efficacy, and the most common side effects of the individual agent. Side-effect monitoring is especially important because side effects can occur before therapeutic effects and negatively impact adherence.
- All antidepressants are contraindicated with the concomitant use of *monoamine oxidase* inhibitors (MAOIs) or sibutramine and use within 14 days of MAOI therapy
- Concomitant use of multiple agents that increase serotonin, such as SSRIs, SNRIs, and TCAs, should be avoided due to the risk for serotonin syndrome, a serious and potentially life-threatening reaction. If this combination is utilized, patients should be educated on the signs and symptoms of serotonin toxicity (see previous discussion). Other medications that can increase the risk for serotonin syndrome when used with antidepressants include triptans, linezolid, dextromethorphan, meperidine, and OTC treatments for depression, such as 5-HTP, SAMe, and St. John's wort.

Members of the Drug Class

In this section: Amitriptyline, doxepin, nortriptyline
Others: Amoxapine, clomipramine, desipramine, imipramine, protriptyline, trimipramine

◉ Amitriptyline

Brand Name
Elavil

Generic Name
Amitriptyline

Rx Only

Dosage Forms
Tablet, injection

Usage
Depression, neuropathic pain syndromes,* migraine prophylaxis*

Pregnancy Category C

Dosing

- Initial dose: 10–25 mg at bedtime
- Dosage adjustment: To prevent severe side effects, the dose should be increased gradually. Adjustments should be made every 2–3 days at 10–25 mg increments. It may take weeks to get a response after leveling off at approximately 150 mg daily. The dose may need to be increased gradually to 200 mg or more.
- Maximum dose: 300 mg daily
- Renal dosage adjustment: No specific dose adjustment recommended. Use with caution and monitor plasma levels and patient response.
- Hepatic dosage adjustment: No specific dose adjustment recommended. Use with caution and monitor plasma levels and patient response.

Pharmacokinetic Monitoring

Therapeutic levels: 100–250 ng/mL

Adverse Reactions: Most Common

Anticholinergic effects (dry mouth, constipation, urinary hesitancy, blurred vision), orthostatic hypotension, sedation (tolerance to these effects is common)

Adverse Reactions: Rare/Severe/Important

AV conduction changes, heart block, myocardial infarction

Major Drug Interactions

- Major substrate of CYP2D6
- Contraindicated with thioridazine, ziprasidone, and cisapride

Drugs Affecting Amitriptyline

- CYP2D6 inhibitors (e.g., quinidine, protease inhibitors, SSRIs, valproic acid, cimetidine, tramadol): Increase effects
- Carbamazepine, barbiturates, rifamycins: Decrease effects

Amitriptyline's Effect on Other Drugs

CNS depressants, anticholinergic drugs, alpha-1 agonists, quinidine, tramadol, thioridazine, and antiarrhythmics: Increases effects

Contraindication

Acute recovery phase post myocardial infarction

Essential Monitoring Parameters

ECG in older adults and patients with cardiac disease, blood pressure and pulse rate prior to and during initial therapy. Amitriptyline is one of the few antidepressants where blood level data is sometimes used, although in the average clinical practice levels are not frequently drawn because they do not always correlate with clinical effectiveness. Therapeutic levels of amitriptyline and its active metabolite, nortriptyline, should be in the range of 100–250 ng/mL and 50–150 ng/mL, respectively. Toxicity can be seen at concentrations > 0.5 µg/mL.

Key Points

- Start elderly patients at half the usual initial doses
- Monitor glucose closely in diabetic patients because this medication can cause hyperglycemia
- Amitriptyline, a tertiary TCA, is metabolized to the active metabolite nortriptyline, a secondary TCA that is marketed as a separate agent. Compared to tertiary TCAs, secondary TCAs have a slightly more favorable side-effect profile (e.g., fewer anticholinergic effects).

◉ Doxepin

Brand Names

Sinequan, Prudoxin, Zonalon, Silenor, Adapin

Generic Name

Doxepin

Rx Only

Dosage Forms

Capsule, tablet, cream, oral solution

Usage

Depression,* insomnia characterized by difficulty with sleep maintenance, pruritic skin conditions (topical cream)

Pregnancy Category C

Dosing

- Initial dose: 25–50 mg at bedtime
- Dosage adjustment: Dose may be increased very gradually to 150–300 mg over 2–3 weeks
- Maximum dose: A single dose should not exceed 150 mg
- Silenor (insomnia):
  - 3–6 mg once daily 30 minutes prior to bedtime
  - Maximum dose: 6 mg daily
- Topical cream: Apply as a thin film four times daily
- Hepatic dosage adjustment: Use a lower dose and adjust gradually in hepatic impairment

Adverse Reactions: Most Common (Oral)

Anticholinergic effects (dry mouth, constipation, urinary hesitancy, blurred vision), orthostatic hypotension, sedation

Adverse Reactions: Rare/Severe/Important (Oral)

AV conduction changes, heart block, myocardial infarction

Major Drug Interactions

- Major substrate of CYP2D6
- Contraindicated with thioridazine and ziprasidone

Drugs Affecting Doxepin

- CYP2D6 inhibitors (e.g., quinidine, protease inhibitors, SSRIs, valproic acid, tramadol): Increase effects
- Carbamazepine: Decreases effects

Doxepin's Effect on Other Drugs

CNS depressants, anticholinergic drugs, alpha-1 agonists, quinidine, tramadol: Increases effects

Contraindications

Narrow-angle glaucoma, urinary retention

Key Points

- Administration should be limited to bedtime to make use of its sedative effects
- Elderly patients more prone to experiencing the "hangover effect." Start elderly patients at half the usual initial dose.

◉ Nortriptyline

Brand Names

Pamelor, Aventyl

Generic Name

Nortriptyline

Rx Only

Dosage Forms

Capsule, solution

Usage

Depression*

Pregnancy Category Not Defined

Dosing

- Initial dose: 25–50 mg daily
- Dosage adjustment: Increase slowly to a maximum dose of 150 mg daily
- Hepatic dosage adjustment: Use lower doses with slower titration in hepatic impairment

Pharmacokinetic Monitoring

Therapeutic levels of nortriptyline should be in the range of 50–150 ng/mL. Toxicity can be seen with levels > 500 ng/mL.

Adverse Reactions: Most Common

Anticholinergic effects (dry mouth, constipation, urinary hesitancy, blurred vision), orthostatic hypotension, sedation. These effects are less than that of the parent compound, amitriptyline.

Adverse Reactions: Rare/Severe/Important

AV conduction changes, heart block, myocardial infarction

Major Drug Interactions

- Major substrate of CYP2D6
- Contraindicated with thioridazine and ziprasidone

Drugs Affecting Nortriptyline

- CYP2D6 inhibitors (e.g., quinidine, protease inhibitors, SSRIs, valproic acid, tramadol): Increase effects
- Carbamazepine: Decreases effects

Nortriptyline's Effect on Other Drugs

CNS depressants, anticholinergic drugs, alpha-1 agonists, quinidine, tramadol: Increases effects

Contraindication

Acute recovery phase post myocardial infarction

Essential Monitoring Parameters

ECG in older adults and patients with cardiac disease; blood pressure and pulse rate prior to and during initial therapy; weight. Nortriptyline is one of the few antidepressants where blood level data is sometimes used, although in the average clinical practice levels are not commonly drawn because they do not always correlate with clinical efficacy.

Key Points

- Nortriptyline, a secondary TCA, is the active metabolite of amitriptyline
- It has a slightly more favorable side-effect profile compared to amitriptyline, especially with regard to sedation
- Like amitriptyline, nortriptyline is also used sometimes in the treatment of chronic pain syndromes
- Start elderly patients at half the usual initial dose

ANTIMANIC AGENTS, MOOD STABILIZERS

Introduction

This class of psychiatric agents is essentially made up of lithium and valproic acid (and its congeners). Valproic acid is covered in the section on anticonvulsant agents. These drugs are mainstays in the acute and maintenance therapy of the bipolar disorders.

Mechanism of Action for Lithium

Lithium produces multiple effects on CNS neurotransmitters via altered cation transport across cell membranes, which influences the reuptake of serotonin and/or norepinephrine

Members of the Drug Class

In this section: Lithium carbonate
Others: Valproic acid

◉ Lithium Carbonate

Brand Names

Eskalith, Eskalith CR, Lithobid

Generic Names

Lithium carbonate, lithium citrate (liquid formulations)

Rx Only

Dosage Forms

Capsule, tablet, extended-release capsule, extended-release tablet, oral solution

Usage

Bipolar disorder,* mania, augmenting agent for refractory depression

Pregnancy Category D

Dosing

- Initial dose:
  - 600–1,200 mg daily (in 2–3 divided doses)
  - Extended-release: 900–1,800 mg daily in 2 doses
- Dosage adjustments are made based on serum levels
- Renal dosage adjustment:
  - CrCl 10–50 mL/min: Administer 50–75% of dose
  - CrCl < 10 mL/min: Administer 25–50% of dose
  - Severe renal impairment: Should not be used

Pharmacokinetic Monitoring

Trough levels should be drawn 8–12 hours after the previous dose. Levels for acute mania (0.6–1.2 mEq/L) are slightly higher than maintenance levels (0.5–0.9 mEq/L). Levels should be drawn twice weekly until levels and clinical status are stable, then every 1–3 months thereafter.

Adverse Reactions: Most Common

GI complaints, dizziness, polydipsia, tremor, sedation, leucocytosis

Adverse Reactions: Rare/Severe/Important

Hypothyroidism, arrhythmias

Major Drug Interactions

Drugs Affecting Lithium

- Diuretics, NSAIDs, tetracyclines, angiotensin receptor antagonists: Decrease excretion of lithium, increasing lithium levels
- High sodium intake: Increases excretion of lithium, decreasing lithium levels

Lithium's Effect on Other Drugs

- MAOIs: Possibility of severe CNS reactions
- CNS neurotoxicity has been rarely reported when lithium is added to some antipsychotic agents, SSRIs, TCAs, and phenytoin

Contraindications

Severe cardiovascular or renal disease, severe debilitation, dehydration, sodium depletion, pregnancy

Essential Monitoring Parameters

Lithium levels, renal, thyroid, and cardiovascular function, fluid status, serum electrolytes, CBC with differential, urinalysis, pregnancy test for nonsterile females, symptoms of toxicity (GI complaints, tremors, confusion, somnolence, seizures)

Counseling Points

- Drug concentration monitoring is frequently performed
- Do not crush or chew extended-release products
- Maintain adequate hydration unless otherwise restricted
- Avoid changes in sodium content because reduction in sodium can increase lithium toxicity
- Inform your healthcare provider before taking new medications, including OTC products, because many can interact with lithium
- Decreased appetite, altered taste, drowsiness, and dizziness may occur, especially early in therapy. Immediately report unresolved diarrhea, abrupt changes in weight, muscular tremors, lack of coordination, fever, or changes in urinary volume.

Key Points

- Lithium is one of the first-line treatments for the bipolar disorders
- Lithium is contraindicated in severe renal or cardiac disease and in pregnancy
- After long-term use, hypothyroidism may develop in up to 10% of patients. Treat with levothyroxine.
- Lithium is not metabolized. It is excreted through the kidneys unchanged. Monitoring renal function and electrolytes throughout therapy is prudent.
- Lithium will be reabsorbed when extra sodium is excreted due to diuretic therapy, heavy perspiration, etc.
- Diuretics, ACE inhibitors, and NSAIDs increase lithium concentrations. Use with caution or decrease lithium dose and monitor concentrations.

ANTIPSYCHOTIC AGENTS, ATYPICAL

Introduction

Atypical agents have replaced the older, typical antipsychotics, such as haloperidol, as first-line treatment of psychotic diagnoses, especially for chronic management in the outpatient setting. Compared to typical agents, atypicals have fewer extrapyramidal symptoms (EPS), a collection of drug-induced movement disorders. The incidence of other adverse effects, such as anticholinergic effects, may also be somewhat lower. The tradeoff is that atypicals can cause significant weight gain, which can lead to increases in glucose, lipids, and diabetes mellitus. Some of the agents are approved as adjunctive treatments for depression.

Mechanism of Action for the Drug Class

These agents have effects on multiple CNS neurotransmitter systems. Dopamine inhibition (D_1, D_2, and D_4 receptors) and serotonin antagonism (5-HT_2), along with unknown effects on glutamate and GABA, lead to the therapeutic effects in the treatment of schizophrenia and other psychotic states.

Counseling Points for the Drug Class

- When appropriate, suggest to patients that they speak to their physician about receiving their entire daily dose at bedtime
- Patients must not use alcohol or other CNS depressants. Patients also should avoid drugs of abuse because they will worsen symptoms.
- Advise caution with driving and operating heavy machinery, especially for the more sedating agents
- Patients should use caution in hot weather due to the potential for thermoregulatory changes. Maintain adequate hydration unless otherwise restricted.
- Diabetic patients need to closely monitor blood glucose and report any changes
- Report changes in weight and psychiatric status
- Immediately report chest pain, palpitations, persistent GI effects, tremors, altered gait, changes in vision, fever, and hyperpyrexia, especially when associated with muscle rigidity and altered mental status (signs of neuroleptic malignant syndrome [NMS], a rare but severe and life-threatening condition)
- The risks of extrapyramidal reactions should be explained. Patients should be told to report abnormal involuntary body movements or abnormal muscle contractions. If there is an acute problem, they should contact their physician immediately or go to the emergency department of their local hospital.
- If a dose is missed, do not double the dose. Resume the regular schedule the following day.
- When possible, explain to patients that their illness is a biological problem, which should be treated like any other medical diagnosis requiring treatment
- Do not stop the medication or stop regular visits to a healthcare provider

Key Points for the Drug Class

- All antipsychotics have a black box warning that patients with dementia-related behavioral disorders treated with atypical antipsychotics are at an increased risk of death compared to placebo
- Metabolic complications should be monitored with all atypical antipsychotic agents. Monitor weight prior to treatment, at 4 weeks, 8 weeks, 12 weeks, and then quarterly. Monitor waist circumference, BMI, and vital signs. Consider switching agents if there is a 5% or greater increase in weight from baseline. Monitor fasting lipids and glucose/Hgb A1c prior to treatment, at 3 months, and then annually.
- Monitor for EPS with use of the abnormal involuntary movement scale (AIMS)

Members of the Drug Class

In this section: Aripiprazole, olanzapine, quetiapine, risperidone, ziprasidone
Others: Clozapine, paliperidone, asenapine, lurasidone

⊙ Aripiprazole

Brand Names
Abilify, Abilify Discmelt

Generic Name
Aripiprazole

Rx Only

Dosage Forms
Tablet, oral dissolving tablet (ODT), oral solution, injection solution

Usage
Schizophrenia,* bipolar disorder,* augmenting agent in treatment of major depressive disorder (MDD), treatment of irritability associated with autistic disorder, agitation associated with schizophrenia or bipolar I disorder (injection)

Pregnancy Category C

Dosing
- Initial dose: 10–15 mg daily, which may be increased over a few weeks to a maximum of 30 mg daily
- Bipolar disorder: Acute treatment may use higher doses
- Depression: Lower doses used as adjunct to treatment
- Renal dosage adjustment: No dosage adjustments are needed
- Hepatic dosage adjustment: No dosage adjustments are needed

Adverse Effects: Most Common

Agitation, insomnia, headache, akathisia, and other extrapyramidal effects

Adverse Effects: Rare/Severe/Important

NMS, hyperglycemia, drug-induced diabetes mellitus

Major Drug Interactions

Major substrate of CYP2D6 and 3A4

Drugs Affecting Aripiprazole

- Inhibitors of CYP450 such as fluoxetine, paroxetine, quinidine, azole antifungals, and clarithromycin: Increase effects
- Inducers of CYP450 such as carbamazepine, phenobarbital, and phenytoin: Decrease effects

Aripiprazole's Effect on Other Drugs

CNS depressants: Additive effects

Counseling Point

Take at the same time each day without regard to meals

Key Points

- There is a black box warning that all antidepressants can increase the risk of suicidal thinking and behavior in children, adolescents, and young adults (18–24 years of age) with depression and other psychiatric disorders. Note that aripiprazole is not approved for adjunctive treatment of depression in children.
- This drug is usually used as a long-term agent
- This agent may have a slightly different mechanism of action than the other atypical antipsychotic agents. It may have more and various effects on serotonin receptors than any of the other atypical agents.
- This agent may cause minimal or less weight gain compared to other atypical agents. It is often used for this reason.
- Akathisia is common with this agent
- Medication errors have occurred because the drug's generic name has confused some healthcare professionals who thought this drug was a proton pump inhibitor or an antifungal agent

⊚ Olanzapine

Brand Names

Zyprexa, Zyprexa IntraMuscular, Zyprexa Zydis, Zyprexa Relprevv

Generic Name

Olanzapine

Rx Only

Dosage Forms

Tablet, oral dissolving tablet (ODT), injection, long-acting injection

Usage

Schizophrenia,* bipolar disorder,* in combination with fluoxetine for treatment-resistant or bipolar I depression, psychosis/agitation associated with Alzheimer's disease

Pregnancy Category C

Dosing

- Initial dose: 5–10 mg daily
- Dosage adjustment: May be increased by 5 mg daily at weekly intervals to 15–20 mg daily
- Maximum dose: 20 mg daily, is often exceeded up to 30 mg daily
- Hepatic dosage adjustment: No specific dosing recommendations are given for hepatic impairment, although adjustment may be necessary

Adverse Effects: Most Common

Somnolence, headache, weight gain, glucose and lipid abnormalities

Adverse Effects: Rare/Severe/Important

NMS, hyperglycemia, drug-induced diabetes mellitus, extrapyramidal effects

Major Drug Interactions

Major substrate of CYP1A2

Drugs Affecting Olanzapine

- CYP1A2 inhibitors (e.g., fluvoxamine, ketoconazole, others): Increase levels
- CYP inducers (e.g., rifampin, carbamazepine, omeprazole): Decrease levels

Olanzapine's Effect on Other Drugs

CNS depressants: Increases effects

Counseling Points

- Olanzapine frequently causes drowsiness. These effects are more common at the beginning of therapy.
- Remove the ODT from the foil blister by peeling back the foil. Do not push the tablet through the foil. Place tablet in mouth immediately upon removal. Tablet dissolves rapidly in saliva and may be swallowed with or without liquid.
- Olanzapine comes coformulated with fluoxetine (Symbyax)

Key Points

- There is a black box warning for the injection Zyprexa Relprevv warning of sedation (including coma) and delirium (including agitation, anxiety, confusion, and disorientation) following the use of this product
- This drug is usually used as a long-term agent
- Of the atypicals, olanzapine is one of the worst at causing weight gain and subsequent metabolic complications

Quetiapine

Brand Names

Seroquel, Seroquel XR

Generic Name

Quetiapine

Rx Only

Dosage Forms

Tablet, extended-release tablet

Usage

Schizophrenia,* bipolar disorder,* bipolar depression, adjunctive treatment of depression

Pregnancy Category C

Dosing

- Initial dose: 25–50 once or twice daily
- Dosage adjustment: Dose may be increased by 50–100 mg daily every few days to usual target dose of 400–500 mg daily
- Maximum dose: 800 mg daily
- Hepatic dosage adjustment: Caution in hepatic impairment. Use smaller dose increases (25–50 mg daily)

Adverse Effects: Most Common

Somnolence, headache, sedation, weight gain, lipid and glucose abnormalities

Adverse Effects: Rare/Severe/Important

Neuroleptic malignant syndrome, hyperglycemia, drug-induced diabetes mellitus, extrapyramidal effects

Major Drug Interactions

Major substrate of CYP3A4

Drugs Affecting Quetiapine

- Strong CYP3A4 inducers (e.g., carbamazepine, phenytoin, phenobarbital): Decrease levels
- CYP3A4 inhibitors (e.g., azole antifungals, protease inhibitors): Increase levels

Quetiapine's Effect on Other Drugs

CNS depressants: Increases effects

Counseling Points

- Extended-release capsules should be swallowed whole and not split, chewed, or crushed. Take the medication without food or with a light meal.
- This agent will cause drowsiness. These effects are more common at the beginning of therapy.

Key Points

- There is a black box warning that all antidepressants can increase the risk of suicidal thinking and behavior in children, adolescents, and young adults (18–24 years of age) with depression and other psychiatric disorders
- This drug is usually used as a long-term agent
- This agent has been used in low doses (25–50 mg) as a hypnotic agent. This suboptimal practice should be discouraged because the risks do not justify the benefits.

Risperidone

Brand Names

Risperdal, Risperdal Consta, Risperdal M-tab

Generic Name

Risperidone

Rx Only

Dosage Forms

Tablet, solution, oral dissolving tablet (ODT), extended-release injection

Usage

Schizophrenia,* bipolar disorder,* treatment of irritability or aggression in autism, Tourette syndrome

Pregnancy Category C

Dosing

- Initial dose: 1 mg twice daily
- Dosage adjustment: Increase dose every 1–2 days to target dose of 4–6 mg daily
- Maximum dose: 16 mg daily
- Renal dosage adjustment: Initial doses should be halved in patients with renal impairment
- Hepatic dosage adjustment: Initial doses should be halved in patients with hepatic impairment
- Careful monitoring is required for continued therapy

Adverse Effects: Most Common

Somnolence, headache, sedation, weight gain, lipid abnormalities, extrapyramidal side effects

Adverse Effects: Rare/Severe/Important

Neuroleptic malignant syndrome, hyperglycemia, drug-induced diabetes mellitus

Major Drug Interactions

Major substrate for CYP2D6

Drugs Affecting Risperidone

- Carbamazepine and other CYP inducers: Decrease levels
- CYP2D6 inhibitors such as paroxetine, quinidine, and some protease inhibitors: Increase levels

Risperidone's Effect on Other Drugs

CNS depressants: Increases effects

Counseling Point

Risperidone may cause drowsiness. This effect is more common at the beginning of therapy.

Key Points

- This drug is usually used as a long-term agent
- It may prolong the QT interval
- The orthostatic hypotensive effects of this agent are due to alpha-adrenergic blockade and are most commonly seen at initiation of therapy
- Out of all the atypicals, risperidone has the highest incidence of extrapyramidal symptoms, particularly at doses > 4–5 mg daily

◉ Ziprasidone

Brand Name

Geodon

Generic Name

Ziprasidone

Rx Only

Dosage Forms

Capsule, injection

Usage

Schizophrenia,* bipolar disorder,* acute agitation in patients with schizophrenia (injection)*

Pregnancy Category C

Dosing

- Initial oral: 20–40 mg twice daily that can be rapidly increased to target dose of 80 mg twice daily. It should be given with morning and evening meals because administration on an empty stomach reduces absorption by ~40%.
- IM dosing for acute agitation: 10–20 mg/dose up to 40 mg daily. Oral therapy should replace continual IM injections.

- Renal dosage adjustment: No dosage recommendations for renal impairment. The IM formulation should be used with caution in renal impairment because it contains cyclodextrin, an excipient that is renally cleared.
- Hepatic dosage adjustment: No dosage recommendations for hepatic impairment

Adverse Effects: Most Common

Headache, somnolence, extrapyramidal side effects

Adverse Effects: Rare/Severe/Important

QT-prolongation, NMS, hyperglycemia, drug-induced diabetes mellitus

Major Drug Interactions

Minor substrate of CYP3A4 and 1A2

Drugs Affecting Ziprasidone

Azole antifungals and ciprofloxacin: Increase effects

Ziprasidone's Effect on Other Drugs

- CNS depressants: Increases effects
- Use with caution with drugs that prolong the QTc interval because additive prolongation can occur

Contraindications

History of or current prolonged QT, congenital long QT syndrome, recent myocardial infarction, uncompensated heart failure, concurrent use of other QT-prolonging agents, such as class Ia or class III antiarrhythmics

Counseling Points

- Drowsiness can occur and is more common at the beginning of therapy
- This agent must be taken with food in order to be properly absorbed

Key Point

This drug is usually used as a long-term agent and must be taken with food to be effective. The IM formulation is also used acutely in the inpatient setting.

ANTIPSYCHOTIC AGENTS, TYPICAL

Introduction

The first-generation antipsychotic agents, sometimes called "typical" antipsychotic agents, were the first class of medications used to treat schizophrenia and related psychoses. The newer atypical agents have essentially replaced their use in chronic management, although typical agents such as haloperidol are still widely used in the inpatient setting to treat acute psychoses. Haloperidol is also used in palliative care to treat nausea, vomiting, and delirium. In fact, haloperidol is a drug of choice for the management of delirium. Typical antipsychotics have a high incidence of extrapyramidal symptoms (EPS), a collection of drug-induced movement disorders that can have a profound negative impact on daily functioning and quality of life. One type of EPS, tardive dyskinesia, is irreversible and untreatable.

Mechanism of Action for the Drug Class

These agents block postsynaptic mesolimbic dopaminergic D_1 and D_2 receptors, improving positive symptoms associated with schizophrenia and other psychotic states. Dopamine blockade in other areas of the brain is responsible for typical antipsychotic toxicity, including EPS, and increases in serum prolactin.

Counseling Points for the Drug Class

- When appropriate, suggest to patients that they speak to their physician about receiving their entire daily dose at bedtime
- Patients must not use alcohol or other CNS depressants. Patients should also avoid drugs of abuse because they can worsen symptoms.
- Advise caution with driving and operating heavy machinery, especially for the more sedating agents
- Patients should use caution in hot weather due to the potential for thermoregulatory changes. Maintain adequate hydration unless restricted.
- Diabetic patients need to closely monitor blood glucose and report any changes
- Report changes in weight and psychiatric status
- Immediately report chest pain, palpitations, persistent GI effects, tremors, altered gait, changes in vision or mental status, fever, and hyperpyrexia, especially when associated with muscle rigidity and altered mental status (signs of neuroleptic malignant syndrome [NMS], a rare but severe and life-threatening condition)
- The risks of extrapyramidal reactions should be explained. Patients should be told to report abnormal involuntary body movements or abnormal muscle contractions. If there is an acute problem, they should contact their physician immediately or go to the emergency department of their local hospital.
- If a dose is missed, do not double the dose. Resume the regular schedule the following day.
- When possible, explain that their illness is a biological problem, which should be considered like any other medical diagnosis requiring treatment
- Do not stop the medication or stop regular visits to healthcare providers

Key Points for the Drug Class

- There is a black box warning for all antipsychotics that patients with dementia-related behavioral disorders treated with antipsychotics are at an increased risk of death compared to placebo
- Monitor for EPS with use of the abnormal involuntary movement scale (AIMS)

Members of the Drug Class

In this section: Haloperidol
Others: Chlorpromazine, fluphenazine, loxapine, molindone, perphenazine, thioridazine, thiothixene, trifluoperazine

◉ Haloperidol

Brand Names
Haldol, Haldol Decanoate

Generic Name
Haloperidol

Rx Only

Dosage Forms
Tablet, oral solution, injection solution, injection oil

Usage
Schizophrenia,* nonschizophrenia psychoses,* delirium,* postoperative nausea and vomiting, Tourette disorder

Pregnancy Category C

Dosing
- Psychoses:
  - Oral:
    - Initial dose: 0.5–5 mg two to three times daily
    - Maximum dose: 30 mg daily
  - IM
    - As lactate: 2–5 mg every 4–8 hours as needed
    - As decanoate: 10–15 times the daily oral dose given at 4-week intervals (maintenance dose: 10–15 times initial oral dose)
- Note: QTc prolongation may occur with cumulative doses ≥ 35 mg, and torsade de pointes has been reported with single doses of ≥ 20 mg

Pharmacokinetic Monitoring
Therapeutic levels for psychotic disorders: 5–20 ng/mL (less for Tourette syndrome and mania). Toxicity can be seen at levels > 42 ng/mL. Note that levels are rarely drawn in clinical practice.

Adverse Effects: Most Common
Agitation, insomnia, headache, akathisia, and other extrapyramidal effects

Adverse Effects: Rare/Severe/Important
NMS, severe EPS, cardiac changes such as QT prolongation

Major Drug Interactions
- Major substrate of CYP2D6 and 3A4
- Moderate inhibitor of 2D6 and 3A4

Drugs Affecting Haloperidol
- CYP2D6 and 3A4 inhibitors: Increase levels
- CYP2D6 and 3A4 inducers (e.g., rifampin): Decrease levels

Haloperidol's Effect on Other Drugs
CNS depressants: Additive effects

Contraindications
Parkinson's disease, severe CNS depression, coma

Essential Monitoring Parameters
Vital signs, lipids, glucose, BMI, ECG with off-label IV administration, EPS, serum concentrations

Counseling Points
- The IM formulation may take 2–3 weeks to achieve desired results
- Dilute oral concentration with juice or water
- Avoid skin contact with medication because it may cause contact dermatitis

Key Points

- Typical antipsychotic agents are used primarily for management of acute psychoses in the inpatient setting. Haloperidol is also the drug of choice for delirium management. For the most part, chronic management of psychotic disorders has been replaced by the atypical agents due to their lesser incidence of EPS, although some patients will still be on typical agents long term.
- EPS is an important side effect of typical antipsychotics. Patients should be counseled on the signs and symptoms of EPS and to report to their local ER immediately if such symptoms occur. EPS monitoring using the AIMS should be employed throughout therapy.
- Although haloperidol is used for inpatients due to its favorable cardiovascular effects compared to other typical agents, negative cardiac and ECG changes can occur, specifically QT prolongation, which can lead to torsades de pointes.

CHOLINESTERASE INHIBITORS

Introduction

Donepezil and rivastigmine are reversible inhibitors of acetylcholinesterase used for the treatment of mild to moderate Alzheimer's disease (AD). The rationale for use of these agents in AD is to increase CNS acetylcholine concentrations, which can be deficient in patients with AD.

Mechanism of Action for the Drug Class

The therapeutic effects from donepezil and rivastigmine in AD is primarily due to an increase in the concentration of acetylcholine through the reversible inhibition of hydrolysis by acetylcholinesterase. Donepezil, a piperidine derivative, is a centrally active, reversible inhibitor of acetylcholinesterase and is structurally unrelated to other anticholinesterase agents (i.e., tacrine, physostigmine). Rivastigmine, a carbamate derivative, is an intermediate-acting, reversible acetylcholinesterase inhibitor that is structurally related to physostigmine, but unrelated to donepezil or tacrine.

Members of the Drug Class

In this section: Donepezil, rivastigmine
Others: Galantamine, tacrine

⊙ Donepezil

Brand Names
Aricept, Aricept ODT

Generic Name
Donepezil

Rx Only

Dosage Forms
Film-coated tablet, orally disintegrating tablet (ODT)

Usage

Treatment of mild, moderate, or severe dementia of the Alzheimer's type,* behavioral syndromes in dementia, mild to moderate dementia associated with Parkinson's disease, Lewy body dementia

Pregnancy Category C

Dosing

Alzheimer's disease:
- Mild to moderate: 5 mg daily at bedtime; may increase to 10 mg daily at bedtime after 4–6 weeks
- Moderate to severe: 5 mg daily at bedtime; may increase to 10 mg daily at bedtime after 4–6 weeks; may further increase to 23 mg daily after ≥ 3 months

Adverse Reactions: Most Common

Nausea, vomiting, diarrhea, bradycardia, hypertension, dizziness, headache, insomnia, fatigue

Adverse Reactions: Rare/Severe/Important

Atrioventricular block, torsades de pointes, GI hemorrhage

Major Drug Interactions

Drugs Affecting Donepezil
- Cholinergic agents: Additive cholinergic side effects
- Anticholinergic agents, St. John's wort: Decrease effect
- Gingko biloba: Increases adverse effects/toxicity

Donepezil's Effect on Other Drugs
Nondepolarizing neuromuscular-blocking agents: Exaggerated muscle relaxation

Counseling Points

- Administer at bedtime without regard to food
- Allow ODT tablet to dissolve completely on tongue and follow with water
- Donepezil is not a cure, but it may help reduce symptoms of Alzheimer's disease
- Improvement associated with donepezil therapy is not maintained following discontinuance of the drug. Contact prescriber before discontinuing medication.
- Report severe nausea, vomiting, diarrhea, anorexia, dehydration, weight loss, insomnia, or signs/symptoms of GI bleeding, especially with current NSAID use
- GI upset is usually transient and occurs at dose titration

Key Points

- Effects will vary from patient to patient but may be observed as subtle improvement in cognition, function, or behavior over time
- Benefits associated with donepezil therapy are not maintained following discontinuance of the drug, suggesting that the underlying disease process of dementia is not altered by this medication
- GI upset generally resolves in 1–3 weeks

◉ Rivastigmine

Brand Name

Exelon

Generic Names

Rivastigmine (topical), rivastigmine tartrate (oral)

Rx Only

Dosage Forms

Capsule, solution, transdermal patch

Usage

Treatment of mild to moderate dementia associated with Alzheimer's or Parkinson's disease,* severe dementia associated with Alzheimer's disease, Lewy body dementia

Pregnancy Category B

Dosing

- Mild to moderate dementia associated with Alzheimer's disease:
  - Oral:
    - Initial dose: 1.5 mg twice daily with meals
    - Dosage adjustment: If tolerated, increase dose every 2 weeks by 1.5 mg twice daily
    - Maximum dose: 6 mg twice daily
  - Transdermal:
    - Initial: 4.6 mg/24-hour patch once daily
    - Dosage adjustment: After a minimum of 4 weeks and good tolerability, increase to 9.5 mg/24-hour patch once daily
- Mild to moderate dementia associated with Parkinson's disease:
  - Oral:
    - Initial dose: 1.5 mg twice daily with meals
    - Dosage adjustment: If tolerated, increase dose by 1.5 mg/dose up to 6 mg twice daily, with a minimum of 4 weeks at each dose
  - Transdermal:
    - Initial: 4.6 mg/24-hour patch once daily
    - Dosage adjustment: After a minimum of 4 weeks and good tolerability, increase to 9.5 mg/24-hour patch once daily
- Conversion from oral therapy:
  - Oral daily dose < 6 mg: Switch to 4.6 mg/24-hour patch. Apply patch on the next day following last oral dose.
  - Oral daily dose 6–12 mg: Switch to 9.5 mg/24-hour patch. Apply patch on the next day following last oral dose.
- Renal dosage adjustment: No dosage adjustment necessary; titrate to tolerability
- Hepatic dosage adjustment: No dosage adjustment necessary; titrate to tolerability
- Low body weight (< 50 kg): Use particular caution when titrating above the recommended dose of 9.5 mg/24 hour

Adverse Reactions: Most Common

Diarrhea, nausea, vomiting, weight loss, indigestion, dizziness, loss of appetite, skin irritation

Adverse Reactions: Rare/Severe/Important

Cardiac arrest, supraventricular tachycardia, tachyarrhythmia, GI hemorrhage, bronchospasm

Major Drug Interactions

Drugs Affecting Rivastigmine

- Gingko biloba: Increases effect
- Cholinergic agents: Additive cholinergic effects
- Anticholinergic agents, dipyridamole, nicotine (increased rivastigmine clearance): Decrease effect

Rivastigmine's Effect on Other Drugs

- Nondepolarizing neuromuscular-blocking agents: Exaggerated muscle relaxation
- Antipsychotics: Neurotoxicity
- Beta blockers: bradycardia
- Corticosteroids: Muscle weakness

Contraindications

Other carbamate derivatives (neostigmine, pyridostigmine, physostigmine)

Counseling Points

- Administration in the morning and evening with food is recommended because the incidence of adverse GI effects may be related to high peak plasma concentrations

- Antiemetics may be used to control GI symptoms
- The oral solution and capsules may be interchanged at equal doses; the oral solution should be administered using the oral dosing syringe according to the patient instructions provided by the manufacturer
- The capsule should be swallowed whole; do not crush or chew. The oral solution can be swallowed directly from the syringe or mixed with water, soda, or cold fruit juice. Stir well and drink within 4 hours of mixing.
- The transdermal system is applied topically to a dry, hairless area of intact skin. Remove and discard the protective liner and firmly press the patch with the adhesive side touching the skin. Placement on the back is recommended to reduce the risk of removal by the patient, but the upper arm or chest may be used as well.
- The transdermal system is worn continuously for 24 hours. Rotate application site. Do not apply to the same site within 14 days. Remove existing patch prior to applying new patch. Store patches in a cool dry place; avoid exposure to heat sources.
- Report persistent abdominal discomfort, diarrhea, or constipation; significantly increased salivation, sweating, tearing, or urination; chest pain or palpitations; acute headache; CNS changes, increased muscle, joint, or body pain; vision changes or blurred vision; shortness of breath, coughing, or wheezing; skin rash.

Key Points

- Rivastigmine is not a cure for Alzheimer's disease, but it may reduce the symptoms
- Titrate to target doses based on GI tolerability; adverse GI effects can be severe at higher than recommended doses
- Advise against sudden discontinuation of drug. Patients who miss doses for several days in a row should contact a healthcare professional, as the drug may need to be restarted at a lower dose.

ANTI-PARKINSON'S AGENTS, DOPAMINE AGONISTS

Introduction

These pharmacologically dissimilar agents affect dopamine receptors. Carbidopa/levodopa is a combination product used primarily for the treatment of Parkinson's disease (PD). Ropinirole hydrochloride is a nonergoline dopamine agonist that has a higher specificity to D_3 subtypes of dopamine receptors. Normal motor function depends on the synthesis and release of dopamine by neurons projecting from the substantia nigra to the corpus striatum. The progressive degeneration of these neurons that occurs in PD disrupts this pathway and results in decreased levels of dopamine. Striatal dopamine levels in symptomatic PD are decreased by 60–80%.

Mechanism of Action for the Drug Class

Levodopa circulates in the plasma to the blood–brain barrier (BBB), where it crosses and is converted to dopamine in the CNS; carbidopa inhibits peripheral decarboxylation of levodopa, decreasing the conversion to dopamine in peripheral tissues. This results in higher plasma levels of levodopa available at the BBB. The proposed mechanism of action of ropinirole is due to stimulation of postsynaptic dopamine D_2-type receptors within the caudate putamen in the brain. Ropinirole also has moderate in vitro affinity for opioid receptors.

Adverse Reactions for the Drug Class: Most Common

Loss of appetite, nausea, vomiting, constipation, abdominal pain, dizziness, headache, fatigue

Adverse Reactions for the Drug Class: Rare/Severe/Important

Heart disease, orthostatic hypotension, dose-related dyskinesia, somnolence, hallucinations, psychotic disorders, neuroleptic malignant syndrome

Counseling Points for the Drug Class

- Take exactly as directed; do not change dosage or discontinue without consulting the prescriber. Do not crush the sustained-release form.
- When administering the ODT, use dry hands to gently remove the tablet from the bottle and immediately place tablet on top of tongue and swallow with saliva after it dissolves. Administration with a liquid is not necessary.
- Take with meals if GI upset occurs, before meals if dry mouth occurs, and after eating if drooling or nausea occur
- Do not use alcohol and prescription/OTC sedatives or CNS depressants without consulting prescriber. Urine or perspiration may appear darker.
- Use caution when driving, climbing stairs, or engaging in tasks requiring alertness
- Use caution when rising from sitting or lying position
- Report exacerbation of underlying depression or psychosis
- Report unresolved constipation or vomiting, CNS changes, increased muscle spasticity or rigidity, unusual skin changes, or significant worsening of condition

Members of the Drug Class

In this section: Carbidopa/levodopa, ropinirole
Others: Amantadine, apomorphine, bromocriptine, entacapone, pramipexole, rotigotine

⊙ Carbidopa/Levodopa

Brand Names

Sinemet, Sinemet CR, Parcopa (orally disintegrating tablet)

Generic Name

Carbidopa/levodopa

Rx Only

Dosage Forms

Immediate-release tablet, sustained-release tablet, orally disintegrating tablet (ODT)

Usage

Idiopathic Parkinson's disease,* postencephalitic parkinsonism, symptomatic parkinsonism from carbon monoxide and/or manganese intoxication, restless leg syndrome, amblyopia

Pregnancy Category C

Dosing

- Parkinson's disease:
  - Immediate-release tablet:
    - Initial: Carbidopa 25 mg/levodopa 100 mg three times a day titrated to desired effects. Use of more than one dosage strength or dosing four times a day may be required.
    - Maximum dose: 8 tablets of any strength per day or 200 mg carbidopa and 2,000 mg levodopa
  - Sustained-release tablet:
    - Initial: Carbidopa 50 mg/levodopa 200 mg two times a day, at intervals not < 6 hours
    - Dosage adjustment: May adjust every 3 days; intervals should be between 4 and 8 hours during the waking day
    - Maximum dose: 8 tablets per day
- Renal dosage adjustment: Use with caution; no specific dosing recommendation in manufacturer labeling
- Hepatic dosage adjustment: Use with caution; no specific dosing recommendation in manufacturer labeling

Major Drug Interactions

Drugs Affecting Carbidopa/Levodopa

- Nonselective MAOIs (phenelzine, tranylcypromine): Increase effect
- Antipsychotics, iron salts, metoclopramide, phenytoin, pyridoxine: Decrease effect
- Herbal considerations: Avoid kava kava

Contraindications

Narrow-angle glaucoma, history of melanoma, nonselective MAOI use concurrently or < 2 weeks prior, suspicious and undiagnosed skin lesions

Key Points

- Therapeutic effects may take several weeks or months to achieve and frequent monitoring may be needed during first weeks of therapy
- Do not use MAOIs concurrently or within 2 weeks of carbidopa/levodopa
- Patients using concomitant antihypertensives may be at an increased risk for orthostatic hypotension
- Avoid high-protein diets and high doses (> 200 mg daily) of vitamin B_6 (pyridoxine)
- False-positive or false-negative urinary glucose results may occur with certain testing agents; false-positive urine ketone results may occur with certain testing agents

⊙ Ropinirole

Brand Names

Requip, Requip XL

Generic Name

Ropinirole

Rx Only

Dosage Forms

Immediate-release tablet, extended-release tablet

Usage

Idiopathic Parkinson's disease,* early Parkinson's disease not receiving concomitant levodopa therapy, advanced Parkinson's disease on concomitant levodopa therapy, moderate to severe primary restless leg syndrome*

Pregnancy Category C

Dosing

- Parkinson's disease:
  - Immediate-release tablets:
    - Initial dose: 0.25 mg three times daily
    - Dosage adjustment: Titrate weekly to therapeutic response in an ascending dose schedule from the initial dose to a maximum dose of 24 mg daily in divided doses
    - Discontinuation taper: Should be gradually tapered over 7 days
  - Extended-release tablets:
    - Initial dose: 2 mg once daily orally
    - Dosage adjustment: Titrate at a weekly or longer interval to therapeutic response at 2 mg daily increments to a maximum dose of 24 mg daily
    - Discontinuation taper: Gradually taper over 7 days

- Restless leg syndrome:
  - Initial dose: 0.25 mg once daily
  - Dosage adjustment: Titrate as needed to a maximum of 4 mg
  - All doses are once daily 1–3 hours before bedtime; doses should be titrated weekly when appropriate, based on clinical response and efficacy
  - Doses up to 4 mg per day may be discontinued without tapering
- Renal dosage adjustment: Use with caution in cases of severe renal impairment (CrCl < 30 mL/min); has not been studied in this population
- Hepatic dosage adjustment: Titrate with caution; has not been studied in this population

Major Drug Interactions

Drugs Affecting Ropinirole

- Ciprofloxacin, CYP1A2 inhibitors, estrogen derivatives, MAOIs: Increase effect
- Antipsychotics, CYP1A2 inducers, metoclopramide: Decrease effect
- Herbal considerations: Avoid kava kava, gotu kola, valerian, St. John's wort

Ropinirole's Effect on Other Drugs

Warfarin: May enhance the anticoagulant effect

Key Points

- Titrate dosing to achieve desired clinical response
- If therapy with a potent inhibitor of CYP1A2 is stopped or started during treatment with ropinirole, adjustment of ropinirole dose may be required
- May switch directly from immediate-release ropinirole; start an extended-release dose that matches most closely with the total daily immediate-release dose

N-METHYL-D-ASPARTATE RECEPTOR ANTAGONISTS

Introduction

Glutamate is an excitatory amino acid present in the CNS. It is thought to contribute to the pathogenesis of Alzheimer's disease by overstimulating glutamate receptors, leading to excitotoxicity and neuronal cell death. Memantine blocks the NMDA type of glutamate receptor, and during excessive receptor activation can affect magnesium and calcium ion influx and efflux. Memantine does not appear to affect normal neurotransmission but is most effective as a receptor blocker under conditions of excessive stimulation.

Mechanism of Action for the Drug Class

Memantine hydrochloride is a low to moderate affinity, noncompetitive NMDA receptor agonist that binds to NMDA receptor–operated cation channels. Memantine also blocks the 5-hydroxytryptamine-3 receptor and nicotinic acetylcholine receptors at various potencies.

Members of the Drug Class

In this section: Memantine

◉ Memantine

Brand Names
Namenda, Namenda XR

Generic Name
Memantine

Rx Only

Dosage Forms

Film-coated tablet, oral solution

Usage

Palliative treatment of moderate to severe dementia of the Alzheimer's type,* mild to moderate vascular dementia

Pregnancy Category B

Dosing

- Immediate-release:
  - Initial: 5 mg once daily
  - Increase dose by 5 mg daily to a target dose of 20 mg daily
- Wait ≥ 1 week between dosing changes
- Doses > 5 mg daily should be given in 2 divided doses
- Titration schedule: 5 mg daily for ≥ 1 week; 5 mg twice daily for ≥ 1 week; 15 mg daily given in 5 mg and 10 mg separated doses for ≥ 1 week; then 10 mg twice daily
- Memantine tablets and oral solution are equivalent on a mg-per-mg basis
- Renal dosage adjustment
  - Mild to moderate impairment: If CrCl 30–80 mL/min, no adjustment needed
  - Severe impairment: If CrCl 5–29 mL/min, then 5 mg twice daily
- Hepatic dosage adjustment: None needed for mild to moderate hepatic impairment

Adverse Reactions: Most Common

Dizziness, confusion, headache, diarrhea, constipation, vomiting, hypertension, back pain, cough, hallucination, somnolence, dyspnea, fatigue

Adverse Reactions: Rare/Severe/Important

Stevens-Johnson syndrome, deep venous thrombosis (DVT), hepatitis, liver failure, cerebral vascular accident (CVA), seizure, transient ischemic attack (TIA), acute renal failure, neuroleptic malignant syndrome

Major Drug Interactions

Drugs Affecting Memantine

- Alkalinizing agents (carbonic anhydrase inhibitors, sodium bicarbonate) that increase urine pH may decrease memantine clearance, resulting in elevated serum memantine concentrations and increased risk of adverse effects
- Trimethoprim may enhance the adverse/toxic effect of memantine. The risk of myoclonus and/or delirium may be increased. Trimethoprim may increase the serum concentration of memantine.

Memantine's Effect on Other Drugs

Trimethoprim may enhance the adverse/toxic effect of memantine. The risk of myoclonus and/or delirium may be increased. Memantine may increase the serum concentration of trimethoprim.

Counseling Points

- Report any dizziness, headache, confusion, diarrhea, constipation, or hypertension
- Take as directed; follow the titration schedule until target dose of 10 mg twice daily is reached
- The oral solution should be administered using the dosing device with oral syringe provided by the manufacturer. Do not mix with any other liquid.

Key Points

- Avoid coadministration with drugs that can increase urine pH. Use caution under certain conditions that can increase urine pH (diet changes to vegetarian diet, renal tubular acidosis, severe urinary tract infections); these may decrease the clearance of memantine, resulting in increased concentrations and increased risk of adverse effects.
- Avoid coadministration with trimethoprim
- The tablet and oral solution formulations are interchangeable

---

SEDATIVE-HYPNOTIC AGENT, NONBENZODIAZEPINES

Introduction

A newer drug class of sedative-hypnotic medications has supplanted much of the use of benzodiazepines for treatment of insomnia. Although the nonbenzodiazepines do not resemble the benzodiazepines structurally, they do function in a similar fashion and have very similar side-effect profiles and patient counseling points. As with all sleep agents, caution needs to be exercised to prevent habitual use and disturbance of a patient's natural sleep pattern. With the exception of ramelteon, a hypnotic with a unique mechanism of action, these agents are Schedule IV medications and may be habit forming. Use should be limited in duration to prevent potential abuse, addiction, and increased reliance on higher dosing at bedtime.

Mechanism of Action for the Drug Class

Although not benzodiazepines, they also facilitate the activity of the inhibitory neurotransmitter GABA. Ramelteon is a potent agonist of melatonin receptors, which play a role in circadian rhythms and the sleep–wake cycle.

Counseling Points for the Drug Class

- Sleep hygiene is the preferred first-line treatment for insomnia and should always be combined with pharmacologic therapy
- The failure of insomnia to remit after 7–10 days of therapy may indicate the presence of a primary psychiatric and/or other medical condition that should be evaluated
- Alcohol use while taking these medications can be dangerous and should be avoided
- Do not abruptly discontinue these drugs. A gradual taper is required to avoid rebound, relapse, and withdrawal symptoms. Insomnia is common after abruptly stopping sleeping aids.
- Only use when needed and for the shortest duration possible
- Take just before going to sleep and monitor for daytime alertness

Members of the Drug Class

In this section: Zolpidem, eszopiclone
Others: Ramelteon, zaleplon

⊙ Zolpidem

Brand Names
Ambien, Ambien CR, Edluar, Intermezzo, Zolpimist

Generic Name
Zolpidem

Rx Only
Class IV controlled substance

Dosage Forms
Tablet, sublingual tablet, spray

Usage
Short- and long-term treatment of insomnia

Pregnancy Category C

Dosing
- Initial dose:
  - Immediate-release tablet, sublingual, and spray: 10 mg at bedtime
  - Extended-release tablet: 12.5 mg at bedtime (1 spray = 5 mg)
- Hepatic dosage adjustment: Use with caution in patients with hepatic impairment:
  - Immediate-release tablet and spray: 5 mg at bedtime
  - Extended-release tablet: 6.25 mg at bedtime

Adverse Reactions: Most Common
Sedation, somnolence, dizziness, emergence of complex behavior ("sleep driving"), headache, diarrhea

Adverse Reactions: Rare/Severe/Important
Withdrawal syndromes and respiratory depression (especially with other CNS depressants or alcohol; use with caution in patients with mild to moderate COPD or sleep apnea), CNS depression, depression, anaphylaxis reactions (angioedema)

Major Drug Interactions
Major substrate of CYP3A4

Drugs Affecting Zolpidem
- Azole antifungal agents, ritonavir, and SSRIs: Increase serum concentrations
- Rifampin: Decreases serum concentrations

Zolpidem's Effect on Other Drugs
CNS depressants: Additive CNS depression

Counseling Points
- Do not crush controlled-release tablets
- Place sublingual tablets under the tongue and do not swallow or administer with water

Key Points
- Use at the lowest effective dose for the shortest duration possible to minimize the potential for dependence and abuse that can occur with long-term use
- Reevaluate patient needs after 7–10 days of use. Zolpidem has been studied for use up to 35 days.
- Elderly patients are the most susceptible to side effects. Starting doses of the immediate-release, sublingual, and spray should be 5 mg at bedtime. The starting dose for the extended-release tablet should be 6.25 mg at bedtime.
- Use the immediate-release tablets for patients who require medication to initiate sleep. Use the extended-release tablets for patients who require medication to maintain sleep throughout the night.

⊙ Eszopiclone

Brand Name
Lunesta

Generic Name
Eszopiclone

Rx Only
Class IV controlled substance

Dosage Form
Tablet

Usage
Insomnia

Pregnancy Category C

Dosing
- Initial dose: 2 mg at bedtime
- Hepatic dosage adjustment: Use with caution in patients with mild to moderate hepatic impairment. For severe hepatic impairment, initial dose should be 1 mg (maximum 2 mg).

Adverse Reactions: Most Common
Headache, sedation, somnolence, dizziness, abnormal dreams, memory impairment, emergence of complex behavior ("sleep driving"), decreased inhibition, dry mouth, impaired coordination, unpleasant taste

Adverse Reactions: Rare/Severe/Important
Withdrawal syndromes and respiratory depression (especially with other CNS depressants or alcohol; use with caution in patients with compromised lung function), CNS depression, depression, anaphylaxis reactions (angioedema, throat closing, dyspnea), chest pain, peripheral edema

Major Drug Interactions

Major substrate of CYP3A4

Drugs Affecting Eszopiclone

Potent 3A4 inhibitors such as azole antifungal agents, clarithromycin, and ritonavir: Increase serum concentrations

Eszopiclone's Effect on Other Drugs

CNS depressants: Additive CNS depression

Key Points

- Use at the lowest effective dose for the shortest duration possible to minimize the potential for dependence and abuse that can occur with long-term use
- Reevaluate patient needs after 7–10 days of use. Eszopiclone has been studied for use up to 6 months.
- Elderly patients are the most susceptible to side effects. The starting dose should be 1 mg at bedtime.

SKELETAL MUSCLE RELAXANTS

Introduction

Centrally acting skeletal muscle relaxants are used for the short-term treatment of skeletal muscle pain and discomfort

Mechanism of Action for the Drug Class

The exact mechanism of action is unclear, but the clinical effects of this class may be associated with general depression of the CNS. These agents typically have no direct effect on skeletal muscle. Baclofen exerts its effects as an agonist at presynaptic GABA$_B$ receptors, acting mainly at the spinal cord level to inhibit the transmission of both monosynaptic and polysynaptic reflexes, with resultant relief of muscle spasticity. Cyclobenzaprine is structurally related to the tricyclic antidepressants (TCAs). It acts primarily at the brainstem within the CNS. Carisoprodol is metabolized to meprobamate, which has anxiolytic and sedative effects. Tizanidine is an imidazole derivative chemically related to clonidine, exhibiting alpha-2 adrenergic agonist properties.

Members of the Drug Class

In this section: Baclofen, carisoprodol, cyclobenzaprine, metaxalone, methocarbamol, tizanidine
Others: Chlorzoxazone, dantrolene, orphenadrine

◉ Baclofen

Brand Names
Gablofen, Lioresal

Generic Name
Baclofen

Rx Only

Dosage Forms
Injection, tablet

Usage
Treatment of muscle spasm associated with acute painful musculoskeletal conditions,* treatment of reversible spasticity associated with multiple sclerosis or spinal cord lesions, intractable hiccups, intractable pain relief, bladder spasticity, trigeminal neuralgia, cerebral palsy, Huntington's chorea

Pregnancy Category C

Dosing

- Oral: 5 mg three times a day, may increase 5 mg/dose every 3 days to a maximum of 80 mg daily
- Intrathecal:
  - Test dose: 50–100 µg, doses > 50 µg should be given in 25 µg increments, separated by 24 hours, until a 4- to 8-hour positive clinical response is seen. Patients not responding to screening dose of 100 µg should not be considered for chronic infusion/implanted pump.
  - Maintenance: After positive response to test dose, a maintenance intrathecal infusion can be administered via an implanted intrathecal pump. Initial pump dose: Infusion at a 24-hourly rate dosed at twice the test dose.
- Renal dosage adjustment: May be necessary to reduce dosage; no specific guidelines have been established
- Geriatric dosing:
  - Use the lowest effective dose
  - Oral, initial: 5 mg two to three times daily, increasing gradually as needed; if no benefits are seen, withdraw drug slowly

Adverse Reactions: Most Common
Nausea, vomiting, drowsiness, dizziness, headache, poor muscle tone, weakness, hypotension

Adverse Reactions: Rare/Severe/Important
Constipation (significant with intrathecal use), withdrawal reactions with abrupt discontinuation (more severe with intrathecal use), coma, seizure

Major Drug Interactions
Avoid concomitant use with azelastine, methadone, paraldehyde

Droperidol, hydroxyzine: Increase effect

Baclofen's Effect on Other Drugs

- Alcohol, azelastine, buprenorphine, CNS depressants, SSRIs, zolpidem: Increased effects
- Herbal considerations: Avoid valerian, St. John's wort, kava kava, gotu kola

Contraindications

Injectable product is for intrathecal use only; IV, epidural, SUB-Q, or IM administration is not recommended

Counseling Points

- Take as prescribed. Do not discontinue this medicine without consulting prescriber.
- Do not take any prescription or OTC sleep-inducing drugs, sedatives, or antispasmodics without consulting prescriber. Avoid alcohol use.
- Use caution when driving or engaging in tasks requiring alertness until response to drug is known
- Frequent small meals or lozenges may reduce GI upset

Key Points

- Avoid abrupt withdrawal of drug. Encourage consistent and early refills of medication to minimize the risk of significant sequelae of withdrawal.
- Avoid alcohol and other CNS depressants

◉ Carisoprodol

Brand Name

Soma

Generic Name

Carisoprodol

Rx Only

Class IV controlled substance

Dosage Form

Tablet

Usage

Short-term treatment of muscle spasm associated with acute painful musculoskeletal conditions,* pain associated with TMJ disorder

Pregnancy Category C

Dosing

- 250–350 mg three times daily and at bedtime
- Renal dosage adjustment: Use with caution in cases of renal impairment; not studied in this population
- Hepatic dosage adjustment: Use lower initial doses in cases of hepatic impairment and increase gradually as needed and tolerated

Adverse Reactions: Most Common

Dizziness, headache, somnolence

Adverse Reactions: Rare/Severe/Important

Paradoxical CNS stimulation, seizure, drug abuse/dependence, withdrawal symptoms

Major Drug Interactions

Avoid Concomitant Use

Azelastine, methadone, paraldehyde

Drugs Affecting Carisoprodol

- CYP2C19 inhibitors (moderate and strong), droperidol, hydroxyzine: Increase effect
- CYP2C19 inducers (strong): Decrease effect

Carisoprodol's Effect on Other Drugs

Ethanol, CNS depressants, buprenorphine, methadone, SSRIs, zolpidem: Additive CNS depression

Contraindications

Not recommended for use in geriatric patients. Acute intermittent porphyria. Hypersensitivity reaction to a carbamate, such as meprobamate.

Counseling Points

- Do not use alcohol, prescription/OTC sedatives, CNS depressants, or psychotropic agents without consulting prescriber
- Use caution when driving, climbing stairs, or engaging in tasks requiring alertness
- Use caution when rising from sitting or lying position
- Report syncope, tachyarrhythmia, or excessive somnolence
- Report signs/symptoms of seizures when withdrawing from prolonged therapy
- Avoid meprobamate while on carisoprodol therapy
- Do not discontinue abruptly; taper dosage slowly to reduce risk of withdrawal symptoms

Key Points

- Carisoprodol should only be used for short periods (2–3 weeks) due to lack of evidence of effectiveness with prolonged use
- Carisoprodol is metabolized to meprobamate, which has anxiolytic and sedative effects. Avoid concurrent use of these two agents.

◉ Cyclobenzaprine

Brand Names

Amrix, Fexmid, Flexeril

Generic Name

Cyclobenzaprine

Rx Only

Dosage Forms

Extended-release capsule, tablet

Usage

Treatment of muscle spasm associated with acute painful musculoskeletal conditions,* treatment of muscle spasm associated with acute TMJ

Pregnancy Category B

Dosing

- Extended-release capsule: 15 mg once daily; some patients may require up to 30 mg once daily
- Immediate-release tablet: 5 mg three times a day; may increase to 7.5–10 mg three times a day if needed
- Hepatic dosage adjustment:
  - Extended-release capsule: Not recommended in mild to severe impairment
  - Immediate-release tablet:
    - Mild impairment: Initial dose of 5 mg; use with caution; titrate slowly, and consider less frequent dosing
    - Moderate to severe impairment: Use not recommended
- Geriatric dosing:
  - Extended-release capsule: Use not recommended
  - Immediate-release tablet: Initiate with a 5 mg dose and increase gradually as needed

Adverse Reactions: Most Common

Palpitations, nervousness, confusion, dizziness, headache, somnolence, bad taste in mouth, constipation, indigestion, nausea, dry mouth, blurred vision

Adverse Reactions: Rare/Severe/Important

Cholestasis, hepatitis, jaundice, cardiac dysrhythmia, anaphylaxis, immune hypersensitivity reaction

Major Drug Interactions

Consider all drug interactions with TCAs as possible interactions with cyclobenzaprine

Avoid Concomitant Use

Azelastine, methadone, paraldehyde

Drugs Affecting Cyclobenzaprine

- Antipsychotics, CYP1A2 inhibitors, hydroxyzine, pramlintide: Increase level/effect
- Acetylcholinesterase inhibitors, peginterferon α-2b: Decrease level/effect

Cyclobenzaprine's Effect on Other Drugs

- Ethanol, anticholinergic drugs, CNS depressants, MAOIs: Increase level/effect
- Acetylcholinesterase inhibitors: Decrease level/effect
- Herbal considerations: Avoid valerian, kava kava, gotu kola (increased risk of CNS depression)

Contraindications

Arrhythmias, cardiac conduction disturbances, heart failure, heart block, acute recovery period following myocardial infarction, hyperthyroidism. Concomitant use with MAOI or use of MAOI within past 14 days may cause hyperpyretic crisis, seizure, and death.

Counseling Points

- Avoid activities requiring mental alertness or coordination until drug effects are realized
- Watch for potential anticholinergic side effects
- Report signs/symptoms of decreased hepatic function, especially with preexisting hepatic disease
- Report lack of symptom improvement within 2–3 weeks of therapy
- Avoid alcohol and other CNS depressants while taking this drug
- Avoid concomitant use of TCAs during therapy with this drug

Key Points

- Not intended for long-term use. Do not use for > 2–3 weeks.
- Use caution in geriatric patients and in those with hepatic impairment
- Not effective for spasticity associated with cerebral palsy
- Given structural similarity to TCAs, advise patients of anticholinergic side effects and precautions. Avoid concomitant use with MAOIs.

⊚ Metaxalone

Brand Name

Skelaxin

Generic Name

Metaxalone

Rx Only

Dosage Form

Tablet

Usage

Treatment of muscle spasm associated with acute painful musculoskeletal conditions

Pregnancy Category Not Established/ Use Not Recommended

Dosing

- Adults and children > 12 years: 800 mg three to four times a day
- Renal dosage adjustment: Use caution in mild to moderate impairment; no specific dosage recommendations
- Hepatic dosage adjustment: Use caution in mild to moderate impairment; no specific dosage recommendations

Adverse Reactions: Most Common

Drug-induced GI disturbances, nausea, vomiting, dizziness, headache, somnolence, nervousness

Adverse Reactions: Rare/Severe/Important

Hemolytic anemia, leukopenia, jaundice, hypersensitivity

Major Drug Interactions

Avoid Concomitant Use

Azelastine, methadone, paraldehyde

Drugs Affecting Metaxalone

- Droperidol, hydroxyzine: Increases CNS depressant effect
- Peginterferon alfa-2b: Decreases level/effect

Metaxalone's Effect on Other Drugs

- Ethanol, CNS depressants, psychotropics, SSRIs: Increase level/effect
- Herbal considerations: Avoid valerian, St. John's wort, kava kava, gotu kola
- Food: Bioavailability may be increased; unclear clinical relevance

Test Interactions

False positive for urine glucose determinations utilizing cupric sulfate, but the drug does not interfere with glucose tests using glucose oxidase (Benedict's solution)

Contraindications

History of drug-induced, hemolytic or other anemias. Severe impairment in hepatic or renal function.

Counseling Points

- Avoid activities requiring mental alertness or coordination until drug effects are realized
- Inform diabetic patients that metaxalone may cause false-positive results for certain urine glucose tests
- Avoid alcohol and other CNS depressants while taking this drug
- If the next dose is > 1 hour past regular dosing time, skip the missed dose
- Report signs/symptoms of decreased hepatic function, especially with preexisting hepatic disease

Key Points

- Use caution in patients with significant renal or hepatic impairment
- May cause leukopenia; use caution with clozapine and carbamazepine
- Monitor relevant laboratory values for renal and hepatic function

⊙ Methocarbamol

Brand Names

Robaxin, Robaxin-750

Generic Name

Methocarbamol

Rx Only

Dosage Forms

Injection, tablet

Usage

Adjunctive treatment of muscle spasm associated with acute painful musculoskeletal conditions,* supportive therapy in tetanus

Pregnancy Category C

Dosing

- Muscle spasm:
  - Oral: 1.5 g four times a day for 2–3 days (up to 8 g daily for severe conditions), then decrease to 4–4.5 g daily in 3–6 divided doses
  - IM, IV:
    - 1 g every 8 hours if oral not possible
    - Maximum dose: 3 g daily for no more than 3 consecutive days
    - If condition persists, may repeat course of therapy after a drug-free interval of 48 hours
- Tetanus:
  - IV initial dose: 1–2 g by direct IV injection
  - Additional doses via infusion to maximum of 3 g total
  - May repeat dose every 6 hours until oral dosing is possible; injection should not be used for more than 3 consecutive days
- Renal dosage adjustment: Use lower initial oral doses in cases of renal impairment and increase gradually as needed and tolerated
- Hepatic dosage adjustment:
  - Specific dosing guidelines are not available; plasma protein binding and clearance are decreased; half-life is increased
  - Use lower initial oral doses and increase gradually as needed and tolerated

Adverse Reactions: Most Common

Flushing, pruritus, rash, urticaria, indigestion, nausea, vomiting, dizziness, headache, nystagmus, somnolence, vertigo, nervousness, blurred vision, conjunctivitis

Adverse Reactions: Rare/Severe/Important

Bradyarrhythmia, hypotension, syncope, leukopenia, anaphylaxis, seizure (IV formulation)

Major Drug Interactions

Avoid Concomitant Use

Azelastine, methadone, paraldehyde

Drugs Affecting Methocarbamol

Droperidol, hydroxyzine: Increase level/effect

Methocarbamol's Effect on Other Drugs

- Ethanol, CNS depressants, SSRIs: Increases levels/effects
- Pyridostigmine: Decreases level/effect
- Herbal considerations: Avoid valerian, St. John's wort, kava kava, gotu kola

Test Interactions

May cause color interference in certain screening tests for urinary 5-HIAA using nitrosonaphthol reagent and in screening tests for urinary VMA using the Gitlow method

Contraindications

Injectable methocarbamol contains polyethylene glycol and is contraindicated in patients with renal dysfunction

Counseling Points

- Do not increase dose or discontinue without consulting prescriber. Take as directed.
- Avoid alcohol and other CNS depressants while taking this drug
- Avoid activities requiring mental alertness or coordination until drug effects are realized
- Drug may color urine brown, black, or green
- Report excessive drowsiness or mental agitation, chest pain, skin rash, swelling of mouth/face, difficulty speaking, or vision changes
- If the next oral dose is > 1 hour late, skip the missed dose

Key Points

- Do not use the injection formulation for more than 3 consecutive days
- Use caution in patients with renal and hepatic impairment
- Use injectable product with caution in patients with history of seizure
- Injectable product is *not* recommended in patients with renal dysfunction

◉ Tizanidine

Brand Name

Zanaflex

Generic Name

Tizanidine

Rx Only

Dosage Forms

Capsule, tablet

Usage

Treatment of muscle spasm associated with acute painful musculoskeletal conditions,* tension headaches, low back pain,* trigeminal neuralgia

Pregnancy Category C

Dosing

- Initial dose: 4 mg, may increase by 2–4 mg as needed for satisfactory reduction of muscle tone every 6–8 hours to a maximum of 3 doses totaling 36 mg in any 24-hour period
- Renal dosage adjustment: Reduce dose with a CrCl < 25 mL/min; clearance reduced > 50%
- Hepatic dosage adjustment: Avoid use if possible. If drug is necessary, use lowest possible doses while monitoring for hypotension. Extensive first-pass hepatic metabolism.
- Geriatric dosing: Clearance is decreased; dose cautiously. No specific dosing guidelines exist.

Adverse Reactions: Most Common

Hypotension, dry mouth, vomiting, constipation, abnormal liver function tests, dizziness, somnolence, nervousness, muscle weakness, speech or vision disturbances

Adverse Reactions: Rare/Severe/Important

Orthostatic hypotension, angina, heart failure, myocardial infarction, syncope, leukopenia, thrombocytopenia, hepatitis

Major Drug Interactions

Avoid Concomitant Use

Azelastine, ciprofloxacin, fluvoxamine, paraldehyde

Drugs Affecting Tizanidine

- Beta blockers, ciprofloxacin, CYP1A2 inhibitors, fluvoxamine, herbal products with hypotensive properties, hydroxyzine, MAOIs, estrogens, phosphodiesterase 5 inhibitors, pentoxifylline: Increase effects
- Antidepressants (alpha-2 antagonists), herbal products with hypertensive properties, methylphenidate, SSRIs/SNRIs, TCAs: Decrease effects

Tizanidine's Effect on Other Drugs

- Ethanol, CNS depressants, antihypertensives (ACE inhibitors), QTc-prolonging agents, SSRIs: Increase effects
- Herbal considerations: Avoid valerian, St. John's wort, kava kava, gotu kola (increase CNS depression); avoid black cohosh, hawthorn, mistletoe, periwinkle, poppy, quinine (increase hypotensive effects)

Contraindications

Concomitant therapy with ciprofloxacin or fluvoxamine (potent CYP1A2 inhibitors)

Essential Monitoring Parameters

Hepatic function (aminotransferase): Measure at baseline, then at 1, 3, and 6 months of therapy, and periodically thereafter, based on clinical status

Counseling Points

- Avoid activities requiring mental alertness until drug effects are realized
- Rise slowly from a lying/seated position because this drug may cause hypotension
- Although this drug may be taken with or without food, take the drug the same way every time. Inconsistent administration with regards to food may enhance or delay onset and change the adverse-effect profile.
- Do not discontinue the drug suddenly
- Do not drink alcohol while taking this drug

Key Points

- Tizanidine is chemically related to clonidine and has alpha-2 adrenergic agonist properties
- Use with caution in the elderly
- Discuss risks of sudden discontinuation of drug
- Follow maximum daily dosing guidelines

STIMULANTS

Introduction

The CNS stimulants are primarily used for ADHD, narcolepsy, and excessive daytime sleepiness (EDS). Stimulants increase alertness and prevent sleep, but their side-effect profile includes insomnia, heart palpitations, hypertension, irritability, and, in more severe cases, serious cardiac events, including sudden death. In addition to their side-effect profile, another downside to stimulants is that they are controlled substances with the potential for abuse and addiction. The goal of using these agents is to improve quality of life while finding a balance between benefit and risk.

Mechanism of Action for the Drug Class

Although the mechanism of action for modafinil is unknown, the other drugs covered in this class are thought to mediate CNS stimulation through either the release of norepinephrine and dopamine (amphetamine/dextroamphetamine) or through blocking the reuptake of norepinephrine and dopamine (methylphenidate)

Counseling Points for the Drug Class

- Avoid alcohol and caffeine
- Avoid evening doses to prevent insomnia
- Consult physician before discontinuing the medication
- Counsel patients about the potential adverse effects on sleep, mood, and appetite. Counsel on the black box warning for both addiction and serious cardiac events. Tell patient to report chest pain, difficulty breathing, fainting, abnormal thinking or behavior, increased aggression, hallucinations, and weight loss.

Key Points for the Drug Class

- With the exception of modafinil, all stimulant medications have two black box warnings, one for abuse/addiction potential and one for serious cardiac events, including sudden death. It is therefore prudent to screen and monitor cardiovascular risk, blood pressure, heart rate, psychiatric status, growth parameters, weight gain, appetite, and signs of tolerance, abuse, or addiction. These same monitoring parameters should also be employed for modafinil.
- When using stimulants for the treatment of ADHD, consider obtaining an ECG prior to therapy. The clinical role of routine ECG monitoring has yet to be determined.
- When using stimulants for non-ADHD indications, monitor for daytime alertness
- Drug holidays may be given to children to determine the need for continued treatment and to allow for "catch-up" growth

Members of the Drug Class

In this section: Amphetamine/dextroamphetamine, methylphenidate, lisdexamfetamine, modafinil
Others: Armodafinil, dextroamphetamine, methamphetamine

⊙ Amphetamine/Dextroamphetamine

Brand Names
Adderall, Adderall XR

Generic Name
Amphetamine/dextroamphetamine

Rx Only
Class II controlled substance

Dosage Forms
Immediate-release tablet, extended-release capsule

Usage
ADHD,* narcolepsy*

Pregnancy Category C

Dosing
- ADHD:
  - Adults:
    - Immediate-release tablet:
      - Initial dose: 5 mg one to two times a day
      - Maximum dose: 40 mg daily
    - Extended-release capsule:
      - Initial dose: 20 mg daily in the morning
      - Maximum dose: 60 mg daily (lack of adequate data that doses this high provide additional benefit)
  - Children:
    - Initial dose:
      - 3–5 years of age:
        - Immediate-release tablet: 2.5 mg daily; maximum 30 mg daily
      - 6 years or older:
        - Immediate-release tablet: 5 mg daily one to two times a day
        - Extended-release capsule: 5–10 mg daily; maximum 30 mg daily
    - Give the first dose on awakening
    - Multiple doses of immediate-release tablets should be dosed at intervals of 4–6 hours
- Narcolepsy:
  - Adults:
    - Initial dose: Immediate release 10 mg daily
    - Maximum dose: 60 mg daily
  - Children:
    - 6–12 years of age: Initial dose 5 mg daily
    - > 12 years of age: Refer to adult dosing

Adverse Reactions: Most Common
Insomnia, headache, weight loss, loss of appetite, nervousness, abdominal pain

Adverse Reactions: Rare/Severe/Important
Cardiac adverse effects, including sudden death; drug abuse/dependency; sudden death in children; suppression of growth in children with long-term use; exacerbation of preexisting or emergence of new psychiatric disorders; worsening of motor and vocal tics; aggression; seizures; visual disturbances; dependency

Major Drug Interactions
Contraindicated with concomitant use of MAOIs or within 14 days of MAOI use

Drugs Affecting Amphetamine/Dextroamphetamine
- Antacids, acetazolamide, thiazides: Increase levels
- Urinary alkalinizing agents: Increase levels
- Urinary acidifying agents: Decrease levels
- Norepinephrine and other stimulants: Increase effects

Amphetamine/Dextroamphetamine's Effect on Other Drugs
Other CNS stimulants: Additive effects

Contraindications
Advanced arteriosclerosis, symptomatic cardiovascular disease, cardiac structure abnormalities, moderate to severe hypertension, hyperthyroidism, glaucoma, agitated states, history of drug abuse, hypersensitivity or idiosyncratic reactions to the sympathomimetic amines

Counseling Point
Do not crush or chew sustained-release formulations. The contents of the capsules may be sprinkled on applesauce.

Key Points
- Amphetamine/dextroamphetamine has many contraindications (see above) due to the possibility of serious cardiac complications including sudden cardiac death as well as the potential for abuse and addiction. There is a black box warning for both abuse potential and serious cardiovascular events with this agent.
- Screen and monitor cardiovascular risk, blood pressure, heart rate, psychiatric history, growth parameters, weight gain, and signs of abuse

⊙ Methylphenidate

Brand Names
Ritalin, Ritalin SR, Ritalin LA, Concerta, Methylin, Methylin ER, Metadate ER, Metadate CD, Daytrana

Generic Name
Methylphenidate

Rx Only
Class II controlled substance

Dosage Forms
Immediate-release, sustained-release, and extended-release tablets; extended-release capsule; chewable tablet; transdermal system; solution

Usage
ADHD,* narcolepsy,* depression, fatigue, traumatic brain injury

Pregnancy Category C

Dosing

- ADHD:
  - Adults:
    - Immediate-release: Initial dose of 10–60 mg daily in 2–3 divided doses
    - Extended-release:
      - Initial dose: 20 mg daily in the morning
      - Maximum dose: 60 mg daily
  - Sustained- and extended-release tablets have an 8-hour duration of action. Administer the 8-hour dose of the regular release tablets.
  - Concerta: Initial dose 18–36 mg once a day
  - Metadate CD: Initial dose 20 mg once a day
  - Daytrana 10 mg patch: Apply to hip 2 hours before effect is needed; remove 9 hours after application
  - Children > 6 years of age: Immediate-release 5 mg twice a day
- Narcolepsy:
  - Initial dose: Immediate-release 10 mg two to three times a day
  - Maximum dose: 60 mg daily

Adverse Reactions: Most Common

Insomnia, headache, anorexia, loss of appetite, nervousness, dizziness, hyperhidrosis, nausea

Adverse Reactions: Rare/Severe/Important

Serious cardiac-adverse events, abuse/addiction/dependency, sudden death in children, suppression of growth in children with long-term use, exacerbation of preexisting or emergence of new psychiatric disorders, worsening of motor and vocal tics, aggression, seizures, visual disturbances, contact dermatitis with transdermal application

Major Drug Interactions

Concomitant use with MAOIs or halogenated anesthetics is contraindicated

Methylphenidate's Effect on Other Drugs

SSRIs and warfarin: Increases serum concentrations

Contraindications

- Structure cardiac abnormalities, advanced arteriosclerosis, symptomatic heart disease, moderate to serve hypertension, history of drug abuse, hypersensitivity or idiosyncratic reactions to sympathomimetic amines, glaucoma, anxiety and agitated states, motor tics, family history or diagnosis of Tourette syndrome
- Metadate CD and Metadate ER have additional contraindications of severe hypertension, heart failure, arrhythmias, hyperthyroidism, recent myocardial infarction or angina, and concomitant use of halogenated anesthetics

Counseling Points

- Do not crush or chew sustained- or extended-release formulations. The contents of the capsules may be sprinkled on applesauce.
- Take immediate-release tablets, chewable tablets, and solution 30–45 minutes before meals
- Drink at least 8 ounces of water with chewable tablets to avoid choking

Key Points

- Methylphenidate has many contraindications due to the potential for serious cardiac complications, including sudden cardiac death and the potential for abuse (see previous discussion)
- There is a black box warning for the potential for drug dependency, and abrupt discontinuation should be avoided in patients receiving prolonged therapy
- Screen and monitor cardiovascular risk, psychiatric history, growth parameters, weight changes, and signs of abuse

◉ Lisdexamfetamine

Brand Name

Vyvanse

Generic Name

Lisdexamfetamine

Rx Only

Class II controlled substance

Dosage Form

Capsule

Usage

ADHD

Pregnancy Category C

Dosing

- Adults and children 6 years and older:
  - Initial dose: 30 mg once daily in the morning
  - Dosage adjustment: May increase by 10–20 mg daily at weekly intervals until optimal response
  - Maximum dose: 70 mg daily
- Administer at lowest effective dose and individualize based on patient response

Adverse Reactions: Most Common

Headache, insomnia, irritability, decreased appetite and weight, xerostomia, abdominal pain, nausea, vomiting

Adverse Reactions: Rare/Severe/Important

Cardiac adverse effects, including sudden death; drug abuse/addiction/dependency; sudden death in children; suppression of growth in children with long-term use; exacerbation of preexisting or emergence of new psychiatric disorders; worsening of motor and vocal tics; aggression; seizures; visual disturbances

Major Drug Interactions

Contraindicated with concomitant use of MAOIs or within 2 weeks of MAOI use

Drugs Affecting Lisdexamfetamine

- Urinary alkalinizing agents: Increase levels
- Urinary acidifying agents: Decrease levels
- Norepinephrine and other stimulants: Increase effects

Lisdexamfetamine's Effect on Other Drugs

- Adrenergic blockers, antihistamines, antihypertensives, phenobarbital, phenytoin: May reduce effects
- TCAs and meperidine: May potentiate effects

Contraindications

Advanced arteriosclerosis, symptomatic cardiovascular disease, cardiac structure abnormalities, moderate to severe hypertension, hyperthyroidism, glaucoma, agitated states, history of drug abuse, hypersensitivity or idiosyncratic reactions to the sympathomimetic amines

Counseling Points

- May be taken with or without food
- Capsules can be taken whole or they can be opened and the entire contents of the capsule can be dissolved in a glass of water. The solution must be drunk immediately and not stored.
- The dose of a single capsule should not be divided
- The patient should not take less than one capsule per day

Key Points

- Lisdexamfetamine has many contraindications (see above) due to the possibility of serious cardiac complications, including sudden cardiac death, as well as the potential for abuse and addiction. There is a black box warning for both abuse potential and serious cardiovascular events with this agent.
- Screen and monitor cardiovascular risk, blood pressure, heart rate, psychiatric status, abuse potential, growth parameters, and weight changes

◉ Modafinil

Brand Name
Provigil

Generic Name
Modafinil

Rx Only
Class IV controlled substance

Dosage Form
Tablet

Usage
Improve wakefulness in patients with EDS associated with narcolepsy or shift-work sleep disorder,* adjunctive therapy for obstructive sleep apnea/hypopnea syndrome,* ADHD, fatigue

Pregnancy Category C

Dosing
- ADHD: Initial dose of 100–300 mg
- Narcolepsy and obstructive sleep apnea/hypopnea syndrome: Initial dose of 200 mg daily taken in the morning
- Shift-work sleep disorder: Initial dose of 200 mg daily taken 1 hour prior to shift work
- Doses of up to 400 mg daily have been well tolerated, but there is no evidence that this dose confers additional benefit
- Hepatic dosage adjustment: Reduce dose by 50% in patients with severe hepatic impairment

Adverse Reactions: Most Common
Insomnia, headache, nervousness, dizziness, nausea, anxiety, decreased appetite and abdominal pain in children

Adverse Reactions: Rare/Severe/Important
Hypertension, rash, Stevens-Johnson syndrome, multiorgan hypersensitivity reaction, angioedema, anaphylaxis, psychiatric symptoms

Major Drug Interactions
- Major substrate of CYP3A4
- Strong inhibitor of CYP2C19
- Weak/moderate inducer of CYP1A2, 2B6, and 3A4

Drugs Affecting Modafinil
- CYP3A4 inhibitors: Increase concentrations
- CYP3A4 inducers: Decrease concentrations

Modafinil's Effect on Other Drugs
Oral contraceptives: Decreases serum concentrations

Counseling Point
If using oral contraceptives, consider an additional or alternative method of birth control

Key Point
Modafinil is a Schedule IV medication that can produce psychoactive and euphoric effects, which can lead to abuse and addiction. Because it is a C-IV and not a C-II, the abuse potential is slightly less compared to other CNS stimulants.

NONSTIMULANT ADHD AGENT, ALPHA-2 ADRENERGIC AGONIST

Introduction

As a treatment for ADHD, guanfacine is a unique medication that works differently than traditional stimulants or modafinil. It is primarily used (extended-release tablets) for the management of ADHD, although it is also indicated for the management of hypertension (immediate-release tablets). It is used infrequently for hypertension, given the availability of safer and better tolerated agents. In contrast to most ADHD medications, guanfacine is a noncontrolled substance. It has not been shown to cause abuse or addiction, making it a good option for patients with a history of drug abuse. Guanfacine also differs from other ADHD medications in that it is not a CNS stimulant and can in fact cause marked CNS depression. It can be used alone or in combination with stimulants, but prolonged use for maintenance treatment greater than 9 weeks duration has not been studied.

Mechanism of Action for the Drug Class

Guanfacine is a selective alpha-2A adrenoreceptor agonist, which reduces sympathetic nerve impulses, resulting in reduced sympathetic outflow and a subsequent decrease in vasomotor tone and heart rate. In addition, guanfacine preferentially binds postsynaptic alpha-2A adrenoreceptors in the prefrontal cortex and has been theorized to improve delay-related firing of prefrontal cortex neurons. As a result, underlying working memory and behavioral inhibition are affected, thereby improving symptoms associated with ADHD.

Members of the Drug Class

In this section: Guanfacine

⊙ Guanfacine

Brand Names
   Intuniv, Tenex

Generic Name
   Guanfacine

Rx Only

Dosage Forms
   Immediate- and extended-release tablets

Usage
   ADHD,* as monotherapy or adjunctive therapy to stimulants

Pregnancy Category B

Dosing

- Extended-release tablets for the treatment of ADHD in patients 6 years and older:
  - Initial dose: 1 mg once daily
  - Dosage adjustment: Dose may be adjusted by increments no larger than 1 mg/week as tolerated, based on clinical response (doses > 4 mg daily have not been studied). Note that in clinical trials significant adverse events were dose- and exposure-related, thus consideration should be given to dosing on a mg/kg basis (initial: 0.05–0.08 mg/kg, if tolerated can increase to 0.12 mg/kg, with a max of 4 mg).
- If a patient misses 2 or more consecutive doses, repeat titration of dose should be considered
- Discontinuation: Taper the dose in decrements of no more than 1 mg every 3–7 days
- Do not substitute extended-release tablets for immediate-release tablets on a mg-per-mg basis because of differing pharmacokinetic profiles
- Renal dosage adjustment: No specific dose adjustments are recommended in renal dysfunction, although adjustments may be required based off clinical response
- Hepatic dosage adjustment: No specific dose adjustments are recommended in hepatic dysfunction, although adjustments may be required based off clinical response

Adverse Reactions: Most Common

Somnolence, sedation, dizziness, headache, fatigue, xerostomia, constipation, abdominal pain, hypotension, bradycardia, syncope

Adverse Reactions: Rare/Severe/Important

Severe hypotension, bradycardia, syncope, sedation, somnolence, atrioventricular block, sinus arrhythmia, abnormal liver function tests

Major Drug Interactions

Major substrate of CYP3A4

Drugs Affecting Guanfacine
- CYP3A4/5 inhibitors such as ketoconazole: Increase concentrations
- CYP3A4/5 inducers such as rifampin: Decrease concentrations

Guanfacine's Effect on Other Drugs
- Valproic acid: Increases concentrations
- Warning of concomitant use with MAOIs due to risk of hypertensive crisis
- Antihypertensives (hypotension) or CNS depressants (CNS depression): Additive effects

Counseling Points

- Avoid excessive alcohol
- Do not crush or chew extended-release tablets
- Take with a full glass of water and maintain adequate hydration unless otherwise restricted
- Do not take with a high-fat meal because of increased absorption
- Sedation can occur, especially after therapy initiation or dose escalation
- Report excessive drowsiness or dizziness, respiratory difficulty, or GI changes
- Do not stop abruptly without tapering

Key Points

- Guanfacine is a noncontrolled medication used to treat ADHD. Abuse potential is nil compared to traditional stimulant medications.
- Guanfacine is a nonstimulant medication that can cause significant, dose-dependent CNS depression, hypotension, and bradycardia
- Doses should be escalated gradually and tapered for discontinuation. If a patient misses 2 or more doses, dose retitration should be employed.
- For ADHD, guanfacine can be used alone or in combination with stimulants, although its use as maintenance treatment for longer than 9 weeks has not been evaluated

1. Which of the following seizure medications is commonly used to treat diabetic neuropathy?

   a. Phenytoin
   b. Gabapentin
   c. Phenobarbital
   d. Carbamazepine

2. Which of the following antiepileptic drugs is available in an orally disintegrating tablet?

   a. Lamotrigine
   b. Levetiracetam
   c. Oxcarbazepine
   d. Topiramate

3. The target serum concentration for valproic acid is:

   a. 4–12 μg/mL.
   b. 10–20 μg/mL.
   c. 10–40 μg/mL.
   d. 50–100 μg/mL.

4. Which of the following has a black box warning for teratogenicity?

   a. Gabapentin
   b. Valproic acid
   c. Lamotrigine
   d. Levetiracetam

5. Which of the following has a black box warning for the risk of life-threatening serious rashes, especially in the pediatric population and when doses are escalated too quickly?

   a. Lamotrigine
   b. Oxcarbazepine
   c. Topiramate
   d. Valproic acid

6. Which of the following antiepileptic drugs is used for migraine prophylaxis?

   a. Phenobarbital
   b. Phenytoin
   c. Topiramate
   d. Lamotrigine

7. Which of the following drugs induces its own metabolism?

   a. Keppra
   b. Lamictal
   c. Tegretol
   d. Trileptal

8. Which of the following antiepileptic drugs is a C-IV medication?

   a. Gabapentin
   b. Pregabalin
   c. Phenobarbital
   d. Levetiracetam

9. Which of the following antidepressants would be the best choice for a patient experiencing sexual dysfunction from an SSRI?

   a. Fluoxetine
   b. Bupropion
   c. Amitriptyline
   d. Citalopram

10. Which of the following antidepressants causes a fair amount of sedation at the recommended starting dose and should always be given at bedtime?

    a. Fluoxetine
    b. Duloxetine
    c. Mirtazapine
    d. Sertraline

11. Which of the following situations would cause a *decrease* in lithium levels?

    a. Concomitant use of ibuprofen
    b. Concomitant use of lisinopril
    c. Excessive loss of sodium during perspiration
    d. Excess sodium in the diet

12. Which of the following psychiatric agents is available in an IM formulation?

    a. Quetiapine
    b. Ziprasidone
    c. Citalopram
    d. Fluoxetine

13. The maximum daily dose for citalopram is:

    a. 40 mg.
    b. 60 mg.
    c. 10 mg.
    d. 80 mg.

14. The therapeutic serum concentration for lithium when treating acute mania is:

    a. 0.8–1.2 mEq/L.
    b. 0.5–0.9 mEq/L.
    c. 600–1,200 mEq/L.
    d. 1–2 mEq/L.

15. Which of the following atypical antipsychotics is the *worst* at causing extrapyramidal symptoms?

    a. Clozaril
    b. Geodon
    c. Zyprexa
    d. Risperdal

16. Which of the following atypical antipsychotics is the *worst* at causing metabolic complications?

    a. Aripiprazole
    b. Olanzapine
    c. Quetiapine
    d. Ziprasidone

17. Which of the following antianxiety agents *cannot* be used for acute treatment due to its delayed onset of action?

    a. Buspirone
    b. Alprazolam
    c. Clonazepam
    d. Diazepam

18. Which of the following ADHD medications is *not* a stimulant?

    a. Concerta
    b. Vyvanse
    c. Adderall
    d. Intuniv

19. Which of the following ADHD medications has the potential to decrease the effectiveness of oral contraceptives?

    a. Lisdexamfetamine
    b. Guanfacine
    c. Adderall XR
    d. Modafinil

20. Which of the following statements is correct regarding counseling for Vyvanse?

    a. The capsule can be opened and the contents dissolved in water, to be drunk at any time during the day.
    b. The patient should not split the dose of the capsule and should not take less than one capsule per day.
    c. Vyvanse should be taken 30 minutes before bedtime.
    d. Vyvanse is a safe medication to use in patients with a history of drug abuse.

21. Which of the following statements is true regarding therapy for ADHD?

    a. Intuniv cannot be taken with Adderall.
    b. Metadate is a C-IV substance.
    c. Stimulants can cause growth suppression in children when used for prolonged periods of time.
    d. All stimulant medications are C-II substances.

22. Which of the following is *not* a first-line treatment for depression?

    a. Amitriptyline
    b. Sertraline
    c. Mirtazapine
    d. Duloxetine

23. Which of the following antidepressants is commonly used to treat neuropathic pain?

    a. Lexapro
    b. Cymbalta
    c. Prozac
    d. Desyrel

24. Which of the following side effects is more common with SNRIs compared to SSRIs?

    a. Hypertension
    b. Dry mouth
    c. Bleeding
    d. Sexual dysfunction

25. Which of the following antidepressants is available co-formulated with an atypical antipsychotic?

    a. Sertraline
    b. Paroxetine
    c. Citalopram
    d. Fluoxetine

26. Which of the following SSRIs is *not* pregnancy category C?

    a. Sertraline
    b. Paroxetine
    c. Fluoxetine
    d. Escitalopram

27. Which of the following antidepressants should be used with caution in the elderly due to its extremely long half-life, which can be prolonged in this patient population?

    a. Sertraline
    b. Fluoxetine
    c. Paroxetine
    d. Escitalopram

28. Haloperidol is the drug of choice for:

    a. outpatient management of chronic schizophrenia.
    b. depression.
    c. delirium.
    d. anxiety.

29. Which of the following statements is true regarding antipsychotic agents?

    a. Haloperidol has a black box warning for metabolic complications such as weight gain.
    b. Atypical agents have a higher affinity for dopamine receptors than typical agents.
    c. Most antipsychotics are metabolized by the kidneys.
    d. Typical agents have a higher rate of EPS than atypical agents.

30. Which of the following antipsychotics must be taken with food?

    a. Quetiapine
    b. Risperidone
    c. Aripiprazole
    d. Ziprasidone

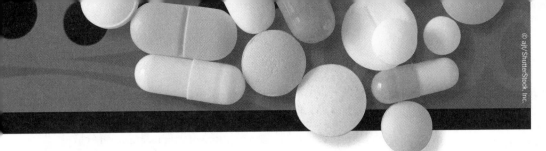

Endocrine Agents

Mirza Perez, PharmD, BCPS

BISPHOSPHONATES

Introduction

Bisphosphonates are used in the treatment and prevention of osteoporosis. The specific dosing instructions provided can prevent the common GI side effects from these medications. Many of them have multiple dosing options, often for the same indications, such as osteoporosis.

Mechanism of Action for the Drug Class

Bisphosphonates have two phosphonate groups that mimic the action of pyrophosphate, an endogenous inhibitor of bone resorption. This leads to decreased osteoclast activity and the prevention of bone destruction. All bisphosphonates become incorporated into the bone, giving them very long half-lives.

Usage for the Drug Class

Osteoporosis,* Paget's disease, hypercalcemia, bone metastasis from solid tumors

Adverse Reactions for the Drug Class: Most Common

Abdominal pain, dyspepsia, nausea, hypocalcemia

Adverse Reactions for the Drug Class: Rare/Severe/Important

Bone/muscle pain, esophagitis, gastritis, esophageal ulcers, osteonecrosis of the jaw

Major Drug Interactions for the Drug Class

Drugs Affecting Bisphosphonates

- Aspirin: Increases risk of adverse GI events
- Nonsteroidal anti-inflammatory drugs (NSAIDs): Increase risk of GI irritation
- Antacids: Decrease absorption of oral bisphosphonates

Contraindications for the Drug Class

Patients with abnormalities of the esophagus, such as strictures or achalasia. Inability to sit upright or stand for at least 30 minutes.

Counseling Points for Oral Bisphosphonates

- Take at least 30 minutes before eating or drinking first thing in the morning. Take with 6–8 oz of plain water only.
- Do not lie down for 30 minutes after taking the medication and until after the first meal of the day
- Do not chew or crush on tablets
- Notify your physician if new symptoms of heartburn or difficulty or pain on swallowing develop
- Take supplemental calcium and vitamin D if dietary intake is inadequate

Key Points for the Drug Class

- Bisphosphonates are first line for the treatment of osteoporosis
- Special administration techniques for oral bisphosphonates are needed in order to prevent GI problems
- Hypocalcemia must be corrected before therapy is initiated
- Osteonecrosis of the jaw, usually related to tooth extraction and/or local infection with delayed healing, has been observed with the use of bisphosphonates. Bisphosphonate-associated osteonecrosis has been reported primarily in cancer patients receiving intravenous bisphosphonates. However, some cases have also been reported in patients receiving treatment for postmenopausal osteoporosis. The known risk factors for osteonecrosis include a cancer diagnosis, poor oral hygiene, concomitant therapies (i.e., radiotherapy, chemotherapy, corticosteroids), and comorbid diseases (i.e., preexisting dental disease, anemia, infection, coagulopathy). Patients who develop osteonecrosis of the jaw should be referred to an oral surgeon for care.
- Patients with GERD or other GI problems may be better candidates for intravenous administration of bisphosphonates (such as zoledronic acid)

* Throughout the text, an asterisk (*) is used to indicate the most common uses of a drug.

Members of the Drug Class

In this section: Alendronate, risedronate, ibandronate, zoledronic acid

Others: Etidronate, pamidronate, clodronate, tiludronate

⊙ Alendronate

Brand Names
Fosamax, Fosamax Plus D

Generic Name
Alendronate

Rx Only

Dosage Form
Tablet

Pregnancy Category C

Dosing
- Treatment of osteoporosis in men and postmenopausal women:
  - 70 mg once a week *or*
  - 10 mg daily
- Prevention of postmenopausal osteoporosis:
  - 35 mg once a week *or*
  - 5 mg daily
- Treatment of glucocorticoid-induced osteoporosis: 5 mg daily (10 mg daily in postmenopausal women not on hormone replacement therapy)
- Treatment of Paget's disease: 40 mg daily for 6 months
- Renal dosage adjustment: Not recommended in patients with CrCl < 35 mL/min

⊙ Risedronate

Brand Name
Actonel

Generic Name
Risedronate

Rx Only

Dosage Form
Tablets

Pregnancy Category C

Dosing
- Treatment and prevention of osteoporosis in postmenopausal women:
  - 5 mg daily or
  - 35 mg once weekly
- Treatment and prevention of glucocorticoid-induced osteoporosis: 5 mg once daily

- Treatment of Paget's disease: 30 mg once daily for 2 months. Retreatment may be necessary after 2 months of observation.
- Renal dosage adjustment: Not recommended in patients with CrCl < 30 mL/min

⊙ Ibandronate

Brand Name
Boniva

Generic Name
Ibandronate

Rx Only

Dosage Forms
Tablet, injection

Usage
Treatment and prevention of osteoporosis,* hypercalcemia of malignancy,* metastatic bone disease*

Pregnancy Category C

Dosing
- Treatment of postmenopausal osteoporosis:
  - Oral:
    - 2.5 mg once daily *or*
    - 150 mg once a month
  - IV: 3 mg every 3 months
- Prevention of postmenopausal osteoporosis:
  - 2.5 mg PO once daily or
  - 150 mg PO once a month
- Hypercalcemia of malignancy (unlabeled use): 2–4 mg IV over 2 hours
- Metastatic bone disease:
  - Oral: 50 mg once daily
  - IV: 6 mg over 1 hour every 3–4 weeks
- Renal dosage adjustment: Avoid in CrCl < 30 mL/min

⊙ Zoledronic Acid

Brand Names
Zometa, Reclast

Generic Name
Zoledronic acid

Rx Only

Dosage Form
Injection

Pregnancy Category D

Dosing

- Treatment of osteoporosis: Reclast 5 mg IV once a year
- Prevention of osteoporosis: Reclast 5 mg IV every 2 years
- Treatment of Paget's disease: Reclast 5 mg IV given as a single dose (no data on retreatment)
- Hypercalcemia of malignancy: Zometa 4 mg IV given as a single dose (may consider retreatment after 7 days)
- Multiple myeloma or metastatic bone disease from solid tumors: Zometa 4 mg IV every 3–4 weeks
- Renal dosage adjustment: Not recommended in patients with CrCl < 35 mL/min for Reclast or < 30 mL/min for Zometa

CALCITONIN-SALMON

Introduction

Calcitonin-salmon is a synthetic version of the hormone calcitonin found in salmon, which ironically is more active in humans than human calcitonin. Calcitonin is used for treating postmenopausal osteoporosis, Paget's disease, and hypercalcemia. It is most commonly given intranasally. Calcitonin is less effective than bisphosphonates for the treatment of osteoporosis. It is therefore usually considered as third-line therapy.

Mechanism of Action for the Drug Class

Directly inhibits osteoclastic bone resorption; promotes the renal excretion of calcium, phosphate, sodium, magnesium, and potassium by decreasing tubular reabsorption. This drug also increases the jejunal secretion of water, sodium, potassium, and chloride.

Members of the Drug Class

In this section: Calcitonin

◉ Calcitonin

Brand Names

Miacalcin, Fortical

Generic Name

Calcitonin-salmon

Rx Only

Dosage Forms

Solution (intranasal spray), injection

Usage

Osteoporosis,* treatment of Paget's disease, hypercalcemia

Pregnancy Category C

Dosing

- Treatment of osteoporosis in postmenopausal women: Use one intranasal spray per day in one nostril; alternate nostrils daily
- Treatment of Paget's disease:
  - Initial IM or SUB-Q: 100 units/day
  - Maintenance IM or SUB-Q:
    - 50 units/day *or*
    - 50–100 units every 1–3 days
- Treatment of hypercalcemia:
  - Initial IM or SUB-Q: 4 units/kg every 12 hours
  - Maximum IM or SUB-Q: 8 units/kg every 6 hours

Adverse Reactions: Most Common

Allergic reactions, nasal mucosal alterations, rhinitis

Adverse Reactions: Rare/Severe/Important

Epistaxis, sinusitis

Counseling Points (nasal spray)

- Allow the medication to reach room temperature before priming or using a new bottle
- To prime the pump, hold the bottle upright and press the two white side arms of the pump toward the bottle until a full spray is produced
- To administer the medication, place the nozzle into the nostril with the head in the upright position
- The pump should not be primed before each dose
- Take supplemental calcium and vitamin D if dietary intake is inadequate
- Store new unassembled bottles in the refrigerator
- Once the pump has been activated, store bottle at room temperature in an upright position for up to 35 days

Key Point

- Usually used when bisphosphonates are not tolerated
- Patient instructions on how to administer the nasal spray are important to ensure appropriate administration

SEX HORMONES: ESTROGENS, PROGESTINS, ESTROGEN AND PROGESTIN COMBINATIONS, ESTROGEN AND ANDROGEN COMBINATIONS

Introduction

These medications are used mainly for the treatment of vasomotor symptoms associated with menopause and the prevention of osteoporosis. However, their use has decreased since the Women's Health Initiative (WHI) trial in 2002. This trial was terminated prematurely because of an increased risk of coronary heart disease and thromboembolic events in patients receiving the estrogen/progesterone combination. The interpretation of this study has been controversial based on the risk profile of the women included in the study, but it led to a significant decrease in the use of these drugs.

Mechanism of Action for the Drug Class

Estrogens (estradiol, conjugated estrogen, esterified estrogen) are important in developing and maintaining the female reproductive system and secondary sex characteristics, promoting growth and development of the vagina, uterus, fallopian tubes, and breasts. Estrogens are also involved in shaping the skeleton and inhibiting bone resorption. Progestins (medroxyprogesterone) inhibit the secretion of gonadotropins, which, in turn, prevent follicular maturation and ovulation and results in endometrial thinning.

Adverse Reactions for the Drug Class: Most Common

- Estrogen-containing products: Vaginal bleeding, breast tenderness, nausea and vomiting
- Progestin-containing products: Breakthrough bleeding, nausea

Adverse Reactions for the Drug Class: Rare/Severe/Important

- Estrogen-containing products: Weight gain, edema, headache, migraines
- Progestin-containing products: Insomnia, somnolence

Major Drug Interactions for the Drug Class

Drugs Affecting Estrogen

Barbiturates, rifampin, phenytoin, carbamazepine, and other agents that induce hepatic microsomal enzymes (CYP450 3A4): May lower estrogen levels

Estrogen's Effect on Other Drugs

Corticosteroids: May increase the pharmacologic and toxicologic effects

Contraindications for the Drug Class

Known or suspected pregnancy; undiagnosed abnormal vaginal bleeding; known or suspected breast cancer, except for selected patients treated for metastatic disease; active thromboembolic disorders; severe liver disease

Counseling Points for the Drug Class (Estrogens)

- Estrogens have been reported to increase the risk of endometrial carcinoma in postmenopausal women
- Do not use estrogens with or without progestins to prevent heart disease, heart attacks, or strokes
- Do not use estrogens and progestins during pregnancy
- Notify a healthcare provider if any of the following occur: pain in the groin or calves, sharp chest pain or sudden shortness of breath, abnormal vaginal bleeding, missed menstrual period, lumps in the breast, sudden severe headache, vision or speech disturbance, weakness or numbness in an arm or leg, severe abdominal pain, yellowing of the skin or eyes, or severe depression
- Women with an intact uterus should also receive monthly progestins, not estrogen-only products
- While taking estrogens, you should visit your doctor at least once a year for appropriate follow-up

Members of the Drug Class (Estrogens)

In this section: Estradiol, estradiol transdermal system, conjugated estrogen
Others: Esterified estrogens, estrone, estropipate

Members of the Drug Class (Progestins)

In this section: Medroxyprogesterone
Others: Hydroxyprogesterone, norethindrone acetate, progesterone

◉ Estradiol

Brand Name
Estrace

Generic Name
Estradiol

Rx Only

Dosage Form
Tablet

Usage
Treatment of moderate to severe vasomotor symptoms,* vulvar and vaginal atrophy associated with menopause, female hypoestrogenism, breast cancer (palliation only),

androgen-dependent carcinoma of the prostate, prevention of osteoporosis,* abnormal uterine bleeding due to hormonal imbalance

Pregnancy Category X

Dosing

- Treatment of moderate to severe vasomotor symptoms, vulvar and vaginal atrophy associated with menopause:
  - Initial dose: 1–2 mg daily adjusted to control symptoms
  - Administration should be cyclic, 3 weeks on, 1 week off
  - Discontinuation/tapering: Attempts to discontinue or taper should be considered at 3- to 6-month intervals
- Treatment of female hypoestrogenism: Initial dose of 1–2 mg daily adjusted to control symptoms
- Treatment of breast cancer for palliation only: Initial dose of 10 mg three times daily
- Treatment of advanced androgen-dependent carcinoma of the prostate: Initial dose of 1–2 mg three times daily adjusted to control symptoms
- Prevention of osteoporosis: Initial dose of 0.5 mg administered cyclically (23 days on and 5 days off), dose adjusted to control menopausal symptoms

⊙ Estradiol Transdermal System

Brand Names
Climara, Estraderm, Vivelle-Dot

Generic Name
Estradiol transdermal system

Rx Only

Dosage Form
Patch

Usage
Treatment of moderate to severe vasomotor symptoms and vulvar and vaginal atrophy; prevention of postmenopausal osteoporosis

Pregnancy Category X

Dosing
- Climara: 0.025–0.05 mg/day applied to the skin once weekly, adjusted based on symptoms
- Estraderm: 0.05 mg/day applied to the skin twice weekly, adjusted based on symptoms
- Vivelle-Dot: 0.025–0.05 mg applied to skin twice weekly, adjusted based on symptoms

Counseling Points
Guidelines for applying the transdermal system:
- Place the adhesive side on a clean, dry area of the lower abdomen or the upper quadrant of the buttock. The area selected should not be oily, damaged, or irritated
- Do not apply the transdermal system to the breasts
- Rotate the sites of application
- Press the system firmly in place for at least 10 seconds
- If a system falls off, apply a new one for the remainder of the treatment duration
- Only one system should be worn at a time
- Swimming, bathing, or using a sauna may decrease the adhesion of the system

Key Points
- In women who are taking oral estrogens, the transdermal system can be initiated 1 week after withdrawal of oral therapy
- Therapy may be given continuously in women who do not have an intact uterus. In patients with an intact uterus, therapy may be given on a cyclic schedule (3 weeks on, 1 week off)
- Climara is a continuous transdermal system for once-weekly administration; Estraderm, and Vivelle-Dot are continuous-transdermal systems for twice-weekly administration

⊙ Conjugated Estrogen

Brand Name
Premarin

Generic Name
Conjugated estrogen

Rx Only

Dosage Form
Tablet

Usage
Treatment of moderate to severe vasomotor symptoms,* vulvar and vaginal atrophy, female hypoestrogenism, prevention of osteoporosis*

Pregnancy Category X

Dosing
0.3–1.25 mg daily

Key Points
- Conjugated estrogens may be given continuously with no interruption in therapy or in cyclic regimens (regimens such as 25 days on drug followed by 5 days off)
- Attempts to discontinue or taper medication should be made at 3- to 6-month intervals

⊙ Medroxyprogesterone

Brand Names

Cycrin, Provera, Depo-Provera, Depo-Sub-Q Provera 104

Generic Name

Medroxyprogesterone

Rx Only

Dosage Forms

Tablet, injection

Usage

Management of endometriosis-associated pain (Depo-Sub-Q Provera only), secondary amenorrhea, abnormal uterine bleeding due to hormonal imbalance, reduction of endometrial hyperplasia in postmenopausal women receiving estrogens, prevention of pregnancy*

Pregnancy Category X

Dosing

- Management of endometriosis-associated pain: 104 mg SUB-Q every 3 months (13 weeks)
- Secondary amenorrhea: 5 or 10 mg tablets daily for 5–10 days
- Abnormal uterine bleeding due to hormonal imbalance: 5 or 10 mg tablets daily for 5–10 days beginning on day 16 or day 21 of the menstrual cycle
- Reduction of endometrial hyperplasia in postmenopausal women receiving 0.625 mg of conjugated estrogens: 5 or 10 mg tablets daily for 12–14 consecutive days per month, either beginning on day 1 of the menstrual cycle or day 16 of the menstrual cycle
- Prevention of pregnancy:
  - IM injection: 150 mg every 3 months (13 weeks)
  - SUB-Q injection: 104 mg every 3 months (13 weeks)

Counseling Points

- Advise patients that at the beginning of Depo-Provera therapy their menstrual cycle may be disrupted and irregular and unpredictable bleeding or spotting may occur
- Progestin withdrawal bleeding usually occurs within 3–7 days after discontinuing oral therapy
- Depo-Sub-Q Provera should be given by SUB-Q injection into the anterior thigh or abdomen

Key Point

Women who use Depo-Provera Contraceptive Injection (IM or SUB-Q) may lose significant bone mineral density. Bone loss is greater with increasing duration of use and may not be completely reversible. Depo-Provera Contraceptive Injection should be used as a long-term birth control method (e.g., > 2 years) only if other birth control methods are inadequate.

⊙ Conjugated Estrogen/ Medroxyprogesterone Acetate

Brand Names

Prempro, Premphase

Generic Name

Conjugated estrogen/medroxyprogesterone acetate

Rx Only

Dosage Form

Tablet

Usage

Treatment of moderate to severe vasomotor symptoms,* vulvar and vaginal atrophy, prevention of postmenopausal osteoporosis*

Pregnancy Category X

Dosing

- Prempro: Start with 0.3 mg/1.5 mg, with subsequent dosage adjustments based on patient response and symptoms
- Premphase: 0.625 mg tablet daily on days 1–14 and 0.625 mg/5 mg daily on days 15–28

Counseling Point

Take as directed by prescriber

Key Point

This medication (combination of estrogen and progesterone) is the drug of choice in women with an intact uterus

⊙ Esterified Estrogens and Methyltestosterone

Brand Names

Covaryx HS, EEMT

Generic Name

Esterified estrogens and methyltestosterone

Rx Only

Dosage Form

Tablet

Usage

Treatment of moderate to severe vasomotor symptoms associated with menopause

Pregnancy Category X

Dosing

1 tablet daily (3 weeks on and 1 week off)

Counseling Point

Take as directed by prescriber

COMBINED ORAL CONTRACEPTIVES, MONOPHASIC

Introduction

The administration of combined oral contraceptives is a contraceptive method that includes a combination of an estrogen and a progestin. When taken daily they inhibit ovulation. They are currently the most common form of pharmacologic birth control. **Table 7-1** summarizes the available monophasic combined oral contraceptives.

Mechanism of Action for the Drug Class

The agents deliver a fixed dosage of estrogen and progestin throughout the cycle that inhibits ovulation by suppressing the gonadotropins, follicle-stimulating hormone (FSH), and luteinizing hormone (LH). Additionally, alterations in the genital tract, including the cervical mucus, which inhibits sperm penetration, and the endometrium, which reduces the likelihood of implantation, may contribute to contraceptive effectiveness.

Members of the Drug Class

In this section: Combinations of ethinyl estradiol and levonorestrel/norethindrone/desogestrel/drospirenone/ norgestimate
Others: Combinations of ethinyl estradiol and ethynodiol or mestranol

TABLE 7-1 Combined Oral Contraceptives (Monophasic)

Brand Name	Generic Name and Dosage
Alesse	Levonorgestrel: 0.1 mg Ethinyl estradiol: 20 µg for 21 days
Desogen	Desogestrel: 0.15 mg Ethinyl estradiol: 30 µg for 21 days
Loestrin FE 1/20, Loestrin 24 FE	Norethindrone acetate: 1 mg Ethinyl estradiol: 20 µg for 21 days Ferrous fumarate: 75 mg for 7 days
Ocella	Drospirenone: 3 mg Ethynyl estradiol: 30 µg for 21 days
Lo-Ovral	Norgestrel: 0.3 mg Ethinyl estradiol: 30 µg for 21 days
Ortho-Cyclen	Norgestimate: 0.25 mg Ethinyl estradiol: 35 µg for 21 days
Yasmin	Drospirenone: 3 mg Ethinyl estradiol: 30 µg for 21 days
Yaz	Drospirenone: 3 mg Ethinyl estradiol: 20 µg for 24 days
Seasonale	Levonorgestrel: 0.15 mg Ethinyl estradiol: 30 µg for 84 days

Rx Only for the Drug Class

Dosage Forms for the Drug Class

Tablet

Usage for the Drug Class

Prevention of pregnancy in women, treatment of menorrhagia, pain associated with endometriosis, dysmenorrhea

Pregnancy Category X for the Drug Class

Dosing for the Drug Class

- 21-day regimen: Day 1 of cycle is the first day of menstrual bleeding. Take 1 tablet daily for 21 days, beginning on day 5 of cycle. Then, no tablets are taken for 7 days. Whether bleeding has stopped or not, start a new course of 21 days.
- 24-day regimen: Take 24 days of active pills and 4 days of inert or iron tablets on the last 4 days of cycle
- 28-day regimen: To eliminate the need to count the days between cycles, some products contain 7 inert or iron-containing tablets to permit continuous daily dosage during the entire 28-day cycle

Adverse Reactions for the Drug Class: Most Common

Nausea, vomiting, bloating, migraine headaches, edema, breast tenderness, breakthrough bleeding (most often in first few cycles of pills), change in menstrual flow, weight gain, tiredness, fatigue, depression

Adverse Reactions for the Drug Class: Rare/Severe/Important

Myocardial infarction, thromboembolism, cerebral hemorrhage, hypertension, gallbladder disease

Major Drug Interactions for the Drug Class

Drugs Affecting Combined Oral Contraceptives

- Antibiotics: Menstrual irregularities and possible contraceptive failure
- Barbiturates, carbamazepine, griseofulvin, phenytoin, rifampin, protease inhibitors: Decreased efficacy via metabolic induction

Combined Oral Contraceptives' Effects on Other Drugs

Tricyclic antidepressants, beta blockers, theophylline, benzodiazepines: Increase effect via decreased metabolism

Contraindications for the Drug Class

History of myocardial infarction, coronary artery disease, known or suspected breast carcinoma or estrogen-dependent neoplasm, hepatic adenomas/carcinomas, undiagnosed abnormal genital bleeding, thromboembolic disorder, pregnancy, acute liver disease

Endocrine Agents

Counseling Points for the Drug Class

- Take oral contraceptive pills at exactly the same time every day for maximum effectiveness and do not exceed dosing intervals > 24 hours
- Missing pills may reduce the effectiveness of the birth control and cause spotting or light bleeding
- Continue to take pills throughout all bleeding episodes
- Use an additional method of birth control for the first week of pills during the initial cycle of oral contraceptive pills
- Spotting or breakthrough bleeding may occur during the first few months of therapy. Talk to your healthcare provider if bleeding lasts more than a few days and occurs in more than one cycle.
- Notify your healthcare provider if pregnancy is suspected or if any of the following occur: Sudden severe headache, visual disturbances, numbness in an arm or leg, severe abdominal pain, prolonged episodes of bleeding, or amenorrhea
- Appropriate action if one or more pills are missed:
  - If 1 pill is missed anytime in the cycle, take the pill as soon as you remember and the next pill at its regular time
  - If 2 pills are missed during the first 2 weeks of the cycle, take 2 pills daily for 2 days; then resume taking pills on their regular schedule. Use additional contraception (e.g., condom) for the remainder of the cycle.
  - If 2 pills are missed during the third week of the cycle and you are a day 1 starter, throw out the rest of the pack and start a new pack that same day. If you are a Sunday starter, keep taking 1 pill every day until Sunday. On Sunday throw out the rest of the pack and start a new pack that same day. Use additional contraception until the new pack of pills is started and for the first 7 days of the new cycle.
  - If 3 or more pills are missed and you are a day 1 starter, throw out the rest of the pack and start a new pack that same day. If you are a Sunday starter, keep taking 1 pill every day until Sunday. On Sunday throw out the rest of the pack and start a new pack that same day. Use additional contraception until the new pack of pills is started and for the first 7 days of the new cycle.

Key Points for the Drug Class

- Combined oral contraceptives are the most common type of pharmacologic contraception
- Combined oral contraceptives should be prescribed with caution, if ever, to smokers and/or > 35 years of age
- Smokers < 30 years of age who are otherwise healthy generally can use combined oral contraceptives
- Special instructions exist if one or more doses are missed
- Seasonale is a combined oral contraceptive that provides continued estrogen and progesterone for 3 months

COMBINED ORAL CONTRACEPTIVES, BIPHASIC

Mechanism of Action for the Drug Class

These drugs inhibit ovulation (as explained in the monophasic drug class section). In this drug class, the amount of estrogen remains the same for the first 21 days of the cycle and decreases at the end of the cycle.

Members of the Drug Class

In this section: Combinations of ethinyl estradiol and desogestrel
Others: Combinations of ethinyl estradiol and norethindrone

◉ Desogestrel/Ethinyl Estradiol

Brand Name
Mircette

Generic Name
Desogestrel/ethinyl estradiol

Rx Only

Dosage Form
Tablet

Usage
Prevention of pregnancy in women

Pregnancy Category X

Dosing
Desogestrel 0.15 mg/ethinyl estradiol 20 μg for 21 days, placebo for 2 days, and then ethinyl estradiol 10 μg for 5 days

COMBINED ORAL CONTRACEPTIVES, TRIPHASIC

Mechanism of Action for the Drug Class

This drug inhibits ovulation (as explained in the monophasic drug class section). In this drug class, the estrogen amount remains the same or varies throughout the cycle; the progestin amount varies. **Table 7-2** summarizes the available triphasic combined oral contraceptives.

Members of the Drug Class

In this section: Combinations of ethinyl estradiol and levonorgestrel/norethindrone/desogestrel/norgestimate

Dosage Form for the Drug Class
Tablet

Usage for the Drug Class
Prevention of pregnancy in women, treatment of moderate acne vulgaris in women > 15 years

Pregnancy Category X for the Drug Class

TABLE 7–2 Combined Oral Contraceptives (Triphasic)

Brand Name	Generic Name and Dosage
Ortho-Novum 7/7/7	Norethindrone: 0.5 mg/ethinyl estradiol: 35 µg for 7 days Norethindrone: 0.75 mg/ethinyl estradiol: 35 µg for 7 days Norethindrone: 1 mg/ethinyl estradiol: 35 µg for 7 days
Ortho Tri-Cyclen, TriNessa, Tri-Sprintec	Norgestimate: 0.18 mg/ethinyl estradiol: 35 µg for 7 days Norgestimate: 0.215 mg/ethinyl estradiol: 35 µg for 7 days Norgestimate: 0.25 mg/ethinyl estradiol: 35 µg for 7 days
Ortho Tri-Cyclen-Lo	Norgestimate: 0.18 mg/ethinyl estradiol: 25 µg for 7 days Norgestimate: 0.215 mg/ethinyl estradiol: 25 µg for 7 days Norgestimate: 0.25 mg/ethinyl estradiol: 25 µg for 7 days
Triphasil, Trivora	Levonorgestrel: 0.050 mg/ethinyl estradiol: 30 µg for 6 days Levonorgestrel: 0.075 mg/ethinyl estradiol: 40 µg for 5 days Levonorgestrel: 0.125 mg/ethinyl estradiol: 30 µg for 10 days

---

ESTROGEN AND PROGESTERONE VAGINAL RING

Mechanism of Action for the Drug Class

The vaginal ring contains the combination of ethinyl estradiol and etonogestrel. It inhibits ovulation by decreasing the amount of gonadotropin hormones, similar to the mechanism of combined oral contraceptives.

Members of the Drug Class

In this section: Ethinyl estradiol and etonogestrel

⦿ Ethinyl Estradiol 0.015 mg/day and Etonogestrel 0.12 mg/day

Brand Name
NuvaRing

Generic Name
Ethinyl estradiol 0.015 mg/day and etonogestrel 0.12 mg/day

Rx Only

Dosage Form
Vaginal ring device

Usage
Contraception

Pregnancy Category X

Dosing
Insert one ring vaginally and leave in place for 3 weeks, then remove for 1 week to allow for breakthrough bleeding

Counseling Points
- Administration: Press sides of the ring together between the fingers and insert folded into the vagina. Specific placement is not required.
- Do not dispose of the ring in the toilet

- A different contraceptive method should be used if the ring is expelled for > 3 hours. If < 3 hours, it should be washed and reinserted.
- A new ring is inserted 7 days after the last one was removed. It should be inserted at approximately the same time.

Key Points
- The efficacy of the vaginal ring is similar to that of combined oral contraceptives
- Side effects and precautions are the same as for combined oral contraceptives
- May have the advantage of better compliance

PROGESTIN-ONLY ORAL CONTRACEPTIVES

Mechanism of Action for the Drug Class

Progestins prevent conception by suppressing ovulation in approximately 50% of users. They thicken the cervical mucus to inhibit sperm penetration, lower the midcycle LH and FSH peaks, slow the movement of the ovum through the fallopian tubes, and alter the endometrium.

Members of the Drug Class

In this section: Norethindrone
Others: Norgestrel

◉ Norethindrone

Brand Name
Micronor

Generic Name
Norethindrone

Rx Only

Dosage Form
Tablet

Pregnancy Category X

Counseling Points
- Effectiveness may be reduced dramatically when progestin-only pills are taken > 3 hours late. Use a backup nonpharmacologic method of contraception (such as condoms) for the next 48 hours whenever pills are taken ≥ 3 hours late.
- Appropriate action if one or more progestin-only pills are missed:
  - If the pill is taken ≥ 3 hours late, take the pill as soon as remembered and use additional contraception for 48 hours
  - If 1 or more pills are missed, take it as soon as remembered. Take today's pill at its regular time, even if that means taking 2 pills in 1 day. Use additional contraception for 48 hours.

SELECTIVE ESTROGEN RECEPTOR MODULATORS

Introduction

Raloxifene is one of the medications in the family of selective estrogen receptor modulators (SERMs). It is more selective in its action than tamoxifen and is used in the treatment of osteoporosis and in the prevention of breast cancer in high-risk women. Note that it is not as effective as bisphosphonates for the treatment and prevention of osteoporosis.

Mechanism of Action for the Drug Class

It is a mixed estrogen agonist/antagonist. It has estrogenic agonist action in the bones and estrogenic antagonistic action in the breast and uterine tissue. It inhibits bone resorption and reduces biochemical markers of bone turnover.

Members of the Drug Class

In this section: Raloxifene

◉ Raloxifene

Brand Name
Evista

Generic Name
Raloxifene

Rx Only

Dosage Form
Tablet

Usage

Prevention and treatment of postmenopausal osteoporosis,* risk reduction for invasive breast cancer in postmenopausal women with osteoporosis and in postmenopausal women with high risk for invasive breast cancer

Pregnancy Category X

Dosing

- 60 mg daily
- Renal dosage adjustment: In cases of moderate to severe renal dysfunction, the dose may be reduced. However, the safety and efficacy in such patients have not been established.
- Hepatic dosage adjustment: Dose may be reduced in cases of hepatic dysfunction. However, safety and efficacy in such patients have not been established.

Adverse Reactions: Most Common

Hot flashes, nausea

Adverse Reactions: Rare/Severe/Important

Muscle aches, vaginal bleeding, abdominal pain, thromboembolism

Major Drug Interactions

Drugs Affecting Raloxifene

Cholestyramine: Reduces raloxifene absorption

Raloxifene's Effect on Other Drugs

- Levothyroxine: Decreases absorption
- Warfarin: May decrease prothrombin time by 10%

Contraindications

Women who are or may become pregnant; history of venous thromboembolic events

Counseling Points

- Discontinue raloxifene at least 72 hours prior to and during prolonged immobilization to prevent clot formations
- Avoid prolonged restrictions of movement during travel because of the increased risk of blood clots
- Take supplemental calcium and vitamin D if daily intake is inadequate

Key Points

- Used for the prevention and treatment of postmenopausal women osteoporosis and for the prevention of breast cancer in high-risk women
- Avoid in patients with a history of thromboembolic disorders

GLUCOCORTICOIDS

Introduction

Glucocorticoids are anti-inflammatory, immunosuppressant agents used in the treatment of a variety of diseases, including those of allergic, dermatologic, endocrine, hematologic, inflammatory, neoplastic, nervous system, renal, respiratory, rheumatic, and autoimmune origin. They may be used in the management of cerebral edema and chronic swelling; as a diagnostic agent, such as in the case of Cushing's syndrome; as an antiemetic; and for many other uses. They have significant adverse effects that can be dose and duration limiting. Converting from one glucocorticoid to another is a common practice. Approximate conversions are listed in **Table 7-3**.

Mechanism of Action for the Drug Class

The exact mechanism of glucocorticoids is unknown. They inhibit interleukin-1 and various other cytokines that mediate inflammatory responses. They also decrease inflammation by suppressing migration of polymorphonuclear leukocytes and decreasing capillary permeability.

Members of the Drug Class

In this section: Methylprednisolone and prednisone, dexamethasone

Others: Betamethasone, cortisone, hydrocortisone, prednisolone, triamcinolone (these are other systemic glucocorticoids)

Usage for the Drug Class

Treatment of multiple inflammatory conditions;* acute asthma;* rheumatoid arthritis (RA); dermatologic lesions, such as keloids; autoimmune disorders, such as multiple sclerosis; adrenogenital syndrome; adjunctive therapy for *Pneumocystis jiroveci* pneumonia (PCP)

TABLE 7-3 Glucocorticoid Conversion	
Glucocorticoid	**Equivalent Anti-Inflammatory Dose**
Cortisone	25 mg
Hydrocortisone	20 mg
Prednisone	5 mg
Prednisolone	5 mg
Methylprednisolone	4 mg
Triamcinolone	4 mg
Betamethasone	0.75 mg
Dexamethasone	0.75 mg

Adverse Reactions for the Drug Class: Most Common

GI irritation, increased appetite, nervousness/restlessness, weight gain, acne, glucose intolerance (transient), lipid abnormalities (transient)

Adverse Reactions for the Drug Class: Rare/Severe/Important

Infections, adrenal suppression, rounding out of the face, hirsutism, glaucoma, osteoporosis, peptic ulceration

Major Drug Interactions for the Drug Class

Drugs Affecting Glucocorticoids

- Alcohol/NSAIDs: Increase risk of gastric ulceration
- Estrogens: May increase toxicity

Glucocorticoids' Effects on Other Drugs

Insulin/oral hypoglycemic agents: Increase glucose levels

Contraindications for the Drug Class

Systemic fungal infections, concomitant administration of live vaccines

Counseling Point for the Drug Class

Take oral tablets with food and preferably in the morning

Key Points for the Drug Class

- Used for many inflammatory conditions
- Too rapid withdrawal of therapy, especially after prolonged use, may cause acute, possibly life-threatening adrenal insufficiency. If course of therapy is > 10–14 days, therapy must be tapered when discontinuing.
- The prescribed dosages of glucocorticoids vary depending on the compound used and the nature of the patient's condition. Depending on these factors, the dose may be taken once a day, spaced evenly throughout the day, or even taken every other day.

◉ Methylprednisolone and Prednisone

Brand Names

Medrol and Medrol Dosepak, Depo-Medrol, Solu-Medrol

Generic Name

Methylprednisolone

Dosage Forms

Tablet, injection

Brand Names

Deltasone, Orasone

Generic Name

Prednisone

Rx Only

Dosage Forms

Tablet, oral solution

Pregnancy Category C

Dosing

- Treatment of acute asthma, including status asthmaticus and allergic rhinitis:
  - Oral: 4–48 mg/day (methylprednisolone) or 40–60 mg/day (prednisone) for 3–10 days; individualize dose based on response
  - Alternate-day oral therapy: Twice the daily dose may be administered every other day
  - Dosepak: Taper each day according to manufacturer's instructions (6-day therapy starting with 24 mg day 1; decrease by 4 mg every day and finish with 4 mg on day 6)
  - IV (sodium succinate): Loading dose: 2 mg/kg/dose then 0.5: 1 mg/kg/dose every 6 hours for 5 days
- Treatment of rheumatoid arthritis:
  - Intra-articular (acetate):
    - Large joints (such as knees and ankles): 20–80 mg
    - Medium joints (such as elbows and wrists): 10–40 mg
    - Small joints (such as metacarpophalangeal): 4–10 mg
  - Oral: < 10 mg/day
- Dermatologic lesions (chronic): 40–120 mg IM (acetate) weekly
- Anti-inflammatory or immunosuppression: 10–40 mg daily oral or IV (sodium succinate) in divided doses
- Acute exacerbation of multiple sclerosis:
  - IV: 500–1,000 mg daily for 3–5 days, with or without a short prednisone taper
  - Oral: 200 mg (prednisone) daily for 1 week then 80 mg every other day for 1 month

◉ Dexamethasone

Brand Names

Decadron, DexPak

Generic Name

Dexamethasone

Rx Only

Dosage Forms

Tablet, oral solution, injection

Usage

Treatment of a variety of diseases, including those of allergic, dermatologic, endocrine, hematologic, inflammatory, neoplastic, nervous system, renal, respiratory, rheumatic, and autoimmune origin; management of cerebral edema and chronic inflammation; diagnosis of Cushing's syndrome; antiemetic

Pregnancy Category C

Dosing

- Anti-inflammatory:
  - Oral, IM, IV: 0.75–9 mg daily in divided doses every 6–12 hours
  - Intra-articular, intralesional, or soft tissue: 0.4–6 mg daily
- Cerebral edema: 10 mg IV stat, then 4 mg IM/IV (should be given as sodium phosphate) every 6 hours until response is maximized

PARATHYROID HORMONE ANALOGS

Introduction

Teriparatide is a recombinant form of parathyroid hormone. It has been shown to decrease osteoporosis fractures. This agent is usually reserved for severe osteoporosis or for patients who are intolerant to bisphosphonates.

Mechanism of Action of the Drug Class

As a parathyroid hormone agonist it stimulates osteoblast function, increases calcium absorption from the GI tract, and increases calcium reabsorption from the kidneys

Members of the Drug Class

In this section: Teriparatide

⊚ Teriparatide

Brand Name
Forteo

Generic Name
Teriparatide

Rx Only

Dosage Form
Injection

Usage

Osteoporosis* and glucocorticoid-induced osteoporosis in people at high risk

Pregnancy Category C

Dosing

20 mg SUB-Q daily

Adverse Reactions: Most Common

Transient hypercalcemia

Adverse Reactions: Rare/Severe/Important

Osteosarcomas, orthostatic hypotension

Major Drug Interactions

No known significant interactions

Counseling Points

- The prefilled pen needs to be kept refrigerated
- Inject subcutaneously in the thigh or abdomen. Patients may need to be shown how to do this.

Key Points

- Because of its significant cost, subcutaneous administration, and limited long-term safety data, teriparatide is reserved for patients with severe osteoporosis and for those intolerant to bisphosphonates
- Administration of teriparatide needs to be combined with calcium and vitamin D supplements

Introduction

Thyroid hormones are chemical compounds that are essential for the function of every cell in the body. They help regulate growth and the body's metabolism. The two most important thyroid hormones are thyroxine (T4) and triiodothyronine (T3).

Mechanism of Action for the Drug Class

The effect of thyroid hormones is believed to be exerted through control of DNA transcription and protein synthesis. Their principal effect is to increase the metabolic rate of body tissues, as noted by increased respiratory rate; cardiac output; heart rate; and protein, fat, and carbohydrate metabolism. They exert a profound effect on every organ system, particularly CNS development. Levothyroxine is a synthetic form of T4.

Members of the Drug Class

In this section: Levothyroxine sodium
Others: Liothyronine, liotrix, thyroid (desiccated)

◉ Levothyroxine Sodium

Brand Names
Levothroid, Levoxyl, Synthroid, Unithroid, Tirosint

Generic Name
Levothyroxine sodium

Dosage
Rx only

Dosage Forms
Tablet, injection

Usage
Hypothyroidism,* myxedema coma

Pregnancy Category A

Dosing
- Hypothyroidism:
  - Oral: 100–125 µg daily
  - Initial dose in patients > 50 years or with underlying cardiac disease: 25–50 µg daily
  - Maximum dose: 300 µg daily
- Myxedema coma:
  - Initial dose: 200–500 µg IV
  - Maintenance dose: 75–100 µg IV daily until stable

Adverse Reactions: Most Common
Fatigue, increased appetite, weight loss, heat intolerance, hyperhidrosis

Adverse Reactions: Rare/Severe/Important
Hair loss, menstrual irregularities, nervousness, irritability, insomnia

Major Drug Interactions
Drugs Affecting Levothyroxine
- Cholestyramine: Impairs absorption
- Estrogens: Increase serum thyroxine-binding globulin, thus decreasing free thyroxine concentrations
- Iron and calcium: Decrease absorption (separate administration)
- Raloxifene: Decreases absorption

Levothyroxine's Effect on Other Drugs
Warfarin: Increased prothrombin time/international normalized ratio

Essential Monitoring Parameters
Thyroid-stimulating hormone, T3, and T4 blood concentrations should be obtained every 6–8 weeks initially until stable, every 8–12 weeks after dose adjustments, and annually thereafter

Contraindications
Untreated thyrotoxicosis, uncorrected adrenal insufficiency

Counseling Points
- Report any signs and symptoms of thyroid hormone toxicity, such as chest pain, increased pulse rate, palpitations, excessive sweating, heat intolerance, and nervousness
- Take oral tablets first thing in the morning on an empty stomach at least half hour before any other food
- If receiving concomitant therapy with cholestyramine and levothyroxine, take doses at least 4–5 hours apart

Key Points
- Used in the treatment of hypothyroidism
- Doses should be adjusted in 12.5–25 µg increments

REVIEW QUESTIONS

1. Which of the following statements about NuvaRing is *false*?
   a. It needs to be replaced every week.
   b. It contains estrogen and progesterone.
   c. The ring should not be disposed of in the toilet.
   d. None of the above

2. Which of the following statements about teriparatide is *false*?
   a. It is indicated for the treatment of osteoporosis.
   b. It is given as a subcutaneous injection once a month.
   c. It is a parathyroid hormone analog.
   d. It increases calcium absorption from the GI tract.

3. Which of the following is a common adverse reaction of Fosamax?
   a. Abdominal pain
   b. Esophageal ulcers
   c. Bone pain
   d. Hypercalcemia

4. Which of the following is an appropriate dose of risedronate for the treatment of osteoporosis?
   a. 5 mg daily
   b. 70 mg weekly
   c. 35 mg weekly
   d. Both A and C

5. Which of the following is *not* an adverse reaction to calcitonin?
   a. Nasal irritation
   b. Esophagitis
   c. Rhinitis
   d. Epistaxis

6. Which of the following is *not* an indication for Estradiol?
   a. Treatment of vasomotor symptoms
   b. Prevention of osteoporosis
   c. Treatment of osteoporosis
   d. Treatment of abnormal uterine bleeding

7. Which of the following is a contraindication for use of estrogen-containing products?
   a. Active thromboembolic disorders
   b. History of diabetes
   c. Severe liver disease
   d. Both A and C

8. Which of the following medications interact with Vivelle?
   a. Rifampin
   b. Phenytoin
   c. Carbamazepine
   d. All of the above

9. What do Miacalcin and Fosamax have in common?
   a. They are both used for the treatment of osteoporosis.
   b. Abdominal pain is the most common adverse reaction to both medications.
   c. They both have an oral formulation.
   d. Antacids may decrease the absorption of both medications.

10. Ibandronate is used for which of the following indications?
    a. Treatment of osteoporosis
    b. Hypercalcemia of malignancy
    c. Metastatic bone disease
    d. All of the above

11. Which of the following medications does *not* contain estrogen?
    a. Climara
    b. Premarin
    c. Depo-Provera
    d. Estraderm

12. Which of the following is *not* a common adverse reaction to estrogen-containing products?
    a. Vaginal bleeding
    b. Breast tenderness
    c. Nausea
    d. Vasomotor symptoms

13. Which of the following is an example of a biphasic combined oral contraceptive?
    a. Desogen
    b. Lo-Ovral
    c. Mircette
    d. Ortho-Novum 7/7/7

14. Which of the following is the appropriate dose of Evista for the treatment of osteoporosis?
    a. 30 mg twice daily
    b. 60 mg daily
    c. 90 mg daily
    d. 120 mg twice daily

15. Which of the following is a common adverse reaction to high-dose glucocorticoids?
    a. GI irritation
    b. Weight gain
    c. Glucose intolerance
    d. All of the above

16. Which of the following is a side effect of rapid withdrawal of high-dose glucocorticosteroids?
    a. Hyperglycemia
    b. Adrenal insufficiency
    c. Thrombocytopenia
    d. Weight gain

17. Which of the following is *not* an important counseling point about the use of transdermal systems containing estrogen?

   a. The transdermal system should be applied to the breasts and thigh.

   b. Only one transdermal system should be worn at any one time.

   c. Using a sauna may decrease the adhesion of the system.

   d. Climara is a continuous transdermal system for once weekly administration.

18. What is the appropriate dose of Depo-Provera for the prevention of pregnancy?

   a. 5–10 mg daily

   b. 150 mg IM every 3 months

   c. 150 mg SUB-Q every 6 months

   d. 104 mg SUB-Q every month

19. Which of the following is a conjugated estrogen and progesterone formulation?

   a. Prempro

   b. Premarin

   c. Premphase

   d. Both A and C

20. Which of the following bisphosphonates is only given intravenously?

   a. Risedronate

   b. Alendronate

   c. Zoledronic acid

   d. Ibandronate

21. Which of the following is *not* a common adverse reaction to Synthroid?

   a. Fatigue

   b. Weight gain

   c. Heat intolerance

   d. Increase appetite

22. Which of the following is a parathyroid hormone analog?

   a. Fosamax

   b. Forteo

   c. Actonel

   d. Zometa

23. Which of the following is a common adverse effect of raloxifene?

   a. Dyspepsia

   b. Hot flashes

   c. Increase in appetite

   d. Lipid abnormalities

24. Which of the following is an estradiol transdermal formulation?

   a. Vivelle

   b. Estrace

   c. Prempro

   d. Provera

25. In which of the following patient populations should one use caution when dispensing combined oral contraceptives?

   a. Noncompliant patients

   b. Smokers

   c. Women > 35 years

   d. All of the above

26. Which of the following is a progestin-only oral contraceptive?

   a. Micronor

   b. Depo-Provera

   c. Yasmin

   d. Lo-oval

27. Which of the following medications will decrease the absorption of Synthroid?

   a. Warfarin

   b. Iron

   c. Antibiotics

   d. Phenytoin

28. Which of the following is *not* a common adverse reaction to prednisone?

   a. Transient glucose intolerance

   b. Weight loss

   c. GI irritation

   d. Nervousness

29. Which of the following is a contraindication for the use of Evista?

   a. History of thrombosis

   b. Pregnancy

   c. History of peptic ulcer disease

   d. Both A and B

30. Which of the following statements about Levoxyl is *false*?

   a. Oral and IV formulations are available.

   b. Increase in appetite is a common adverse reaction.

   c. It can increase the INR in patients receiving warfarin.

   d. It should be taken with antacids to improve absorption.

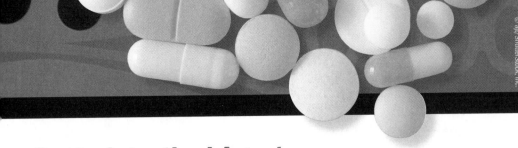

Gastrointestinal Agents

Jamila Stanton Seibel, PharmD, BCPS

5-HT$_3$ RECEPTOR ANTAGONISTS

Introduction

Serotonin subtype-3 (5-HT$_3$) receptor antagonists are commonly used in the treatment of nausea and vomiting caused by moderate to highly emetogenic chemotherapy regimens, radiation therapy, and postoperatively. They are frequently given in combination with one or more additional agents and are most effective when used on a scheduled basis to prevent nausea and vomiting, rather than as needed, or "prn." With the exception of palonosetron, which differs from the other drugs in this class by having a longer half-life and stronger receptor affinity, these agents have not been consistently effective in preventing delayed chemotherapy-induced nausea and vomiting. Of note, alosetron, a 5-HT$_3$ antagonist approved in 2000, is only indicated for the treatment of severe diarrhea-predominant irritable bowel syndrome in women; this agent should not be used for antiemetic purposes.

Mechanism of Action for the Drug Class

Act as a selective antagonist of serotonin subtype-3 (5-HT$_3$) receptors that are present peripherally on vagal nerve terminals and centrally in the chemoreceptor trigger zone of the brain. Drugs in this class bind to the 5-HT$_3$ receptors, blocking the signal to the vomiting center in the brain, thus preventing nausea and vomiting.

Members of the Drug Class

In this section: Ondansetron, palonosetron
Others: Alosetron, dolasetron, granisetron

⦿ Ondansetron

Brand Names
Zofran, Zofran ODT, Zuplenz

Generic Name
Ondansetron

Rx Only

Dosage Forms

Injection, oral solution, tablet, orally disintegrating tablet (ODT), oral soluble film

Usage

Prevention of chemotherapy-induced nausea and vomiting,* prevention of radiation-induced nausea and vomiting,* prevention and treatment of postoperative nausea and vomiting,* hyperemesis gravidum

Pregnancy Category B

Dosing

- Prevention of chemotherapy-induced nausea and vomiting:
  - IV: 8 mg or 0.15 mg/kg/dose (maximum of 16 mg) over 15 minutes for 3 doses, beginning 30 minutes prior to chemotherapy, followed by subsequent doses 4 and 8 hours after the first dose
  - Oral: 24 mg given 30 minutes prior to chemotherapy or 8 mg 30 minutes prior to chemotherapy and repeat in 8 hours, then 8 mg every 12 hours for 1–2 days postchemotherapy (dosing regimen dependent on chemotherapy emetogenicity potential)
- Prevention of radiation-induced nausea and vomiting: 8 mg orally 1–2 hours prior to radiotherapy; may repeat every 8 hours after radiotherapy for 1–2 days after completion of radiotherapy
- Prevention of postoperative nausea and vomiting:
  - IV, IM: 4 mg as a single dose (over 2–5 minutes if giving IV) administered 30 minutes before the end of anesthesia. Alternatively, the dose may be given immediately before the induction of anesthesia, however this has been shown to be less effective
  - Oral: 16 mg given 1 hour before induction of anesthesia
- Hyperemesis gravidum:
  - Oral: 8 mg every 12 hours
  - IV: 8 mg administered over 15 minutes every 12 hours
- Hepatic dosage adjustment: For Child-Pugh Class C, maximum daily dose of 8 mg (IV and PO)

* Throughout the text, an asterisk (*) is used to indicate the most common uses of a drug.

Adverse Reactions: Most Common

Headache, constipation, dizziness, malaise/fatigue, drowsiness, itching

Adverse Reactions: Rare/Severe/Important

EKG changes (QT prolongation, tachycardia, bradycardia), hypotension, elevated liver function tests

Major Drug Interactions

Ondansetron's Effect on Other Drugs

- Apomorphine: Enhances hypotensive effect
- Additive effect on QT prolongation when combined with other agents known to prolong the QT interval

Contraindication

Concomitant use of apomorphine

Essential Monitoring Parameters

EKG in patients with electrolyte abnormalities, heart failure, bradyarrhythmias, or with concomitant use of QT prolonging medication(s)

Counseling Points

- Do not remove the ODT from the blister pack until you are ready to take the medication. Peel the backing off; do not push through the backing. Using dry hands, place the tablet on the tongue and swallow with saliva.
- Do not remove the orally disintegrating film from the package until immediately before use. Using dry hands, place the film on top of tongue and allow it to dissolve; swallow with or without liquid.

Key Points

- 5-HT$_3$ receptor antagonists are frequently used in combination with one or more agents to prevent chemotherapy-associated nausea and vomiting
- In general, the 5-HT$_3$ receptor antagonists should be taken on a scheduled basis and not as needed because they are more effective in prevention of nausea and vomiting rather than treatment of existing symptoms
- Some agents, particularly dolasetron, have been associated with a dose-dependent increase in EKG intervals (PR, QRS, QT/QT$_c$). In patients with underlying QT prolongation, electrolyte imbalances, or those taking medications known to prolong the QT interval, this could result in torsades de pointes. All 5-HT$_3$ receptor antagonists should be used with caution in patients at risk.

⊙ Palonosetron

Brand Name
Aloxi

Generic Name
Palonosetron

Rx Only

Dosage Form
Injection

Usage

Prevention of chemotherapy-induced nausea and vomiting* (including highly emetogenic therapy and acute or delayed moderately emetogenic therapy), prevention and treatment of postoperative nausea and vomiting*

Pregnancy Category B

Dosing

- Prevention of chemotherapy-induced nausea and vomiting: 0.25 mg IV 30 minutes prior to the start of chemotherapy
- Prevention of postoperative nausea and vomiting: 0.075 mg IV given immediately prior to anesthesia induction

Adverse Reactions: Most Common

Headache, dizziness, constipation, weakness, anxiety, hyperkalemia

Adverse Reactions: Rare/Severe/Important

EKG changes (QT prolongation, tachycardia, bradycardia), hypotension

Major Drug Interactions

Palonosetron's Effect on Other Drugs

- Apomorphine: Enhances hypotensive effect
- Additive effect on QT prolongation when combined with other agents known to prolong the QT interval

Key Points

- 5-HT$_3$ receptor antagonists are frequently used in combination with one or more agents to prevent chemotherapy-associated nausea and vomiting. Due to its long half-life, palonosetron is the only 5-HT$_3$ antagonist that is effective for delayed nausea and vomiting.
- In general the 5-HT$_3$ receptor antagonists should be taken on a scheduled basis and not as needed because they are more effective in prevention of nausea and vomiting rather than treatment of existing symptoms
- Some agents, particularly dolasetron, have been associated with a dose-dependent increase in EKG intervals (PR, QRS, QT/QT$_c$). In patients with underlying QT prolongation, electrolyte imbalances, or those taking medications known to prolong the QT interval, this could result in torsades de pointes. All 5-HT$_3$ antagonists should be used with caution in patients at risk.

ANTACIDS

Introduction

The class of antacid agents encompasses a variety of aluminum, magnesium, and calcium products generally used to neutralize gastric acidity. Drugs in this class are available as single and combination therapy preparations in multiple dosage forms, including liquids, gelcaps, tablets, and chewable tablets. Most of these preparations are available over the counter; therefore, healthcare providers should pay particular attention to the use of these products in patients with renal dysfunction, duration of use > 2 weeks, and those taking prescription drugs known to interact with antacid compounds.

Mechanism of Action for the Drug Class

Neutralize gastric acid, inactivate pepsin, and bind bile salts

Members of the Drug Class

In this section: Magnesium hydroxide/aluminum hydroxide (Maalox), calcium carbonate (Tums)
Others: Numerous preparations of single-ingredient or combinations of aluminum hydroxide, magnesium hydroxide, calcium carbonate, and simethicone are available

⊙ Magnesium Hydroxide/ Aluminum Hydroxide

Brand Names

Maalox, Alamag, Mag-Al, Mag-Al Ultimate, Mylanta

Generic Names

Magnesium hydroxide/aluminum hydroxide ± simethicone; chewable products may also contain calcium carbonate

OTC

Dosage Forms

Oral suspension, tablet, chewable tablet

Usage

Acid indigestion,* heartburn,* short-term treatment of hyperphosphatemia in renal failure; aluminum hydroxide may also be used for prevention of GI bleeding and as an adjunctive agent in peptic ulcer disease

No Official Pregnancy Category

Dosing

- Oral suspension: 10–20 mL every 4–6 hours as needed before meals and at bedtime (see product-specific dosing)
- Tablets/chewable tablets: 1–2 tablets every 4–6 hours as needed before meals and at bedtime (see product-specific dosing)

- Renal dosage adjustment: Use caution; aluminum and magnesium may accumulate (no specific dosing requirements)

Adverse Reactions: Most Common

Constipation, diarrhea, chalky taste, abdominal cramps, nausea, vomiting

Adverse Reactions: Rare/Severe/Important

Hypermagnesemia, aluminium intoxication, hypophosphatemia, metabolic alkalosis, intestinal obstruction, dehydration

Major Drug Interactions

Drugs Affecting Magnesium Hydroxide/Aluminum Hydroxide
Vitamin D analogs: May increase the absorption of aluminum, leading to toxicity

Magnesium Hydroxide/Aluminum Hydroxide's Effect on Other Drugs
Antacid preparations have been reported to decrease the pharmacologic effect/exposure of many drugs when concomitantly administered. Monitor for therapeutic efficacy and failure. Good evidence supports a significant interaction with iron salts, tetracyclines, itraconazole, ketoconazole, rilpivirine, fluoroquinolones, quinine, and thyroid hormones.

Counseling Points

- Separate administration of antacid medications by at least 2 hours from other medications
- Use with caution if you have renal insufficiency. Contact a physician immediately if irregular heartbeat, severe stomach pain, or excessive weakness or tiredness occurs.
- For self-medication, antacids should not be taken for longer than 2 weeks. Contact a physician if symptoms are not relieved promptly or symptoms return often.

Key Points

- Because of easy OTC access to these agents, patients should be assessed for potential drug interactions and renal impairment that may result in toxicity
- Symptoms that recur and persist beyond 2 weeks may be a sign of more serious disease; these patients should be referred to a physician

⊙ Calcium Carbonate

Brand Names

Tums, Maalox Regular Chewable, Calci-Chew, Rolaids, Chooz, Alka-Mints

Generic Name

Calcium carbonate

OTC

Dosage Forms

Chewable tablet, gum tablet, lozenge, liquid

Usage

Acid indigestion,* heartburn,* treatment/prevention of calcium deficiency,* hyperphosphatemia in renal failure

No Official Pregnancy Category

Dosing

- Acid indigestion, heartburn:
  - Liquid:
    - 5–10 mL every 2 hours (see product-specific dosing)
    - Maximum of 7,000 mg calcium carbonate/24 hours
  - Tablets/chewable tablets:
    - 1–2 tablets every 2 hours (see product-specific dosing)
    - Maximum of 7,000 mg calcium carbonate/24 hours
- Treatment/prevention of calcium deficiency: 1–2 g of elemental calcium daily in 2–3 divided doses with meals (variable based on serum calcium and clinical condition)

Adverse Reactions: Most Common

Constipation, bloating, gas, nausea, vomiting, abdominal pain, xerostomia

Adverse Reactions: Rare/Severe/Important

Hypercalcemia, hypophosphatemia, milk-alkali syndrome

Major Drug Interactions

Calcium Carbonate's Effect on Other Drugs

Calcium carbonate antacid preparations have been reported to decrease the pharmacologic effect/exposure of many drugs when concomitantly administered. Monitor for therapeutic efficacy and failure. Good evidence supports a significant interaction with iron salts, tetracyclines, fluoroquinolones, ketoconazole, itraconazole, rilpivirine, and thyroid hormones.

Counseling Points

- Separate administration of antacid medications by at least 2 hours from other medications
- Chew tablets completely before swallowing; do not swallow whole
- For self-medication, antacids should not be taken for > 2 weeks. Contact a physician if symptoms are not relieved promptly or symptoms return often.

Key Points

- Because of easy OTC access to these agents, it is important to assess patients for potential drug interactions and more serious symptoms that require a physician's care
- Symptoms that recur and persist beyond 2 weeks may be a sign of more serious disease; these patients should be referred to a physician
- Calcium-containing antacids may be safely used during pregnancy; however, special consideration should be taken to ensure that the addition of calcium to other daily vitamins does not exceed the upper limit of 2,500 mg of calcium per day.

ANTIDIARRHEAL/ANTISECRETORY AGENTS

Introduction

Bismuth subsalicylate possesses antisecretory, anti-inflammatory, and antibacterial effects. Available over the counter, it is commonly used to self-treat a variety of indications, including indigestion, upset stomach, and diarrhea. Bismuth subsalicylate may also be used in combination with antibacterial and acid suppressive therapy to treat *Helicobacter pylori*. It is important to remember that an active component of this agent is salicylate, an aspirin derivative that may lead to toxicities in excessive doses or an inappropriate patient population.

Mechanism of Action for the Drug Class

The exact mechanism of action has not been determined. The salicylate moiety provides an antisecretory effect, and bismuth moiety exhibits antimicrobial activity directly against bacterial and viral GI pathogens. Bismuth also has some antacid properties.

Members of the Drug Class

In this section: Bismuth subsalicylate/bismuth subgallate
Others: None

⊙ Bismuth Subsalicylate/ Bismuth Subgallate

Brand Names

Pepto-Bismol, Kaopectate, Bismatrol

Generic Names

Bismuth subsalicylate, bismuth subgallate

OTC

Dosage Forms

Oral suspension, tablet, chewable tablet

Usage

Indigestion,* diarrhea,* upset stomach,* abdominal cramps, prevention and treatment of traveler's diarrhea, treatment of *H. pylori*–associated gastritis/ulcer (in combination only)

Pregnancy Category C/D

Dosing

- Diarrhea:
  - 524–1,050 mg every 30–60 minutes as needed (see product-specific dosing)
  - Maximum of 4–8 doses (4,200 mg) every 24 hours
- *H. pylori*: 524 mg four times a day (in combination)

Adverse Reactions: Most Common

Constipation, diarrhea, nausea, grayish-black tongue discoloration, grayish-black vomiting, grayish-black discoloration of stool

Adverse Reactions: Rare/Severe/Important

Persistent tinnitus, hearing loss, nausea, vomiting, neurotoxicity with excessive doses (confusion, slurred speech, severe headache, muscle weakness, seizure)

Major Drug Interactions

Bismuth Subsalicylate/Bismuth Subgallate's Effect on Other Drugs

- Tetracycline, doxycycline: Decrease absorption and effectiveness
- Aspirin/anticoagulants: Use of multiple salicylates may lead to toxicity and increase risk of bleeding

Contraindications

Children or teenagers with influenza or chickenpox due to the risk of Reye's syndrome, hypersensitivity to salicylates (including aspirin), coagulopathy, severe GI bleeding

Counseling Points

- Medication may temporarily darken the tongue and/or stools (nonharmful)
- Chew tablet well or shake suspension well before use
- Report any changes in hearing or ringing in your ears
- If diarrhea is accompanied by high fever, blood/mucus in the stool, or continues for > 2 days, consult a physician

Key Points

- Bismuth subsalicylate is a commonly used OTC drug for a variety of GI indications
- This medication may be harmful in large doses; neurotoxicity has been reported. Any symptoms of encephalopathy should be reported to a physician.
- Bismuth subsalicylate should be avoided in children and teenagers with viral symptoms or chickenpox

ANTIDIARRHEALS

Introduction

Antidiarrheals are widely available over the counter and are commonly used in the symptomatic treatment of diarrhea, including symptoms of mild or uncomplicated cases of travelers' diarrhea. Concurrent fluid and electrolyte replacement is often necessary in all age groups depending on the severity of diarrhea. Importantly, patients with bacterial enteritis should not use these agents; similarly, they should not be used if diarrhea is accompanied by high fever or blood in stool.

Mechanism of Action for the Drug Class

Antidiarrheals act peripherally on intestinal opioid receptors, inhibiting peristalsis and prolonging transit time, reducing fecal volume, increasing viscosity, and diminishing fluid and electrolyte losses. They demonstrate antisecretory activity.

Members of the Drug Class

In this section: Loperamide
Others: Bismuth subsalicylate (see section on antidiarrheal/antisecretory agents), diphenoxylate/atropine, multiple formulations of kaolin pectin ± activated attapulgite ± bismuth salts

⊚ Loperamide

Brand Name
Imodium

Generic Name
Loperamide

OTC

Dosage Forms
Capsule, caplet, chewable tablet, oral liquid

Usage

Symptomatic relief and control of acute nonspecific diarrhea (including traveler's diarrhea),* treatment of chronic diarrhea associated with inflammatory bowel disease,* antineoplastic agents, bowel resection

Pregnancy Category C

Dosing

- Acute diarrhea: 4 mg orally, followed by 2 mg after each loose stool, up to 16 mg/day
- Chronic diarrhea: 4 mg orally, followed by 2 mg after each loose stool until symptoms are controlled; dosage should then be slowly titrated down to the minimum dose required to control symptoms (average dose 4–8 mg/day in divided doses)
- Self-medication: 4 mg orally, followed by 2 mg after each loose stool, up to 8 mg/day

Adverse Reactions: Most Common

Abdominal pain, constipation, dizziness, drowsiness, dry mouth

Adverse Reactions: Rare/Severe/Important

Toxic megacolon, ileus, necrotizing enterocolitis

Major Drug Interactions

Loperamide's Effect on Other Drugs

CNS depressants, phenothiazines, and tricyclic antidepressants: Potentiates adverse effects

Counseling Points

- May cause drowsiness or dizziness; exercise caution while driving or performing hazardous tasks
- Consult physician if acute diarrhea lasts > 48 hours or is accompanied by blood, severe abdominal pain, distention, or fever
- Maintain adequate hydration during treatment

Key Points

- Do not use in acute diarrhea associated with bacterial enteritis or *Clostridium difficile* or for diarrhea associated with high fever or bloody stool
- Loperamide is not recommended for use in cases of acute flares of ulcerative colitis because it may increase the risk of developing toxic megacolon
- Use with caution in treatment of AIDS patients. Stop therapy at the sign of abdominal distention; cases of toxic megacolon have occurred in AIDS patients with infectious colitis.

ANTIFLATULENTS

Introduction

Simethicone has been used as an adjunct in the treatment of various clinical conditions in which gas retention may be a problem, including postoperative gaseous distention, air swallowing, dyspepsia, infant colic, peptic ulcer, spastic or irritable colon, and diverticulitis

Mechanism of Action for the Drug Class

Decreases the surface tension of gas bubbles, thereby dispersing and preventing gas pockets in the GI system

Members of the Drug Class

In this section: Simethicone
Others: None

⊙ Simethicone

Brand Names

Gas-X, Mylanta Gas, Mylicon, Phazyme

Generic Name

Simethicone

OTC

Dosage Forms

Capsule, chewable tablet, oral suspension (drops), oral disintegrating strip

Usage

Relief of bloating, pressure, and discomfort of gas;* adjunctively in upper abdominal ultrasound to enhance delineation by reducing gas shadowing

Pregnancy Category C

Dosing

40–125 mg orally four times daily after meals and at bedtime as needed

Adverse Reactions: Most Common

None

Counseling Points

- This medication works best when taken after meals and at bedtime
- Avoid drinking carbonated beverages or eating foods that may cause an increase in stomach gas

Key Points

- Simethicone is a frequently used OTC medication for people of various ages, ranging from infants to adults. It may be used as needed for gas pain and discomfort.
- It works optimally when taken after meals
- Simethicone is not absorbed by the GI tract; it does not have well-documented side effects, contraindications, or drug interactions

LAXATIVES, BULK-FORMING

Introduction

Bulk-forming laxatives are fiber derivatives used in addition to dietary modifications for the treatment and prevention of constipation; they are often considered first-line therapy for treatment of simple constipation. They can also be used to increase the bulk of stool in patients with chronic, watery diarrhea. Bulk-forming laxatives usually have an effect within 12–24 hours and reach a maximum effect after several days. This class of medications includes several fiber products, including methylcellulose, polycarbophil, and psyllium; most agents are available over the counter.

Mechanism of Action for the Drug Class

Bulk-forming laxatives dissolve or swell in water to form an emollient gel or viscous solution that promotes peristalsis and reduces transit time

Members of the Drug Class

In this section: Psyllium
Others: Methylcellulose, polycarbophil, wheat dextrin

◉ Psyllium

Brand Names

Fiberall, Genfiber, Konsyl, Metamucil, Reguloid

Generic Name

Psyllium

OTC

Dosage Forms

Capsule, powder, wafer

Usage

Dietary fiber supplement,* treatment of occasional and chronic constipation, irritable bowel syndrome, inflammatory bowel disease, diverticular disease, adjunctive agent for cholesterol lowering

No Official Pregnancy Category

Dosing

- Daily fiber recommended intake for adults 19–50 years:
  - Male: 38 g per day
  - Female: 25 g per day
- Up to 30 g orally daily given in divided doses of 2.5–7.5 g per dose

Adverse Reactions: Most Common

Abdominal pain and cramping, constipation, diarrhea, flatulence

Adverse Reactions: Rare/Severe/Important

Bronchospasm (following inhalation of powder), bowel obstruction/impaction, esophageal obstruction

Major Drug Interactions

Psyllium may affect how other drugs are absorbed from the GI tract; separate medications from psyllium by 1–2 hours

Contraindications

Intestinal obstruction, fecal impaction

Counseling Points

- Powder: Mix in large glass of water or juice (≥ 8 oz) and drink immediately. Maintain adequate hydration and fiber intake during therapy. Do not inhale powder.
- Capsules and wafers: Take each dose with ≥ 8 oz of water
- Separate this medication from other medications by at least 1–2 hours
- Results may begin in 12 hours; full results may take 2–3 days
- Report persistent constipation; watery diarrhea; difficulty, pain, or choking with swallowing; do not use for > 1 week without consulting a physician

Key Points

- For most patients, treatment of constipation should consist of bulk-forming agents in addition to dietary modifications to increase fiber intake. Considering most agents in this class are extremely well tolerated, they can likely be continued for daily use if directed by a physician.
- Bulk-forming laxatives must be taken with plenty of fluids (8 oz per dose) to prevent bowel/esophageal obstruction and fecal impaction; elderly patients not receiving enough fluids may be at particularly high risk for these adverse effects
- Bulk-forming laxatives are the common first-line choice to treat constipation in pregnant women if dietary changes are ineffective
- Due to the potential adsorption of concomitantly administered medications, separate administration by at least 1–2 hours
- Specific formulations (sugar-free, sodium-free) are available for particular patient populations with dietary restrictions

LAXATIVES, STOOL SOFTENERS

Introduction

Stool softeners are a preferred type of laxative in patients who have conditions in which straining at defecation should be avoided, such as recent myocardial infarction, recent rectal surgery, painful hemorrhoids, and hernias. Docusate is used to treat constipation associated with hard, dry stools and is considered safe to use in geriatric patients and pregnant women. Because the main effect of docusate is stool softening, not stimulation, it is better at preventing constipation than treating it; to treat constipation, docusate may be combined with a stimulant laxative.

Mechanism of Action for the Drug Class

Stool softeners reduce surface tension at the oil–water interface of the feces, allowing water and lipids to penetrate the stool, resulting in stool softening

Members of the Drug Class

In this section: Docusate
Others: None

◉ Docusate

Brand Names

Colace, Correctol, Doc-Q-Lace, Dulcolax

Generic Name

Docusate

OTC

Dosage Forms

Capsule, oral solution, tablet

Usage

Constipation;* promotes easy passage of stool in patients who should avoid straining;* constipation with dry, hard stool*

Pregnancy Category C

Dosing

50–360 mg daily divided into two to three doses (usual dose is 100 mg 1–2 times per day)

Adverse Reactions: Most Common

Abdominal pain and cramping

Major Drug Interactions

No known significant interactions

Contraindication

Intestinal obstruction

Counseling Points

- Maintain adequate hydration
- Do not chew or break capsules; swallow whole
- Report persistent constipation

Key Points

- Docusate works by hydrating the stool to facilitate easy passage through the intestinal tract in patients with dry, hard bowel movements. It is probably more effective at preventing constipation in patients who should avoid straining rather than treating acute episodes.
- For opiate-induced constipation, docusate should be combined with a stimulant agent
- Docusate is available in several different salt forms that are interchangeable; the amount of sodium, potassium, and calcium per dosage unit is clinically irrelevant

LAXATIVES, STIMULANT

Introduction

For patients with acute constipation, stimulant laxatives are generally considered safe and effective for short-term intermittent use. If laxative treatment is required for > 1 week, the patient should consult a physician to determine whether there is an underlying condition that requires additional treatment. Because the stimulant agents may commonly cause defecation urgency, abdominal cramping, and fluid and electrolyte imbalances, they are not recommended as first-line agents in geriatric patients or those requiring therapy for chronic constipation. Commonly, these agents are used to effectively treat and prevent opiate-induced constipation. At one time it was thought that chronic use of these agents could lead to physical dependence, but currently there is no data to support this theory; the main concern with chronic use is generally the risk of fluid and electrolyte imbalance.

Mechanism of Action for the Drug Class

Directly stimulates the smooth muscle of the intestine at the colonic nerve plexus, causing peristalsis; may also alter intestinal water and electrolyte secretion

Members of the Drug Class

In this section: Bisacodyl, senna
Others: None

◉ Bisacodyl

Brand Names

Biscolax, Correctol, Dulcolax, Fleet Bisacodyl

Generic Name

Bisacodyl

OTC

Dosage Forms

Tablet, suppository, enema

Usage

Constipation,* bowel evacuation/bowel preparation for colonoscopy*

No Official Pregnancy Category

Dosing

- Oral: 5–15 mg as a single dose (up to 30 mg may be given for complete bowel evacuation)
- Rectal: 10 mg as a single dose

Adverse Reactions: Most Common

Abdominal pain and cramps, nausea, vomiting, rectal burning

Adverse Reactions: Rare/Severe/Important

Electrolyte and fluid imbalance

Major Drug Interaction

Antacids may diminish the therapeutic effect of bisacodyl by causing early dissolution of the tablet

Contraindication

Bowel obstruction

Counseling Points

- Usually produces a bowel movement in 6–12 hours when taken orally; 15–60 minutes when given rectally
- Not for chronic use, consult a physician if constipation persists or if symptoms of nausea, pain, or abdominal distention become severe
- Maintain adequate fluid intake

Key Points

- Bisacodyl is recommended for intermittent, short-term use in acute constipation. It is also frequently prescribed as part of bowel preparation regimens prior to colonoscopy.
- Stimulant laxatives are not recommended for routine or chronic use in elderly patients due to their adverse event profile. Agents that are preferred in this patient population include bulk-forming stool softeners and osmotic agents.

◉ Senna

Brand Names

Senokot, Senexon, Senna-Lax, ex-lax

Generic Name

Senna

OTC

Dosage Forms

Tablet, oral liquid, oral disintegrating strip, chewable tablet

Usage

Constipation,* bowel evacuation/bowel preparation for colonoscopy*

Pregnancy Category C

Dosing

- Constipation: 15 mg once daily up to a maximum of 70–100 mg daily divided into 2 doses
- Bowel evacuation: Doses and regimens are variable; doses of up to 130 mg may be used

Adverse Reactions: Most Common

Abdominal cramping, diarrhea, nausea, vomiting

Adverse Reactions: Rare/Severe/Important

Electrolyte and fluid imbalance

Contraindications

Bowel obstruction, acute intestinal inflammation, abdominal pain of unknown origin

Counseling Points

- Usually produces a bowel movement in 6–12 hours
- Not for chronic use, consult a physician if constipation persists or if symptoms of nausea, pain, or abdominal distention become severe
- Maintain adequate fluid intake

Key Points

- Senna is recommended for intermittent, short-term use in acute constipation. It is also frequently prescribed as part of bowel preparation regimens prior to colonoscopy.
- Stimulant laxatives are not recommended for routine or chronic use in elderly patients due to their adverse event profile. Agents that are preferred in this patient population include bulk-forming stool softeners and osmotic agents.

LAXATIVES, OSMOTIC/HYPEROSMOLAR

Introduction

Osmotic laxatives are commonly recommended to treat occasional constipation. Because they are hyperosmolar, these agents draw water into the bowel, softening the stool and facilitating movement through the GI tract. Polyethylene glycol 3350, discussed in this chapter, is one of the most commonly used osmotic laxatives. It is used in small doses for relief of constipation and in large doses for GI procedures to evacuate the bowel. Polyethylene glycol 3350 is particularly well known because it is available over the counter and has a benign side-effect profile. Unlike many of the other agents in this class, it generally does not cause cramping, bloating, urgency, or flatulence.

Mechanism of Action for the Drug Class

Polyethylene glycol is a hyperosmolar agent that causes retention of water in the stool, resulting in a softer stool and more frequent bowel movements

Members of the Drug Class

In this section: Polyethylene glycol 3350 (MiraLAX)
Others: Glycerin, lactulose, sorbitol

⊙ Polyethylene Glycol 3350

Brand Name
MiraLAX

Generic Name
Polyethylene glycol 3350

OTC

Dosage Form
Powder for oral solution

Usage
Constipation (occasional and chronic)*

Pregnancy Category C

Dosing
17 g of powder (1 capful filled to line) dissolved in 4–8 oz of water daily; speak to a physician regarding use > 7 days

Adverse Reactions: Most Common
Nausea, abdominal fullness, diarrhea, flatulence, stomach cramps

Adverse Reactions: Rare/Severe/Important
Dermatitis, rash, urticaria

Major Drug Interactions
None reported

Contraindication
Bowel obstruction, known or suspected

Counseling Points
- Mix 17 g of powder (1 capful filled to line) in 4–8 oz of water and drink immediately. May take 2–4 days to produce a bowel movement.
- Maintain adequate fluid intake throughout use
- If used as self-medication, do not use this medicine for > 1 week unless directed by your healthcare provider
- Consult your healthcare provider if you have nausea, vomiting, abdominal pain, renal dysfunction, diarrhea, or blood in stools. Discontinue use if severe pain, cramping, or nausea persists.

Key Points
- Prolonged, frequent, or excessive use could lead to dehydration and electrolyte imbalance
- MiraLAX may be better tolerated than other laxatives with regard to adverse GI effects (i.e., gas, cramping, bloating); however, it can take up to 2–4 days to see results
- MiraLAX has been shown to be safe and effective for up to 6 months in trials treating chronic constipation; however, patients should consult their physician prior to use beyond 1 week

LAXATIVES, BOWEL PREPARATION/BOWEL EVACUANTS

Introduction

Several agents and combinations of agents are commonly prescribed to evacuate the bowel in preparation for a colonoscopy. Although some products are available over the counter, the newest agents are available by prescription only. In order to clearly view the colon during the colonoscopy, all solid waste must be evacuated; therefore, it is extremely important that patients understand the directions for completing a bowel preparation regimen. The newer agents, discussed in this section, require less volume than the traditional 4 liter polyethylene glycol 3350 preparation product known as GoLYTELY; lower volume preps are generally preferred by patients. Of note, sodium phosphate preparation products have been associated with acute phosphate nephropathy, a condition resulting from phosphate crystal deposits in the renal tubules, possibly leading to permanent kidney damage.

Mechanism of Action for the Drug Class

Mechanism dependent on product

Members of the Drug Class

In this section: Polyethylene glycol 3350 (MoviPrep), polyethylene glycol 3350 and bisacodyl (HalfLytely Bowel Prep Kit)

Others: Polyethylene glycol 3350 (GoLYTELY), sodium phosphate

◉ Polyethylene Glycol 3350

Brand Name

MoviPrep

Generic Name

Polyethylene glycol 3350

Rx Only

Dosage Form

Powder for oral solution

Usage

Bowel evacuation/bowel preparation for colonoscopy*

Pregnancy Category C

Dosing

- MoviPrep: Administer 2 L total with an additional 1 L of clear fluid prior to colonoscopy as follows:
  - Split dose: The evening before the colonoscopy consume 240 mL (8 oz) every 15 minutes until 1 L is consumed. Then drink 16 oz of clear liquid. On the morning of the colonoscopy, repeat process with second liter over 1 hour and then drink 16 oz of clear liquid at least 1 hour before the procedure.
  - Full dose: The evening before the colonoscopy (~ 6 P.M.), consume 240 mL (8 oz) every 15 minutes until 1 L is consumed; 90 minutes later (~7:30 P.M.), repeat dose. Then drink 32 oz of clear liquid.

Adverse Reactions: Most Common

Abdominal pain and distension, nausea, vomiting, anal irritation, malaise, rigors, thirst, dizziness, headache, dyspepsia

Adverse Reactions: Rare/Severe/Important

Aspiration, upper GI bleed from Mallory-Weiss tear, electrolyte imbalance, ischemic colitis

Major Drug Interactions

Oral medications administered within 1 hour of the start of administration of this product may be flushed from the GI tract and not absorbed

Contraindications

Bowel obstruction, ileus, gastric retention, bowel perforation, toxic megacolon

Counseling Points

- Each powder pouch must be diluted in water before ingestion
- Oral medications may not be absorbed properly if taken within 1 hour of starting prep
- MoviPrep will make you have watery stools. Stay hydrated before, during, and after the use of MoviPrep. No solid food should be consumed from the start of the prep until after the colonoscopy.
- The first bowel movement may occur approximately 1 hour after starting the prep. Abdominal bloating and discomfort is common; if pain is severe, stop drinking MoviPrep temporarily or drink each portion over a longer time interval until symptoms diminish. If severe symptoms persist, contact your healthcare provider.

Key Points

- MoviPrep is a newer, lower-volume polyethylene glycol 3350 bowel preparation agent. It is equally effective and may cause fewer GI side effects compared to the older polyethylene glycol 3350 agent, GoLYTELY. MoviPrep does not contain sodium phosphate and has not been associated with acute phosphate nephropathy.
- Patients will experience diarrhea and the stool should have a watery consistency; this is necessary to clean the colon for optimal visualization during the colonoscopy. Blood in the stool is not expected; the patient should be advised to contact a healthcare provider if this occurs.
- Encourage patients to remain hydrated because extreme fluid loss can lead to dehydration, electrolyte imbalances, seizures, and renal dysfunction

◉ Polyethylene Glycol 3350/Bisacodyl

Brand Name

HalfLytely Bowel Prep Kit

Generic Name

Polyethylene glycol 3350/bisacodyl

Rx Only

Dosage Form

Powder for oral solution (polyethylene glycol 3350)/tablet (bisacodyl)

Usage

Bowel evacuation/bowel preparation for colonoscopy*

Pregnancy Category C

Dosing

- HalfLytely Bowel Prep Kit consists of a powder for oral solution and tablet. Both agents should be used as part of the bowel preparation:
  - Bisacodyl: 5 mg as a single dose taken first
  - Polyethylene glycol-electrolyte solution: Dilute with 2 L of water. Initiate solution after first bowel movement or 6 hours (whichever occurs first). Drink 8 oz every 10 minutes until 2 L are consumed.

Adverse Reactions: Most Common

Flatus, cramping, nausea, overall discomfort, vomiting

Adverse Reactions: Rare/Severe/Important

Aspiration, upper GI bleed from Mallory-Weiss tear, electrolyte imbalance, ischemic colitis

Major Drug Interactions

- Oral medications administered within 1 hour of the start of administration of this product may be flushed from the GI tract and not absorbed
- Antacids may diminish the therapeutic effect of bisacodyl by causing early dissolution of the tablet

Contraindications

Bowel obstruction, ileus, gastric retention, bowel perforation, toxic megacolon

Counseling Points

- Administer bisacodyl tablet with water; do not chew or crush tablet. Do not take antacids within 1 hour of taking bisacodyl. Rapidly drinking the polyethylene glycol-electrolyte solution is preferred to drinking small amounts continuously. If severe bloating, distention, or abdominal pain occurs, administration should be slowed or temporarily discontinued until symptoms resolve.
- May add flavor packet provided in kit to the solution; no other ingredients should be added to the solution. Shake well.
- Drink only clear liquids the day of and during the bowel preparation. After consuming the solution, avoid drinking large quantities of clear liquids until after the colonoscopy.
- Oral medications may not be absorbed properly if taken within 1 hour of starting prep
- HalfLytely will make you have watery stools. Stay hydrated before, during, and after the use of HalfLytely.

Key Points

- HalfLytely is a newer, lower volume polyethylene glycol 3350 bowel preparation agent. Compared to the older agent, GoLYTELY, the volume consumed is decreased by half. It does not contain sodium phosphate and has not been associated with acute phosphate nephropathy.
- Patients will experience diarrhea and the stool should have a watery consistency; this is necessary to clean the colon for optimal visualization during the colonoscopy. Blood in the stool is not expected; contact a healthcare provider if this occurs.
- Encourage patients to remain hydrated, as extreme fluid loss can lead to dehydration, electrolyte imbalances, seizures, and renal dysfunction.

H_2 RECEPTOR ANTAGONISTS

Introduction

H_2 receptor antagonists are used for the treatment of GI disorders where acid suppression is desired or for prevention of ulcers in critically ill patients. These agents are available as prescription products, and several agents are also available in over-the-counter doses, making access to them widespread. They are commonly used for mild gastroesophageal reflux disease (GERD); however, they have been shown to be less effective than other acid-suppressive therapies in moderate to severe disease. In the treatment of peptic ulcer disease, H_2 receptor blockers are effectively used to heal ulcers and maintain ulcer healing; however, their efficacy in NSAID-induced gastric ulcers is variable and therefore not usually recommended. These agents are generally very safe and well-tolerated, with an adverse event profile similar to placebo in many studies.

Mechanism of Action for the Drug Class

Competitive inhibition of histamine at H_2 receptors of the gastric parietal cells, which ultimately reduces gastric acid secretion

Members of the Drug Class

In this section: Cimetidine, famotidine, ranitidine
Others: Nizatidine

◉ Cimetidine

Brand Name

Tagamet

Generic Name

Cimetidine

Rx and OTC

Dosage Forms

Injectable solution, tablet, oral solution

Usage

Treatment of GERD,* prevention or relief of heartburn,* acid indigestion,* or sour stomach;* prevention of upper GI bleeding in critically ill patients; short-term treatment and maintenance therapy of active duodenal ulcers; short-term treatment of gastric ulcers and gastric hypersecretory states; part of a multidrug regimen for *H. pylori* eradication

Pregnancy Category B

Dosing

- Oral:
  - Rx: 300–800 mg one to four times daily (dose- and frequency-dependent on indication)
  - OTC: 200 mg twice daily
- IM/IV: 300 mg every 6–8 hours; infusion: 37.5 mg/hour
- Renal dosage adjustment:
  - CrCl 10–50 mL/min: Administer 50% of normal dose
  - CrCl < 10 mL/min: Administer 25% of normal dose
- Hepatic dosage adjustment: Dosing adjustment in severe liver disease may be required; however, no specific recommendations are available

Adverse Reactions: Most Common

Diarrhea, dizziness, headache, somnolence, gynecomastia

Adverse Reactions: Rare/Severe/Important

Agranulocytosis, thrombocytopenia, altered mental status/confusion, necrotizing enterocolitis in fetus/newborn, cardiac arrhythmias and hypotension (following rapid IV administration)

Major Drug Interactions

Cimetidine's Effect on Other Drugs

- Dofetilide, lidocaine, amiodarone, procainamide, quinidine, calcium channel blockers (except amlodipine), warfarin, theophylline, tricyclic antidepressants, SSRIs, phenytoin, carbamazepine, cyclosporine, sulfonylureas: Increases effect/toxicity
- Iron salts, itraconazole, ketoconazole, posaconazole, atazanavir, rilpivirine, cefditoren, dasatinib, erlotinib, clopidogrel: Decreases effect/absorption

Counseling Points

- If using cimetidine to prevent heartburn, take oral formulations 30–60 minutes prior to meals
- If used for self-medication, do not use if you have difficulty swallowing, are vomiting blood, or have bloody or black stools; seek medical attention
- If used for self-medication, consult a physician for heartburn or stomach pain that continues or worsens or if use is required for > 14 days

Key Points

- Cimetidine is an effective and inexpensive option for the treatment of multiple GI disorders requiring acid suppression. However, of the H$_2$ antagonists available it has the most significant inhibition of multiple CYP enzymes, and therefore the most drug interactions; it is also associated with the highest incidence of adverse CNS effects.
- Patients with renal and severe liver dysfunction should receive an adjusted dose to prevent adverse effects, such as confusion; this is particularly true for elderly patients
- Rapid IV administration has been associated with cardiac arrhythmias and hypotension; therefore intermittent or continuous infusions are preferred when IV administration is necessary

◉ Famotidine

Brand Names

Pepcid, Pepcid AC, Pepcid Complete (combination famotidine/calcium carbonate/magnesium hydroxide)

Generic Name

Famotidine

Rx and OTC

Dosage Forms

Oral suspension, tablet, chewable tablet, injectable solution

Usage

Treatment of GERD,* relief of heartburn and acid indigestion,* stress ulcer prophylaxis in critically ill patients,* maintenance therapy and treatment of duodenal ulcer, acute treatment of gastric ulcer, pathologic hypersecretory conditions, part of a multidrug regimen for *H. pylori* eradication, symptomatic relief in gastritis

Pregnancy Category B

Dosing

- Oral:
  - Rx: 20–40 mg daily or twice daily (dose and frequency depends on indication; higher doses up to 160 mg every 6 hours have been used for hypersecretory conditions)
  - OTC: 10–20 mg daily or twice daily
- IV: 20–40 mg daily or twice daily (dose- and frequency-dependent on indication; higher doses up to 160 mg every 6 hours have been used for hypersecretory conditions)
- Renal dosage adjustment: If CrCl < 50 mL/min, then administer 50% of normal dose or increase dosing interval to every 36–48 hours

Adverse Reactions: Most Common

Constipation, diarrhea, dizziness headache

Adverse Reactions: Rare/Severe/Important

Thrombocytopenia, altered mental status/confusion, necrotizing enterocolitis in fetus/newborn

Major Drug Interactions

Famotidine's Effect on Other Drugs

Decreased effect/absorption of iron salts, itraconazole, ketoconazole, posaconazole, atazanavir, rilpivirine, cefditoren, erlotinib, dasatinib

Counseling Points

- If using to prevent heartburn, take oral formulations 15–60 minutes prior to meals
- Do not use for self-medication if you have difficulty swallowing, are vomiting blood, or have bloody or black stools; seek medical attention
- If used for self-medication, consult a physician for heartburn or stomach pain that continues or worsens or if use is required for > 14 days

Key Points

- Famotidine is an effective option for the treatment of multiple GI disorders requiring acid suppression and is commonly used for stress ulcer prophylaxis in the ICU setting. It is very well tolerated and has a mild adverse event profile.
- Unlike cimetidine, famotidine it is not an inhibitor of the CYP enzyme system; therefore, drug interactions are limited to those drugs with decreased absorption in the altered gastric pH
- Patients with renal dysfunction should receive dosing adjustments to prevent adverse effects, such as confusion; this is particularly true for elderly patients

◉ Ranitidine

Brand Name

Zantac

Generic Name

Ranitidine

Rx and OTC

Dosage Forms

Effervescent tablet, injectable solution, oral syrup, tablet, capsule

Usage

Treatment of GERD,* relief of heartburn,* indigestion,* short-term and maintenance therapy of duodenal and gastric ulcers, erosive esophagitis, pathologic hypersecretory conditions, part of a multidrug regimen for *H. pylori* eradication, prevention of stress-induced ulcers in critically ill patients

Pregnancy Category B

Dosing

- Oral:
  - Rx: 150 mg one to four times daily (frequency-dependent on indication) or 300 mg daily (depending on indication)
  - OTC: 75 mg twice daily
- IV/IM: 50 mg every 6–8 hours; continuous infusion: 6.25 mg/hour
- Renal dosage adjustment:
  - Oral: If CrCl < 50 mL/min, then 150 mg every 24 hours
  - IM/IV: If CrCl < 50 mL/min, then 50 mg every 24 hours
- Hepatic dosage adjustment: Minor changes in half-life, distribution, clearance, and bioavailability are possible; however, dosage adjustments are not necessary

Adverse Reactions: Most Common

Abdominal pain, diarrhea, constipation, headache, fatigue

Adverse Reactions: Rare/Severe/Important

Anemia, thrombocytopenia, altered mental status/confusion, necrotizing enterocolitis in fetus or newborn, pancreatitis

Major Drug Interactions

Ranitidine's Effect on Other Drugs

- Procainamide (at doses > 300 mg): Increases effect/toxicity
- Iron salts, atazanavir, dasatinib, delavirdine, erlotinib, gefitinib, cefditoren, itraconazole, ketoconazole, po-saconazole: Decreases effect/absorption

Counseling Points

- If using to prevent heartburn, take 30–60 minutes before having foods/drinks that cause heartburn
- Do not use for self-medication if you have difficulty swallowing, are vomiting blood, or have bloody or black stools; seek medical attention
- If used for self-medication, consult a physician for heartburn or stomach pain that continues or worsens or if use is required for > 14 days
- Ranitidine effervescent granules should not be chewed, swallowed whole, or dissolved on tongue. Dissolve in at least 1 teaspoon of water; swallow when completely dissolved.

Key Points

- Because ranitidine is a weak inhibitor of CYP1A2 and 2D6, it has the potential to cause drug interactions, although to much less extent than cimetidine
- Ranitidine is generally very well tolerated and an effective treatment option for mild GERD symptoms and heartburn relief, especially in the outpatient setting
- Patients with renal dysfunction should receive dosage adjustments to prevent adverse effects, such as confusion; this is particularly true for elderly patients

PROKINETIC AGENTS

Introduction

Metoclopramide is classified as both an antiemetic and prokinetic agent. It is frequently used in the treatment of gastroparesis and chemotherapy-induced nausea and vomiting. Although metoclopramide is generally well tolerated, recent data have led to an FDA black box warning regarding chronic metoclopramide use and an increased risk of developing tardive dyskinesia.

Mechanism of Action for the Drug Class

Metoclopramide has a dual mechanism of action. It blocks dopamine receptors in the chemoreceptor zone in the CNS and also enhances the response of acetylcholine in the upper GI tract, causing enhanced motility and accelerating gastric emptying.

Members of the Drug Class

In this section: Metoclopramide
Others: None

◉ Metoclopramide

Brand Names
Reglan, Metozolv ODT

Generic Name
Metoclopramide

Rx Only

Dosage Forms
Injectable solution, tablet, syrup, orally disintegrating tablet (ODT)

Usage
Diabetic gastroparesis,* prevention/treatment of nausea and vomiting associated with chemotherapy,* generalized nausea and vomiting,* gastroesophageal reflux disease (GERD), postpyloric placement of enteral feeding tubes

Pregnancy Category B

Dosing
- GERD, gastroparesis: 10–15 mg PO/IV/IM four times daily, with meals and at bedtime
- Chemotherapy-induced nausea/vomiting:
  - IV: 1–2 mg/kg 30 minutes before chemotherapy, and repeated every 2 hours for 2 doses, then every 3 hours for 3 doses
  - Alternate dosing for low-risk chemotherapy: 10–40 mg PO/IV every 4–6 hours
- Renal dosage adjustment: If CrCl ≤ 40 mL/min, then administer 50% of the normal dose

Adverse Reactions: Most Common
Drowsiness, fatigue, restlessness, insomnia, headache, dizziness, nausea, extrapyramidal reactions (generally in the form of dystonic reactions or Parkinson-like symptoms)

Adverse Reactions: Rare/Severe/Important
Depression, neuroleptic malignant syndrome (NMS), tardive dyskinesia (long-term use)

Major Drug Interactions
Drugs Affecting Metoclopramide

Succinylcholine, anticholinergics: Antagonize effects

Metoclopramide's Effect on Other Drugs
- Anti-Parkinson's agents: Diminishes therapeutic effect secondary to opposite mechanisms of action
- Antipsychotic agents: Increases risk of EPS, tardive dyskinesia
- Serotoninergic antidepressants: Increases risk of serotonin syndrome

Contraindications
GI obstruction, perforation, or hemorrhage; pheochromocytoma; history of seizures or concomitant use of other agents likely to increase extrapyramidal reactions

Counseling Points
- Do not remove ODT from packaging until time of administration. Do not use if tablet is broken or crushed. Using dry hands, place tablet on tongue and allow to dissolve. Swallow with saliva.
- If used for gastroparesis, take 30 minutes prior to meals
- Notify your physician if you experience any spastic or involuntary movements, altered mental status, or palpitations
- Drowsiness and dizziness may occur. Use caution while driving or performing tasks that require alertness.

Key Points
- Use of metoclopramide remains widespread despite well-known side effects; this is likely because options to treat gastroparesis are limited and metoclopramide is recommended as a first-line therapy. The most common side effects are drowsiness, restlessness, and insomnia. Rare but serious side effects include EPS, NMS, and the risk of serotonin syndrome with concomitant agents that affect serotonin. Depression, ranging from mild to severe, has also occurred in patients without a previous history of depression.
- Dystonic reactions are more common in elderly patients and young children/adults. They occur more frequently with higher doses.
- In 2009, the FDA issued a black box warning for the risk of tardive dyskinesia with high doses and prolonged use of metoclopramide

8

Gastrointestinal Agents

Introduction

Proton pump inhibitors (PPIs) are well tolerated and a relatively safe option for the treatment of GI disorders requiring acid-suppression therapy. They are considered first-line therapy in the treatment of moderate to severe GERD symptoms, erosive esophagitis, and treatment of NSAID-induced ulcers in the setting of continued NSAID use. A PPI-based multidrug regimen is also the first-line treatment for eradication of *H. pylori*–associated ulcers because PPIs have been shown to be more effective than H_2 antagonist–based regimens. With such widespread use in recent years, data have emerged linking the use of these agents to an increased risk of pneumonia, *C. difficile* infection, osteoporosis-related bone fractures, and hypomagnesemia.

Mechanism of Action of the Drug Class

PPIs must be activated within the gastric parietal cell. Once activated, they bind to the H^+/K^+-ATPase, inactivate the acid pump, and stop the secretion of hydrochloric acid into the stomach.

Usage for the Drug Class

Acute treatment and maintenance therapy for erosive esophagitis;* treatment of GERD;* part of a multidrug regimen for *H. pylori* eradication;* prevention of gastric ulcers associated with continuous NSAID therapy;* long-term treatment of pathologic hypersecretory conditions, including Zollinger-Ellison syndrome;* stress ulcer prophylaxis in critically ill patients;* relief of heartburn and indigestion*

Adverse Reactions for the Drug Class: Most Common

Headache, dizziness, somnolence, diarrhea, constipation, nausea

Adverse Reactions for the Drug Class: Rare/Severe/Important

- Associated with the following (causality currently under investigation): *C. difficile*-associated diarrhea, community-acquired pneumonia, and hospital-acquired pneumonia
- Long-term use (> 1 year): Possible risk of osteoporosis-related bone fracture, hypomagnesemia, and vitamin B_{12} deficiency

Major Drug Interactions for the Drug Class

Drugs Affecting Proton Pump Inhibitors

Rifampin, St. John's wort: Decrease efficacy/concentration of omeprazole

Proton Pump Inhibitors' Effects on Other Drugs

- Itraconazole, ketoconazole, posaconazole, atazanavir, nelfinavir, cefditoren, dasatinib, erlotinib, mesalamine derivatives, mycophenolate mofetil: Decrease efficacy/absorption
- Tacrolimus (except pantoprazole), citalopram, possibly escitalopram, cilostazol: Increase efficacy/concentration
- Clopidogrel: Omeprazole may decrease efficacy

Counseling Points for the Drug Class

- Take 1 hour before meal, usually recommended to take before breakfast
- Do not crush or chew tablets
- Do not use for self-medication if you have difficulty swallowing, are vomiting blood, or have bloody or black stools; seek medical attention
- If used for self-medication, consult a physician if heartburn or stomach pain continues or worsens or if use is required for > 14 days

Key Points for the Drug Class

- For short-term use, PPIs are very well tolerated with few serious side effects. For this reason, they are often overprescribed by physicians and overused by patients. It may take up to 72 hours to achieve optimal effectiveness and symptom improvement.
- Overuse of these agents has led to concern regarding the potential for adverse effects, such as increased risk of pneumonia, *C. difficile* infection, bone fractures, and hypomagnesemia. These adverse effects have not been evaluated in a prospective study and are currently under review. Limit use to the lowest effective dose for the shortest duration.
- PPIs are generally considered interchangeable; selection of agent is usually based on cost and formulary considerations. IV formulations are generally more expensive than oral and not more efficacious; if a patient is able to take medications by mouth, oral therapy usually is preferred.
- Multiple PPIs are available over the counter; thus healthcare providers should assess patients for prolonged use, potential drug interactions, or symptoms of more serious disease that require a physician's attention

Members of the Drug Class

In this section: Esomeprazole, lansoprazole, omeprazole, pantoprazole, rabeprazole
Others: Dexlansoprazole, omeprazole/sodium bicarbonate (combination agent)

⊙ Esomeprazole

Brand Name
  Nexium

Generic Name
  Esomeprazole

Rx Only

Dosage Forms

Capsules, oral granules for suspension, injectable solution

Pregnancy Category B

Dosing

- Oral/IV: 20–40 mg one to two times daily (dose- and frequency-dependent on indication)
- IV infusion: 80 mg bolus, followed by 8 mg/hour
- Hepatic dosage adjustment: In cases of severe hepatic impairment (Child-Pugh Class C), maximum dose is 20 mg per day

Administration Points

- If using granules, empty granules into container with 1 tablespoon of water and stir; leave 2–3 minutes to thicken. Stir and drink within 30 minutes.
- The esomeprazole capsule can be opened and contents mixed with 1 tablespoon of applesauce. Swallow immediately; mixture should not be chewed or warmed.

⊙ Lansoprazole

Brand Name

Prevacid

Generic Name

Lansoprazole

Rx and OTC

Dosage Forms

Capsule, orally disintegrating tablet (ODT), suspension

Pregnancy Category B

Dosing

- Oral:
  - Rx: 15–30 mg one to three times daily (dose- and frequency-dependent on indication)
  - OTC: 15 mg daily for 14 days; treatment may be repeated after 4 months

Administration Points

- Do not swallow ODTs whole and do not chew. Place tablet on tongue and allow to dissolve (with or without water) until particles can be swallowed.
- Lansoprazole capsules may be opened and the intact granules sprinkled on 1 tablespoon of applesauce, pudding, cottage cheese, yogurt, or strained pears. The granules should then be swallowed immediately. They may also be opened and emptied into about 60 mL orange juice, apple juice, or tomato juice; mix and swallow immediately.

⊙ Omeprazole

Brand Name

Prilosec

Generic Name

Omeprazole

Rx and OTC

Dosage Forms

Capsule, tablet, granules for suspension, powder for suspension

Pregnancy Category C

Dosing

- Oral:
  - Rx: 20–40 mg one to two times daily (dose- and frequency-dependent on indication)
  - OTC: 20 mg daily for 14 days; treatment may be repeated after 4 months

Administration Points

- Capsules may be opened and contents added to 1 tablespoon of applesauce, use immediately; do not chew or warm
- Granules for oral suspension: Empty the contents of the 2.5 mg packet into 5 mL of water (or 10 mg packet into 15 mL of water); stir. Note that the suspension should be left to thicken for 2–3 minutes prior to administration.
- Granules for oral suspension: For NG tube administration, add 5 mL of water into a catheter-tipped syringe, and then add the contents of a 2.5 mg packet (15 mL water for the 10 mg packet); shake. Note that the suspension should be left to thicken for 2–3 minutes prior to administration.
- Oral suspension: Reconstitute in a catheter-tipped syringe, shake well, allow 2–3 minutes to thicken. Administer within 30 minutes of reconstitution. Use NG tube or gastric tube that is a size 6 French or larger; flush the syringe and tube with water.

⊙ Pantoprazole

Brand Name

Protonix

Generic Name

Pantoprazole

Rx Only

Dosage Forms

Tablet, injectable solution, granules for suspension

Pregnancy Category B

Dosing

- Oral/IV push: 40–80 mg one to two times daily (dose- and frequency-dependent on indication)
- IV infusion: 80 mg bolus, followed by 8 mg/hour IV drip

Administration Point

The delayed-release oral suspension should only be administered in apple juice or applesauce and taken about 30 minutes before a meal. Do not administer with any other liquid or food.

⊚ Rabeprazole

Brand Name

AcipHex

Generic Name

Rabeprazole

Rx Only

Dosage Form

Tablet

Pregnancy Category B

Dosing

20 mg one to two times daily, up to 60 mg twice daily (dose- and frequency-dependent on indication)

ANTICHOLINERGIC/ANTISPASMODIC AGENTS

Introduction

Anticholinergic agents such as dicyclomine are used in the treatment of GI motility disorders such as irritable bowel syndrome (IBS) and urinary incontinence. The use of anticholinergic agents is generally limited by their side effects, including dizziness, drowsiness, blurry vision, and dry mouth. Dicyclomine and oxybutynin are two of the most common agents in this class, likely because they have fewer anticholinergic effects and act mostly as antispasmodic agents. Limited data support the efficacy of these agents, and many patients are unable to tolerate therapeutic doses; therefore, they are not considered first-line therapy for IBS or urinary incontinence.

Mechanism of Action for the Drug Class

Anticholinergic agents block the action of acetylcholine at parasympathetic sites in smooth muscle, secretory glands, and the CNS

Members of the Drug Class

In this section: Dicyclomine
Others: GI anticholinergics: Hyoscyamine, scopolamine, belladonna, propantheline, atropine; urinary anticholinergics/antispasmodics: oxybutynin, tolterodine, trospium, solifenacin, darifenacin

⊚ Dicyclomine

Brand Name

Bentyl

Generic Name

Dicyclomine

Rx Only

Dosage Forms

Capsule, tablet, syrup, injectable solution

Usage

Irritable bowel syndrome,* urinary incontinence, infant colic, acute enterocolitis

Pregnancy Category B

Dosing

- Oral: 20–40 mg four times a day
- IM: 20 mg four times day; maximum of 1–2 days
- IV: Do not administer IV

Adverse Reactions: Most Common

Dry mouth, dizziness, drowsiness, blurred vision, nausea, constipation, weakness, nervousness, light-headedness (parenteral administration), local irritation (parenteral administration)

Adverse Reactions: Rare/Severe/Important

Decreased sweating, tachyarrhythmia, psychosis, difficulty breathing

Major Drug Interactions

Dicyclomine's Effect on Other Drugs

- Anticholinergic drugs: Belladonna/belladonna alkaloids may have additive anticholinergic effects/toxicities
- Acetylcholinesterase inhibitors: Theoretical interaction because they would likely antagonize the therapeutic effect of each other

Contraindications

Obstructive diseases of the GI tract, severe ulcerative colitis, reflux esophagitis, unstable cardiovascular status in acute hemorrhage, obstructive uropathy, narrow-angle glaucoma, myasthenia gravis, infants < 6 months of age

Counseling Points

- This drug may impair mental alertness; use caution when driving or engaging in tasks that require alertness

- Dicyclomine may cause constipation; increasing exercise, fluids, fruit, or fiber may help if patients experience this side effect

Key Point

Dicyclomine is not considered a first-line therapy for urinary incontinence or IBS due to a lack of data supporting its efficacy over alternative agents and high incidence of side effects. Notable side effects are dizziness, drowsiness, dry mouth, blurry vision, nausea, and nervousness.

ANTIEMETICS, PHENOTHIAZINE, TYPICAL ANTIPSYCHOTICS

Introduction

Phenothiazines are among the most commonly prescribed antiemetic agents available. They come in a wide variety of preparations for oral, rectal, and IV/IM administration, and are generally less expensive than newer antiemetics on the market. They are particularly effective for treatment of drug-induced nausea. Adverse effects such as extrapyramidal reactions, tardive dyskinesia, orthostatic hypotension, and drug-induced Parkinson's syndrome are relatively common and are more likely to develop in elderly patients and young children. This class of drugs is also approved to treat psychiatric conditions such as schizophrenia and anxiety; however, the drugs are no longer recommended as first-line therapy for these conditions due to their questionable efficacy and potential for significant adverse events.

Mechanism of Action for the Drug Class

These drugs have an antiemetic effect through central inhibition of dopamine receptors in the medullary chemoreceptor trigger zone. The antipsychotic effect stems from the ability of phenothiazines to block postsynaptic mesolimbic dopaminergic (D_1 and D_2) receptors in the brain.

Members of the Drug Class

In this section: Prochlorperazine
Others: Chlorpromazine, perphenazine, promethazine

⊙ Prochlorperazine

Brand Names
Compazine, Compro

Generic Name
Prochlorperazine

Rx Only

Dosage Forms
Tablet, suppository, injection solution

Usage

Nausea/vomiting* (including chemotherapy-induced nausea and vomiting and postoperative nausea and vomiting), schizophrenia, anxiety, psychosis/agitation related to Alzheimer's dementia (not recommended for this use), migraines and associated nausea and vomiting

Pregnancy Category C

Dosing

- Antiemetic:
  - Oral (immediate release):
    - 5–10 mg three to four times a day
    - Maximum: 40 mg daily
  - Rectal: 25 mg twice daily
  - IV/IM (deep):
    - 2.5–10 mg every 3–4 hours
    - Maximum: 10 mg/dose, 40 mg/day
- Postoperative:
  - IV: 5–10 mg 15–30 minutes before anesthesia induction; may repeat once
  - IM: 5–10 mg 1–2 hours before anesthesia induction; may repeat once
- Hepatic dosage adjustment: Guidelines not provided by the manufacturer; however, prochlorperazine is primarily eliminated hepatically. Caution is advised because drug accumulation may occur.

Adverse Reactions: Most Common

Hypotension (IV administration), constipation, dry mouth, dizziness, extrapyramidal reactions (akathisia, dystonia, parkinsonian symptoms)

Adverse Reactions: Rare/Serious/Important

Agranulocytosis, leukopenia, thrombocytopenia, ineffective thermoregulation, neuroleptic malignant syndrome, cholestatic jaundice, seizure (lower seizure threshold), tardive dyskinesia (long-term use), QT prolongation (mostly associated with other agents in this class)

Major Drug Interactions

Prochlorperazine's Effect on Other Drugs

- Dofetilide: Increases serum concentration
- Antagonistic action against dopaminergic agents used to treat Parkinson's disease
- CNS depressants/sedatives: Enhances CNS depression

Contraindications

Children < 2 kg or < 9 kg, pediatric surgery, presence of large amounts of CNS depressants

Counseling Points

- This drug may impair mental alertness; use caution when driving or engaging in tasks that require alertness
- Notify your physician if feelings of restlessness or involuntary/spastic muscle movements occur or if you experience fever, muscle rigidity, or altered mental status

Key Points

- Prochlorperazine should not be given SUB-Q because of local irritation. If giving IV, do not administer as a bolus; give as a slow IV push (max rate of 5 mg/min) or infusion. Hypotension may occur with IV administration.
- Prochlorperazine is most commonly used for the acute treatment of generalized nausea and vomiting and nausea and vomiting related to chemotherapy. It is particularly effective for postoperative nausea and vomiting and drug- or toxin-induced nausea and vomiting.
- Although the class of phenothiazines has been associated with a significant number of adverse effects, many of these effects are seen at high doses, with chronic therapy, and in combination with other psychiatric agents. As an antiemetic, especially with short-term as needed use, prochlorperazine is generally well tolerated.
- Prochlorperazine has fallen out of favor as an antipsychotic agent and is rarely used for this purpose any longer

ANTIEMETICS, PHOSPHORATED CARBOHYDRATE SOLUTIONS

Introduction

Phosphorated carbohydrate solution is a mixture of fructose, dextrose, and phosphoric acid. It has been available over the counter for many years; however, clinical data supporting its efficacy are lacking. Importantly, this solution is the only antiemetic available over the counter with the exception of medications used for motion sickness. If phosphorated carbohydrate solution is being used to treat nausea *not* related to motion sickness, medical advice may be warranted because nausea can be a sign of a more serious underlying condition.

Mechanism of Action for the Drug Class

The combination of the hyperosmolar solution and phosphoric acid is hypothesized to act locally on the GI tract, decreasing smooth muscle contractions and delaying gastric emptying time

Members of the Drug Class

In this section: Phosphorated carbohydrate solution
Others: None

⊙ Phosphoric Acid/Dextrose/Fructose

Brand Names

Emetrol, Formula EM, Nausetrol

Generic Name

Phosphoric acid/dextrose/fructose

OTC

Dosage Form

Liquid

Usage

Treatment of nausea associated with upset stomach that occurs with intestinal or stomach flu and food indiscretions

No Official Pregnancy Category

Dosing

15–30 mL; repeat dose every 15 minutes until symptoms subside (do not take for > 1 hour or > 5 doses)

Adverse Reactions: Most Common

Abdominal pain, diarrhea

Contraindication

Hereditary fructose intolerance

Counseling Points

- Do not dilute solution
- May chill in refrigerator to improve palatability
- Do not consume other liquids for 15 minutes after taking each dose

Key Points

- It is important to remember that nausea, unless related to motion sickness, may be symptom of a more serious underlying condition. If nausea does not resolve, the patient should seek medical attention from a physician.

- Phosphorated carbohydrate solution has been used off-label for motion sickness and morning sickness; however, it is recommended that all pregnant women speak with a physician before self-medicating
- This product contains a significant amount of sugar, thus it is not recommended for use in diabetics

CHLORIDE CHANNEL ACTIVATORS

Introduction

Lubiprostone is a single agent in a new class of drugs used to treat chronic idiopathic constipation and irritable bowel syndrome with constipation (IBS-C) in women. It has a novel mechanism of action, affecting chloride channels in the intestine responsible for regulating fluid balance, without any clinically significant changes in serum electrolyte concentrations. Because the vast majority of patients enrolled in the IBS-C studies were women, lubiprostone has not been approved to use for IBS-C in men due to a lack of clinical data.

Mechanism of Action for the Drug Class

Activates ClC-2 chloride channels in the intestine, promoting a chloride-rich fluid secretion into the intestine, thereby improving motility and passage of stools

Members of the Drug Class

In this section: Lubiprostone
Others: None

◉ Lubiprostone

Brand Name

Amitiza

Generic Name

Lubiprostone

Rx Only

Dosage Form

Capsule

Usage

Treatment of chronic idiopathic constipation,* IBS-C in women*

Pregnancy Category C

Dosing

- Chronic idiopathic constipation: 24 µg twice a day (dose may be decreased to once a day if poorly tolerated due to nausea)
- IBS-C: 8 µg twice a day

- Hepatic dosage adjustment:
  - Moderate hepatic impairment (Child-Pugh class B):
    - Chronic idiopathic constipation: 16 µg twice daily; may increase to 24 mcg twice daily if tolerated and an adequate response has not been obtained with lower dosage
    - IBS-C in women: No dosage adjustment required
  - Severe hepatic impairment (Child-Pugh class C):
    - Chronic idiopathic constipation: 8 µg twice daily; may increase to 16–24 µg twice daily if tolerated and an adequate response has not been obtained with lower dosage
    - IBS-C: 8 µg once daily; may increase to 8 µg twice daily if tolerated and an adequate response has not been obtained at lower dosage

Adverse Reactions: Most Common

Nausea, diarrhea, headache, dizziness, abdominal pain and distention, flatulence, vomiting, dyspepsia

Adverse Reactions: Rare/Severe/Important

Dyspnea, which may also be described as chest tightness or discomfort. Usually occurs within 30–60 minutes after the first dose and resolves after several hours; may occur again after subsequent doses. Not an allergic reaction. Therapy can be continued if tolerated; however, it may lead to therapy discontinuation in some patients.

Contraindications

Known or suspected mechanical GI obstruction

Counseling Points

- This medication may be taken with meals to decrease nausea
- Swallow whole, do not break or chew
- Dyspnea, also referred to as chest discomfort, may occur following the first dose. This is not an allergic reaction and generally resolves within 3 hours, but may recur with subsequent doses.
- Notify your doctor if experiencing severe nausea, severe diarrhea, or dyspnea

REVIEW QUESTIONS

1. Which of the following brand:generic name pairs do *not* match?

   a. Bentyl: dicyclomine
   b. Prilosec: esomeprazole
   c. Reglan: metoclopramide
   d. Pepcid: famotidine

2. Which of the following counseling points concerning calcium carbonate (Tums) tablets is *false*?

   a. Patients should consult their doctors if symptoms persist for > 2 weeks.
   b. Calcium carbonate may be used during pregnancy.
   c. Tums may be taken at the same time as ciprofloxacin.
   d. Tablets should be chewed before swallowing.

3. Which of the following is the correct indication for simethicone?

   a. Acid reflux
   b. Diarrhea
   c. Gas
   d. Nausea

4. Which of the following serious adverse effects is *not* associated with loperamide?

   a. Ileus
   b. Necrotizing enterocolitis
   c. Toxic megacolon
   d. Vancomycin-resistant *Enterococcus* (VRE) super-infection

5. Which of the following is *not* one of the available dosage forms of psyllium?

   a. Capsules
   b. Powder
   c. Suppository
   d. Wafers

6. Which of the following medications requires adjustment for renal insufficiency?

   a. Loperamide
   b. Ondansetron
   c. Pantoprazole
   d. Ranitidine

7. Which of the following is the mechanism of action of Bentyl?

   a. It acts peripherally on opioid receptors.
   b. It blocks H^+/K^+-ATPase in the gastric parietal cells.
   c. It blocks the action of acetylcholine at parasympathetic sites.
   d. It competitively inhibits histamine at H_2 receptors.

8. Which of the following is a contraindication for Mira-LAX therapy?

   a. Aspirin allergy
   b. Baseline QT prolongation
   c. Bone marrow depression
   d. Bowel obstruction

9. Prochlorperazine has fallen out of favor due to a high incidence of adverse effects. Which of the following adverse effects has been associated with prochlorperazine?

   a. Drug-induced Parkinson's syndrome
   b. Hypotension
   c. Tardive dyskinesia
   d. All of the above

10. Which of the following proton pump inhibitors is available over the counter?

    a. Esomeprazole
    b. Lansoprazole
    c. Pantoprazole
    d. Rabeprazole

11. Which of the following agents may be used as a prokinetic agent in patients with diabetic gastroparesis *and* as an antiemetic for chemotherapy-induced nausea and vomiting?

 a. Dicyclomine
 b. Metoclopramide
 c. Prochlorperazine
 d. Simethicone

12. A patient approaches the pharmacy counter to ask for advice regarding over-the-counter laxatives. He recently had surgery and has been taking chronic opioid analgesics for the past 3 weeks. He is currently nauseous and hasn't eaten for the last 4 days due to vomiting. His last bowel movement was 7 days ago, he is not passing any gas, and complains of abdominal pain and distension; he is concerned that he may have a bowel obstruction. What is the best recommendation for this patient?

 a. Metamucil
 b. Metoclopramide
 c. MiraLAX
 d. Refer him to a physician

13. Which of the following agents is an antidiarrheal?

 a. Bismuth subsalicylate
 b. Calcium carbonate
 c. Magnesium hydroxide/aluminum hydroxide
 d. Simethicone

14. Which of the following counseling statements regarding antacids is true?

 a. Aluminum-containing compounds may accumulate in patients with renal dysfunction.
 b. Contact a physician if prolonged use (> 2 weeks) is required.
 c. Patients should separate administration of antacids from other medications by 1–2 hours.
 d. All of the above

15. Which of the following agents would not require a dosage adjustment in an 86-year-old woman with a CrCl < 30 mL/min?

 a. Pepcid
 b. Reglan
 c. Imodium
 d. Zantac

16. Which of the following statements regarding docusate sodium is true?

 a. Docusate sodium contains a high amount of sodium and is contraindicated in patients with heart failure.
 b. Docusate sodium is commonly used to prevent constipation in patients who should avoid straining during defecation.
 c. Docusate sodium is considered an effective stimulant laxative for treatment of opiate-induced constipation.
 d. The dose of docusate sodium must be renally adjusted in patients with a CrCl < 30 mL/min.

17. Which of the following statements regarding 5-HT$_3$ antagonists is *false*?

 a. Aloxi has a longer half-life than other agents in this class.
 b. Zofran may be used for severe nausea and vomiting during pregnancy.
 c. Aloxi is better at treating acute episodes of nausea and vomiting than preventing them.
 d. Dolasetron may prolong the QT interval; monitor EKG in select patients.

18. Bisacodyl is best described as what kind of laxative?

 a. Bulk-forming laxative
 b. Osmotic laxative
 c. Stimulant laxative
 d. Stool softener

19. Which of the following agents is most likely to decrease the efficacy of clopidogrel?

 a. Famotidine
 b. Omeprazole
 c. Pantoprazole
 d. Ranitidine

20. Which of the following counseling points is pertinent to MoviPrep?

 a. Contact your healthcare provider if you experience diarrhea.
 b. Do not consume solid food during the prep.
 c. Do not crush or chew tablets.
 d. Other medications should be administered 1–2 hours after starting the prep.

21. Which of the following statements is true regarding Tagamet?

 a. Tagamet has been associated with adverse CNS effects.
 b. Tagamet may be used for ulcer prophylaxis in critically ill patients.
 c. Tagamet should be taken 30–60 minutes before an offending meal to prevent heartburn.
 d. All of the above

22. Which of the following statements regarding Amitiza is *false*?

    a. Amitiza does not have a significant effect on serum electrolytes.
    b. Amitiza has been associated with feelings of dyspnea and chest discomfort.
    c. Amitiza was found to be ineffective in men.
    d. The most common side effect of Amitiza is nausea.

23. Which of the following products contain simethicone?

    a. Dulcolax
    b. Imodium
    c. Mylicon
    d. Pepto-Bismol

24. Reglan has been associated with all of the following serious adverse effects, *except*:

    a. extrapyramidal reactions.
    b. hyperkalemia.
    c. neuroleptic malignant syndrome.
    d. serotonin syndrome.

25. Which of the following is *false* regarding Metamucil?

    a. Metamucil is a stimulant laxative and should be avoided in elderly patients.
    b. Metamucil is considered a first-line agent for treatment of simple constipation.
    c. Metamucil should be separated from other medications by at least 1–2 hours.
    d. Metamucil should be taken with at least 8 oz of fluids per dose.

26. Which of the following patients should avoid Pepto-Bismol?

    a. A 14-year-old child with chickenpox
    b. A 46-year-old female with an allergy to aspirin
    c. An 88-year-old male with a recent GI bleed
    d. All of the above

27. Emetrol is primarily used for which of the following purposes?

    a. Heartburn
    b. Constipation
    c. Gas
    d. Nausea

28. Which of the following is the appropriate dosing for oral prochlorperazine?

    a. 10 mg PO every 6 hours
    b. 25 mg PO every 12 hours
    c. 25 mg PO every 6 hours
    d. 100 mg PO every 12 hours

29. Bentyl may be used for which of the following indications?

    a. Bowel evacuation prior to colonoscopy
    b. Gastroesophageal reflux disease
    c. Inflammatory bowel disease
    d. Urinary incontinence

30. Which of the following agents is most effective at controlling gastric acid in patients with severe GERD?

    a. Calcium carbonate chewable tablets
    b. H_2 receptor antagonists
    c. Magnesium hydroxide/aluminum hydroxide suspension
    d. Proton pump inhibitors

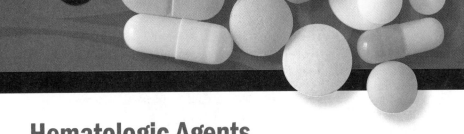

CHAPTER

9

Hematologic Agents

Michael C. Barros, PharmD, BCPS, BCACP
Deborah DeEugenio-Mayro, PharmD, BCPS, CACP

ANTICOAGULANTS, COUMARIN DERIVATIVES

Introduction

Warfarin is an oral anticoagulant used to reduce the formation of pathologic clots. Its exceptional efficacy is tempered by its narrow therapeutic index and significant drug–drug, drug–diet, drug–disease interactions and need for intensive monitoring to ensure safety and efficacy. Its major adverse effect is bleeding.

Mechanism of Action for the Drug Class

Warfarin inhibits the carboxylation (activation) of the vitamin K-dependent clotting factors II, VII, IX, and X, thereby increasing the time it takes for blood to clot

Members of the Drug Class

In this section: Warfarin
Others: Acenocoumarol

⊙ Warfarin

Brand Names
  Coumadin, Jantoven

Generic Name
  Warfarin

Rx Only

Dosage Forms
  Tablet, injection available for IV use (rarely used clinically)

Usage
  Prophylaxis and treatment of deep venous thrombosis (DVT) and its extension and/or pulmonary embolism (PE);* prophylaxis and treatment of stroke in high-risk patients with atrial fibrillation;* prophylaxis and treatment of the thromboembolic complications associated with cardiac valve replacement;* reduces risk of death, recurrent myocardial infarction, and thromboembolic events, such as stroke and systemic embolization, after myocardial infarction*

Pregnancy Category X

Dosing
  - Initial dose: Warfarin therapy should generally begin with the average dose requirement of 5 mg per day for the first few days, with subsequent dosing based on the INR response
  - Dosage adjustments: Patients expected to have lower dosage requirements (i.e., malnourished, active liver disease, on interacting medications) should be initiated on 2.5 mg per day

Pharmacokinetic Monitoring
  INR goal is usually 2–3 for most indications, but 2.5–3.5 for most mechanical cardiac valve replacements

Adverse Reactions: Most Common
  Bleeding

Adverse Reactions: Rare/Severe/Important
  Intracranial, retroperitoneal, or intraocular bleeding, purple toe syndrome, skin necrosis

Major Drug Interactions
  Drugs Affecting Warfarin
  - Amiodarone, fluconazole, metronidazole, ciprofloxacin, erythromycin, prednisone, sulfamethoxazole/trimethoprim: Potentiate INR
  - Carbamazepine, rifampin: Decrease INR
  - Aspirin, NSAIDs, concomitant anticoagulants: Increase risk of bleeding

---

* Throughout the text, an asterisk (*) is used to indicate the most common uses of a drug.

Contraindications

Hemorrhagic tendencies (e.g., patients bleeding from the GI, respiratory, or GU tract; aneurysm; cerebrovascular hemorrhage; following spinal puncture and other diagnostic or therapeutic procedures with potential for significant bleeding; history of bleeding diathesis); recent or potential surgery of the eye or CNS; major regional lumbar block anesthesia or surgery resulting in large, open surfaces; blood dyscrasias; severe uncontrolled or malignant hypertension; pericarditis or pericardial effusion; subacute bacterial endocarditis; history of warfarin-induced necrosis; an unreliable, noncompliant patient; alcoholism; patient who has a history of falls or is a significant fall risk; unsupervised senile or psychotic patient; eclampsia/preeclampsia, threatened abortion, pregnancy

Counseling Points

- Explain importance of blood test monitoring; INR testing required every 3 days to every 4 weeks
- Risk of bleeding: Monitor for blood in urine, stool, nosebleeds, hemoptysis
- Drug–drug, drug–herbal interactions: Inform your doctor when initiating or discontinuing any medication
- Drug–food interaction: Keep vitamin K intake consistent
- Alcohol: Binge drinking will increase INR
- Avoid or take precautions (e.g., helmet, protective clothing) when participating in contact sports or activities with high risk of trauma
- Have an ID card in your wallet or a medical bracelet noting that you are taking warfarin in case of emergency
- Warfarin is pregnancy category X: Discuss with your doctor before attempting to become pregnant or use appropriate contraception

Key Points

- Generally stop 5 days before surgical procedure
- Vitamin K is the antidote
- Warfarin is pregnancy category X
- Always review a patient's concomitant medications and disease states prior to initiating or adjusting warfarin therapy

FACTOR Xa INHIBITORS

Introduction

Rivaroxaban is an oral factor Xa inhibitor used for stroke prevention in atrial fibrillation, prevention of *venous thromboembolism* in patients who have undergone knee/hip replacement, and for treatment of deep vein thrombosis (DVT), and pulmonary embolism (PE). It requires no therapeutic monitoring, but significant drug–drug interactions do exist. Its major adverse effect is bleeding.

Mechanism of Action for the Drug Class

Rivaroxaban inhibits platelet activation and fibrin clot formation by selectively and reversibly inhibiting factor Xa

Members of the Drug Class

In this section: Rivaroxaban
Others: Apixiban, fondaparinux

⊙ Rivaroxaban

Brand Name
Xarelto

Generic Name
Rivaroxaban

Rx Only

Dosage Form
Tablet

Usage

Postoperative prophylaxis in patients who have undergone hip or knee replacement surgery,* prevention of stroke and systemic embolism in patients with nonvalvular atrial fibrillation*, treatment of DVT and PE*

Pregnancy Category C

Dosing

- Thromboprophylaxis following knee/hip replacement: 10 mg PO once daily. Avoid use if CrCl < 30 mL/min.
- Nonvalvular atrial fibrillation: 20 mg PO once daily. 15 mg PO once daily if CrCl 15–50 mL/min and avoid use if CrCl < 15 mL/min.
- DVT and PE: Initial 15 mg PO twice daily for three weeks, followed by 20 mg PO once daily. Avoid use if CrCl < 30 mL/min.
- Conversion from warfarin: Discontinue warfarin and initiate rivaroxaban when INR falls to < 3.0
- Conversion to warfarin: Initiate warfarin and a parenteral anticoagulant 24 hours after discontinuing rivaroxaban
- Conversion from continuous infusion unfractionated heparin: Initiate rivaroxaban at the time of heparin discontinuation
- Conversion to continuous infusion unfractionated heparin: Initiate continuous infusion unfractionated heparin 24 hours after discontinuation of rivaroxaban

Pharmacokinetic Monitoring

None. However, measurement of prothrombin time may be used to detect presence of rivaroxaban.

Adverse Reactions: Most Common

Bleeding

Adverse Reactions: Rare/Severe/Important

Agranulocytosis, hemorrhage (cerebral, retroperitoneal), Stevens-Johnson syndrome

Major Drug Interactions

Drugs Affecting Rivaroxaban

- Aspirin, NSAIDs, concomitant anticoagulants: Increase risk of bleeding, use cautiously
- Clarithromycin, conivaptan, itraconazole, ketoconazole, ritonavir: Increase risk of bleeding and should be avoided
- Carbamazepine, phenytoin, rifampin, St. John's Wort: Decrease efficacy and should be avoided

Contraindication

Active pathological bleeding

Counseling Points

- Risk of bleeding: Monitor for blood in urine, stool, nosebleeds, hemoptysis
- For hip or knee replacement surgery: 10 mg dose may be taken with or without food
- For atrial fibrillation and DVT/PE: 20 mg dose should be taken with food
- Inform your doctor if you start taking any new medications

Key Points

- Prothrombin complex concentrate (PCC) may be used as an antidote
- 10 mg dose may be taken with or without food and 20 mg dose should be taken with food

---

ANTIPLATELETS, ASPIRIN

Introduction

Aspirin is an oral antiplatelet agent used as an analgesic, antipyretic, anti-inflammatory, and, most commonly, for prevention of cardiovascular events. Aspirin is most commonly used to reduce arterial thrombosis, which may lead to myocardial infarction or stroke in high-risk patients. Aspirin's benefits are tempered by its dose-dependent risk of bleeding, especially gastrointestinal.

Mechanism of Action for the Drug Class

Aspirin irreversibly inhibits the cyclo-oxygenase enzyme, blocking the synthesis of cyclic prostanoids, such as thromboxane A2, prostacyclin, and other prostaglandins. Aspirin's antiplatelet effects are due to the inhibition of thromboxane A2 synthesis, a potent mediator of platelet aggregation and vasoconstriction.

Members of the Drug Class

In this section: Aspirin
Others: None

⊙ Aspirin

Brand Names

Various

Generic Name

Aspirin

OTC

Dosage Forms

Tablet, chewable tablet, enteric-coated tablet, suppository

Usage

Pain;* fever;* various inflammatory conditions, such as rheumatic fever, rheumatoid arthritis, and osteoarthritis; cardioprotection (prevention of cerebrovascular accident [CVA] and myocardial infarction [MI]) in high-risk primary prevention patients and in secondary prevention of MI, CVA, or transient ischemic attack (TIA), or following percutaneous coronary intervention (PCI) or *coronary artery bypass grafting* (CABG),* prevention of in-stent thrombosis following PCI or graft thrombosis following CABG

Pregnancy Category D

Dosing

- Pain, fever: 325–650 mg PO every 4–6 hours as needed
- Inflammation: 3.6–5.4 g PO daily in divided doses
- TIA/CVA: 75–100 mg PO daily
- MI/post-PCI/post-CABG: 81–325 mg PO daily

Adverse Reactions: Most Common

Dyspepsia, bleeding

Adverse Reactions: Rare/Severe/Important

GI bleeding (dose dependent)

Major Drug Interactions

Drugs Affecting Aspirin

- Diuretics, uricosurics: May decrease effectiveness
- Anticoagulants: Increase bleeding risk
- NSAIDs: Increase bleeding risk and may reduce antiplatelet efficacy

Aspirin's Effect on Other Drugs
- Lithium: Increases levels
- Methotrexate: Increases levels
- ACE inhibitors: Decreases effectiveness

Contraindications

Hypersensitivity to salicylates, other NSAIDs, or any component of the formulation; asthma; rhinitis; nasal polyps; inherited or acquired bleeding disorders (including factor VII and factor IX deficiency); do not use in children (< 16 years of age) for viral infections (chickenpox or flu symptoms), with or without fever, due to a potential association with Reye's syndrome; pregnancy (third trimester especially)

Counseling Points

- There is an increased risk of bleeding: Monitor for blood in urine and stool and watch for nosebleeds
- Take with food or after meals to reduce GI upset
- Limit alcohol intake

Key Points

- Avoid use in children < 16 years of age due to risk of Reye's syndrome
- Generally, stop 1 week before surgical procedure
- Use minimal required dose because GI bleeding is a dose-dependent adverse effect

ANTIPLATELETS, ASPIRIN/DIPYRIDAMOLE

Introduction

Aspirin and dipyridamole are oral antiplatelet agents used in combination to reduce stroke risk in patients who have had a transient ischemic attack (TIA) due to thrombosis. Major adverse effects including bleeding and headache.

Mechanism of Action for the Drug Class

Aspirin and dipyridamole have additive antiplatelet effects. Aspirin irreversibly inhibits the cyclo-oxygenase enzyme, blocking the synthesis of cyclic prostanoids, such as thromboxane A2, prostacyclin, and other prostaglandins. Aspirin's antiplatelet effects are due to the inhibition of thromboxane A2 synthesis, a potent mediator of platelet aggregation and vasoconstriction. Dipyridamole decreases platelet aggregation and platelet activation by increasing endogenous concentrations of adenosine and cyclic adenosine monophosphate (cAMP).

Members of the Drug Class

In this section: Aspirin and dipyridamole
Others: None

⊙ Aspirin and Dipyridamole

Brand Name

Aggrenox

Generic Name

Aspirin and dipyridamole

Rx Only

Dosage Form

Capsule

Usage

Reduce stroke risk in patients who have had a transient ischemic attack (TIA) due to thrombosis*

Pregnancy Category D

Dosing

1 capsule (dipyridamole 200 mg, aspirin 25 mg) orally twice daily

Adverse Reactions: Most Common

Headache, nausea

Adverse Reactions: Rare/Severe/Important

Bleeding

Major Drug Interactions

Drugs Affecting Aspirin

- Diuretics, uricosurics: May decrease effectiveness
- Anticoagulants: Increase bleeding risk
- NSAIDs: Increase bleeding risk and may reduce antiplatelet efficacy of aspirin

Aspirin's Effect on Other Drugs

- Lithium: Increases levels
- Methotrexate: Increases levels
- ACE inhibitors: Decreases effectiveness

Drugs Affecting Dipyridamole

Antiplatelets, anticoagulants, NSAIDs: Increase risk of bleeding

Dipyridamole's Effect on Other Drugs

- Adenosine, beta blockers: Increases effect
- Colchicine: Increases serum concentrations. Avoid if patient has impaired renal or hepatic function.
- Everolimus: Increases serum concentrations

Contraindications

Hypersensitivity to dipyridamole, aspirin, NSAIDs, or any component of the formulation; asthma; rhinitis; nasal polyps; inherited or acquired bleeding disorders (including factor VII and factor IX deficiency); do not use in children (< 16 years of age) for viral infections (chickenpox or flu symptoms), with or without fever, due to a potential association with Reye's syndrome; pregnancy (third trimester especially)

Counseling Points

- Increased risk of bleeding: Monitor for blood in urine and stool and watch for nosebleeds
- Capsule should be swallowed whole; do not crush or chew. May be administered with or without food.

- Limit alcohol intake
- Rise slowly from a sitting/supine position
- This drug may cause a headache. May take up to 1 week for tolerance to headache to develop.

Key Points

- Avoid use in children < 16 years of age due to risk of Reye's syndrome
- Generally, stop 1 week before surgical procedure

ANTIPLATELETS, THIENOPYRIDINES

Introduction

The thienopyridine antiplatelet agents are used predominantly in combination with aspirin to prevent arterial thrombosis, especially following myocardial infarction (MI) or percutaneous coronary intervention (PCI). Ticlopidine has been largely replaced in clinical practice by clopidogrel and prasugrel because of its increased risk of hematologic adverse effects. Clopidogrel is the most commonly used thienopyridine; however, its effectiveness is reduced in patients taking certain medications and in patients who are not able to convert it to the active drug due to genetic variations. Prasugrel is a newly available thienopyridine; however, its efficacy is tempered by its limited use due to contraindications/precautions in patients with a history of stroke, advanced age, and low body weight. The major adverse effects are bleeding.

Mechanism of Action for the Drug Class

Clopidogrel and prasugrel irreversibly inhibit platelet aggregation by selectively blocking adenosine diphosphate's (ADP) binding to its platelet receptor and the subsequent ADP-mediated activation of the glycoprotein GPIIb/IIIa complex, thereby inhibiting platelet aggregation

Members of the Drug Class

In this section: Clopidogrel, prasugrel
Others: Ticlopidine

◉ Clopidogrel

Brand Name
Plavix

Generic Name
Clopidogrel

Rx Only

Dosage Form
Tablet

Usage

Reduction of thrombotic events (MI, stroke, and vascular death) in patients with atherosclerosis documented by recent stroke, recent MI, or established peripheral arterial disease (PAD);* for patients with acute coronary syndromes (unstable angina/MI), including patients who are to be managed medically and those who are to be managed with PCI or CABG*

Pregnancy Category B

Dosing

- Recent MI, recent stroke, or established PAD: 75 mg PO daily
- Acute coronary syndromes, including PCI: 600 mg loading dose PO on day 1, then 75 mg PO daily (administer 300 mg loading dose if fibrinolytic administered within previous 24 hours)

Adverse Reactions: Most Common

Bleeding

Adverse Reactions: Rare/Severe/Important

Agranulocytosis

Major Drug Interactions

Drugs Affecting Clopidogrel
Proton pump inhibitors: May decrease effectiveness

Clopidogrel's Effect on Other Drugs
Anticoagulants, NSAIDs, aspirin: Increases bleeding risk

Contraindication

Active pathological bleeding such as peptic ulcer or intracranial hemorrhage

Counseling Points

- Adherence is critical post-PCI or post-CABG because in-stent thrombosis and graft thrombosis has a high fatality rate
- Report unusual bleeding, symptoms of dark or bloody urine, or petechiae

Key Points

- Stop clopidogrel 5 days before surgical procedure
- Genetic tests are available to determine effectiveness

⊙ Prasugrel

Brand Name
Effient

Generic Name
Prasugrel

Rx Only

Dosage Form
Tablet

Usage
Reduction of thrombotic events (stent thrombosis) in patients who are to be managed with PCI for acute coronary syndromes (unstable angina/MI)*

Pregnancy Category B

Dosing
Acute "coronary syndromes" undergoing PCI: 60 mg loading dose at time of PCI, then 10 mg orally daily (manufacturer suggests to decrease maintenance dose to 5 mg orally once daily in patients weighing < 60 kg; however, data do not exist to support this recommendation)

Adverse Reactions: Most Common
Bleeding

Adverse Reactions: Rare/Severe/Important
Thrombotic thrombocytopenic purpura, hemorrhage (postprocedural, retinal, retroperitoneal)

Major Drug Interactions
Prasugrel's Effect on Other Drugs
Anticoagulants, NSAIDs, aspirin: Increases bleeding risk

Contraindications
Active pathological bleeding, such as peptic ulcer or intracranial hemorrhage; history of TIA; patients ≥ 75 years (may be considered in high-risk situations such as patients with diabetes or history of MI); patients who are likely to undergo urgent CABG surgery

Counseling Points
- Adherence is critical post-PCI or post-CABG because in-stent thrombosis or graft thrombosis has a high fatality rate
- Report unusual bleeding, symptoms of dark or bloody urine, or petechiae

Key Points
- Stop prasugrel 7 days before surgical procedure
- Do not use prasugrel in patients with history of TIA

COLONY-STIMULATING FACTORS

Introduction
Filgrastim and pegfilgrastim are colony-stimulating factors used most commonly for the prevention and treatment of neutropenia in cancer and HIV patients. Pegfilgrastim is a pegylated form of filgrastim with a longer duration of action.

Mechanism of Action for the Drug Class
Filgrastim and pegfilgrastim are human granulocyte colony-stimulating factors (G-CSFs), which are produced by recombinant DNA technology. Endogenous G-CSF is a lineage-specific colony-stimulating factor that is produced by monocytes, fibroblasts, and endothelial cells. G-CSF regulates the production of neutrophils within the bone marrow and affects neutrophil progenitor proliferation, differentiation, and selected end-cell functional activation. Pegfilgrastim has a longer duration of action than filgrastim.

Members of the Drug Class
In this section: Filgrastim, pegfilgrastim
Others: Eltrombopag, peginesatide, romiplostim, sargramostim

⊙ Filgrastim

Brand Name
Neupogen

Generic Name
Filgrastim

Rx Only

Dosage Forms
Injection (IV, SUB-Q)

Usage
- Myelosuppressive chemotherapy: Decreases incidence of infection, as manifested by febrile neutropenia, in patients with nonmyeloid malignancies receiving myelosuppressive anticancer drugs associated with a significant incidence of severe neutropenia and fever*
- Bone marrow transplantation (BMT): Reduces duration of neutropenia and neutropenia-associated sequelae in patients with nonmyeloid malignancies undergoing myeloablative therapy followed by BMT*

- Peripheral blood progenitor cell (PBPC) collection and therapy in cancer patients: Mobilizes hematopoietic progenitor cells into the peripheral blood for leukapheresis collection*
- Patients with severe chronic neutropenia (SCN): Chronic administration reduces the incidence and duration of sequelae of neutropenia in symptomatic patients with congenital, cyclic, or idiopathic neutropenia*
- Treatment of neutropenia in patients with human immunodeficiency virus (HIV)*

Pregnancy Category C

Dosing

- Myelosuppressive chemotherapy: Initial dose of 5 μg/kg per day SUB-Q daily, short IV infusion (15–30 minutes), or continuous SUB-Q or IV infusion
- BMT: 10 μg/kg per day IV infusion of 4 or 24 hours or 24-hour SUB-Q infusion
- PBPC: 10 μg/kg per day SUB-Q, either as a bolus or continuous infusion
- SCN:
  - Congenital neutropenia: 6 μg/kg SUB-Q twice daily
  - Idiopathic or cyclic neutropenia: 5 μg/kg SUB-Q daily
- HIV with neutropenia: 5–10 μg/kg per day SUB-Q for 2–4 weeks

⊙ Pegfilgrastim

Brand Name
Neulasta

Generic Name
Pegfilgrastim

Rx Only

Dosage Form
Injection (SUB-Q)

Usage

- Myelosuppressive chemotherapy: Decreases incidence of infection, as manifested by febrile neutropenia, in patients with nonmyeloid malignancies receiving myelosuppressive anticancer drugs associated with a significant incidence of severe neutropenia and fever
- PBPC collection and therapy in cancer patients: Mobilizes hematopoietic progenitor cells into the peripheral blood for leukapheresis collection*

Pregnancy Category C

Dosing

- Myelosuppressive chemotherapy: Initial dose: 6 mg SUB-Q once per chemotherapy cycle
- PBPC: 6–12 mg SUB-Q

Adverse Reactions: Most Common

Bone pain, reversible elevations in uric acid, lactate hydrogenase, alkaline phosphatase, nausea, vomiting

Adverse Reactions: Rare/Severe/Important

Hypersensitivity, splenic rupture, ARDS, sickle cell crisis

Major Drug Interactions

Drugs Affecting Filgrastim/Pegfilgrastim

Lithium: May potentiate release of neutrophils

Essential Monitoring Parameter

Neutrophil count is monitored to assess response to therapy

Counseling Point

Advise on proper dosage and administration

Key Points

- Nonnarcotic analgesics relieve bone pain
- Round dose to nearest full vial or prefilled syringe
- Do not administer 14 days before to 24 hours after administration of cytotoxic chemotherapy

ERYTHROPOIETINS, RECOMBINANT HUMAN

Introduction

Epoetin alfa and darbepoetin alfa are both injections used to treat anemia. Darbepoetin alfa has a longer duration of action.

Mechanism of Action for the Drug Class

Erythropoietin is a glycoprotein that stimulates red blood cell production. It is produced in the kidneys and stimulates the division and differentiation of committed erythroid progenitors in the bone marrow. Epoetin alfa and darbepoetin alfa are made by recombinant DNA technology and have the same biological effects as endogenous erythropoietin. Darbepoetin alfa has a longer terminal half-life than epoetin alfa.

Members of the Drug Class

In this section: Epoetin alfa, darbepoetin alfa

⊙ Epoetin Alfa

Brand Names

Epogen, Procrit

Generic Name

Epoetin alfa

Rx Only

Dosage Forms

Injection (IV, SUB-Q)

Usage

Treatment of anemia associated with chronic renal failure (CRF),* treatment of anemia in cancer patients on chemotherapy,* treatment of anemia related to zidovudine therapy in HIV,* reduction of allogeneic blood transfusion in surgery patients*

Pregnancy Category C

Dosing

- CRF on dialysis:
  - Initial dose: 50–100 units/kg three times weekly IV or SUB-Q
  - Maintenance dose: Individualize dose to target Hgb (not to exceed 11 g/dL)
- CRF not on dialysis:
  - Initial dose: 50–100 units/kg three times weekly IV or SUB-Q
  - Maintenance dose: Individualize dose to target Hgb (not to exceed 10 g/dL)
- HIV:
  - Initial dose: 100 units/kg IV or SUB-Q three times weekly for 8 weeks
  - Maintenance dose: Increase dosages in 50–100 units/kg increments to achieve target Hgb (not to exceed 12 g/dL)
  - Maximum dose: 300 units/kg dose three times weekly
- Cancer patients:
  - Initial dose: 150 units/kg SUB-Q three times weekly
  - Maximum dose: 300 units/kg dosed three times weekly
- Surgery:
  - 300 units/kg per day SUB-Q for 10 days before surgery and for 4 days after surgery *or*
  - 600 units/kg SUB-Q in once-weekly doses 21, 14, and 7 days before surgery plus a fourth dose on the day of surgery

⊙ Darbepoetin Alfa

Brand Name

Aranesp

Generic Name

Darbepoetin alfa

Rx Only

Dosage Form

Injection (IV or SUB-Q)

Usage

Treatment of anemia associated with CRF,* treatment of anemia in cancer patients on chemotherapy*

Pregnancy Category C

Dosing

- CRF on dialysis:
  - Initial dose: 0.45 µg/kg as single IV or SUB-Q injection once weekly
  - Maintenance dose: Individualize dose to target Hgb (not to exceed 11 g/dL)
- CRF not on dialysis:
  - Initial dose: 0.45 µg/kg SUB-Q once every 4 weeks
  - Maintenance dose: Individualize dose to target Hgb (not to exceed 10 g/dL)
- Cancer patients:
  - Initial dose:
    - 2.25 µg/kg SUB-Q weekly *or*
    - 500 µg SUB-Q every 3 weeks
  - Maximum dose: Individualize dose to maintain a Hgb level sufficient to avoid red blood cell transfusions

Adverse Reactions: Most Common

Hypertension, headache, tachycardia, nausea, vomiting, diarrhea, shortness of breath, hyperkalemia

Adverse Reactions: Rare/Severe/Important

Hypertension, hypersensitivity, thrombosis, seizures

Major Drug Interactions

None

Counseling Points

- Advise of proper dosage and administration
- Be aware of the signs and symptoms of an allergic drug reaction and take appropriate action if necessary
- Do not reuse needles, syringes, or drug products and dispose of them properly

Key Points

- Approximately 2–6 weeks for clinically significant change in Hgb
- Iron stores should be assessed and iron supplementation given, as needed
- Physicians need to be registered in the ESA APPRISE Oncology Program in order to prescribe and/or dispense epoetin alfa or darbepoetin alfa for anemia in cancer patients on chemotherapy

HEPARINS, UNFRACTIONATED

Introduction

Unfractionated heparin (UFH) is an injectable anticoagulant used to prevent and treat arterial and venous thromboses. UFH's use is limited by its short half-life requiring a continuous infusion to maintain therapeutic levels and its propensity to cause the life-threatening adverse effect heparin-induced thrombocytopenia (HIT). UFH has largely been replaced by newer heparin formulations such as low molecular weight heparins and fondaparinux. However, UFH is still the treatment of choice for patients with severe renal dysfunction or those needing invasive procedures that require temporary disruptions in anticoagulation. UFH is often used as a "bridge" to maintenance therapy with warfarin.

Mechanism of Action for the Drug Class

Binds to antithrombin and accelerates antithrombin's ability to inhibit factors IXa, Xa, XIa, XIIa, and IIa

Members of the Drug Class

In this section: Unfractionated heparin
Others: None

◉ Unfractionated Heparin

Brand Names
Various

Generic Names
Heparin, UFH

Rx Only

Dosage Forms
Injection, IV infusion for treatment doses (SUB-Q administration has poor absorption and it is very difficult to maintain therapeutic levels with this route), SUB-Q injection can be used for prophylaxis

Usage
Prophylaxis and treatment of venous thrombosis and its extension, pulmonary embolism (PE), peripheral arterial embolism, atrial fibrillation with high risk of stroke;* diagnosis and treatment of acute and chronic consumption coagulopathies (disseminated intravascular coagulation);* prevention of postoperative deep venous thrombosis (DVT) and PE in high-risk medical and surgical patients;* prevention of clotting in arterial and heart surgery, blood transfusions, extracorporeal circulation, dialysis procedures, and blood samples;* "bridge" to warfarin therapy to prevent cardiovascular accident in patients with cardiac valve replacements*

Pregnancy Category C

Dosing
- IV infusion for treatment of thromboembolism: 80 units/kg (range: 50–100 units/kg) IV bolus, followed by 18 units/kg per hour (range: 15–25 units/kg per hour) continuous IV infusion. Adjust dosage to target aPTT.
- Acute coronary syndrome: 60–70 units/kg IV bolus (maximum 5,000 units), followed by 12–15 units/kg per hour continuous IV infusion (maximum 1,000 units/hour). Adjust dosage to target aPTT.
- Prophylaxis of postoperative thromboembolism: 5,000 units SUB-Q every 8 to 12 hours

Pharmacokinetic Monitoring
- Partial thromboplastin time (PTT) or aPTT: Institution-specific values: Correlates with 0.3–0.7 anti-factor Xa units
- Activated clotting time (ACT) used in cardiac catheterization lab and for CABG

Adverse Reactions: Most Common
Bleeding

Adverse Reactions: Rare/Severe/Important
HIT type I and type II, osteoporosis (with prolonged use), bleeding

Major Drug Interactions
Drugs Affecting Heparin

Anticoagulants, antiplatelets, thrombolytics: Increase bleeding risk

Contraindications
History of HIT, severe thrombocytopenia; uncontrolled active bleeding except when due to disseminated intravascular coagulation (DIC); suspected intracranial hemorrhage; not for IM use; not for use when appropriate blood coagulation tests cannot be obtained at appropriate intervals (applies to full-dose heparin only)

Counseling Point
Note that there is a risk of bleeding. Monitor for blood in urine and stool and watch for nosebleeds.

Key Points
- Does not cross placenta in pregnancy; however, difficult to maintain therapeutic levels with SUB-Q administration
- High risk of osteoporosis with extended use
- Protamine sulfate is antidote
- Half-life is 1 hour when aPTT is therapeutic; however, half-life increases exponentially when supratherapeutic. Usually held for 4 hours before surgery if aPTT is initially therapeutic.
- Monitor platelets frequently to assess for HIT
- Never administer IM due to risk of hematoma

HEPARINS, LOW MOLECULAR WEIGHT

Introduction

Enoxaparin and dalteparin are low molecular weight heparins (LMWH) that have a similar anticoagulant effect to unfractionated heparin (UFH). The LMWHs are largely replacing UFH because of better SUB-Q absorption; a longer half-life, allowing for less frequent dose administration; and a much lower risk of HIT and osteoporosis. The major adverse effect is bleeding.

Mechanism of Action for the Drug Class

Binds to antithrombin and accelerates antithrombin's ability to inhibit factor Xa and IIa. Anti-factor Xa activity is greater than anti-factor IIa activity.

Usage for the Drug Class

Prophylaxis and treatment of deep venous thrombosis (DVT) and pulmonary embolism (PE);* unstable angina/non-Q-wave myocardial infarction*

Members of the Drug Class

In this section: Dalteparin, enoxaparin
Others: Tinzaparin

◉ Dalteparin

Brand Name
Fragmin

Generic Name
Dalteparin

Rx Only

Dosage Form
Injection (SUB-Q)

Usage
Prophylaxis and treatment of deep venous thrombosis (DVT) and pulmonary embolism (PE);* unstable angina/non-Q-wave myocardial infarction*

Pregnancy Category B

Dosing
- DVT/PE prophylaxis:
  - Hip replacement surgery (three dosing strategies exist):
    - Postoperative: 2,500 units SUB-Q 4–8 hours after surgery, followed by 5,000 units SUB-Q once daily for maintenance therapy
    - Preoperative (starting day of surgery): 2,500 units SUB-Q within 2 hours before surgery followed by 2,500 units SUB-Q 4–8 hours after surgery and 5,000 units SUB-Q once daily thereafter for maintenance therapy
    - Preoperative (starting evening prior to surgery): 5,000 units SUB-Q 10–14 hours before surgery. Administer 5,000 units SUB-Q 4–8 hours after surgery followed by 5,000 units SUB-Q once daily thereafter for maintenance therapy.
  - Abdominal surgery:
    - Low risk: 2,500 units SUB-Q 1–2 hours prior to surgery, then once daily
    - High risk: 5,000 units SUB-Q the evening prior to surgery and then once daily
- DVT/PE treatment:
  - 200 units/kg SUB-Q once daily or
  - 100 units/kg SUB-Q twice daily
  - Initiate concomitant warfarin therapy when appropriate and continue dalteparin for a minimum of 5 days and until a therapeutic anticoagulant effect has been achieved (INR: 2–3)
- Unstable angina/non–Q-wave MI: 120 units/kg SUB-Q (maximum dose: 10,000 units) every 12 hours in conjunction with oral aspirin therapy

Pharmacokinetic Monitoring
Generally, no monitoring is required. However, anti-Xa levels may be indicated to monitor effects in patients with obesity or severe renal dysfunction and in pregnancy and pediatric populations. Monitoring also may be used in patients with abnormal coagulation parameters or with bleeding. Goal dalteparin peak anti-Xa levels (drawn 4–6 hours after patient has received 3–4 doses) are usually 0.5–1.5 units/mL for once daily dosing.

◉ Enoxaparin

Brand Name
Lovenox

Generic Name
Enoxaparin

Rx Only

Dosage Forms
Injection (SUB-Q), can be given IV for acute coronary syndrome

Usage
Prophylaxis and treatment of DVT and PE;* unstable angina/non-Q-wave myocardial infarction*

Pregnancy Category B

Dosing

- DVT/PE prophylaxis:
  - Hip or knee replacement surgery:
    - 30 mg every 12 hours SUB-Q with initial dose given within 12–24 hours postoperatively for 7–10 days
    - Renal dosage adjustment: 30 mg SUB-Q every 24 hours for renal insufficiency (estimated CrCl 10–30 mL/min)
  - Abdominal or high-risk surgery: 40 mg once-daily SUB-Q with initial dose given 2 hours prior to surgery for 7–10 days
  - Medically ill/immobility: 40 mg SUB-Q once daily continued for up to 14 days
- DVT/PE treatment:
  - Outpatient DVT treatment: 1 mg/kg SUB-Q every 12 hours
  - Inpatient: DVT with or without PE:
    - 1 mg/kg SUB-Q every 12 hours *or*
    - 1.5 mg/kg SUB-Q once daily
  - Renal dosage adjustment: 1 mg/kg SUB-Q every 24 hours for renal insufficiency (CrCl 10–30 mL/min)
  - Initiate concomitant warfarin therapy when appropriate and continue enoxaparin for a minimum of 5 days and until a therapeutic anticoagulant effect has been achieved (INR: 2–3)
- Unstable angina/non-Q-wave MI:
  - 1 mg/kg SUB-Q every 12 hours in conjunction with oral aspirin therapy (100–325 mg once daily)
  - Renal dosage adjustment: 1 mg/kg SUB-Q every 24 hours for renal insufficiency (CrCl 10–30 mL/min)

Pharmacokinetic Monitoring

Generally no monitoring. However, anti-Xa units should be measured in special populations (pregnant, severe renal dysfunction, pediatrics, morbidly obese). Goal enoxaparin peak anti-Xa levels (drawn 4 hours postdose at steady state) are usually 0.6–1 IU/mL for twice-daily dosing and probably > 1 IU/mL for once-daily dosing.

Adverse Reactions: Most Common

Bleeding, bruising at injection site

Adverse Reactions: Rare/Severe/Important

HIT type I and type II (lower incidence than with UFH), osteoporosis (with prolonged use, but lower incidence than with UFH), bleeding

Contraindications

Thrombocytopenia associated with a positive in vitro test for antiplatelet antibodies in the presence of enoxaparin; hypersensitivity to pork products; active major bleeding; not for IM use

Major Drug Interactions

Anticoagulants, antiplatelets, thrombolytics: Increase bleeding risk

Counseling Points

- Contact physician if experiencing bleeding
- Injections are given around the navel or in the upper thigh or buttocks
- Rotate injection sites daily
- Use proper injection technique: Inject under the skin, not into muscle
- Expect a slight pain during injection and bruising at the injection site

Key Points

- Never administer dalteparin or enoxaparin IM due to risk of hematoma
- Protamine sulfate is antidote but only partially reverses therapeutic effects
  - Protamine sulfate (1%): 1 mg for every 1 mg of enoxaparin
  - Protamine sulfate (1%): 1 mg for every 100 units of dalteparin
- Use enoxaparin cautiously in patients with severe renal impairment or very low or high body weight
- When neuraxial anesthesia or spinal puncture is employed, patients who are anticoagulated or scheduled to be anticoagulated with LMWHs for prevention of thromboembolic complications are at risk of developing an epidural or spinal hematoma that can result in long-term or permanent paralysis. Consider benefit versus risk.
- Discontinue 24 hours prior to surgery
- Safe for home use and often employed as a "bridge" to maintenance anticoagulation with warfarin
- May be used in pregnancy
- Cannot be used in patients with a history of HIT
- Discontinue 24 hours prior to surgery
- For dalteparin, monitor anti-Xa levels if available for patients weighing > 190 kg

Introduction

The thrombin inhibitors are anticoagulants used in various clinical situations. Bivalirudin is available IV and may be used in patients with acute coronary syndromes undergoing percutaneous coronary intervention (PCI) as well as in patients with a history of heparin-induced thrombocytopenia (HIT). Dabigatran is the first orally approved direct thrombin inhibitor, and it is more commonly used for stroke prevention in patients with nonvalvular atrial fibrillation. It does not require therapeutic monitoring, but its use may be limited due to lack of a reversal agent. The major side effect with the thrombin inhibitors is bleeding.

Mechanism of Action for the Drug Class

The thrombin inhibitors reversibly inhibit coagulation by preventing thrombin-mediated effects, such as cleavage of fibrinogen to fibrin monomers and thrombin-induced platelet aggregation

Members of the Drug Class

In this section: Bivalirudin, dabigatran
Others: Argatroban

⊙ Bivalirudin

Brand Name
Angiomax

Generic Name
Bivalirudin

Rx Only

Dosage Forms
Injection, IV

Usage
Unstable angina/non-ST-elevation myocardial infarction (UA/NSTEMI) (moderate-high risk) undergoing early invasive strategy,* STEMI undergoing primary PCI,* HIT

Pregnancy Category B

Dosing
- UA/NSTEMI undergoing early invasive strategy:
  - 0.1 mg/kg IV bolus, followed by 0.25 mg/kg/hour IV. Once PCI is determined to be warranted, give an additional bolus of 0.5 mg/kg IV and increase infusion rate to 1.75 mg/kg/hour IV.
  - Renal dosage adjustment:
    - CrCl 10–29 mL/min: Decrease initial infusion rate to 1 mg/kg/hour IV
    - Dialysis: Begin infusion at 0.25 mg/kg/hour IV

- STEMI undergoing PCI:
  - 0.75 mg/kg IV bolus, followed by initial infusion of 1.75 mg/kg/hour IV
  - Renal dosage adjustment:
    - CrCl 10–29 mL/min: Decrease initial infusion rate to 1 mg/kg/hour IV
    - Dialysis: Initial infusion rate of 0.25 mg/kg/hour IV
- HIT: 0.15–0.2 mg/kg/hour IV; adjust to aPTT 1.5–2.5 times baseline value and overlap with warfarin for at least 5 days until INR is within target range

Pharmacokinetic Monitoring
Depends on indication for use of bivalirudin (ACT or aPTT)

Adverse Reactions: Most Common
Bleeding

Adverse Reactions: Rare/Severe/Important
Anaphylaxis, fatal bleeding

Major Drug Interactions
Aspirin, NSAIDs, concomitant anticoagulants: Increase risk of bleeding

Contraindication
Active bleeding

Counseling Points
- There is a risk of bleeding. Monitor for blood in urine, stool, nosebleeds, hemoptysis.
- Irritation may occur around the IV site
- Watch for signs of anaphylaxis, such as chest tightness; swelling of face, lips, tongue, or throat

Key Point
Only given IV

⊙ Dabigatran

Brand Name
Pradaxa

Generic Name
Dabigatran

Rx Only

Dosage Form
Capsule

Usage
Prevention of stroke and systemic embolism in patients with nonvalvular atrial fibrillation*

Pregnancy Category C

Dosing

- Prevention of stroke and systemic embolism in patients with nonvalvular atrial fibrillation:
  - 150 mg orally twice daily
  - Renal dosage adjustment:
    - ◆ CrCl < 30 mL/min: Dabigatran use has not been studied in clinical trials in this patient population
    - ◆ CrCl 15–30 mL/min: 75 mg orally twice daily
    - ◆ CrCl < 15 mL/min or requiring hemodialysis: Use not recommended
- Conversion from a parenteral anticoagulant:
  - Enoxaparin: Initiate dabigatran ≤ 2 hours prior to the time of the next scheduled dose of the parenteral anticoagulant
  - Heparin: Initiate dabigatran at the time of discontinuation if heparin given continuously
- Conversion to a parenteral anticoagulant:
  - CrCl > 30 mL/min: Wait 12 hours after the last dose of dabigatran before initiating a parenteral anticoagulant
  - CrCl < 30 mL/min: Wait 24 hours after the last dose of dabigatran before initiating a parenteral anticoagulant
- Conversion from warfarin: Discontinue warfarin and initiate dabigatran when INR < 2.0
- Conversion to warfarin:
  - CrCl > 50 mL/min: Initiate warfarin 3 days before discontinuation of dabigatran
  - CrCl 31–50 mL/min: Initiate warfarin 2 days before discontinuation of dabigatran
  - CrCl 15–30 mL/min: Initiate warfarin 1 day before discontinuation of dabigatran
  - CrCl < 15 mL/min: Use not recommended

Pharmacokinetic Monitoring

Not routinely used, but aPTT values > 2.5 may indicate overanticoagulation

Adverse Reactions: Most Common

Bleeding, dyspepsia

Adverse Reactions: Rare/Severe/Important

Serious bleeding rates and acute coronary events have been reported

Major Drug Interactions

- Aspirin, NSAIDs, concomitant anticoagulants: Increase risk of bleeding
- Carbamazepine, phenytoin, rifampin, St. John's wort: Decrease efficacy and should be avoided
- Amiodarone, clarithromycin, quinidine, verapamil: Increase risk of bleeding; should be avoided in patients with CrCl 15–30 mL/min
- Dronedarone, itraconazole: Increase risk of bleeding; dose of dabigatran should be reduced in patients with CrCl 30–50 mL/min

Contraindication

Active bleeding

Counseling Points

- Capsules must be swallowed whole. Do not break, chew, or open capsules.
- Keep medication in original bottle; discard 4 months after opening original container
- May be taken without regards to meals
- Drug–drug interactions: Inform your doctor when initiating or discontinuing any medication
- Risk of bleeding: Monitor for blood in urine, stool, nosebleeds, hemoptysis

Key Points

- No antidote currently exists. May use fresh frozen plasma or packed red blood cells for severe hemorrhage. Use of activated charcoal may be considered if ingestion occurred < 2 hours prior to presentation.
- Multiple drug–drug interactions for dabigatran exist

THROMBOLYTICS

Introduction

Thrombolytics such as alteplase are the only agents available that can dissolve formed pathologic clots. These agents are employed in life-threatening situations such as myocardial infarction (MI), cerebrovascular accident (CVA), and critical limb ischemia where the benefit outweighs the risk of life-threatening bleeding.

Mechanism of Action for the Drug Class

Alteplase is a tissue plasminogen activator produced by recombinant DNA technology. Alteplase has high affinity to fibrin-bound plasminogen that stimulates the conversion of plasminogen to plasmin, which dissolves fibrin clots.

Members of the Drug Class

In this section: Alteplase
Others: Defibrotide, reteplase, tenecteplase

⊙ Alteplase

Brand Name
Activase

Generic Names
Alteplase, recombinant or tissue plasminogen activator (TPA)

Rx Only

Dosage Form
IV injection

Usage
Acute MI,* acute ischemic stroke, pulmonary embolism,* peripheral arterial thromboembolism, central venous catheter occlusion*

Pregnancy Category C

Dosing
- Acute MI:
  - Accelerated infusion:
    - If weight > 67 kg: 15 mg IV bolus, 50 mg infused IV over 30 minutes, then 35 mg infused IV over 60 minutes
    - If weight ≤ 67 kg: 15 mg IV bolus, 0.75 mg/kg infused IV 30 minutes (not to exceed 50 mg), then 0.50 mg/kg infused IV over 60 minutes (not to exceed 35 mg)
  - 3-hour infusion: 100 mg given as 60 mg infused IV in the first hour, 20 mg infused IV over the second hour, and 20 mg infused IV over the third hour. For smaller patients (< 65 kg), use a dose of 1.25 mg/kg infused IV over 3 hours as described.
- Acute ischemic stroke: 0.9 mg/kg (not to exceed 90 mg) infused IV over 60 minutes with 10% of the total dose administered as an initial IV bolus over 1 minute
- Pulmonary embolism: 100 mg infused IV over 2 hours
- Catheter occlusion: 2 mg/2 mL instilled into occluded catheter; up to 2 doses may be used

Adverse Reactions: Most Common
Bleeding

Adverse Reactions: Rare/Severe/Important
Intracranial hemorrhage, life-threatening bleeding

Major Drug Interactions
Drugs Affecting Alteplase/TPA

Anticoagulants, antiplatelets: Increase bleeding risk

Contraindications
Active internal bleeding, history of CVA, recent intracranial or intraspinal surgery or trauma, intracranial neoplasm, arteriovenous malformation or aneurysm, known bleeding diathesis, severe uncontrolled hypertension, suspected aortic dissection

Counseling Point
This medication has a life-threatening bleeding risk, especially intracranial bleeding

Key Points
- Most beneficial if given within 12 hours of onset of MI symptoms or within 3 hours of onset of stroke symptoms. May be given within 3–4.5 hours of onset of stroke symptoms in select patients.
- There is an extensive list of contraindications and precautions that must be considered. These indicate situations where the risk of life-threatening bleeding may outweigh the benefit of therapy.

REVIEW QUESTIONS

1. Which of the following is the antidote for Coumadin?

   a. Vitamin K
   b. Protamine
   c. Folic acid
   d. Potassium

2. Which of the following describes warfarin's mechanism of action?

   a. It inhibits the cyclo-oxygenase enzyme.
   b. It inhibits the carboxylation (activation) of the vitamin K–dependent clotting factors II, VII, IX, and X.
   c. It binds to antithrombin to inactivate thrombin, factor Xa, and other clotting factors.
   d. It regulates the production of neutrophils within the bone marrow.

3. Which of the following describes Xarelto's mechanism of action?

   a. It inhibits platelet activation and fibrin clot formation by selectively and reversibly inhibiting factor Xa.
   b. It inhibits platelet aggregation by directly inhibiting thrombin.
   c. It inhibits the cyclo-oxygenase enzyme.
   d. It regulates the production of neutrophils within the bone marrow.

4. Which of the following is an indication for Xarelto therapy?

   a. Myocardial infarction
   b. Mechanical valve
   c. Nonvalvular atrial fibrillation
   d. Heart failure

5. Which of the following counseling points regarding Xarelto is *false*?

   a. There is a risk of bleeding.
   b. The 20 mg dose should be taken on an empty stomach.
   c. The 10 mg dose may be taken with or without food.
   d. Inform your doctor if you start taking any new medications.

6. Which of the following is the antidote for rivaroxaban?

   a. Vitamin K
   b. Activated charcoal
   c. Prothrombin Complex Concentrate
   d. Protamine

7. Which of the following is *not* an indication for aspirin therapy?

   a. Myocardial infarction
   b. Transient ischemic attack
   c. Post-PCI
   d. Hypertension

8. Aspirin use should be avoided in children < 16 years due to risk of which of the following?

   a. Myocardial infarction
   b. Dyspepsia
   c. Reye's syndrome
   d. Brugada syndrome

9. Patients taking Aggrenox should be counseled that it will take approximately 1 week for which of the following side effects to subside?

   a. Bleeding
   b. Headache
   c. Dyspepsia
   d. Nausea

10. Plavix is available in which dosage form in the United States?

    a. Tablet
    b. IV injection
    c. Tablet and IV injection
    d. Suppository

11. Which of the following is an indication for clopidogrel therapy?

    a. Stroke
    b. Post-PCI
    c. Peripheral vascular disease
    d. All of the above

12. Which of the following classes of medications may reduce the effectiveness of Plavix?

    a. NSAIDs
    b. H_2 blockers
    c. Proton pump inhibitors
    d. Antiplatelets

13. Which of the following are contraindications to prasugrel therapy?

    a. History of a transient ischemic attack
    b. Patients ≥ 75 years with diabetes
    c. Patients ≥ 75 years with history of myocardial infarction
    d. Weight < 60 kg

14. What is the difference between Neupogen and Neulasta?

    a. They have a similar mechanism of action, but Neulasta has a shorter duration of action.
    b. They have a similar mechanism of action, but Neulasta has a longer duration of action.
    c. Neulasta increases production of neutrophils, whereas Neupogen increases production of eosinophils.
    d. They have the exact same mechanism of action.

15. Which of the following is one of the uses for epoetin alfa?

    a. Treatment of neutropenia in HIV patients
    b. Treatment of anemia in chronic renal failure
    c. Treatment of hypertension
    d. Prevention and treatment of deep venous thrombosis and pulmonary embolism

16. Which of the following routes of administration are appropriate for unfractionated heparin?

    a. IV, SUB-Q
    b. IV, IM
    c. PO, IM
    d. IV, PO

17. Which of the following is *not* an adverse effect of unfractionated heparin?

    a. HIT
    b. Osteoporosis
    c. Bleeding
    d. Hypernatremia

18. Which of the following is an appropriate dosing regimen for Lovenox?

    a. 1 mg/kg SUB-Q every 12 hours
    b. 5,000 units SUB-Q every 8 hours
    c. 5 mg PO daily
    d. 81 mg PO daily

19. How long before surgery or invasive procedures must Lovenox be withheld?

    a. 1 week
    b. 5 days
    c. 24 hours
    d. 4 hours

20. How long before surgery must prasugrel be withheld?

    a. 5 days
    b. 7 days
    c. 14 days
    d. 24 hours

21. What medication class includes Pradaxa?

    a. Thrombin inhibitor
    b. Anticoagulant
    c. Thrombolytic
    d. Heparin, Low Molecular Weight

22. Which of the following is an approved use for dabigatran?

    a. Unstable angina
    b. Post-PCI
    c. Deep venous thrombosis
    d. Nonvalvular atrial fibrillation

23. Dabigatran is available in which dosage form in the United States?

    a. IV
    b. SUB-Q
    c. PO
    d. IM

24. How many months after the original container has been opened should Pradaxa be discarded?

    a. 2 months
    b. 4 months
    c. 6 months
    d. 8 months

25. Which drug should not be used in combination with Pradaxa in patients with a CrCl of 15–30 mL/min due to an increased risk of bleeding?

    a. Itraconazole
    b. Carbamazepine
    c. Phenytoin
    d. Amiodarone

26. Which of the following routes of administration is appropriate for dalteparin?

    a. PO
    b. SUB-Q
    c. IM
    d. IV

27. What medication class includes Activase?

    a. Antiplatelet
    b. Anticoagulant
    c. Thrombolytic
    d. Antihypertensive

28. What medication class includes clopidogrel?

    a. Antiplatelet
    b. Anticoagulant
    c. Thrombolytic
    d. Antihypertensive

29. What test is used for monitoring of warfarin therapy?

    a. INR
    b. PTT
    c. Anti-Xa
    d. ACT

30. Which of the following is *not* an adverse effect of Aranesp?

    a. Hypertension
    b. Headache
    c. Seizures
    d. Thrombocytopenia

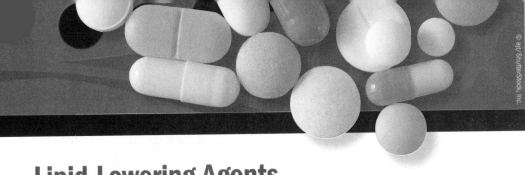

Lipid-Lowering Agents

Nima M. Patel, PharmD, BCPS

HMG-COA REDUCTASE INHIBITORS, STATINS

Introduction

Statins are considered first-line treatment for patients with dyslipidemia, in most patients with atherosclerotic vascular disease, and in patients at risk of developing atherosclerosis. In numerous clinical trials across many patient populations statins have shown significant reduction in morbidity and mortality. Significant toxicities include myalgias that rarely lead to rhabdomyolysis. In February 2012, the Food & Drug Administration approved important safety label changes for statins. The changes included the removal of the guideline regarding routine monitoring of liver enzymes and the addition of information about the potential for generally nonserious and reversible cognitive side effects and reports of increased blood glucose and glycosylated hemoglobin (HbA1c) levels. Statins are contraindicated in patients with active liver disease. Because they are pregnancy category X drugs, they should not be used by women who are pregnant or breast-feeding.

Mechanism of Action for the Drug Class

HMG-CoA reductase inhibitors competitively inhibit hydroxymethylglutaryl-coenzyme A (HMG-CoA) reductase to mevalonate, which is the rate-limiting step in cholesterol biosynthesis. In addition, low-density lipoprotein (LDL) cholesterol receptors are upregulated, enhancing the catabolic rate of LDL and reducing the plasma pool of LDL. The combination of these pharmacologic effects makes statins highly effective LDL-lowering agents. To a lesser extent, they may also increase high-density lipoprotein (HDL) cholesterol and decrease triglycerides (TGs).

Members of the Drug Class

In this section: Atorvastatin, fluvastatin, lovastatin, pravastatin, rosuvastatin, simvastatin
Other: Pitavastatin

Generic and Brand Names for the Drug Class

Atorvastatin (Lipitor), fluvastatin (Lescol), lovastatin (Mevacor) lovastatin ER (Altoprev), pravastatin (Pravachol), simvastatin (Zocor), rosuvastatin (Crestor)

Rx Only for the Drug Class

Dosage Forms for the Drug Class

Tablet

Usage for the Drug Class

- Adjunct to diet and exercise, commonly referred to as therapeutic lifestyle changes (TLCs), for the treatment of various dyslipidemia disorders in patients with no evidence of cardiovascular disease (primary prevention) and in patients with documented coronary artery disease (secondary prevention)*
- Various dyslipidemias are described using the Fredrickson-Levy-Lees classification of hyperlipoproteinemia.* Using this classification system, statins are primarily indicated for treatment of mixed dyslipidemia known as Fredrickson types IIa and IIb.
- Adjunct for treatment of hypertriglyceridemia (Fredrickson type IV hyperlipidemia) and primary dysbetalipoproteinemia (Fredrickson type III hyperlipidemia)

Pregnancy Category X for the Drug Class

---

* Throughout the text, an asterisk (*) is used to indicate the most common uses of a drug.

Dosing for the Drug Class

- Statins should be used in combination with TLCs. **Table 10-1** provides guidelines for statin dosing equivalencies. Patients can be started with the following doses of statins, although doses should be individualized according to the percentage decrease in LDL cholesterol needed, the recommended goal of therapy, and the patient's response:
  - Rosuvastatin: 10 mg daily
  - Atorvastatin: 10 mg daily
  - Pravastatin: 40 mg daily
  - Simvastatin: 10 or 20 mg daily. Note that the use of 80 mg of simvastatin should be restricted to patients who have been receiving long-term therapy (e.g., ≥ 12 months) at this dosage without evidence of muscle toxicity.
  - Fluvastatin: 20 mg daily
  - Lovastatin: 20 mg daily
- Dosage adjustment:
  - Titration should occur 4–6 weeks after initiation to a maximum of 80 mg/day for all statins except rosuvastatin and simvastatin (maximum: 40 mg/day)
  - Several studies have started patients on maximum doses of statins without titration. This is especially noted for atorvastatin (80 mg daily) in the setting of acute coronary syndrome.
- Renal dosage adjustment:
  - Atorvastatin: No adjustment is necessary
  - Fluvastatin: Use with caution in cases of severe renal impairment (doses > 40 mg daily have not been studied)
  - Pravastatin: Initial dose is 10 mg daily in patients with significant impairment
  - Lovastatin: If CrCl < 30 mL/min, then use with caution and carefully consider doses > 20 mg/day
  - Simvastatin: If CrCl < 30 mL/min, then initial dose is 5 mg daily with close monitoring
  - Rosuvastatin: In patients with CrCl < 30 mL/min who are not undergoing hemodialysis, initiate dosage of 5 mg once daily, not to exceed 10 mg once daily
- Hepatic dosage adjustment: All statins are contraindicated in active liver disease

Pharmacokinetic/Pharmacodynamic Properties

- The ability of a statin to lower LDL is very important in the treatment of dyslipidemia. Rosuvastatin and atorvastatin have the greatest ability to lower LDL (by approximately 60%), followed by simvastatin, lovastatin, pravastatin, and fluvastatin.
- The pharmacokinetic property of a particular statin plays an important role in the choice of statin for an individual patient. Increased bioavailability, decreased protein binding, long half-life, lipophilicity, and metabolism are all important characteristics that may influence the risk of developing statin-induced myopathies. Of all the properties just listed, metabolism is considered to be the most important due to the potential for drug interactions.
- Atorvastatin, lovastatin, and simvastatin are metabolized by the CYP3A4 system
- Fluvastatin is metabolized by the CYP2C9 system
- Rosuvastatin is metabolized by the CYP2C9 system to a limited extent
- Pravastatin is not metabolized by the CYP system; instead it is metabolized by hydroxylation, oxidation, and conjugation

Adverse Reactions for the Drug Class: Most Common

GI upset, myalgias (dose-related)

Adverse Reactions for the Drug Class: Rare/Severe/Important

- Myopathy (dose-related), rhabdomyolysis (dose-related)
- Hepatotoxicity (dose-related): Irreversible liver damage resulting from statins is exceptionally rare and is likely idiosyncratic in nature. No data exist that show that routine periodic monitoring of liver biochemistries is effective in identifying the very rare individual who may develop significant liver injury from ongoing statin therapy. If serious liver injury with clinical symptoms and/or hyperbilirubinemia or jaundice occur during treatment, therapy should be interrupted. If an alternate etiology is not found, the statin should not be restarted.

TABLE 10-1 General Guidelines for Statin Dose Equivalency

Atorvastatin	Fluvastatin	Lovastatin	Pravastatin	Rosuvastatin	Vytorin	Simvastatin	% Decrease LDL-C
–	40 mg	20 mg	20 mg	–	–	10 mg	30%
10 mg	80 mg	40 or 80 mg	40 mg	–	–	20 mg	38%
20 mg	–	80 mg	80 mg	5 mg	10/10 mg	40 mg	41%
40 mg	–	–	–	10 mg	10/20 mg	80 mg	47%
80 mg	–	–	–	20 mg	10/40 mg	–	55%
–	–	–	–	40 mg	10/80 mg	–	63%

Source: Data from U.S. Food and Drug Administration. Relative LDL-lowering efficacy of statin and statin-based therapies. Available at: www.fda.gov/Drugs/DrugSafety/ucm256581.htm. Accessed June 29, 2012.

- Cognitive impairment (e.g., memory loss, forgetfulness, amnesia, memory impairment, confusion) associated with statin use has been rarely reported in the postmarketing period. These cognitive issues have been reported for all statins. The reports are generally nonserious and reversible upon statin discontinuation, with variable times to symptom onset (1 day to years) and symptom resolution (median of 3 weeks).
- A small increase in glycosylated hemoglobin (HbA1c) and fasting serum glucose levels (dose-related) have been reported with statin use; however, the benefits of statin therapy far outweigh the risk of dysglycemia

Major Drug Interactions for the Drug Class

- Enhanced toxicity with drugs that inhibit isoenzyme CYP3A4 and statins that are substrates of CYP3A4 (lovastatin, simvastatin, and atorvastatin). Dose limitations exist for certain inhibitors (e.g., simvastatin doses should be limited to 20 mg/day with amiodarone). With strong CYP3A4 inhibitors, including itraconazole, ketoconazole, posaconazole, erythromycin, clarithromycin, telithromycin, nefazodone, gemfibrozil, cyclosporine, human immunodeficiency virus (HIV) protease inhibitors, and the hepatitis C virus (HCV) protease inhibitors boceprevir and telaprevir, the use of lovastatin and simvastatin is contraindicated and/or should be avoided. Atorvastatin up to 20 mg/day can be used with clarithromycin, itraconazole, HIV protease inhibitors (saquinavir plus ritonavir, darunavir plus ritonavir, fosamprenavir, fosamprenavir plus ritonavir) because the extent of interaction between atorvastatin and CYP3A4 inhibitors is less than that with lovastatin and simvastatin.
- Rosuvastatin exposure can be increased via unknown mechanisms with protease inhibitors in combination with ritonavir; therefore, the dose of rosuvastatin in these combinations should be limited to 10 mg/day.
- Statins are substrates for P-glycoprotein; therefore, drugs that inhibit P-glycoprotein (e.g., cyclosporine) may increase statin levels (e.g., in patients receiving cyclosporine limit rosuvastatin dose to 5 mg/day).
- Fibric acid derivatives increase the risk for myopathy/rhabdomyolysis due to additive effects of both drugs. Gemfibrozil can reduce the elimination of a statin by inhibiting glucuronidation, an elimination pathway of all statins except fluvastatin. Therefore, the use of fenofibrate when combination therapy with a statin is required may be a better choice. Dose limitation or avoidance of use is recommended when gemfibrozil is used in combination with a statin (e.g., limit rosuvastatin to 10 mg/day with gemfibrozil).

Essential Monitoring Parameters for the Drug Class

Before starting therapy, check the patient's fasting lipid profile and check baseline liver function tests (LFTs) and repeat as clinically indicated. Baseline creatine phosphokinase (CPK) in high-risk patients may be checked. If the patient has symptoms of myalgia, check CPK.

Counseling Points for the Drug Class

- Report unexplained muscle pain, tenderness, or weakness, particularly if accompanied by malaise or fever
- It is best to take statins with a short half-life, such as lovastatin, simvastatin, pravastatin, and fluvastatin, in the evening because of a greater lipid-lowering effect. Hepatic cholesterol production increases overnight.
- Take lovastatin with an evening meal because fat facilitates absorption
- Atorvastatin and rosuvastatin may be taken anytime during the day without regard to meals because of their longer half-lives and more potent LDL cholesterol–lowering ability
- Avoid drinking grapefruit juice with statins metabolized by the CYP3A4 system

Key Points for the Drug Class

- Statins are first-line drugs of choice for prevention of cardiovascular disease
- When combination therapy of a statin and fibrate is necessary, fenofibrate may be a better choice due to an increased risk of myopathy with gemfibrozil and a statin
- Be vigilant about dose limitation and avoidance of statins with concomitant use of inhibitors of the CYP3A4 system

FIBRIC ACID DERIVATIVES

Introduction

Fibric acid derivatives are mainly used for the treatment of hypertriglyceridemia. Fenofibrate and gemfibrozil belong to this class. Fenofibrate is the preferred agent when used in combination with statins due to the potential for fewer drug interactions. These drugs are contraindicated in patients with severe renal or hepatic disease, including primary biliary cirrhosis, unexplained persistent elevated liver function abnormality, and preexisting gallbladder disease.

Mechanism of Action for the Drug Class

The mechanism of action of fibric acid derivatives is complex and not well understood. These drugs stimulate peroxisome proliferator-activated receptors (PPARα). Activation of PPARα leads to an increase in lipoprotein lipase activity and a reduction in the production of apoprotein CIII (an inhibitor of lipoprotein lipase), causing a decrease in total triglycerides and triglyceride-rich lipoprotein (VLDL). In addition, these drugs upregulate the synthesis of apolipoprotein A-I, the building block of HDL, and therefore cause an increase in HDL.

Members of the Drug Class

In this section: Gemfibrozil, fenofibrate
Others: None

◉ Gemfibrozil

Brand Name

Lopid

Generic Name

Gemfibrozil

Rx Only

Dosage Forms

Tablet

Usage

Treatment of hypertriglyceridemia in Fredrickson types IV and V hyperlipidemia for patients who are at greater risk for pancreatitis and who have not responded to dietary intervention; *to reduce the risk of coronary heart disease (CHD) development in Fredrickson type IIb patients without a history or symptoms of existing CHD who have not responded to dietary and other interventions (including pharmacologic treatment) and who have decreased HDL, increased LDL, and increased triglycerides

Pregnancy Category C

Dosing

- 600 mg twice daily 30 minutes before the morning and evening meals
- Renal dosage adjustment: Use caution in cases of mild to moderate renal impairment. Deterioration of renal function has been reported in patients with baseline serum creatinine > 2 mg/dL.

Adverse Reactions: Most Common

Dyspepsia, GI-related side effects such as nausea, vomiting, diarrhea, constipation

Adverse Reactions: Rare/Severe/Important

Myalgias and more serious muscle-related adverse drug reactions such as myopathy and rhabdomyolysis (risk is increased when gemfibrozil is combined with a statin), hepatotoxicity, cholelithiasis, gallstones

Major Drug Interactions

Gemfibrozil's Effect on Other Drugs

- Warfarin: Increases INR; an empiric reduction in warfarin dosage may be considered to minimize bleeding risk
- HMG-CoA reductase inhibitors: Increases the risk of myopathy and rhabdomyolysis. The risk is greater with gemfibrozil than fenofibrate; thus, fenofibrate is preferred for combination treatment with a statin.
- Repaglinide: Increases hypoglycemic effects. Use with caution in combination.

Essential Monitoring Parameters

- LFT elevations have been observed; however, these are reversible when gemfibrozil is discontinued. Therefore, periodic LFTs are recommended, and gemfibrozil therapy should be terminated if abnormalities persist.
- Worsening renal insufficiency upon the addition of gemfibrozil therapy has been reported in individuals with baseline plasma creatinine > 2 mg/dL. In such patients, the use of alternative therapy should be weighed against the risks and benefits of a lower dose of gemfibrozil.

Counseling Points

- Take 30 minutes before meals
- Avoid alcohol
- Report unexplained muscle pain, tenderness, or weakness, particularly if accompanied by malaise or fever
- Use in conjunction with diet and exercise for optimal therapeutic effect

Key Points

- When combination therapy with a statin and a fibrate is required, fenofibrate may be preferred. The gemfibrozil–statin combination has an increased risk of myalgias, although rarely leading to myopathy and rhabdomyolysis.
- Gemfibrozil can individually increase the INR, and a patient's warfarin dose may be empirically reduced to avoid elevated bleeding risk

◉ Fenofibrate

Brand Names

Antara, Fenoglide, Lipofen, Lofibra, TriCor, Triglide

Generic Name

Fenofibrate

Rx Only

Dosage Forms

Capsule, tablet

Usage

Adjunct to dietary therapy for the treatment of adults with elevations of serum triglyceride levels (types IV and V hyperlipidemia); adjunct to dietary therapy for the reduction of LDL, total cholesterol, TGs, and apolipoprotein B and to increase HDL in adult patients with primary hypercholesterolemia or mixed dyslipidemia (Fredrickson types IIa and IIb)*

Pregnancy Category C

Dosing

- Many different formulations are available, thus doses can range from 50–200 mg daily
- Renal dosage adjustment: Use in severe renal impairment (including patients on dialysis) is contraindicated (see product labeling)

Adverse Reactions: Most Common

Dyspepsia, GI-related side effects such as nausea, vomiting, diarrhea, constipation

Adverse Reactions: Rare/Severe/Important

Myalgias and more serious muscle-related adverse drug reactions such as myopathy and rhabdomyolysis (risk is increased when fenofibrate is combined with a statin), hepatotoxicity, cholelithiasis, gallstones

Major Drug Interactions

Fenofibrate's Effect on Other Drugs

- Bile acid sequestrants: Potential pharmacokinetic interaction due to decreased absorption of fenofibrate. Fenofibrate should be administered 1 hour before or 4–6 hours after a bile acid sequestrant.
- Cyclosporine: Increases risk of cyclosporine-induced nephrotoxicity (i.e., deterioration in renal function). Use with caution.
- Warfarin: Increases INR; an empiric reduction in warfarin dosage may be considered to minimize bleeding risk
- HMG-CoA reductase inhibitors: Increases risk of adverse musculoskeletal effects (i.e., increased creatine kinase, myoglobinuria, rhabdomyolysis). Avoid concomitant use unless potential benefit outweighs risk.

Essential Monitoring Parameters

- Monitor LFTs regularly and discontinue therapy if LFTs remain greater than three times normal limits
- Monitor renal function in patients with renal impairment or in those at increased risk for developing renal impairment. Elevation in serum creatinine returns to baseline following discontinuation of fenofibrate. The clinical significance of these observations is unknown.

Counseling Points

- Report unexplained muscle pain, tenderness, or weakness, particularly if accompanied by malaise or fever
- Use in conjunction with diet and exercise for therapeutic effects

Key Points

- Fenofibrate should be avoided in patients with severe kidney disease
- Fenofibrate can increase a patient's INR; the warfarin dose may be empirically reduced to avoid elevated bleeding risk

NIACIN

Introduction

Niacin is a water-soluble B vitamin that is important for DNA repair and energy metabolism. When used in high doses of 1–2 g per day, niacin is an antilipemic agent. Because it is considered a vitamin, niacin is available as an OTC dietary supplement as well as by prescription. Niacin is available in three main dosage forms: immediate-release, slow/timed-release, and extended-release capsules or tablets. The differences in formulations relate to flushing and hepatotoxicity risk. Niacin is the best-known agent to raise HDL. Niacin should not be used in patients with active liver disease or unexplained transaminase elevations.

Mechanism of Action for the Drug Class

The exact mechanism of action is not fully understood. The process may involve inhibiting mobilization of free fatty acids from peripheral adipose tissue to the liver, resulting in decreased hepatic production of VLDL, ultimately decreasing LDL production. Niacin reduces the amount of apolipoprotein A-I extracted and catabolized from HDL during hepatic uptake, resulting in increased HDL.

Members of the Drug Class

In this section: Niacin
Others: None

⦿ Niacin

Brand Names
Slo-Niacin, Niacor (IR), Niaspan ER (Rx), Niacin-Time

Generic Name
Niacin

Rx and OTC

Dosage Forms

Tablet, capsule

Usage

Adjunctive treatment of dyslipidemias (types IIa and IIb or primary hypercholesterolemia) to lower the risk of recurrent myocardial infarction (MI) and/or slow progression of coronary artery disease;* combination therapy with other antidyslipidemic agents when additional TG-lowering or HDL-increasing effects are desired;* treatment of hypertriglyceridemia in patients at risk of pancreatitis; treatment of pellagra (niacin deficiency)

Pregnancy Category C

Dosing

- Hyperlipidemia:
  - Immediate-release: 1.5–6 g daily in 3 divided doses with or after meals using an upward dosage titration schedule
  - Extended-release: Initial dose is 500 mg once daily at bedtime. Increase dosage by no more than 500 mg at 4-week intervals until desired effect is observed or maximum daily dosage of 2 g is reached.
- Pellagra:
  - 50–100 mg three to four times daily
  - Maximum: 500 mg daily

Adverse Reactions: Most Common

Flushing (prostaglandin-mediated) is most common with immediate-release products and least common with long-acting products; hyperglycemia, hyperuricemia, upper GI distress

Adverse Reactions: Rare/Severe/Important

Rise in serum transaminase values are seen with all niacin formulations, but the worst cases have been reported with slow-release niacin, and there is often a dose-related side effect when doses > 2,000 mg/day are administered. Slow-release products should not be recommended due to increased hepatotoxicity risk. Immediate-release products have the least hepatotoxicity; however, they must be dosed three times daily and can cause significant flushing. Most experts prefer Niaspan (extended-release niacin) because it causes less flushing than immediate-release niacin, is dosed once daily, and is associated with less liver toxicity than sustained-release, controlled-release, or timed-release niacin (e.g., Slo-Niacin).

Major Drug Interactions

Drugs Affecting Niacin

Bile acid sequestrants: May decrease levels (give niacin 1 hour before or 4–6 hours after giving bile acid sequestrant)

Essential Monitoring Parameters

Glucose levels should be closely monitored in diabetic or potentially diabetic patients, particularly during the first few months of use or dose adjustment. Liver function tests should be taken at baseline, every 6 to 12 weeks for the first year, and then periodically thereafter.

Counseling Point

Adherence may be compromised due to the adverse effects of flushing. Proper counseling reduces the incidence of flushing. The flushing occurs because of the release of prostaglandin D_2 from the skin. Taking aspirin or ibuprofen 30 minutes before therapy helps diminish this side effect. Patients should be advised to take niacin on a full stomach and that flushing may be worsened by hot, spicy food; hot beverages; hot baths; and hot showers.

Key Points

- Niacin is the best-known agent to raise HDL. The side effect of flushing may diminish adherence. Patients should be properly counseled on avoiding this side effect.
- The different formulations of niacin relate to the risk of hepatotoxicity and flushing. Products that claim to be "flush-free" or "no flush" are available OTC; however, these products fail to release free niacin, making them ineffective antilipemic agents.

CHOLESTEROL ABSORPTION INHIBITORS

Introduction

Ezetimibe is the only agent available in this class. It is specifically used in combination with a statin to lower LDL. An additional lowering of approximately 25% in LDL can be seen when ezetimibe is combined with a statin, which makes it an attractive add-on agent to reach a lower LDL goal of < 70 mg/dL. Ezetimibe has been proven to be effective in combination with statins in patients unable to achieve or sustain target LDL levels on a statin alone or to reduce the dose of a statin required to achieve target levels.

Evidence is emerging with regard to lowering of cardiovascular events with ezetimibe treatment. (See the Vytorin section.)

Mechanism of Action for the Drug Class

Ezetimibe inhibits absorption of cholesterol at the brush border of the small intestine via the sterol transporter Niemann-Pick C1-Like1, leading to decreased delivery of cholesterol to the liver, reduction of hepatic cholesterol stores, and increased clearance of cholesterol from the blood

Members of the Drug Class

In this section: Ezetimibe
Others: None

◉ Ezetimibe

Brand Name
Zetia

Generic Name
Ezetimibe

Rx Only

Dosage Form
Tablet

Usage
Used as monotherapy or in combination with HMG-CoA reductase inhibitors for primary heterozygous familial and nonfamilial hypercholesterolemia (in combination with dietary therapy),* mixed hyperlipidemia (in combination with fenofibrate), homozygous familial hypercholesterolemia (in combination with atorvastatin or simvastatin), homozygous sitosterolemia

Pregnancy Category C

Dosing
- 10 mg daily without regard to meals
- Renal dosage adjustment: None required for renal insufficiency
- Hepatic dosage adjustment:
  - Mild hepatic insufficiency: No adjustment necessary
  - Moderate to severe hepatic impairment: Use not recommended

Adverse Reactions: Most Common
When compared to placebo, ezetimibe is well tolerated. The most common side effects are abdominal pain, diarrhea, arthralgia, cough, fatigue, and headache.

Adverse Reactions: Rare/Severe/Important
Hypersensitivity reactions (including angioedema and rash), increased LFTs, drug-induced myopathy (very rarely with monotherapy), rhabdomyolysis (very rarely with monotherapy; the risk is increased in combination with a statin)

Major Drug Interactions
Drugs Affecting Ezetimibe
- Bile acid sequestrants: May decrease bioavailability; administer ezetimibe 2 hours before or 4 hours after bile acid sequestrants
- Cyclosporine: May increase serum levels. No monitoring is recommended for ezetimibe.
- Fibrates: May increase cholesterol excretion into the bile, leading to cholelithiasis

Ezetimibe's Effect on Other Drugs
Cyclosporine: May increase serum levels. Cyclosporine levels should be monitored.

Counseling Points
- Take at the same time every day, without regard for meals
- Report allergic reactions: Itching/hives, swelling in the face/hands, trouble breathing (angioedema)
- Report any muscle pain, tenderness, or weakness
- Report nausea, vomiting, loss of appetite, pain in the upper stomach (cholelithiasis)
- Use in conjunction with diet and exercise

Key Points
- In combination with a statin, LDL is lowered by approximately an additional 25%
- Ezetimibe should not be prescribed as a first-line agent

OMEGA-3 FATTY ACIDS

Introduction
Omega-3 fatty acids are polyunsaturated fatty acids derived from marine and plant sources. Omega-3 fatty acids can decrease triglycerides by 50%, although in patients with very high triglycerides (> 500 mg/dL) there is an increase in LDL. Omega-3 fatty acids are available as dietary supplements; however, the amounts of eicosapentaenoic acid (EPA) and docosahexaenoic acid (DHA) are lower compared with the only prescription product, Lovaza. Lovaza is the purest form of omega-3 fatty acids and contains 85% of EPA and DHA in a 1,000 mg capsule.

Mechanism of Action for the Drug Class
The mechanism of action has not been completely defined. Possible mechanisms include inhibition of acyl CoA:1,2-diacyl-glycerol acyltransferase, increased hepatic beta-oxidation, a reduction in the hepatic synthesis of triglycerides, or an increase in plasma lipoprotein lipase activity.

Members of the Drug Class
In this section: Omega-3 fatty acids
Others: None

Omega-3 Fatty Acids

Brand Name

Lovaza

Generic Name

Omega-3 fatty acids

Rx (Lovaza) and OTC

Dosage Form

Capsule

Usage

Adjunct to diet therapy in the treatment of hypertriglyceridemia (≥ 500 mg/dL),* prophylaxis to prevent a myocardial infarction (unlabeled use), treatment of immunoglobulin (Ig)A nephropathy (unlabeled use)

Pregnancy Category C

Dosing

- Hypertriglyceridemia/treatment of IgA nephropathy: 4 g daily as a single dose or in two divided doses
- Prophylaxis to prevent a myocardial infarction: 1 g daily

Adverse Reactions: Most Common

Generally well tolerated. The most common side effect is a "fishy" smelling burp called eructation, fishy aftertaste, and GI upset/nausea. Refrigeration of the capsules may help minimize these side effects.

Adverse Reactions: Rare/Severe/Important

Increase in bleeding time, although this does not appear to exceed the normal range of bleeding time

Major Drug Interactions

Omega-3 Fatty Acids' Effects on Other Drugs

Antiplatelet agents and warfarin: May increase levels/effects. More frequent monitoring may be necessary in patients taking warfarin.

Essential Monitoring Parameters

In patients with hepatic impairment, monitor ALT and AST levels periodically during therapy. Omega-3 fatty acids may increase levels of LDL. Monitor LDL levels periodically during therapy.

Counseling Point

OTC products differ in their EPA/DHA content. It is important to note the total amount of omega-3 fatty acids contained in each capsule rather than the amount of fish oil concentrate. Some products may require consumption of up to 11 capsules to obtain the same amount of omega-3 fatty acid content that is obtained from 4 capsules of Lovaza.

Key Point

Omega-3 fatty acids are increasingly being used for prevention of myocardial infarction at doses of 1 g daily. Higher doses of 2–4 g daily are used to lower TGs. Lovaza is the purest form of omega-3 fatty acids.

BILE ACID SEQUESTRANTS

Introduction

The three bile acid sequestrants (BASs) on the market are cholestyramine, colestipol, and colesevelam. The primary effect of these agents at optimal doses is to reduce LDL by 15–30%. In clinical practice, cholestyramine and colestipol are underused due to GI side effects and classic drug-binding interactions of concomitantly administered drugs. Colesevelam is much better tolerated and has fewer drug-binding interactions and thus is generally the preferred agent in this class. These agents are contraindicated in patients with complete biliary obstruction and bowel obstruction. BASs may increase triglycerides; therefore, these agents should generally be avoided in patients with TGs > 400 mg/dL.

Mechanism of Action for the Drug Class

Cholesterol is the precursor of bile acids, which are needed for emulsifying fat and lipid particles in food. Bile acids are secreted into the intestine through the bile, and most bile acids are reabsorbed into the intestines and returned to the liver by enterohepatic circulation. BASs bind to bile acids in the gut, which interrupts recycling through enterohepatic recirculation. Hepatic cells convert more cholesterol into bile acid, and there is an increased synthesis of LDL receptors, leading to increased hepatic uptake of systemic LDL particles and lowered LDL.

Members of the Drug Class

In this section: Cholestyramine
Others: Colesevelam, colestipol

Cholestyramine

Brand Names

Prevalite, Questran, Questran Light

Generic Name

Cholestyramine

Rx Only

Dosage Form

Powder for oral suspension

Usage

Adjunct to diet in the management of primary hypercholesterolemia,* pruritus associated with elevated levels of bile acids, diarrhea associated with excess fecal bile acids, binding of toxicologic agents, adjunctive therapy for pseudomembranous colitis

Pregnancy Category C

Dosing

- Initial dose: 4 g once or twice daily
- Dosage adjustment: Increase gradually over ≥ 1-month intervals until maintenance dose of 8–16 g a day divided into 2 doses is reached
- Maximum dose: 24 g daily
- Renal dosage adjustment: Because BASs are not systemically absorbed, renal dosage adjustment is not necessary
- Hepatic dosage adjustment: Because BASs are not systemically absorbed, hepatic dosage adjustment is not necessary

Adverse Reactions: Most Common

Constipation (increases with dose and age of the patient); other GI-related adverse reactions include abdominal pain, flatulence, nausea, vomiting, dyspepsia, and steatorrhea

Adverse Reactions: Rare/Severe/Important

Theoretically, patients taking BASs may be at an increased risk of bleeding from hypoprothrombinemia (secondary to vitamin K deficiency)

Major Drug Interactions

Cholestyramine's Effect on Other Drugs

Delays or reduces the absorption of many drugs when administered concomitantly. To avoid this drug interaction, in general give other medications 1 hour before or 4–6 hours after giving BASs. (Note that Colesevelam does have a decreased frequency for causing these interactions.) The absorption of the following drugs may be delayed or reduced by cholestyramine (this list is not all-inclusive): Amiodarone, corticosteroids, digoxin, ezetimibe, fat-soluble vitamins (vitamins A, D, E, and K), gemfibrozil, HMG-CoA inhibitors, methyldopa, methotrexate, niacin, NSAIDs, propranolol (and potentially other beta blockers), sulfonylureas, thyroid hormones, thiazide and loop diuretics, thiazolidinedione, valproic acid, warfarin.

Counseling Points

- Cholestyramine oral suspension packets should be mixed with 4–6 oz of beverage. May also be mixed with highly fluid soups, cereals, applesauce, or pulpy fruits. To decrease the occurrence of flatulence, mix cholestyramine with noncarbonated pulpy juices and swallow it without engulfing air by using a straw.
- Separate the administration of other drugs by 1 hour before or 4–6 hours after cholestyramine

Key Points

- Patients should be counseled on drug-binding interactions and to separate dosing of other drugs from cholestyramine. GI-related adverse effects and the palatability of the drug may limit the use of the drug long term.
- Cholestyramine Light formulations contain 14 g of phenylalanine per 5 g dose of cholestyramine

COMBINATION PRODUCT, VYTORIN

Introduction

The combination product Vytorin contains simvastatin and ezetimibe. Until recently, there was lack of meaningful clinical outcome data regarding the use of Vytorin. With the publication of the Study of Heart and Renal Protection (SHARP) trial, Vytorin has been shown to be effective in reducing the risk of vascular events in patients with moderate to severe chronic kidney disease (CKD) and no history of myocardial infarction (MI) or coronary revascularization.

Mechanism of Action for the Drug Class

See the Ezetimibe and Statin sections

Members of the Drug Class

In this section: Ezetimibe/simvastatin (Vytorin)
Others: None

◉ Ezetimibe/Simvastatin

Brand Name
Vytorin

Generic Name
Ezetimibe/simvastatin

Rx Only

Dosage Form

Tablet

Usage

Used in combination with dietary modification for the treatment of primary hypercholesterolemia and homozygous familial hypercholesterolemia

Pregnancy Category X

Dosing

- Homozygous familial hypercholesterolemia: 10/40 mg ezetimibe/simvastatin once daily in the evening
- Hyperlipidemias:
  - Initial dose:
    - 10/10–20 mg ezetimibe/simvastatin once daily in the evening
    - Patients who require less aggressive reduction in LDL-C: 10/10 mg ezetimibe/simvastatin once daily in the evening
    - Patients who require > 55% reduction in LDL-C: 10/40 mg ezetimibe/simvastatin once daily in the evening
  - Dosing range: 10/10–40 mg ezetimibe/simvastatin once daily
- Dosage adjustment: In Chinese patients on niacin doses ≥ 1 g daily, use caution with simvastatin doses exceeding 20 mg PO daily because of an increased risk of myopathy. Do not administer simvastatin 80 mg.

Adverse Reactions: Most Common

See the Ezetimibe and Statin sections

Adverse Reactions: Rare/Severe/Important

See the Ezetimibe and Statin sections

Major Drug Interactions

- Strong CYP3A4 inhibitors (e.g., itraconazole, ketoconazole, posaconazole, erythromycin, clarithromycin, telithromycin, HIV protease inhibitors, boceprevir, telaprevir, nefazodone), gemfibrozil, cyclosporine, danazol: Concomitant use is contraindicated
- Verapamil, diltiazem: Do not exceed 10/10 mg ezetimibe/simvastatin daily

- Amiodarone, amlodipine, ranolazine: Do not exceed 10/20 mg ezetimibe/simvastatin daily
- Grapefruit juice: Avoid large quantities of grapefruit juice (> 1 quart daily)
- Other lipid-lowering medications: Use with other fibrate products or lipid-modifying doses (≥ 1 g/day) of niacin increases the risk of adverse skeletal muscle effects. Caution should be used when prescribing with ezetimibe/simvastatin.

Essential Monitoring Parameters

Liver function tests are required at baseline and as clinically indicated. Consider creatine kinase at baseline and with dosage increases; closely monitor in those with moderate to severe renal impairment receiving doses higher than 10/20 mg ezetimibe/simvastatin.

Counseling Points

- Report unexplained muscle pain, tenderness, or weakness, particularly if accompanied by malaise or fever
- Report promptly any symptoms that may indicate liver injury, including fatigue, anorexia, right upper abdominal discomfort, dark urine, or jaundice
- Women of childbearing age should be advised to use an effective method of birth control to prevent pregnancy while using ezetimibe/simvastatin

Key Points

- Ezetimibe monotherapy has produced relatively moderate reductions in LDL cholesterol in patients with primary hypercholesterolemia (less than that of statins). However, studies have shown that the addition of ezetimibe to statin therapy produces greater reductions in LDL cholesterol than monotherapy with either agent alone.
- The combination of ezetimibe and simvastatin presents sufficient dose options to achieve desired treatment goals while providing greater convenience to the patient, therefore potentially increasing compliance
- Available in four combinations of ezetimibe/simvastatin: 10/10 mg, 10/20 mg, 10/40 mg, and 10/80 mg

REVIEW QUESTIONS

1. Fibric acid derivatives are most commonly used for which of the following purposes?
   a. To decrease LDL
   b. To decrease total cholesterol
   c. To decrease triglycerides
   d. To increase HDL

2. Which of the following is *not* a common adverse effect of gemfibrozil and fenofibrate?
   a. Diarrhea
   b. Constipation
   c. Dyspepsia
   d. Pancreatitis

3. Gemfibrozil is the preferred agent when used in combination with statins due to the potential for fewer drug interactions.
   a. True
   b. False

4. Which of the following statements is true with regard to cholestyramine?
   a. It can be used for pruritus associated with elevated levels of bile acids.
   b. It can be used for treatment of constipation.
   c. It does not bind to toxicologic agents.
   d. It is not indicated for pseudomembranous colitis.

5. What is the effect of fenofibrate on warfarin?
   a. It increases INR.
   b. It decreases INR.
   c. It increases bleeding risk without affecting INR.
   d. It decreases its anticoagulation effect without affecting INR.

6. Which of the following statements should be included when counseling a patient receiving gemfibrozil?
   a. Take 30 minutes before meals.
   b. Avoid alcohol.
   c. Report unexplained muscle pain, tenderness, or weakness.
   d. All of the above

7. Which of the following is the correct dose of Lovaza for patients with hypertriglyceridemia?
   a. 1 g daily
   b. 2 g daily
   c. 4 g daily
   d. 8 g daily

8. In patients with high triglycerides (> 500 mg/dL), omega-3 fatty acids can:
   a. decrease LDL cholesterol.
   b. increase LDL cholesterol.
   c. increase HDL cholesterol.
   d. decrease HDL cholesterol.

9. Which of the following is a common adverse reaction of omega-3 fatty acids?
   a. Fishy aftertaste
   b. Myopathy
   c. Hyperglycemia
   d. Flushing

10. Vytorin contains:
    a. ezetimibe and lovastatin.
    b. ezetimibe and atorvastatin.
    c. ezetimibe and simvastatin.
    d. ezetimibe and pravastatin.

11. Which of the following is the mechanism of action of ezetimibe?
    a. It increases the breakdown of cholesterol.
    b. It inhibits hepatic production of cholesterol.
    c. It increases the production of HDL cholesterol.
    d. It inhibits the absorption of cholesterol at the small intestine.

12. Myositis is an adverse effect of all of the following agents, *except*:
    a. simvastatin.
    b. pravastatin.
    c. gemfibrozil.
    d. colestipol.

13. Niacin can be toxic to the:
    a. liver.
    b. kidneys.
    c. pancreas.
    d. thyroid.

14. A patient comes into the pharmacy and complains of flushing with use of immediate-release niacin. What should you recommend?
    a. Switch to "flush-free" niacin.
    b. Switch to Slo-Niacin, which causes less flushing.
    c. Ask the doctor for a prescription for Niaspan, which causes less flushing.
    d. Take niacin in the morning with a hot coffee to decrease flushing.

15. Which of the following medications is *not* a bile acid sequestrant?
    a. Questran
    b. Cholecalciferol
    c. Cholestyramine
    d. Colesevelam

16. Through what mechanism does niacin cause flushing?
    a. It causes the release of prostaglandins.
    b. It changes the hypothalamic regulatory point.
    c. It activates the pancreas.
    d. It irritates the dermis of the skin.

17. Which of the following is the best-known agent to increase HDL?

   a. Statins
   b. Niacin
   c. Fish oil
   d. Fibrates

18. What is an important counseling point for patients taking cholestyramine?

   a. Take it at the same time as your other medications for increased efficacy.
   b. Take at bedtime for increased efficacy.
   c. Avoid drinking large quantities of grapefruit juice with the medication.
   d. Take other medications 1 hour before or 4–6 hours after taking cholestyramine.

19. Colesevelam is much better tolerated in terms of GI side effects and has fewer drug-binding interactions as compared to cholestyramine.

   a. True
   b. False

20. What is the clinical benefit of using Vytorin over Zocor alone?

   a. Faster absorption
   b. Beneficial effects on high triglycerides
   c. Less GI upset
   d. Increased reduction in LDL

21. Which of the following statements is true regarding the clinical use of fish oils?

   a. At high doses it is an adjunctive therapy for hypertriglyceridemia.
   b. At low doses it is a prophylaxis to prevent myocardial infarction.
   c. It is a treatment for immunoglobulin (Ig)A nephropathy.
   d. All of the above

22. In 2012, the FDA approved which of the following changes in the safety labeling of statins?

   a. Removal of routine liver function test monitoring
   b. Addition of reversible cognitive impairment
   c. Addition of increased blood glucose and glycosylated hemoglobin (HbA1c) levels
   d. All of the above

23. Which of the following is *not* true of atorvastatin?

   a. Renal dosage adjustment is required in patients with impaired kidney function.
   b. It is contraindicated in active liver disease.
   c. It is contraindicated in pregnancy (category X drug).
   d. It has drug–drug interactions with CYP3A4 enzyme inhibitors.

24. The dosage of rosuvastatin should be limited to _____ daily for patients who are concomitantly receiving treatment with ritonavir.

   a. 10 mg
   b. 20 mg
   c. 30 mg
   d. 40 mg

25. Which of the following is *not* an important patient counseling point for lovastatin?

   a. Take in the evening for greater lipid-lowering effect.
   b. Take with an evening meal to increase oral absorption.
   c. Take with grapefruit juice.
   d. Report any experience of unexplained muscle pain, tenderness, or weakness.

26. Which of the following statins is *not* metabolized by CYP enzyme system?

   a. Pravastatin
   b. Atorvastatin
   c. Simvastatin
   d. Lovastatin

27. Patients taking statins should be counseled on which of the following potential side effects?

   a. Myalgia/rhabdomyolysis
   b. Hepatotoxicity
   c. Reversible cognitive impairment
   d. All of the above

28. Which of the following antibiotics is contraindicated with simvastatin?

   a. Erythromycin
   b. Doxycycline
   c. Amoxicillin
   d. Vancomycin

29. Which of the following is *not* a common side effect of niacin?

   a. Prostaglandin-mediated flushing
   b. Hyperglycemia
   c. Hyperuricemia
   d. Hepatotoxicity

30. Which of the following is true regarding simvastatin?

   a. A patient who started simvastatin 80 mg at bedtime 2 months ago may remain on the drug as long as the patient is asymptomatic with regard to muscle pains.
   b. A patient who started simvastatin 80 mg at bedtime 2 years ago may remain on the drug as long as the patient is asymptomatic with regard to muscle pains.
   c. The dose of simvastatin should be reduced to 10 mg at bedtime for patients starting therapy with posaconazole.
   d. Simvastatin should be switched to lovastatin 40 mg at bedtime for patients who are starting therapy with erythromycin.

Miscellaneous Agents

Neela Bhajandas, PharmD
Talitha Pulvino, PharmD, BCPS

5-ALPHA REDUCTASE INHIBITORS

Introduction

The 5-alpha reductase inhibitors are agents that interfere with testosterone's stimulatory effect on the size of the prostate gland. They are used to reduce prostate size and alleviate urinary obstruction and the symptoms associated with benign prostatic hyperplasia (BPH), including urinary hesitancy, urgency, and nocturia. These actions may slow disease progression and decrease the risk of disease complications. The 5-alpha reductase inhibitors also slow the progression of male-pattern hair loss.

Mechanism of Action for the Drug Class

These drugs competitively inhibit 5-alpha reductase in the prostate, liver, and skin, blocking the conversion of testosterone to dihydrotestosterone (DHT). DHT is an androgen that stimulates prostate growth and contributes to male-pattern baldness.

Members of the Drug Class

In this section: Finasteride
Other: Dutasteride

◉ Finasteride

Brand Names
Propecia, Proscar

Generic Name
Finasteride

Rx Only

Dosage Form
Tablet

Usage
Treatment of moderate to severe BPH,* treatment of male-pattern baldness*

Pregnancy Category X

Dosing
- BPH: 5 mg daily
- Male pattern baldness: 1 mg daily

Adverse Reactions: Most Common
Rash, breast tenderness and swelling, reduced libido, ejaculation disturbances, erectile dysfunction

Adverse Reactions: Rare/Severe/Important
Hypersensitivity, testicular pain, neoplasm of male breast, may increase risk of high-grade prostate cancer

Major Drug Interactions
No known significant drug interactions

Contraindications
Known or suspected pregnancy, use in women of child-bearing potential, children

Essential Monitoring Parameter
Finasteride predictably decreases the PSA level; establish a new baseline PSA 6 months postinitiation, then monitor periodically

Counseling Points
- Women of childbearing age should not touch or handle broken tablets due to risk of cutaneous absorption
- Results of therapy may take several months
- This medication can be taken with or without meals

Key Points
- This drug is pregnancy category X because it can cause abnormalities of the external genitalia of the male fetus. Females of childbearing age should not handle broken tablets.
- Typically dispensed in sealed container or unit-dose package to minimize handling
- A minimum of 6 months may be needed to determine effectiveness

---

* Throughout the text, an asterisk (*) is used to indicate the most common uses of a drug.

ACNE PRODUCTS, RETINOIC ACID DERIVATIVES

Introduction

Topical retinoic acid derivatives are commonly used in the treatment of mild to moderate acne; however, the oral retinoic acid derivative isotretinoin is reserved for severe cases of acne that have been unresponsive to conventional therapies, including anti-infectives. Unlike other therapies, the beneficial effect of isotretinoin is prolonged beyond discontinuation of therapy. Isotretinoin requires special monitoring due to its side-effect profile.

Mechanism of Action for the Drug Class

Reduces sebaceous gland size and secretions. Regulates cell proliferation and differentiation.

Members of the Drug Class

In this section: Isotretinoin
Others: Topical tretinoin

◉ Isotretinoin

Brand Names

Accutane, Amnesteem, Claravis, Sotret, Absorica, Myorisan

Generic Name

Isotretinoin

Rx Only

Dosage Form

Capsule

Usage

Treatment of severe recalcitrant nodular acne that is unresponsive to conventional therapy*

Pregnancy Category X

Dosing

Adults and children ≥ 12 years of age: 0.5–1 mg/kg/day in two divided doses given with meals for 15–20 weeks or until the total nodule count decreases by 70%, whichever occurs first; severe scaring may require 2 mg/kg/day

Adverse Reactions: Most Common

Cheilitis, conjunctivitis, hair thinning, elevated triglycerides, dry skin, photosensitivity, pruritus, xerostomia, arthralgia, backache, dry nasal mucosa, epistaxis

Adverse Reactions: Rare/Severe/Important

Pancreatitis, neutropenia, hepatotoxicity, anaphylaxis, visual disturbances, hearing loss, aggressive behavior, depression, violent behavior, skeletal hyperostosis, osteoporosis, pseudotumor cerebri

Major Drug Interactions

Drugs Affecting Isotretinoin

- Vitamin A derivatives: Additive toxicity (i.e., dry skin and mucous membranes)
- Ethanol: Increases risk of elevated triglycerides

Isotretinoin's Effect on Other Drugs

- Tetracyclines: May increase the risk of pseudotumor cerebri
- Contraceptives: May decrease effectiveness of progestin-only oral contraceptives

Essential Monitoring Parameters

Lipid panel with serum triglycerides, liver function tests, CBC, pregnancy tests

Contraindications

Patients who are pregnant or who may become pregnant

Counseling Points

- Avoid pregnancy during treatment with isotretinoin
- Counsel men about the risks associated with impregnating a woman on isotretinoin
- Take with meals; failing to take isotretinoin with food can significantly reduce drug absorption (except Absorica)
- Exacerbations of acne can occur during first week of treatment
- Immediately report any of the following to your healthcare provider: Visual difficulties, abdominal pain, rectal bleeding, feelings of depression, and/or suicidal ideation
- Avoid prolonged sun exposure, use sunscreen, and wear protective clothing
- Manage cheilitis (dry mouth, cracked skin around lips, nose, and eyes) with lip balms, sugarless candy, saline nasal spray, and artificial tears
- The capsule should be swallowed whole with a full glass of water

Key Points

- Last line therapy for severe nodular acne
- This drug is pregnancy category X; it can cause craniofacial, cardiovascular, thymus, parathyroid gland, and CNS structure malformations in a developing fetus
- All patients (male and female), prescribers, wholesalers, and dispensing pharmacists must register and be active in the iPLEDGE risk management program designed to eliminate fetal exposure to isotretinoin
  - Female patients:
    - No woman should be pregnant or become pregnant when prescribed isotretinoin
    - No woman should become pregnant for at least 1 month following isotretinoin treatment

- Female patients must have two negative pregnancy tests before a prescription for isotretinoin is written. Additionally, they are required to have a pregnancy test each month during treatment.
- Women must have selected and committed to use two forms of contraception for 1 month prior, during, and for 1 month after isotretinoin treatment
- Women should not donate blood while taking isotretinoin

- Male patients:
  - Male patients should be aware of the possibility of birth defects in an unborn child exposed to isotretinoin
  - Male patients should not donate blood while taking isotretinoin
- No more than a 30-day supply of isotretinoin should be dispensed
- Prescriptions for isotretinoin can only be filled within 7 days of the date of the "qualification"
- No refills are permitted

ANTIMALARIALS, AMINOQUINOLINES

Introduction

Hydroxychloroquine is an antimalarial that is also used to treat rheumatoid arthritis (RA) and autoimmune conditions that are not related to malaria. It is important to be familiar with the side-effect profile of this medication to know how to minimize the adverse effects.

Mechanism of Action for the Drug Class

Hydroxychloroquine interferes with digestive vacuole function within sensitive malarial parasites. With regard to RA, it inhibits locomotion of neutrophils and chemotaxis of eosinophils and impairs complement-dependent antigen–antibody reactions.

Members of the Drug Class

In this section: Hydroxychloroquine
Others: Chloroquine, primaquine

⊙ Hydroxychloroquine

Brand Name
Plaquenil

Generic Name
Hydroxychloroquine

Rx Only

Dosage Form
Tablet

Usage
Treatment of systemic lupus erythematosus (SLE),* treatment of RA,* suppression and treatment of malaria, Q fever, porphyria cutanea tarda, polymorphous light eruption

Pregnancy Category D

Dosing
- Malaria:
  - Chemoprophylaxis: 400 mg once weekly beginning 2 weeks before exposure and continuing for 4 weeks after leaving endemic area. If suppressive therapy is not begun before the exposure, double the initial dose and give in 2 doses 6 hours apart and continue treatment for 8 weeks.
  - Acute attack: Initial dose of 800 mg followed by 400 mg at 6, 24, and 48 hours
- Rheumatoid arthritis:
  - Initial dose: 400–600 mg daily; increase dose gradually until optimum response level is reached
  - Maintenance dose: After 4–12 weeks, the dose should be reduced by half to a maintenance dose of 200–400 mg/day
- SLE:
  - Initial dose: 400 mg once or twice daily until remission
  - Maintenance dose: 200–400 mg once daily
- Renal dosage adjustment: Use with caution in patients with renal impairment
- Hepatic dosage adjustment: Use with caution in patients with hepatic impairment

Adverse Reactions: Most Common

Skin pigmentation changes (blue/back), nausea, vomiting, diarrhea, myopathy, headache, corneal changes

Adverse Reactions: Rare/Severe/Important

Stevens-Johnson syndrome, agranulocytosis, aplastic anemia, thrombocytopenia, retinopathy, loss of visual acuity, night blindness, blurred vision, neuromyopathy, cardiomyopathy

Major Drug Interactions

Drug Affecting Hydroxychloroquine

Dapsone: Additive risk of hemolytic reactions such as blood dyscrasias

- Digoxin: Increases serum concentrations
- Mefloquine: Increases risk of seizures and QT interval prolongation
- Metoprolol: Increases plasma levels

Contraindication

Retinal or visual field changes attributable to 4-aminoquinoline derivatives or to any other etiology

Counseling Points

- Obtain ophthalmic examinations every 3 months if using this medication over extended periods
- This medication may increase sensitivity to sunlight. Therefore, wear dark glasses and protective clothing, use sunblock, and avoid direct exposure to sunlight.
- GI side effects are short lived and typically managed by taking the medication with food

Key Points

- Monitoring is needed to avoid severe side effects (e.g., CBC, liver function tests)
- This is not the preferred first-line agent in the prevention and treatment of malaria
- Use with caution in patients with G6PD deficiency because it can be associated with hemolysis
- Use with caution in patients with psoriasis because psoriasis can be exacerbated by hydroxychloroquine

ANALGESICS, OPIOID PARTIAL AGONISTS

Introduction

Buprenorphine/naloxone is used to treat opioid addiction. Buprenorphine in combination with naloxone reduces the parenteral misuse of buprenorphine/naloxone by producing withdrawal symptoms if injected.

Mechanism of Action for the Drug Class

Buprenorphine is a mixed agonist–antagonist medication. It is a mu-opioid receptor partial agonist and a kappa-opioid receptor antagonist. It binds to the CNS opiate receptors, where it produces an analgesic effect. Naloxone is a mu-opioid receptor antagonist, which also competes for the mu and kappa receptors in the CNS.

Members of the Drug Class

In this section: Buprenorphine/naloxone
Others: Buprenorphine, butorphanol, nalbuphine, pentazocine, pentazocine/acetaminophen, pentazocine/naloxone

◉ Buprenorphine/Naloxone

Brand Name

Suboxone

Generic Name

Buprenorphine/naloxone

Rx Only

Class III controlled substance

Dosage Forms

Sublingual film, sublingual tablet

Usage

Maintenance treatment for opioid dependence*

Pregnancy Category C

Dosing

- Target dose: 16 mg daily
- Dosage adjustment: Adjust by adding 2–4 mg tablets
- Usual dosage range: 4–24 mg/day
- Hepatic dosage adjustment: Use caution in cases of moderate to severe hepatic impairment

Adverse Reactions: Most Common

Drowsiness, dizziness, headache, CNS depression

Adverse Reactions: Rare/Severe/Important

Hepatitis, orthostatic hypotension

Major Drug Interactions

Drugs Affecting Buprenorphine/Naloxone

Sedatives and alcohol: Increase CNS depression

Buprenorphine/Naloxone's Effect on Other Drugs

- Opioid analgesics: Decreases the therapeutic effect of opioids; can precipitate withdrawal in opioid-dependent patients
- Selective serotonin reuptake inhibitors (SSRIs): Increases serotonergic effect; may cause serotonin syndrome

Counseling Points

- Avoid activities that require mental alertness (e.g., driving, operating machinery) until the effects of the medication are known and comfortable. Follow this advice whenever the dose is increased.
- Place the sublingual film under the tongue until it dissolves completely; it should not be swallowed, chewed, or moved after placement. If more than one film is needed, the additional film should be placed under the tongue to the opposite side.
- Place the sublingual tablet under the tongue until it dissolves completely; it should not be swallowed. If two or more tablets are needed per dose, all can

be placed under the tongue together or they can be placed two at a time. Subsequent doses should be taken the same way.

Key Points

- Obtain baseline liver function tests and monitor periodically during treatment
- The same dose should be used when switching between sublingual tablets and sublingual film. Caution should be exercised because the sublingual film has a potential for greater bioavailability; monitor

patients closely when changing formulations for changes in mental (respiratory) status or withdrawal.
- Only physicians with a registered DEA number for buprenorphine/naloxone can prescribe for it
- Buprenorphine sublingual tablets are preferred during the induction phase. Buprenorphine/naloxone can be used during the induction phase for short-acting opioids. When using buprenorphine/naloxone, prior to induction, the last dose of opioids should be taken > 12–24 hours prior to induction therapy.

ANTICHOLINERGICS, ANTI-PARKINSON'S AGENTS

Introduction

Anticholinergic agents are used in the treatment of Parkinson's disease and to relieve the parkinsonian signs of antipsychotic agent–induced extrapyramidal symptoms (EPS). Their use in the treatment of EPS has decreased since the introduction of atypical antipsychotic agents. These agents should be used with caution due to the risk of anticholinergic adverse effects.

Mechanism of Action for the Drug Class

These agents decrease the activity of acetylcholine to balance out the production of dopamine and acetylcholine. They may inhibit the reuptake and storage of dopamine, thereby prolonging the action of dopamine.

Members of the Drug Class

In this section: Benztropine
Others: Trihexyphenidyl, procyclidine

⊙ Benztropine

Brand Name
Cogentin

Generic Name
Benztropine

Rx Only

Dosage Forms
Tablet, injection

Usage
Adjunctive treatment of Parkinson's disease,* treatment of drug-induced EPS (except tardive dyskinesia)*

Pregnancy Category B

Dosing

- Parkinsonism:
  - Oral/IM/IV: 1–2 mg/day (range: 0.5–6 mg/day)
  - Initiate at lower dosage and increase gradually until relief or a maximum dose of 6 mg/day
  - Given as a single daily dose or up to four times daily
- Drug-induced EPS: Oral/IM/IV dose is 1–4 mg once or twice daily
- May be given IV, but typically administered IM in patients who cannot take orally

Adverse Reactions: Most Common

Tachyarrhythmia, constipation, nausea, xerostomia, blurred vision, urinary retention

Adverse Reactions: Rare/Severe/Important

Heat stroke, anhidrosis, hyperthermia, paralytic ileus, confusion, increased intraocular pressure, mood or mental changes, visual hallucinations

Major Drug Interactions

Drugs Affecting Benztropine

- Agents with anticholinergic activity: Additive anticholinergic side effects
- Ethanol: Increases CNS depression

Benztropine's Effect on Other Drugs
Potassium chloride: Increases risk of GI lesions

Contraindications

Pyloric or duodenal obstruction, stenosing peptic ulcers, bladder neck obstructions, achalasia, myasthenia gravis, closed-angle glaucoma, children < 3 years of age

Counseling Points

- This drug may impair heat regulation; use caution when engaging in activities that lead to increased body temperature
- May cause drowsiness, dizziness, and blurry vision
- Avoid alcohol use

ANTICHOLINERGICS, ANTIHISTAMINE ANTIEMETICS

Introduction

The medications in this drug class are antihistamines used to treat and prevent nausea and vomiting due to motion sickness. Meclizine is readily available over the counter for patient self-treatment.

Mechanism of Action for the Drug Class

Centrally acting agents with anticholinergic, antihistaminic, and antiemetic activity; decrease the excitability of the labyrinth of the middle ear and block conduction of the middle ear vestibular pathways

Members of the Drug Class

In this section: Meclizine
Others: Cyclizine, dimenhydrinate, promethazine, hydroxyzine, cetirizine, levocetirizine

⊙ Meclizine

Brand Names

Antivert, Bonine (OTC), Dramamine Less Drowsy Formula (OTC), Trav-L-Tabs (OTC)

Generic Name

Meclizine

Rx and OTC

Dosage Forms

Tablet, chewable tablet

Usage

Prevention and treatment of motion sickness* and vertigo*

Pregnancy Category B

Dosing

- Motion sickness: For adults and children ≥ 12 years of age, 12.5–25 mg 1 hour before travel; repeat if necessary at 24-hour intervals. Doses of up to 50 mg may be needed.
- Vertigo: 25–100 mg daily in divided doses, depending on clinical response

Adverse Reactions: Most Common

Drowsiness, somnolence, dry mouth, constipation

Adverse Reactions: Rare/Severe/Important

Cholestatic jaundice, blurred vision, auditory and visual hallucinations

Major Drug Interactions

Drugs Affecting Meclizine

- CNS depressant agents: Additive sedation
- Anticholinergic agents: Additive anticholinergic effects

Counseling Points

- Meclizine may impair the ability to perform hazardous activities requiring mental alertness or physical coordination, including driving and operating heavy machinery
- Avoid alcohol and other CNS depressants while using meclizine

Key Points

- Meclizine should only be used for mild to moderate motion sickness because other medications are more effective for severe conditions
- Meclizine is more effective for prevention rather than treatment of motion sickness
- Drowsiness is a common side effect of meclizine

ANTICHOLINERGICS

Introduction

Scopolamine is a naturally occurring anticholinergic agent used for the prevention of nausea and vomiting from motion sickness or following anesthesia.

Mechanism of Action of the Drug Class

Blocks the action of acetylcholine in smooth muscle, secretory glands, and the CNS. Also antagonizes histamine and serotonin.

Members of the Drug Class

In this section: Scopolamine

◉ Scopolamine

Brand Name

Transderm-Scop

Generic Name

Scopolamine

Rx Only

Dosage Forms

Transdermal patch (scopolamine hydrobromide given IV, IM, and subcutaneously)

Usage

Prevention of nausea and vomiting associated with motion sickness and recovery from anesthesia and surgery,* breakthrough treatment of nausea and vomiting associated with chemotherapy (off label)

Pregnancy Category C

Dosing

- The transdermal system delivers approximately 1 mg of scopolamine over 72 hours
- Motion sickness: Apply 1 patch to hairless area behind the ear at least 4 hours prior to exposure and every 72 hours as needed
- Preoperative: Apply 1 patch to hairless area behind the ear the night before surgery. Remove 24 hours after surgery.

Adverse Reactions: Most Common

Xerostomia, drowsiness, dizziness, transient impairment of eye accommodation

Adverse Reactions: Rare/Severe/Important

Acute toxic psychosis, glaucoma

Major Drug Interactions

Drugs Affecting Scopolamine

- CNS depressant agents: Additive sedation
- Anticholinergic agents: Additive anticholinergic effects

Contraindication

Narrow angle glaucoma

Counseling Points

- Wipe the area behind the ear dry prior to application
- Wash hands thoroughly after handling the patch
- Wear the patch continuously; avoid removing and reapplying the patch during the 72-hour period
- Dispose of the patch responsibly, avoiding potential contact of the patch with pets and children
- Can be worn during bathing/showering
- Use with caution if participating in underwater sports as disorientation is possible
- May cause dry mouth; may use hard candy or ice chips to alleviate
- May contain metal, remove prior to MRI

Key Points

- The scopolamine patch should be applied at least 4 hours prior to exposure and can be worn for 3 days. A new patch can be applied if ongoing protection is needed.
- Scopolamine also is used preoperatively and then removed following surgery
- Anticholinergic side effects should be expected with additive effects if used with other anticholinergics or CNS depressants

ANTIDOTE, ACETYLCYSTEINE

Introduction

Acetylcysteine is an antidote used to treat acute acetaminophen overdose–induced hepatotoxicity and to prevent contrast-induced nephropathy (CIN). It is utilized for its mucolytic properties.

Mechanism of Action for Acetylcysteine

Acetylcysteine is an antidote for acute acetaminophen toxicity. It is considered to be hepatoprotective by maintaining and restoring hepatic concentrations of glutathione. Glutathione is needed to inactivate a hepatotoxic metabolite of acetaminophen. Its mucolytic action is due to its ability to open disulfide bonds in mucoproteins, therefore decreasing the viscosity of the mucus. The presumed mechanism in preventing CIN is its ability to scavenge oxygen-derived free radicals and improve endothelium-dependent vasodilation.

Members of the Drug Class

In this section: Acetylcysteine
Others: Mucomyst, Dornase alfa

⊙ Acetylcysteine

Brand Name

Acetadote

Generic Name

Acetylcysteine, N-Acetylcysteine

Rx Only

Dosage Forms

Injection, solution, oral inhalation

Usage

Acetaminophen overdose,* prevention of nephropathy associated with radiographic contrast media,* adjunctive mucolytic agent in patients with viscous mucous secretions

Pregnancy Category B

Dosing

- Acetaminophen poisoning:
  - 72-hour PO regimen:
    - Total number of doses: 18 (total dose is 1,330 mg/kg)
    - Loading dose: 140 mg/kg
    - Maintenance dose: 70 mg/kg every 4 hours
  - 21-hour IV regimen:
    - Total number of doses: 3 (total dose is 300 mg/kg)
    - Loading dose: 150 mg/kg (maximum dose: 15 g) infused over 1 hour
    - Second dose: 50 mg/kg (maximum dose: 5 g) infused over 4 hours
    - Third dose: 100 mg/kg (maximum dose: 10 g) infused over 16 hours
- Prevention of CIN: 600–1,200 mg PO twice daily for 2 days (regimen should be started the day before the procedure)

Adverse Reactions: Most Common

Anaphylactoid reaction, flushing, erythema, tachycardia, nausea, vomiting

Adverse Reactions: Rare/Severe/Important

Anaphylaxis, angioedema, bronchospasm, chest tightness

Major Drug Interactions

No known significant drug interactions

Counseling Point

May repeat oral acetylcysteine dose if vomiting occurs within 1 hour of ingestion

Key Points

- Itching, flushing, rash, and anaphylactoid reactions can occur with acetylcysteine. Patients should be continuously monitored in an inpatient setting when initiating acetylcysteine for acetaminophen overdose.
- Benadryl IV (1 mg/kg, max dose of 50 mg IV) can be administered for the treatment of non–life-threatening allergic reactions
- For prevention of CIN, depending on the procedure acetylcysteine (IV or PO) or IV hydration (e.g. 0.9% NaCl) can be used

ANTIDOTE, FLUMAZENIL

Introduction

Flumazenil is a benzodiazepine GABA receptor antagonist used most commonly for benzodiazepine overdose. It antagonizes the CNS effects of benzodiazepines.

Mechanism of Action for Flumazenil

Flumazenil is a benzodiazepine antagonist. It competitively inhibits the receptor site on the GABA/benzodiazepine receptor complex, thus reversing the sedative effects of benzodiazepines.

Members of the Drug Class

In this section: Flumazenil
Others: None

⊙ Flumazenil

Brand Name

Romazicon

Generic Name

Flumazenil

Rx Only

Dosage Form

Injection

Usage

Benzodiazepine overdose,* reversal of general anesthesia, reversal of conscious sedation

Pregnancy Category C

Dosing

Benzodiazepine overdose (IV push doses given over 30 seconds):

- Initial dose: 0.2 mg IV
- If desired consciousness is not achieved 30 seconds after initial dose, give 0.3 mg IV push (over 30 seconds). If desired consciousness is still not achieved, give 0.5 mg IV push at 1-minute intervals for a cumulative dose of 3–5 mg IV.
- If patient partially responds to the cumulative dose of 3 mg IV and desired consciousness is still not achieved, can go up to a maximum cumulative dose of 5 mg IV

Adverse Reactions: Most Common

Dizziness, sweating, headache, blurred vision

Adverse Reactions: Rare/Severe/Important

Seizures, extravasation, cardiac arrhythmias (e.g., ventricular tachycardias), death (has occurred in patients who have ingested large amounts of tricyclic antidepressants as part of the overdose)

Major Drug Interactions

Flumazenil's Effect on Other Drugs

Nonbenzodiazepine hypnotics: May decrease sedative effects

Contraindications

Patients receiving benzodiazepines for potentially life-threatening condition (e.g., status epilepticus, control of intracranial pressure); tricyclic antidepressant overdose

Counseling Points

- Do not participate in activities requiring alertness for at least 24 hours after hospital discharge
- Avoid alcohol

Key Points

- Patients should be continuously monitored in an inpatient setting when receiving flumazenil
- Flumazenil can precipitate benzodiazepine withdrawal, including seizures
- Most patients respond to a cumulative dose of 1–3 mg IV of flumazenil
- Flumazenil does not antagonize the CNS effects of GABA agonists, which are not bound at the GABA/benzodiazepine receptor complex (e.g., ethanol, general anesthetics, barbiturates) or reverse the effects of opioids

ANTIDOTE, NALOXONE

Introduction

Naloxone is an opioid reversal agent that is used as an antidote for opioid overdose

Mechanism of Action for the Drug Class

Naloxone is an opioid antagonist, which has the greatest affinity for mu receptors. It acts by competing for the mu, kappa, and opiate receptor sites in the CNS, therefore antagonizing the analgesic, dysphoric, sedative, and other opioid pharmacologic effects.

Members of the Drug Class

In this section: Naloxone hydrochloride
Others: Naltrexone, alvimopan, methylnaltrexone

◉ Naloxone

Brand Name

Narcan

Generic Name

Naloxone

Rx Only

Dosage Forms

Tablet, injection

Usage

Acute opioid overdose,* opioid-induced respiratory depression,* opioid-induced depression, rapid detoxification in the management of opioid withdrawal, opioid-induced pruritus

Pregnancy Category C

Dosing

- Opioid overdose:
  - Naloxone should be used in combination with ACLS protocols
  - Initial dose: 2 mg (IV, IM, SUB-Q); repeat dose every 2–3 minutes if needed
  - Maximum dose: 10 mg (consider other causes of respiratory depression > 10 mg)
- Reversal of therapeutic opioid-induced respiratory depression: 0.04–0.4 mg (IV, IM, SUB-Q), may repeat to a desired response (if dose > 0.8 mg, consider other causes of respiratory depression)

Adverse Reactions: Most Common

Nausea, vomiting

Adverse Reactions: Rare/Severe/Important

Acute opioid withdrawal (pain, hypertension, sweating, agitation, irritability)

Major Drug Interactions

No known significant drug interactions

Contraindication

Hypersensitivity to naloxone

Key Points

- Naloxone may precipitate symptoms of opioid withdrawal (pain, hypertension, sweating, agitation, irritability)
- When used in the management of acute opiate overdose, because of naloxone's short duration of action resuscitative measures should be available (e.g., maintenance of an adequate airway, ACLS)
- The goal of naloxone treatment in the postoperative setting is to reverse the excessive opioid effect without completely reversing the analgesic effect of the opioid, which could lead to increased pain
- Consider using an IV continuous infusion in patients with an exposures to long-acting opioids (e.g., methadone) or sustained-release products

ANTIGOUT AGENT, COLCHICINE

Introduction

Colchicine is an antimitotic drug that is effective at relieving acute gout attacks. It possesses weak anti-inflammatory and antigout properties.

Mechanism of Action for the Drug Class

The specific mechanism of action of colchicine is unknown. However, it is thought that colchicine binds to beta-tubulin, a microtubular protein, causing its depolymerization and preventing activation and migration of neutrophils associated with mediating some gout symptoms. Its anti-inflammatory property with regard to gout appears to be due to its ability to decrease leukocyte motility, phagocytosis, and lactic acid production, therefore decreasing the deposition of urate crystals in the joints.

Members of the Drug Class

In this section: Colchicine
Others: None

◉ Colchicine

Brand Name

Colcrys

Generic Name

Colchicine

Rx Only

Dosage Form

Tablet

Usage

Treatment and prophylaxis of acute gout attacks,* treatment of familial Mediterranean fever, pericarditis post-STEMI, recurrent autoimmune or idiopathic pericarditis, primary biliary cirrhosis

Pregnancy Category C

Dosing

- Gout:
  - Treatment of acute attacks:
    - Initial dose: 1.2 mg at first sign of a flare, followed by 0.6 mg 1 hour later
    - Maximum dose: 1.8 mg within 1 hour
  - Prophylaxis:
    - Initial dose: 0.6 mg orally twice daily
    - Maximum dose: 1.2 mg/day
- Familial Mediterranean fever: 1.2–2.4 mg daily
- Renal dosage adjustment:
  - CrCl < 30 mL/min: Initial dose of 0.3 mg/day (use with caution if titrating dose and monitor for adverse effects)
  - Hemodialysis: Avoid chronic use
  - Treatment of gout flare should not be repeated more often than every 14 days, as it is not removed by hemodialysis
  - Treatment of gout flare is not recommended in patients receiving prophylactic colchicine in patients with renal impairment
- Hepatic dosage adjustment:
  - Dose reduction may be considered
  - Treatment for gout flare should not be repeated more often than every 14 days
  - Treatment of gout flare is not recommended in patients receiving prophylactic colchicine who have hepatic impairment

Adverse Reactions: Most Common
Nausea, vomiting, diarrhea

Adverse Reactions: Rare/Severe/Important
Myelosuppression, neuromyopathy, aplastic anemia, hepatotoxicity

Major Drug Interactions
Drugs Affecting Colchicine

- CYP3A4 and P-glycoprotein inhibitors (i.e., azole antifungals, cyclosporine, macrolides, diltiazem, verapamil, protease inhibitors): Increase concentrations and increase risk of toxicity
- Digoxin: Increases concentration
- P-glycoprotein inducers: Decrease concentration and effectiveness

Colchicine's Effect on Other Drugs

- HMG-CoA reductase inhibitors: Increases risk of myopathy and rhabdomyolysis
- Fibric acid derivatives: Increases risk of myopathy rhabdomyolysis

Contraindications
Concomitant use of P-glycoprotein or strong CYP3A4 inhibitors in the presence of hepatic or renal impairment

Counseling Points
- A low purine diet and adequate hydration is recommended to decrease the frequency of gout attacks
- Avoid grapefruit juice; it can increase the concentration of colchicine

Key Points
- Dose needs to be adjusted in patients with hepatic and renal dysfunction. Renal and hepatic function and CBCs should be monitored periodically.
- Doses need to be adjusted if used in combination with CYP3A4 inhibitors and p-glycoprotein inhibitors. Concurrent use with strong CYP3A4 inhibitors and p-glycoproteins are contraindicated in renal and hepatic impairment.
- The most common side effect of colchicine is diarrhea. Lower doses may help to decrease GI side effects.

ANTIHYPERURICEMIC AGENTS, ANTIGOUT AGENTS

Introduction
Allopurinol is a xanthine oxidase inhibitor used to treat primary hyperuricemia of gout and hyperuricemia secondary to high uric acid levels in patients receiving chemotherapy. It also is used to prevent gout attacks.

Mechanism of Action for the Drug Class
Allopurinol decreases the production of uric acid by blocking the action of xanthine oxidase, an enzyme that converts hypoxanthine to xanthine and then xanthine to uric acid

Members of the Drug Class
In this section: Allopurinol
Other: Febuxostat

◉ Allopurinol

Brand Names
Zyloprim, Aloprim

Generic Name
Allopurinol

Rx Only

Dosage Forms
Tablet, injection

Usage
Prevention of gout attacks,* treatment of secondary hyperuricemia associated with chemotherapy (tumor lysis syndrome), prevention of recurrent calcium oxalate calculi

Pregnancy Category C

Dosing
- Gout:
  - Mild gout: 100–300 mg PO daily as a single or divided dose
  - Moderate to severe gout:
    - 400–600 mg PO daily
    - Maximum dose: 800 mg PO daily
- Renal dosage adjustment: Doses are adjusted when CrCl < 20 mL/min and are individualized based on serum uric acid levels

Adverse Reactions: Most Common
Maculopapular rash and pruritus

Adverse Reactions: Rare/Severe/Important
Rash, Stevens-Johnson syndrome, toxic epidermal necrolysis (TEN), agranulocytosis, aplastic anemia, eosinophilia, myelosuppression, thrombocytopenia, hepatitis, renal failure

Major Drug Interactions

Drugs Affecting Allopurinol

- ACE inhibitors and thiazide diuretics: Increase risk of hypersensitivity
- Uricosurics: Decrease effectiveness
- Antacids: Decrease absorption

Allopurinol's Effect on Other Drugs

- Azathioprine: Inhibits metabolism; dose of azathioprine must be reduced by 50–75% to prevent severe myelosuppression
- Mercaptopurine: Inhibits metabolism; increases risk of myelosuppression
- Didanosine: Inhibits metabolism, leading to increased concentrations
- Cyclosporine: Increases levels
- Amoxicillin/ampicillin: Increases risk of rash
- Warfarin: Enhances anticoagulant effect

Contraindication

Concomitant use of didanosine

Counseling Points

- Immediately report any skin rash to your healthcare provider
- Maintain adequate hydration while taking allopurinol
- Avoid alcohol, caffeine, and large amounts of vitamin C during therapy (large amounts of vitamin C may acidify urine, thus increasing chance of kidney stone formation)
- Take allopurinol with food to minimize GI upset
- Report any fever, sore throat, painful urination, blood in urine, and/or swelling of mouth or lips to your healthcare provider
- Periodic blood tests (e.g., CBC, LFTs, uric acid level, renal function) may be ordered to monitor for effectiveness and side effects

Key Points

- Rash is a common adverse reaction that can occur any time during therapy
- Reduce dosage in renal failure

ELECTROLYTE SUPPLEMENTS

Introduction

Potassium is a major intracellular electrolyte that is essential for the conduction of nerve impulses and contraction of skeletal, cardiac, and smooth muscle. The body requires appropriate amounts of potassium to function properly. Potassium chloride is the most common potassium formulation used when replenishing potassium.

Mechanism of Action for the Drug Class

Potassium is the major intracellular cation and is essential for the conduction of nerve impulses in the heart, brain, and skeletal muscle. Potassium maintains intracellular tonicity; contractility of cardiac, skeletal, and smooth muscle; acid–base balance; gastric secretion; and carbohydrate metabolism.

Members of the Drug Class

In this section: Potassium chloride

◉ Potassium Chloride

Brand Names

Klor-Con, Micro-K, K-Tab, Epiklor

Generic Name

Potassium chloride

Dosage Forms

Tablet, capsule, powder, liquid, injection

Rx Only

Usage

Treatment and prevention of hypokalemia*

Pregnancy Category C

Dosing

- Prevention of hypokalemia due to diuretic therapy: 20–40 mEq PO daily in 1–2 divided doses
- Treatment of hypokalemia:
  - Oral:
    - Limit to 20–40 mEq/dose to minimize adverse GI effects
    - Asymptomatic, mild: 40–100 mEq/day in divided doses
    - Mild to moderate: 120–240 mEq/day in divided in doses
  - Intermittent IV infusion:
    - Continuous ECG monitoring recommended in > 10 mEq/hour. Frequent lab monitoring should occur after repletion to avoid hyperkalemia, and dosing recommendations should be patient specific and based on institutional guidelines.
    - Serum potassium > 2.5 mEq/L:
      - Maximum infusion rate: 10 mEq/hour
      - Maximum concentration: 40 mEq/L
      - Maximum 24-hour dose: 200 mEq
    - Serum potassium < 2 mEq/L and symptomatic:
      - Maximum infusion rate: 40 mEq/hour (via central line)
      - Maximum 24-hour dose: 400 mEq

Adverse Reactions: Most Common

Nausea, vomiting, diarrhea, flatulence (more common with oral repletion), hyperkalemia

Adverse Reactions: Rare/Severe/Important

Cardiac arrest, ECG abnormalities, heart block, asystole, ventricular arrhythmias, abdominal pain, GI ulcer, extravasation (IV)

Major Drug Interactions

Drugs Affecting Potassium Chloride

ACE inhibitors, angiotensin II receptor blockers, potassium-sparing diuretics, salt substitutes containing potassium: Increase risk of hyperkalemia

Contraindications

Hyperkalemia; structural, pathologic, and/or pharmacologic GI delay or immobility (solid oral dosage form)

Counseling Points

- Oral potassium repletion: Doses should be taken with meals with a full glass of water to minimize GI irritation
- Sustained-release and wax-matrix products: Do not crush. These products should be swallowed whole.
- Powder formulations: May be diluted in water or juice
- Capsule formulations (e.g., Micro-K): Should be swallowed whole; however, capsules can be opened and sprinkled on applesauce or pudding

Key Points

- The potassium chloride concentrate for injections must be diluted before use. Numerous fatalities have occurred when patients were accidentally given undiluted potassium chloride concentrate. Potassium chloride concentrate should only be stored in a pharmacy and diluted to appropriate volume before dispensing.
- It is generally recommended to limit oral doses of potassium to 20–40 mEq/dose to avoid GI discomfort and adverse effects
- IV doses of potassium in an inpatient setting can be incorporated into the patient's maintenance IV fluids
- Intermittent IV potassium administration should be reserved for patients with severe depletion. ECG monitoring is recommended for peripheral or central infusions > 10 mEq/hour.
- Patients should receive IV potassium chloride via a central line when receiving ≥ 20 mEq/hour
- Dosing recommendations should be patient specific and based on institutional guidelines

ANTICHOLINERGICS AND ANTISPASMODICS, OVERACTIVE BLADDER AGENTS

Introduction

Anticholinergic and antispasmodic agents are used to suppress premature detrusor contractions, enhance bladder storage, and relieve urge urinary incontinence symptoms and complications. These agents are recommended second-line for the treatment of overactive bladder after behavioral therapies. The extended-release products are associated with lower rates of dry mouth than the immediate-release.

Mechanism of Action for the Drug Class

Anticholinergic agents for overactive bladder antagonize muscarinic receptors in the bladder smooth muscle, which reduces bladder contractions and enhances bladder storage.

Members of the Drug Class

In this section: Darifenacin, oxybutynin, tolterodine
Others: Fesoterodine, solifenacin, trospium

◉ Darifenacin

Mechanism of Action

Acts as a selective antagonist of the M3 cholinergic receptor, limiting bladder contractions

Brand Names

Enablex

Generic Name

Darifenacin

Rx Only

Dosage Form

Tablet

Usage

Overactive bladder*

Pregnancy Category C

Dosing

- Extended-release tablet: 7.5 mg once daily; if inadequate response after 2 weeks, may increase to 15 mg once daily
- Hepatic dosage adjustment:
    - Moderate impairment (Child-Pugh class B): Do not exceed 7.5 mg/day
    - Severe impairment (Child-Pugh class C): Use is not recommended
- Dosage adjustment with concomitant potent CYP3A4 inhibitors: Do not exceed 7.5 mg/day

Adverse Reactions: Most Common

Constipation, xerostomia, headache

Adverse Reactions: Rare/Severe/Important

Anaphylactoid reaction, angioedema

Major Drug Interactions

Drugs Affecting Darifenacin

- Anticholinergic agents: Additive anticholinergic side effects
- CYP3A4 inhibitors: May increase levels
- CYP3A4 inducers: May decrease levels
- Thioridazine: Avoid concomitant use

Darifenacin's Effect on Other Drugs

Medications metabolized by CYP2D6 that have a narrow therapeutic index: May increase levels

Contraindications

Urinary retention, gastric retention, uncontrolled narrow-angle glaucoma

Counseling Points

- Swallow tablets whole
- May cause constipation, headache, dizziness, dry mouth, abdominal discomfort, and heat prostration
- Drink water or eat sugarless candy to lessen effects of dry mouth

Key Points

- Anticholinergic side effects are common
- Limit the dose with potent CYP3A4 inhibitors

◉ Oxybutynin

Mechanism of Action

An antispasmodic that inhibits the action of acetylcholine on bladder smooth muscle; direct antispasmodic effect on smooth muscle

Brand Names

Ditropan, Ditropan XL, Oxytrol, Gelnique

Generic Name

Oxybutynin

Rx Only

Dosage Forms

Gel, transdermal patch, syrup, tablet, extended-release tablet

Usage

Overactive bladder,* neurogenic bladder*

Pregnancy Category B

Dosing

- Immediate-release tablet:
    - Initial dose: 5 mg two to three times daily
    - Maximum dose: 5 mg four times a day
- Extended-release tablet:
    - Initial dose: 5–10 mg once daily
    - Dosage adjustment: Adjust dose in 5 mg increments at weekly intervals
    - Maximum dose:
        - Adults: 30 mg daily
        - Children ≥ 6 years: 20 mg
- 10% topical gel: Apply contents of 1 sachet (100 mg/g) to dry, intact skin on the abdomen, upper arms/shoulders, or thighs once daily
- Transdermal patch: Apply one 3.9 mg/day patch twice weekly (every 3–4 days)

Adverse Reactions: Most Common

Dry mouth, xerophthalmia, blurred vision, constipation, delirium, headache, dizziness, sedation

Adverse Reactions: Rare/Severe/Important

Tachycardia, hallucinations, mydriasis

Major Drug Interactions

Drugs Affecting Oxybutynin

Anticholinergics: Additive anticholinergic side effects

Contraindications

Uncontrolled narrow-angle glaucoma, urinary retention, gastric retention or conditions with severely decreased GI motility

Counseling Points

- Common side effects include dry mouth and constipation
- Extended-release tablet: Patient may see tablet-like substance in the stool
- Transdermal patch: Apply to clean, dry skin on abdomen, hip, or buttocks. Select a new site for each new system. Avoid reapplication to the same site within 7 days.
- Topical gel: Apply to clean, dry, intact skin on abdomen, thighs, or upper arms/shoulders. Rotate sites. Do not apply to the same site on consecutive days. Wash hands after use. Cover treated area with clothing after gel has dried to prevent transfer of medication to others. Do not bathe, shower, or swim until 1 hour after gel has been applied.

Key Point

Anticholinergic side effects are common

⊙ Tolterodine

Mechanism of Action
An anticholinergic that competitively antagonizes muscarinic receptors, causing the detrusor muscle to relax, thus reducing the frequency and intensity of bladder contractions

Brand Names
Detrol, Detrol LA

Generic Name
Tolterodine

Dosage Forms
Tablet, capsule, extended-release capsule

Uses
Overactive bladder*

Pregnancy Category C

Dosing
- Extended-release capsule:
  - 4 mg/day, may reduce to 2 mg/day based on tolerability
  - Renal dosage adjustment:
    - CrCl = 10–30 mL/min: 2 mg/day
    - CrCl < 10 mL/min: Use is not recommended
  - Hepatic dosage adjustment:
    - Mild to moderate hepatic impairment (Child-Pugh class A or B): 2 mg/day
    - Severe hepatic impairment (Child-Pugh class C): Use is not recommended
  - Dosage adjustment with concomitant potent CYP3A4 inhibitors: 2 mg/day

- Immediate-release tablet:
  - 2 mg twice daily; may reduce to 1 mg twice daily based on tolerability
  - Renal dosage adjustment: Reduce dose to 1 mg twice daily
  - Hepatic dosage adjustment: Reduce dose to 1 mg twice daily
  - Dosage adjustment with potent CYP3A4 inhibitors: Reduce dose to 1 mg twice daily

Adverse Reactions: Most Common
Constipation, xerostomia, headache

Adverse Reactions: Rare/Severe/Important
Anaphylactoid reaction, dementia, memory impairment, angioedema

Major Drug Interactions
Drugs Affecting Tolterodine
- Anticholinergic agents: Additive anticholinergic side effects
- CYP3A4 and 2D6 inhibitors: Increase anticholinergic side effects
- CYP3A4 and 2D6 inducers: Increase metabolism

Tolterodine's Effect on Other Drugs
Warfarin: May increase effects

Contraindications
Urinary retention, gastric retention, uncontrolled narrow-angle glaucoma

Counseling Points
- Do not crush or chew extended-release capsules
- Drink water or eat sugarless candy to lessen effects of dry mouth
- Exercise caution with driving because this medication may cause sedation

Key Points
- Anticholinergic side effects are common
- Tolterodine is a major substrate of CYP3A4 and 2D6

PHOSPHODIESTERASE INHIBITORS, ERECTILE DYSFUNCTION AGENTS

Introduction
Phosphodiesterase inhibitors are used as first-line treatment of erectile dysfunction. They have a convenient route of administration, low incidence of side effects, and are effective.

Mechanism of Action for the Drug Class
The agents in this class inhibit phosphodiesterase 5 (PDE5), leading to increased levels of cyclic guanosine monophosphate and enhancing smooth muscle relaxation in the corpus cavernosum of the penis and smooth muscle of the pulmonary vasculature. Overall, these agents enhance the nitric oxide–induced relaxation of penile vascular smooth muscle. Some have complex dosing schedule adjustments for renal and hepatic impairment as well as concurrent medications.

Usage for the Drug Class
Erectile dysfunction, pulmonary arterial hypertension, benign prostatic hyperplasia (BPH)

Adverse Reactions for the Drug Class: Most Common

Headache, flushing, dizziness, rhinitis, visual abnormalities (inability to distinguish between blue and green)

Adverse Reactions for the Drug Class: Rare/Severe/Important

Chest pain, myocardial infarction, prolonged QT interval, seizure, optic neuropathy, decreased hearing, sudden hearing loss, priapism

Major Drug Interactions for the Drug Class

Drugs Affecting Phosphodiesterase Inhibitors

- Potent CYP3A4 inhibitors (i.e., protease inhibitors, erythromycin, azole antifungals): Increase levels
- Nitrates: Potentiate vasodilation, potentially causing fatal hypotension
- Antihypertensives: Potentiate antihypertensive effect

Contraindication for the Drug Class

Concomitant use of organic nitrates of any kind

Counseling Points for the Drug Class

- PDE5 inhibitors offer no protection against sexually transmitted infections
- These agents are ineffective in the absence of sexual arousal
- Do not take if you are using any form of nitrate
- Be aware of signs of low blood pressure, such as dizziness and unsteadiness
- Report sudden decrease or loss of hearing or vision
- Priapism (prolonged erection > 6 hours) is a medical emergency. Seek immediate medical attention.
- Do not engage in sexual activity if clinically inadvisable

Key Point for the Drug Class

Nitrates are contraindicated while using phosphodiesterase inhibitors

Members of the Drug Class

In this section: Sildenafil, tadalafil, vardenafil
Other: Avanafil

◉ Sildenafil

Brand Names
Viagra, Revatio

Generic Name
Sildenafil

Usage
Erectile dysfunction,* pulmonary arterial hypertension*

Pregnancy Category B

Dosage Form
Tablet

Dosing

- Erectile dysfunction: 50 mg 30 minutes to 4 hours before anticipated sexual activity; may increase to 100 mg or decrease to 25 mg
- Pulmonary arterial hypertension (Revatio only): 20 mg three times daily
- Renal dosage adjustment: If CrCl < 30 mL/min, consider initial dose of 25 mg
- Hepatic dosage adjustment: If mild to moderate impairment (Child-Pugh class A or B), consider starting dose of 25 mg
- Concomitant use of potent CYP3A4 inhibitors: Initial dose of 25 mg
- Concomitant alpha-blocker dose adjustment: Initial dose of 25 mg

◉ Tadalafil

Brand Names
Cialis, Adcirca

Generic Name
Tadalafil

Usage
Erectile dysfunction,* pulmonary arterial hypertension,* BPH*

Pregnancy Category B

Dosage Form
Tablet

Dosing

- Erectile dysfunction:
  - As-needed dosing: 10 mg at least 30 minutes before anticipated sexual activity (range 5–20 mg)
  - Once daily dosing: 2.5 mg daily; may increase to 5 mg/day
  - Renal dosage adjustment:
    - As-needed dosing: If CrCl < 50 mL/min, then initial dose is 5 mg
    - Once daily dosing: If CrCl < 30 mL/min, then use is not recommended
  - Hepatic dosage adjustment:
    - As-needed dosing:
      - Mild to moderate impairment (Child-Pugh class A or B): 10 mg maximum dose
      - Severe hepatic impairment (Child-Pugh class C): Use not recommended
  - Dosage adjustment with concomitant potent CYP3A4 inhibitors:
    - As-needed dosing: 10 mg maximum dose in a 72-hour period
    - Once daily dosing: 2.5 mg/day starting and maximum dose

- Pulmonary arterial hypertension (Adcirca only):
  - 40 mg daily
  - Renal dosage adjustment:
    - CrCl < 80 mL/min: Reduce dosage
    - Severe renal impairment: Avoid use
  - Hepatic dosage adjustment:
    - Mild to moderate hepatic impairment: Use with caution. Reduce dosage.
    - Severe hepatic impairment (Child-Pugh class C): Avoid use
- BPH:
  - 5 mg once daily
  - Renal dosage adjustment:
    - CrCl = 30–50 mL/min: Initial dose is 2.5 mg
    - CrCl < 30 mL/min: Use not recommended
  - Hepatic dosage adjustment:
    - Mild to moderate hepatic impairment: Reduce dosage. Use with caution.
    - Severe hepatic impairment (Child-Pugh class C): Avoid use
- Dosage adjustment with concomitant alpha blockers: Initiate at the lowest possible dose
- Concomitant protease inhibitor regimen: Higher initial dose of 20 mg/day required

⊙ Vardenafil

Brand Names
Levitra, Staxyn

Generic Name
Vardenafil

Usage
Erectile dysfunction*

Pregnancy Category B

Dosage Forms
Tablet, orally disintegrating tablet (ODT)

Dosing
- 10 mg approximately 60 minutes before anticipated sexual activity
- Dosage adjustments: May be increased up to a maximum dose of 20 mg or decreased to 5 mg
- Maximum dosing frequency is once daily
- Renal dosage adjustment: None
- Hepatic dosage adjustment:
  - Mild hepatic impairment: No dosage adjustment needed
  - Moderate hepatic impairment (Child-Pugh class B): Initial dose of 5 mg is recommended; may increase cautiously to maximum of 10 mg
  - Severe hepatic impairment (Child-Pugh class C): Use not recommended
- Dosage adjustment with concomitant CYP3A4 inhibitors: Maximum dose of 2.5–5 mg in a 24-hour period
- Dosage adjustment with concomitant alpha blockers:
  - Tablet: Initial dose of 5 mg
  - ODT: Do not initiate with vardenafil ODTs

SMOKING CESSATION AIDS

Introduction
The most commonly used smoking cessation aids in this class are the nicotine replacement agents. These are available in different dosage forms to allow for better compliance based on patients' preferences. Other smoking cessation aids include Wellbutrin and Varenicline, which are prescription medications.

Mechanism of Action for Nicotine Replacement Therapy
Nicotine replacement agents provide smaller amounts of nicotine than that found in cigarettes in an effort to prevent or reduce withdrawal symptoms

Member of the Drug Class
In this section: Nicotine
Others: None

⊙ Nicotine

Brand Names
Nicorette (gum), Thrive (gum), Commit (lozenge), Nico-Derm CQ (patch), Nicotrol OTC (patch), Nicotrol NS (nasal spray), Nicotrol Inhaler (inhaler)

Generic Name
Nicotine

Rx and OTC
Rx: Nicotrol NS, Nicotrol Inhaler
OTC: Nicotine gum, nicotine lozenge, nicotine patch

Dosage Forms
Gum, lozenge, patch, nasal spray, oral inhaler

Usage
Smoking cessation aid for the relief of nicotine withdrawal symptoms and cravings*

Pregnancy Category D

Dosing

- Nicorette gum:
  - Chew 1 piece of gum every 1–2 hours for 6 weeks, decrease to 1 piece every 2–4 hours for 3 weeks, then chew 1 piece every 4–8 hours for 3 weeks, then discontinue:
    - ≥ 25 cigarettes daily: 4 mg gum
    - < 25 cigarettes daily: 2 mg gum
  - Maintenance dose:
    - 4 mg gum: 9–12 pieces a day
    - 2 mg gum: 9–12 pieces a day; may use 4 mg gum in patients not responding to the 2 mg gum
  - Duration of therapy: 2–6 months; attempt to wean and stop therapy by month 4–6
  - Maximum dose:
    - 4 mg gum: 24 pieces a day
    - 2 mg gum: 30 pieces a day
- Commit lozenge:
  - Take 1 lozenge every 1–2 hours for weeks 1–6, decrease to 1 piece every 2–4 hours for weeks 7–9, then 1 lozenge every 4–8 hours for weeks 10–12, then discontinue:
    - Patients who normally smoke 30 minutes after awakening in the morning: 2 mg lozenge
    - Patients who normally smoke within 30 minutes of awakening: 4 mg lozenge
  - Maintenance dose: ≥ 9 lozenges/day
  - Maximum dose: 5 lozenges within 6 hours, 20 lozenges/day
- NicoDerm CQ patch:
  - ≥ 10 cigarettes/day: One 21 mg patch applied daily for 6 weeks, then one 14 mg patch daily for 2 weeks, then one 7 mg patch daily for 2 weeks, then discontinue
  - < 10 cigarettes/day: One 14 mg patch applied daily for 6 weeks, then one 7 mg patch daily for 2 weeks, then discontinue
- Nicotrol nasal spray (NS): Each dose (2 sprays; 1 spray in each nostril) contains 1 mg of nicotine):
  - Initial dose: 1–2 doses (sprays)/hour
  - Maintenance dose: Individualized for a duration of 3 months
  - Maximum dose: 5 mg (10 sprays)/hour, 40 mg (80 sprays)/day
- Nicotrol Inhaler:
  - Initial dose: 6–16 cartridges daily for up to 12 weeks
  - Maintenance dose: Individualized for 12 weeks, then tapered over an additional 6–12 weeks
  - Maximum dose: 16 cartridges/day for 12 weeks before tapering

Adverse Reactions: Most Common

- Palpitations, tachycardia, insomnia, headache, hypertension
- Gum and lozenge: Mouth soreness, throat irritation, dyspepsia, nausea, gingivitis, taste perversion
- Transdermal patch: Local skin reaction (skin), insomnia, vivid dreams

- Nicotrol NS: Nasal irritation
- Nicotine Inhaler: Local irritation of mouth and throat

Major Drug Interactions

Drugs Affecting Nicotine

Cimetidine: May increase serum concentration. If patient is taking > 600 mg PO of cimetidine with a nicotine patch, decrease the dose of the nicotine patch to the next lower patch dose.

Contraindications

Patients immediately postmyocardial infarction, life-threatening arrhythmias, worsening or unstable angina

Counseling Points

- Nicorette gum:
  - Start on quit date
  - Chew gum slowly until a tingling sensation or "peppery taste" occurs, then "park" between the gum and the cheek. When tingling subsides, re-chew again until tingling returns. Repeat process until most of tingling sensation is gone (~30 minutes).
  - Avoid eating or drinking 15 minutes before chewing gum and while gum is in mouth
  - Do not use nicotine gum if you have dental problems
- Commit lozenge:
  - Start on quit date
  - Avoid eating or drinking 15 minutes before and while using the lozenge
  - Suck on the lozenge and move it from side to side; suck each piece until it dissolves
  - Do not chew or swallow the lozenge. Minimize swallowing while dissolving the lozenge.
- Nicotine patch:
  - Start on quit date
  - Apply new patch every 24 hours to clean, hairless, dry skin without cuts or scratches on upper body; rotate sites
  - Wash site of application with water only; soap will increase absorption
  - Dispose of patches and gum carefully and out of reach of children and pets
  - If sleep disruption or vivid dreams occur, remove at night before bedtime and apply a new patch upon awakening
  - Do not smoke when using the patch
- Nicotrol NS:
  - Start on quit date
  - Tilt head back slightly; do not sniff, inhale through nose, or swallow while spraying
- Nicotrol Inhaler:
  - Start on quit date
  - Inhale like smoking a cigarette
  - Avoid eating or drinking 15 minutes before and during use
  - Delivery decreases if < 40°F in winter; therefore, in winter do not keep in car

Key Points

- Use with caution in patients with GI ulcers because nicotine may delay healing
- Avoid use in patients immediately postmyocardial infarction, with life-threatening arrhythmias, and/or with worsening or unstable angina
- Nicotrol NS: Not recommended for patients with chronic nasal disorders (e.g., sinusitis, nasal polyps, allergic rhinitis) because nasal mucosa irritation can occur. Avoid use in severe reactive airway disease.
- Nicotrol inhaler: Avoid use in cases of bronchospastic disease

◉ Varenicline

Brand Name
Chantix

Generic Name
Varenicline

Mechanism of Action

Varenicline is a partial neuronal alpha-4 beta-2 nicotinic receptor agonist, thus producing agonist activity at the nicotinic receptor but at a lower level than nicotine. Varenicline also prevents nicotine from binding to this receptor, preventing stimulation of the central nervous mesolimbic dopamine system, which is responsible for the reinforcement-and-reward experience associated with smoking.

Rx Only

Dosage Form
Tablet

Usage
Treatment of smoking cessation*

Pregnancy Category C

Dosing

- 0.5 mg once daily on days 1–3, 0.5 mg twice daily on days 4–7, and then 1 mg twice daily (start 1 week before quit date) for 12–24 weeks
- Renal dosage adjustment: If CrCl < 30 mL/min, then 0.5 mg once daily to a maximum dose of 0.5 mg twice daily

Adverse Reactions: Most Common

Insomnia, vivid dreams, constipation, flatulence, nausea (dose dependent), vomiting, headache

Adverse Reaction: Rare/Severe/Important

Abnormal behavior, changes in mood, suicidal ideation, hypersensitivity reactions (Stevens-Johnson syndrome, angioedema)

Major Drug Interactions

Drugs Affecting Varenicline

Alcohol may increase the risk of adverse psychiatric events. H2-antagonists (i.e., cimetidine), quinolone antibiotics (i.e., levofloxacin), and trimethoprim may increase serum concentrations especially in patients with severe renal impairment.

Contraindications

Specific contraindications have not been established

Counseling Points

- Start medication 1 week before quit date
- Report changes in mood (e.g., depression, suicide ideation, emotional/behavioral changes) to your healthcare provider
- Take with food to reduce nausea
- Take evening dose with dinner instead of at bedtime if insomnia occurs

Key Points

- Patients with a history of psychiatric disorders should not receive this medication
- Use with caution in patients with cardiovascular disease. Varenicline has not been studied in patients with unstable cardiovascular disease and patients experiencing recent cardiovascular events < 2 months prior to varenicline treatment.

URINARY ANALGESICS

Introduction

The urinary analgesic phenazopyridine is an azo dye that has analgesic or local anesthetic action on the urinary tract mucosa. It is used short-term to ease symptoms of urinary tract infections (UTIs).

Mechanism of Action for the Drug Class

The azo dye exerts local anesthetic or analgesic action on the urinary tract mucosa through an unknown mechanism

Members of the Drug Class

In this section: Phenazopyridine
Others: None

◉ Phenazopyridine

Brand Names

Pyridium, Azo-Standard, Prodium

Generic Name

Phenazopyridine

Rx and OTC

Rx: Pyridium
OTC: Azo-Standard, Prodium

Dosage Form

Tablet

Usage

Symptomatic relief of urinary burning, itching, frequency, and urgency associated with UTIs or following urologic procedures*

Pregnancy Category B

Dosing

- Adults: 100–200 mg three times daily after meals until pain and discomfort are relieved. Should not be used for more than 2 days when used concomitantly with an antibiotic. Use for OTC self-medication for up to 2 days.
- Children: 12 mg/kg in 3 divided doses/day given after meals
- Renal dosage adjustment:
  - CrCl = 50–80 mL/min: Change dosing interval to every 8–16 hours
  - CrCl < 50 mL/min: Avoid use

Adverse Reactions: Most Common

Headache, pruritus, GI disturbances, anaphylactoid reaction

Adverse Reactions: Rare/Severe/Important

Hemolytic anemia, hepatotoxicity, nephrotoxicity

Major Drug Interactions

No known significant drug interactions

Contraindications

Impaired renal function, severe hepatic disease, pyelonephritis during pregnancy; avoid with G6PD deficiency

Counseling Points

- Take with food to lessen gastric irritation
- Phenazopyridine may discolor urine and sclera red or orange, leading to staining of contact lenses and undergarments. Tablets also may stain clothing. This discoloration is physically harmless.

Key Points

- Phenazopyridine is only effective for relief of symptoms
- Phenazopyridine will discolor urine and can interfere with urine dipstick tests to diagnose UTIs
- Taking phenazopyridine with food can minimize GI irritation

REVIEW QUESTIONS

1. Which of the following is *not* a common adverse reaction of Proscar?

   a. Erectile dysfunction
   b. Xerostomia
   c. Breast tenderness and swelling
   d. Reduced libido

2. Which of the following tablets, if broken, should *not* be handled by a pregnant woman?

   a. Benztropine
   b. Meclizine
   c. Oxybutynin
   d. Finasteride

3. Which of the following is *not* a brand name of isotretinoin?

   a. Propecia
   b. Accutane
   c. Claravis
   d. Sotret

4. Which of the following is *not* an important monitoring parameter during treatment with isotretinoin?

   a. Creatinine clearance
   b. Pregnancy test
   c. Lipid panel
   d. Liver function tests

5. Which of the following medications requires pharmacist participation in the iPLEDGE risk management program?

   a. Cialis
   b. Enablex
   c. Claravis
   d. Propecia

6. Which of the following medications can discolor sclera and contact lenses?

   a. Cogentin
   b. Pyridium
   c. Proscar
   d. Accutane

7. Which of the following is *not* a counseling point for hydroxychloroquine?

   a. You should have an ophthalmic exam every 3 months if using hydroxychloroquine over an extended period of time.
   b. Avoid large amounts of vitamin C because it may acidify the urine, thus increasing the chance of kidney stone formation.
   c. Hydroxychloroquine may increase sensitivity to sunlight. Therefore, you should wear dark glasses and protective clothing, use sunblock, and avoid direct exposure to sunlight.
   d. Take hydroxychloroquine with food to minimize GI upset.

8. Allopurinol is a _____ inhibitor used to prevent gout attacks and treat high uric acid levels.

   a. CYP3A4
   b. CYP1A2
   c. CYP2D6
   d. Xanthine oxidase

9. Which of the following is one of the *most* common adverse effects of Colcrys?

   a. Drowsiness
   b. Dry mouth
   c. Irritability
   d. Diarrhea

10. Which of the following medications is used to treat extrapyramidal symptoms associated with antipsychotic use?

    a. Meclizine
    b. Cogentin
    c. Tolterodine
    d. Oxybutynin

11. Which of the following is an appropriate initial dose of darifenacin?

    a. 1 mg once daily
    b. 5 mg once daily
    c. 7.5 mg once daily
    d. 15 mg once daily

12. Which of the following is *not* an adverse reaction associated with benztropine?

    a. Angioedema
    b. Constipation
    c. Urinary retention
    d. Blurred vision

13. Which of the following is the active ingredient in Dramamine Less Drowsy Formula?

    a. Diphenhydramine
    b. Meclizine
    c. Benztropine
    d. Tolterodine

14. Which of the following is the most appropriate dosing interval for meclizine when used for motion sickness?

    a. Every 8 hours
    b. Every 12 hours
    c. Every 24 hours
    d. Every 48 hours

15. All of the following medications can cause hyperkalemia when used concomitantly with potassium chloride, *except*:

    a. furosemide.
    b. lisinopril.
    c. valsartan.
    d. spironolactone.

16. All of the following agents could potentially interact with Viagra, *except:*

    a. isosorbide dinitrate.
    b. erythromycin.
    c. fluconazole.
    d. amoxicillin.

17. Which of the following is the best starting dose for sildenafil for erectile dysfunction in a patient with a CrCl of 20 mL/min?

    a. 25 mg
    b. 50 mg
    c. 100 mg
    d. 200 mg

18. Tadalafil dosing should be adjusted for which of the following conditions?

    a. Renal impairment
    b. Hepatic impairment
    c. Concomitant CYP3A4 inhibitors
    d. All of the above

19. Which of the following dosing intervals is most appropriate for phenazopyridine in a patient with normal renal function?

    a. Once daily
    b. Twice daily
    c. Three time a day
    d. Four time a day

20. Use of phenazopyridine should be limited to _____ day(s) when used concomitantly with an antibiotic.

    a. 1
    b. 2
    c. 3
    d. 4

21. Taking Detrol LA and meclizine concomitantly would most likely increase the risk of which of the following?

    a. Peripheral edema
    b. QT prolongation
    c. Constipation
    d. Sleep disturbances

22. Which of the following is *not* a counseling point for phosphodiesterase inhibitors?

    a. Be aware of signs of low blood pressure.
    b. Avoid prolonged exposure to the sun.
    c. Seek medical attention for priapism.
    d. Do not take if you are using any form of nitrate.

23. Which of the following is *not* a counseling point for the oxybutynin patch?

    a. May cause dry mouth.
    b. Apply to clean, dry skin on the abdomen, hip, or buttocks.
    c. May cause ringing in the ears.
    d. Avoid reapplication to the same site within 1 week.

24. Which of the following medications does *not* need to be taken with food to reduce adverse GI effects?

    a. K-Dur
    b. Zyloprim
    c. Chloroquine
    d. Commit lozenges

25. What strength nicotine replacement patch should patients start with if they are smoking ≥ 10 cigarettes a day?

    a. 7 mg
    b. 14 mg
    c. 21 mg
    d. 28 mg

26. Which of the following is *not* a common adverse effect of nicotine replace therapy?

    a. Palpitations
    b. Tachycardia
    c. Headache
    d. Drowsiness

27. Which of the following is *not* a counseling point for varenicline?

    a. Varenicline should be started on the patient's quit date.
    b. Patients should report any mood changes to their physician.
    c. Varenicline should be taken with food to reduce symptoms of nausea.
    d. If insomnia occurs the evening dose should be taken with dinner instead of at bedtime.

28. Suboxone contains which of the following?

    a. Buprenorphine and naloxone
    b. Buprenorphine and acetylcysteine
    c. Buprenorphine and flumazenil
    d. Buprenorphine and niacin

29. Flumazenil is used as a(n) _____ reversal agent.

    a. acetaminophen
    b. opioid
    c. benzodiazepine
    d. tricyclic antidepressant

30. Which of the following is *not* an indication for acetylcysteine?

    a. Non–life-threatening allergic reactions
    b. Acetaminophen overdose
    c. Adjunctive mucolytic agent
    d. Prevention of contrast-induced nephropatfhy

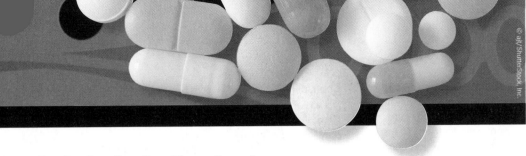

Ophthalmic Products

Jamila Stanton Seibel, PharmD, BCPS

PROPER ADMINISTRATION OF OPHTHALMIC PRODUCTS

Administration of Solutions

Proper instillation of all eye solutions, suspensions, and ointments is necessary for optimal efficacy and prevention of superinfection. Refer to the techniques provided here for all ophthalmic solutions, suspensions, and ointments. Follow these recommended procedures for application of ophthalmic *solutions*:

- Wash hands thoroughly before administration
- Tilt head back or lie down and gaze upward
- Place medication in conjunctival sac and close eyes; do not blink
- Apply light finger pressure on lacrimal sac (corner of eye near nose) for 1 minute following instillation; this is called *nasolacrimal occlusion* (NLO)
- If more than one type of ophthalmic solution is used, wait at least 5 minutes before administering second agent
- To avoid contamination, do not touch tip of container to eye or any surface

Administration of Suspensions

Recommended procedures for application of ophthalmic *suspensions* are as follows:

- Shake bottle before instillation
- Follow steps for application of ophthalmic solution

Administration of Ointments

These are the recommended procedures for application of ophthalmic *ointments*:

- Wash hands thoroughly before administration
- Hold the ointment tube in your hand for a few minutes to warm ointment and facilitate flow
- When opening tube for the first time, squeeze out and discard the first 0.25 inch of ointment
- Tilt head backward or lie down and gaze upward
- Gently pull down lower lid to form a pouch
- Place 0.25–0.5 inch of ointment in sweeping motion inside the lower eyelid
- To avoid contamination, do not touch tip of container to eye or any surface
- Close the eye for 1 or 2 minutes and roll the eyeball in all directions
- If more than one type of ointment is needed, wait at least 10 minutes before administering second agent
- Vision may be blurry for up to 20 minutes following administration of ophthalmic ointments

ANTIBIOTICS, OTHER

Introduction

Ophthalmic antibacterial agents are active against a variety of gram-positive and gram-negative organisms. They are generally used to treat ocular infections involving the conjunctiva or cornea, such as conjunctivitis, keratitis, corneal ulcers, and blepharitis. Many different combination preparations are available on the U.S. market, so particular caution should be exercised when dispensing these products with regard to the selected agent, strength, and formulation. In addition, the dosage and frequency of administration varies with each agent; individual package labeling is a useful reference for pharmacists. In general, the risk of superinfection is high when using topical ophthalmic antibiotics due to contamination of the container (e.g., dropper, tube). Proper administration technique is an important counseling point to help reduce the incidence of superinfection (see the beginning of this chapter for the

---

* Throughout the text, an asterisk (*) is used to indicate the most common uses of a drug.

proper administration technique for ophthalmic products). Patients being treated for bacterial conjunctivitis, the most common indication, should be advised not to wear contact lenses until the infection is completely resolved. Disposable lenses should be thrown away, and a new pair should be started. Nondisposable lenses should be thoroughly cleaned before reinsertion following an eye infection. Using a new contact lens case also is recommended.

Members of the Drug Class

In this section: Neomycin/polymyxin B sulfate/gramicidin (combination product), erythromycin, tobramycin (in combination). See section on Antibiotics, Fluoroquinolones for additional agents.

Others: Multiple mono and combination products are available containing the following antibacterial agents: Chloramphenicol, gentamicin, bacitracin, tetracycline, trimethoprim, sulfisoxazole, sulfacetamide

◉ Neomycin/Polymyxin B Sulfate/Gramicidin

Mechanism of Action

This combination antibiotic product has multiple mechanisms of action. Most commonly described is its ability to interfere with bacterial protein synthesis by binding to 30S ribosomal subunits, resulting in bacterial cell death. In addition, it also alters the permeability of the bacterial cell membrane, causing leakage of intracellular contents, and ultimately cell death.

Brand Name
Neosporin

Generic Name
Neomycin/polymyxin B sulfate/gramicidin

OTC

Dosage Form
Solution

Usage
Superficial ophthalmic infections such as bacterial conjunctivitis and blepharitis due to strains of microorganisms susceptible to the antibiotic*

Pregnancy Category C

Dosing
Instill 1 or 2 drops into the affected eye(s) every 4–6 hours

Adverse Reactions: Most Common
Superinfection, transient burning, stinging, irritation upon instillation

Adverse Reactions: Rare/Severe/Important
Sensitivity reaction, which manifests as itching, reddening, irritation, and edema of the conjunctiva and eyelid or failure to heal; decreased vision

Counseling Points
- For ophthalmic use only
- To avoid contamination, do not touch tip of container to eye or any other surface
- Do not wear contact lenses while using this medication and for the duration of ocular infection

Key Points
- Common adverse effects, including stinging, irritation, and burning, are usually transient and not harmful
- Products containing neomycin have been specifically linked to sensitization reactions, which manifest as itching, reddening, and edema of the conjunctiva and eyelid or failure of infection to heal; contact prescriber if these symptoms occur or if infection persists

◉ Erythromycin

Mechanism of Action
Macrolides bind to the 50S subunit of the bacterial ribosome, inhibiting RNA-dependent bacterial protein synthesis

Brand Name
Ilotycin

Generic Name
Erythromycin

Rx Only

Dosage Form
Ointment

Usage
Treatment of superficial ocular infections involving the conjunctiva or cornea caused by organisms susceptible to the antibiotic,* prophylaxis of ophthalmia neonatorum due to *Neisseria gonorrhoeae**

Pregnancy Category B

Dosing
- Bacterial conjunctivitis: Apply a 0.5-inch ribbon into the conjunctival sac of the affected eye two to six times daily, depending on severity
- Prophylaxis of ophthalmia neonatorum: Apply a 0.5-inch ribbon into the conjunctival sacs of neonates shortly after birth

Adverse Reactions: Most Common
Blurred vision for the first few minutes after instillation, transient minor irritation and redness upon instillation

Adverse Reactions: Rare/Severe/Important
Decreased vision, hypersensitivity

Counseling Points

- For ophthalmic use only
- To avoid contamination, do not touch tip of container to the eye or to any other surface
- Do not wear contact lenses while using this medication and for the duration of ocular infection

Key Points

- Erythromycin ophthalmic ointment is a first-line agent in treating simple cases of bacterial conjunctivitis
- Ointments often are preferred in children and those who have difficulty administering medications. The ointment commonly stays on the lid and lashes, providing a therapeutic effect, even if the medication is not applied directly to the conjunctiva.
- Erythromycin is recommended for routine use in all neonates for prophylaxis of ophthalmia neonatorum due to *N. gonorrhoeae*. Importantly, infants diagnosed with gonococcal ophthalmia or born to mothers with gonorrhea require treatment with systemic (oral) antibiotics because topical erythromycin alone is inadequate. Topical antibiotics are not necessary when oral erythromycin is utilized.
- Topical ophthalmic erythromycin it is not effective for the prevention or treatment of neonatal ocular infections caused by *Chlamydia trachomatis*

ANTIBIOTICS, FLUOROQUINOLONES

Introduction

Fluoroquinolones are among the most commonly prescribed ophthalmic antibiotics on the market. This is likely due to their broad spectrum of action against both gram-positive and gram-negative bacteria. They are used for a variety of ophthalmic infections, including bacterial conjunctivitis and corneal ulcers. They also are considered the agents of choice for conjunctivitis in contact lens wearers.

Mechanism of Action for the Drug Class

Fluoroquinolones work by inhibiting the activity of DNA gyrase and topoisomerase IV, enzymes needed for replication of bacterial DNA. Inhibition of bacterial DNA synthesis results in cell death and accounts for the bactericidal action of these agents.

Usage for the Drug Class

Treatment of ocular infections, including bacterial conjunctivitis and corneal ulcers (keratitis), due to strains of microorganisms susceptible to the antibiotic*

Pregnancy Category C for the Drug Class

Adverse Reactions for the Drug Class: Most Common

- Localized discomfort and irritation; transient burning, pain, or stinging; dry eye; itching; redness; tearing; papillary conjunctivitis; taste disturbance
- During the first 7 intensive days of corneal ulcer treatment, a nonharmful white crystalline precipitate commonly forms on the cornea defect; therapy should be continued. The precipitate usually resolves as the regimen is deescalated (ciprofloxacin).

Adverse Reactions for the Drug Class: Rare/Severe/Important

Prolonged redness, irritation, swelling, pain, or itching; secondary infection; decreased vision; hypersensitivity; keratitis. Prolonged use may result in fungal or bacterial superinfections

Counseling Points for the Drug Class

- For ophthalmic use only
- To avoid contamination, do not touch tip of container to the eye or to any other surface
- Do not wear contact lenses while using this medication and for the duration of ocular infection

Key Points for the Drug Class

- Bacterial conjunctivitis is usually self-limiting; however, use of topical antibiotics is common to help accelerate resolution, decrease spread, and prevent complications
- With a broad spectrum of activity and efficacy against gram-positive and gram-negative bacteria, fluoroquinolones often are overused, leading to bacterial resistance, a common concern among clinicians. They are, however, the drug of choice for treatment of corneal ulcers and conjunctivitis in contact lens wearers due to their activity against *P. aeruginosa*.

Members of the Drug Class

In this section: Ciprofloxacin, gatifloxacin, moxifloxacin, ofloxacin
Others: Besifloxacin, levofloxacin

⦿ Ciprofloxacin

Brand Name
Ciloxan

Generic Name
Ciprofloxacin

Rx Only

Dosage Forms
Solution, ointment

Dosing
- Corneal ulcers:
  - Day 1: Instill 2 drops into the affected eye every 15 minutes for the first 6 hours and then 2 drops into the affected eye every 30 minutes for the remainder of the day
  - Day 2: Instill 2 drops into the affected eye hourly
  - Days 3–14: Instill 2 drops into the affected eye every 4 hours; treatment may be continued > 14 days in some patients
- Bacterial conjunctivitis:
  - Solution:
    - Days 1–2: Instill 1 or 2 drops into the affected eye every 2 hours while awake
    - Days 3–7: Instill 1 or 2 drops into the affected eye every 4 hours
  - Ointment:
    - Days 1–2: Apply a 0.5-inch ribbon into the conjunctival sac three times a day
    - Days 3–7: Apply a 0.5-inch ribbon into the conjunctival sac two times a day

⊙ Gatifloxacin

Brand Names
Zymar, Zymaxid

Generic Name
Gatifloxacin

Rx Only

Dosage Form
Solution

Dosing
- Bacterial conjunctivitis:
  - Gatifloxacin 0.3% (Zymar):
    - Days 1–2: Instill 1 drop into the affected eye every 2 hours while awake, up to a maximum of eight times a day
    - Days 3–7: Instill 1 drop into the affected eye up to four times a day while awake
  - Gatifloxacin 0.5% (Zymaxid):
    - Day 1: Instill 1 drop into the affected eye every 2 hours while awake, up to a maximum of eight times a day
    - Days 2–7: Instill 1 drop into the affected eye 2–4 times a day while awake

⊙ Moxifloxacin

Brand Names
Vigamox, Moxeza

Generic Name
Moxifloxacin

Rx Only

Dosage Form
Solution

Dosing
- Bacterial conjunctivitis:
  - Moxifloxacin (Vigamox): Instill 1 drop into the affected eye three times a day for 7 days
  - Moxifloxacin (Moxeza): Instill 1 drop into the affected eye twice daily for 7 days

⊙ Ofloxacin

Brand Name
Ocuflox

Generic Name
Ofloxacin

Rx Only

Dosage Form
Solution

Dosing
- Bacterial corneal ulcer:
  - Days 1 and 2: Instill 1–2 drops into the affected eye every 30 minutes while awake and every 4–6 hours during normal sleeping time
  - Days 3–7: Instill 1–2 drops into the affected eye every hour while awake
  - Days 7–9 through treatment completion: Instill 1–2 drops into the affected eye four times a day
- Bacterial conjunctivitis:
  - Days 1 and 2: Instill 1–2 drops into the affected eye every 2–4 hours
  - Days 3–7: Instill 1–2 drops into the affected eye four times a day

Introduction

Ophthalmic steroids are applied topically for a variety of inflammatory conditions, including allergic conjunctivitis, uveitis, iritis, and superficial punctate keratitis. In addition, these agents are often used in the setting of chemical, thermal, or foreign body injury to the eye and in the immediate postocular surgical setting to decrease inflammation and scar tissue formation. Steroids may delay wound healing, so they are generally not recommended for minor abrasions or injury. In general, steroids do not have a role in the treatment of simple conjunctivitis and should not be used in most cases of viral conjunctivitis; their use may prolong and exacerbate the severity of viral ocular infections. Prolonged use of ophthalmic steroids may lead to elevated intraocular pressure (IOP) and damage to the optic nerve. Caution is advised when using these agents in patients with primary open-angle glaucoma or elevated IOP.

Mechanism of Action for the Drug Class

The exact mechanism of corticosteroids' action is unknown. Their anti-inflammatory action is likely related to their ability inhibit edema, fibrin deposition, capillary dilation, and leukocyte migration. They are also known to decrease the activity of inflammatory mediators such as prostaglandins and leukotrienes.

Members of the Drug Class

In this section: Loteprednol
Others: Dexamethasone, difluprednate, fluocinolone (ocular implant), fluorometholone, prednisolone, rimexolone, triamcinolone (ocular injection)

◉ Loteprednol

Brand Names
Lotemax, Alrex

Generic Name
Loteprednol

Rx Only

Dosage Forms
Suspension, ointment

Usage
Various ocular inflammatory conditions,* allergic conjunctivitis,* postoperative pain and inflammation following ocular surgery

Pregnancy Category C

Dosing
- Allergic conjunctivitis:
  - Loteprednol 0.2% suspension (Alrex): Instill 1 drop into the affected eye(s) four times a day
- Inflammatory conditions:
  - Loteprednol 0.5% suspension (Lotemax): Instill 1–2 drops into the affected eye(s) four times a day; during initial week of therapy, dose may be increased to a maximum of 1 drop every hour if necessary
- Postoperative inflammation:
  - Loteprednol 0.5% suspension (Lotemax): Instill 1–2 drops into the affected eye(s) four times a day beginning 24 hours after surgery and continuing through the first 2 weeks of the postoperative period
  - Loteprednol 0.5% ointment (Lotemax): Instill 0.5-inch ribbon into the conjunctival sac of the affected eye(s) four times a day beginning 24 hours after surgery and continuing through the first 2 weeks of the postoperative period

Adverse Reactions: Most Common
Transient burning, stinging, irritation upon instillation; foreign body sensation; chemosis; itching; dry eye; excessive tearing; blurry vision; photophobia. Systemic effects include headache, rhinitis, and pharyngitis.

Adverse Reactions: Rare/Severe/Important
Visual changes/decreased vision, elevated IOP, optic nerve damage, glaucoma, secondary infections (bacterial, viral, fungal), cataract formation

Contraindications
Viral, mycobacterial, and fungal infections of the cornea and conjunctiva

Essential Monitoring Parameter
IOP if use is > 10 days

Counseling Points
- For ophthalmic use only
- To avoid contamination, do not touch tip of container to the eye or to any other surface
- Loteprednol contains benzalkonium chloride, which may be absorbed by contact lenses. Remove contact lens before instillation of the solution. You may reinsert contact lenses 15 minutes following loteprednol administration.

Key Points

- Common adverse effects, including stinging, irritation, and burning, are usually transient and not harmful
- Generally, application of ophthalmic corticosteroids does not provide enough systemic absorption to cause severe systemic side effects and is not associated with HPA-axis suppression
- Duration of use > 10 days should only occur under the direct supervision of a physician and with careful monitoring of IOP. Long-term use of these agents has been associated with increased IOP in some patients.
- Ophthalmic dexamethasone is the most frequently reported corticosteroid eye drop to cause elevated IOP.
- Loteprednol was developed as a "site-specific steroid" and has less of an effect on IOP due to its high lipophilicity and rapid metabolism. It is frequently prescribed to prevent and treat seasonal allergies; however, use > 14 days should only occur under the supervision of a medical professional.
- Prolonged use of ocular corticosteroids may increase the incidence of secondary infection, mask acute infection, or prolong or exacerbate viral infections

COMBINATION ANTIBIOTIC/CORTICOSTEROID AGENTS

Introduction

Combination antibiotic/corticosteroid ophthalmic products are used in a variety of conditions in which a corticosteroid is indicated and in which superficial bacterial infection or risk of infection exists. The steroid component suppresses the inflammatory response; however, it is also likely to delay or slow wound healing. Because corticosteroids may inhibit the body's defense mechanisms against infection, a concomitant antimicrobial agent may be used when this inhibition is considered to be clinically significant. Topical ophthalmic steroids are not recommended for long-term use; prolonged use may lead to elevated IOP and the development of glaucoma.

Members of the Drug Class

In this section: Tobramycin/dexamethasone
Others: Multiple combination products are available containing the following antibacterial agents: Neomycin, neomycin/polymyxin B, gentamicin, tobramycin, chloramphenicol, bacitracin, sulfacetamide; multiple combination products are available containing the following steroid components: hydrocortisone, prednisolone, dexamethasone, loteprednol

⊙ Tobramycin/Dexamethasone

Mechanism of Action

Dexamethasone is a potent corticosteroid that inhibits the inflammatory response by inhibiting interleukin-1 and various other cytokines that mediate inflammatory responses. It also decreases inflammation by suppressing the migration of polymorphonuclear leukocytes and decreasing capillary permeability. Tobramycin is an aminoglycoside antibiotic that provides activity against susceptible organisms by irreversibly binding to the 30S ribosomal subunit, disrupting bacterial protein synthesis. This results in cell death.

Brand Name
TobraDex

Generic Name
Tobramycin/dexamethasone

Rx Only

Dosage Forms
Suspension, ointment

Usage
Steroid-responsive inflammatory ocular conditions with infection or risk of infection*

Pregnancy Category C

Dosing

- Suspension:
  - Instill 1 or 2 drops into the affected eye every 4–6 hours
  - Severe infections: Instill 1 or 2 drops every 2 hours for the first 24–48 hours, and then decrease administration to every 4–6 hours
- Ointment:
  - Apply 0.5-inch ribbon to the conjunctival sac every 6–8 hours
  - Severe infections: Apply 0.5-inch ribbon to the conjunctival sac every 3–4 hours for the first 24–48 hours, and then decrease administration to every 6–8 hours

Adverse Reactions: Most Common
Superinfection, itching and swelling

Adverse Reactions: Rare/Severe/Important
Visual changes/decreased vision; hypersensitivity reaction manifested as itching, redness, and edema of the eyelid; optic nerve damage; glaucoma; secondary infections (bacterial, viral, fungal)

Contraindications

Viral, mycobacterial, and fungal infections of the cornea and conjunctiva

Counseling Points

- For ophthalmic use only
- Store suspensions upright and shake well before using
- To avoid contamination, do not touch tip of container to the eye or to any other surface
- Do not wear contact lenses during the use of this product; the suspension contains benzalkonium chloride, which may be absorbed by contact lenses

Key Points

- Prolonged use of ophthalmic corticosteroids is associated with risk of elevated IOP, damage of the optic nerve, development of glaucoma, secondary infections, and thinning/perforation of the cornea or sclera in susceptible patients
- Prolonged use of ophthalmic corticosteroids in combination with antibiotics may increase the incidence of secondary infection, mask acute infection, or prolong or exacerbate viral infections

ANTIGLAUCOMA AGENTS, TOPICAL

Introduction

Glaucoma is the second leading cause of blindness in the world and the leading cause of blindness among African Americans. Of the different types, primary open-angle glaucoma is the most common, accounting for over 90% of all cases. Although glaucoma may occur at normal intraocular pressure (normal tensive glaucoma), it is commonly associated with intraocular hypertension, the only modifiable risk factor that has been identified. As a result, the goal of treatment for open-angle glaucoma and ocular hypertension is lowering of the intraocular pressure (IOP). Multiple classes of agents are used to lower IOP, and patients often will require combination therapy. Adherence is particularly challenging in treating glaucoma; many products are dosed multiple times per day, and elderly patients, who are typically affected, may have difficulty remembering to take their medications or self-administering eye drops. Newer formulations and therapies have the advantage of once-daily dosing; however, these drugs are usually expensive and may not be covered by insurances.

Members of the Drug Class

In this section: Latanoprost, travoprost, timolol, timolol-XE, timolol/brimonidine (combination product)

Others: Multiple mono and combination products are available containing the following antibacterial agents: Bimatoprost, tafluprost, betaxolol, carteolol, levobunolol, metipranolol, brimonidine, apraclonidine, brinzolamide, dorzolamide, phenylephrine, pilocarpine, carbachol, dipivefrin

◉ Latanoprost

Mechanism of Action

Latanoprost is a prostaglandin analog; it effectively reduces IOP by increasing aqueous humor outflow from the eye

Brand Name

Xalatan

Generic Name

Latanoprost

Rx Only

Dosage Form

Solution

Usage

Treatment of elevated IOP in patients with open-angle glaucoma or ocular hypertension*

Pregnancy Category C

Dosing

Instill 1 drop into the affected eye(s) once daily in the evening

Adverse Reactions: Most Common

Increased pigmentation of the iris, eyelash changes, eyelid skin darkening, transient burning and stinging upon instillation, blurred vision, conjunctival hyperemia

Adverse Reactions: Rare/Severe/Important

Excessive tearing, eyelid crusting, pain, discomfort, iritis/uveitis

Counseling Points

- For ophthalmic use only
- To avoid contamination, do not touch tip of container to the eye or to any other surface
- Latanoprost may cause a color change of the iris, increasing the amount of brown pigmentation. This change occurs slowly, may not present for several months to a year, and is likely to be permanent. Latanoprost may cause darkening of the eyelid skin and changes to the eyelashes, including increased thickness, length, and darkening.
- Latanoprost contains benzalkonium chloride, which may be absorbed by contact lenses. Remove contact

lens before instillation of the solution. You may reinsert contact lenses 15 minutes following latanoprost administration.

- Storage considerations: Protect this medication from light. Store unopened bottles in the refrigerator. Once opened, you may store the bottle at room temperature for up to 6 weeks.

Key Points

- Prostaglandin analogs are effective agents for the treatment of elevated IOP and glaucoma and in some studies have demonstrated superior IOP lowering when compared with timolol twice a day. Additionally, with once-daily administration and limited systemic side effects, these drugs have been advocated by some as first-line agents in the management of glaucoma.
- Once-daily dosing should not be exceeded because more frequent administration may decrease the effectiveness of latanoprost
- Although systemic adverse effects are limited, local side effects are notable for changes in iris, eyelid, and eyelash pigmentation

◉ Travoprost

Mechanism of Action

Travoprost is a prostaglandin analog; it effectively reduces IOP by increasing aqueous humor outflow from the eye

Brand Name

Travatan Z

Generic Name

Travoprost

Rx Only

Dosage Form

Solution

Usage

Treatment of elevated IOP in patients with open-angle glaucoma or ocular hypertension*

Pregnancy Category C

Dosing

Instill 1 drop into the affected eye(s) once daily in the evening

Adverse Reactions: Most Common

Darkening of the iris, growth and thickening of the eyelashes, eyelid skin darkening, transient burning and stinging upon instillation, conjunctival hyperemia, itching

Adverse Reactions: Rare/Severe/Important

Excessive tearing, eyelid crusting, pain, discomfort, iritis/uveitis

Contraindications

Hypersensitivity to latanoprost or benzalkonium chloride

Counseling Points

- For ophthalmic use only
- To avoid contamination, do not touch tip of container to the eye or to any other surface
- Travoprost may cause a color change of the iris, increasing the amount of brown pigmentation. This change occurs slowly, may not present for several months to a year, and is likely to be permanent. Travoprost may cause darkening of the eyelid skin and changes to the eyelashes, including increased thickness, length, and darkening.
- Remove contact lens before instillation of the solution. You may reinsert contact lenses 15 minutes following travoprost administration.

Key Points

- Prostaglandin analogs are effective agents for the treatment of elevated IOP and glaucoma and in some studies demonstrated superior IOP lowering when compared with timolol twice a day. Additionally, with once-daily administration and limited systemic side effects, these drugs have been advocated by some as first-line agents in the management of glaucoma.
- Once-daily dosing should not be exceeded because more frequent administration may decrease the effectiveness of travoprost
- Although systemic adverse effects are limited, local side effects are notable for changes in iris, eyelid, and eyelash pigmentation
- Travoprost has been shown to lower IOP more in African American patients than non-African American patients; the reason for this is unknown

◉ Timolol, Timolol-XE

Mechanism of Action

Timolol is a beta-adrenergic blocker. Ophthalmic beta-adrenergic blocking agents decrease IOP by reducing aqueous humor production in the ciliary body of the eye. Nonselective beta blockers (timolol, levobunolol, carteolol, and metipranolol) affect beta-1 and beta-2 receptors, whereas selective beta blockers (betaxolol) affect only beta-1 receptors.

Brand Name

Timoptic, Timoptic-XE, Timoptic GFS, Istalol, Betimol

Generic Names

Timolol, timolol-XE

Rx Only

Dosage Forms

Solution, gel-forming solution

Usage

Treatment of elevated IOP in patients with open-angle glaucoma or ocular hypertension*

Pregnancy Category C

Dosing

- Solution:
  - Timoptic: Instill 1 drop into the affected eye(s) twice a day
  - Timoptic XE: Instill 1 drop into the affected eye(s) once daily
  - Betimol: Instill 1 drop into the affected eye(s) twice a day. If IOP lowering is maintained, administration may be changed to once daily.
  - Istalol: Instill 1 drop into the affected eye(s) once daily in the morning
- Gel-forming solution: Instill 1 drop in the affected eye(s) once daily

Adverse Reactions: Most Common

Temporary burning and stinging following instillation; blurry vision is common for 5–10 minutes following administration of the gel-forming solution

Adverse Reactions: Rare/Severe/Important

Local reactions include uveitis, keratitis, superinfection, dry eye, blepharitis, corneal anesthesia, stinging, tearing. Systemic reactions include bradycardia, hypotension, exacerbation of congestive heart failure, bronchospasm, fatigue, dizziness.

Contraindications

Asthma, severe COPD, bradycardia, second- or third-degree AV block, sinus node dysfunction, uncompensated heart failure, cardiogenic shock

Counseling Points

- This medication is for ophthalmic use only
- To avoid contamination, do not touch tip of container to the eye or to any other surface
- Using proper technique of nasolacrimal occlusion (NLO) is particularly important to optimize efficacy and decrease systemic absorption and toxicities
- Before using, invert gel-forming solution and shake once. Administer other topical ophthalmic medications used concomitantly at least 10 minutes before the gel-forming solution.
- Remove contact lenses before using this medication; wait 15 minutes following administration to reinsert

Key Points

- Ophthalmic beta-adrenergic blockers are generally equally effective in IOP lowering; however, they differ in duration of action, adverse-effect potential, and cost. These agents are generally considered first-line therapy for the treatment of open-angle glaucoma.

- Because of the risk of systemic adverse events, these drugs are contraindicated in patients with severe pulmonary disease, bradycardia, second- or third-degree heart block, overt heart failure, and cardiogenic shock. If used, clinicians should exercise extreme caution, monitor carefully, and use of the lowest effective dose. Patients should practice nasolacrimal occlusion.

◉ Timolol/Brimonidine

Mechanism of Action

Combigan is composed of timolol, a beta-adrenergic blocker, and brimonidine, an alpha-2 agonist. Ophthalmic beta-adrenergic blocking agents decrease IOP by reducing aqueous humor production in the ciliary body of the eye. Ophthalmic alpha-2 agonists also reduce aqueous humor production; however, they also increase aqueous humor outflow via the uveoscleral pathway of the eye.

Brand Name

Combigan

Generic Names

Timolol/brimonidine

Rx Only

Dosage Forms

Solution

Usage

Treatment of elevated IOP in patients with open-angle glaucoma or ocular hypertension*

Pregnancy Category C

Dosing

Instill 1 drop into the affected eye(s) twice a day, approximately 12 hours apart

Adverse Reactions: Most Common

Temporary burning and stinging following instillation, allergic conjunctivitis, itching, conjunctival hyperemia, conjunctival folliculosis, excessive tearing

Adverse Reactions: Rare/Severe/Important

Local adverse reactions include blepharitis, blurred vision, corneal erosion, eye pain, eyelid edema, eyelid erythema, superficial punctuate keratitis. Systemic adverse reactions include hypertension, bradycardia, exacerbation of congestive heart failure, bronchospasm, fatigue, dizziness.

Contraindications

Asthma, severe COPD, bradycardia, second- or third-degree AV block, sinus node dysfunction, uncompensated heart failure, cardiogenic shock

Counseling Points

- Medication is for ophthalmic use only
- To avoid contamination, do not touch tip of container to the eye or to any other surface
- Using proper technique of nasolacrimal occlusion (NLO) is particularly important to optimize efficacy and decrease systemic absorption and toxicities
- Remove contact lenses before using this medication; wait 15 minutes following administration to reinsert

Key Points

- Combigan is a combination product composed of a nonselective beta-adrenergic blocker (timolol) and an alpha-adrenergic agonist (brimonidine)

- Ophthalmic alpha-agonists have been associated with a localized allergic-type reaction characterized by eyelid edema, erythema, itching, discomfort, and foreign object sensation. Among the alpha-agonists, brimonidine has the lowest incidence of this side effect, affecting approximately 5–9% of patients in clinical trials.
- Because of the risk of systemic adverse events with ophthalmic beta blockers, these drugs are contraindicated in patients with severe pulmonary disease, bradycardia, second- or third-degree heart block, overt heart failure, and cardiogenic shock. If used, clinicians should exercise extreme caution, monitor carefully, and use the lowest effective dose. Patients should practice nasolacrimal occlusion.

ANTIHISTAMINES

Introduction

Allergic conjunctivitis is an allergic-type reaction occurring in the conjunctiva of the eye in response to a specific allergen. It is commonly seasonal and is usually associated with exposure to pollen, ragweed, dust, or mold spores. Pharmacotherapy options used to treat acute episodes of allergic conjunctivitis include artificial tears and combination topical antihistamines/topical vasoconstrictor products. For frequent episodes or seasonal and perennial allergies, the agents of choice are topical antihistamines and mast cell stabilizers. It takes 5–14 days to see optimal effects with mast cell stabilizers, thus they are best initiated 2–4 weeks before allergy exposure rather than as treatment for acute symptoms. The agents discussed in this section, ketotifen and olopatadine, possess both antihistamine and mast cell–stabilizing properties. They are considered drugs of choice because they effectively work on both the chronic and acute symptoms of allergic conjunctivitis.

Mechanism of Action for the Drug Class

These agents block the effects of histamine by selectively blocking H1 receptors. They also exhibit mast cell–stabilizing properties, preventing mast cell degranulation, which is the first step in the allergy cascade.

Usage for the Drug Class

Allergic conjunctivitis*

Pregnancy Category C for the Drug Class

Adverse Reactions for the Drug Class: Most Common

Localized discomfort and irritation, transient burning, pain or stinging, dry eye, itching, redness, tearing, foreign body sensation. Systemic adverse reactions include cold syndrome, headache, pharyngitis.

Adverse Reactions for the Drug Class: Rare/Severe/Important

Secondary infection, decreased vision, hypersensitivity, keratitis, photophobia, rash

Counseling Points for the Drug Class

- Medications are for ophthalmic use only
- To avoid contamination, do not touch tip of container to eye or any other surface
- Remove contact lenses before using this medication; wait 15 minutes following administration to reinsert. Should not be used to treat contact lens–related irritation.
- If using a topical antihistamine as a self-care product, seek medical advice if symptoms do not improve within 48–72 hours

Key Points for the Drug Class

- Occasional, acute onset allergic conjunctivitis is best treated with a combination topical antihistamine/vasoconstrictor product, artificial tears and cold compress
- Frequent episodes or seasonal/perennial allergic conjunctivitis are best treated with a dual-action antihistamine/mast cell–stabilizing agents, which are effective at acute relief of symptoms and chronic management of the condition

Members of the Drug Class

In this section: Olopatadine, ketotifen
Others: Azelastine, epinastine, bepotastine, alcaftadine, emedastine, pheniramine
Mast cell stabilizers: Cromolyn sodium, nedocromil sodium, lodoxamide, pemirolast

Ketotifen

Brand Names

Alaway, Claritin Eye, Zaditor, Zyrtec Itchy Eye

Generic Name

Ketotifen

OTC

Dosage Form

Solution 0.025%

Dosing

Instill 1 drop into the affected eye(s) twice a day

Olopatadine

Brand Names

Pataday, Patanol

Generic Name

Olopatadine

Rx Only

Dosage Form

Solution

Dosing

- Pataday 0.2%: Instill 1 drop into the affected eye(s) once a day
- Patanol 0.1%: Instill 1 drop into the affected eye(s) twice a day, 6–8 hours apart

---

REVIEW QUESTIONS

1. Which of the following statements regarding installation of antibiotic ophthalmic products is *false*?

   a. Proper instillation technique begins with washing your hands.
   b. Proper instillation technique helps prevent super-infection.
   c. Proper instillation technique requires cleaning the applicator tip with an alcohol swab before each use.
   d. All of the above

2. Which of the following conditions is *not* a contraindication for the use of ophthalmic beta blockers?

   a. Cardiogenic shock
   b. Severe COPD
   c. Tachycardia
   d. Third-degree AV block

3. Which of the following "generic name—brand name" pairs is *not* correctly matched?

   a. Ciprofloxacin—Ocuflox
   b. Erythromycin—Ilotycin
   c. Latanoprost—Xalatan
   d. Timolol—Timoptic

4. Viral, mycobacterial, and fungal infections of the cornea are contraindications for which of the following agents?

   a. Ciloxan
   b. Neosporin
   c. TobraDex
   d. Xalatan

5. Which of the following agents is available as a gel-forming solution?

   a. Latanoprost
   b. Ofloxacin
   c. Timolol
   d. Tobramycin/dexamethasone

6. Erythromycin ointment belongs to which of the following classes of antibacterial agents?

   a. Aminoglycoside
   b. Beta-lactam
   c. Fluoroquinolone
   d. Macrolide

7. Which of the following statements regarding latanoprost is true?

   a. A well-known adverse effect of latanoprost is eyelash thinning.
   b. Latanoprost is inferior to topical beta blockers when treating glaucoma.
   c. Twice daily dosing is more effective than once daily dosing.
   d. Unopened bottles that are not in use should be stored in the refrigerator.

8. Which of the following statements is *false*?

   a. Always avoid contact of the applicator tip to the surface of the eye.
   b. Generally, contact lenses should be removed during treatment for conjunctivitis.
   c. Nasolacrimal occlusion is most useful for ophthalmic ointments.
   d. Ophthalmic suspensions should be shaken before use.

9. Which of the following drug: mechanism of action pairs is *incorrect*?

   a. Erythromycin: Inhibits RNA dependent protein synthesis
   b. Latanoprost: Decreases aqueous humor outflow from the eye
   c. Ofloxacin: Inhibits activity of DNA gyrase
   d. Timolol: Reduces aqueous humor production in the ciliary body of the eye

10. Which of the following is *not* a common adverse reaction to TobraDex?

    a. Eyelid itching
    b. Eyelid swelling
    c. Hypersensitivity reaction
    d. Superinfection

11. Which of the following agents should be used to treat an infected corneal ulcer?

    a. Neosporin
    b. Ofloxacin
    c. Timolol
    d. Travoprost

12. Which of the following statements regarding ophthalmic beta blockers is *false*?

    a. Nasolacrimal occlusion is particularly important to help decrease the incidence of systemic side effects.
    b. Ophthalmic beta blockers are generally considered first-line therapy for open-angle glaucoma.
    c. Timolol is a selective beta-1 receptor blocker.
    d. Ophthalmic beta blockers are among the most commonly used medications to treat glaucoma.

13. Which of the following agents may be used for long-term treatment of ocular hypertension?

    a. Combigan
    b. Dexamethasone
    c. Erythromycin
    d. Lotemax

14. Which of the following ophthalmic agents is most likely to have systemic adverse effects potentially limiting its use?

    a. Erythromycin ointment
    b. Latanoprost
    c. Gatifloxacin solution
    d. Timolol

15. Which of the following statements is true regarding ophthalmic erythromycin ointment?

    a. Erythromycin ointment is commonly used for prophylaxis of ophthalmia neonatorum.
    b. Erythromycin ointment is the drug of choice for uncomplicated conjunctivitis.
    c. Temporarily blurred vision is common following administration.
    d. All of the above

16. Neosporin ointment contains which of the following ingredients?

    a. Gramicidin
    b. Polymyxin B
    c. Neomycin
    d. All of the above

17. Which of the following statements is true regarding Lotemax?

    a. Lotemax has the greatest effect on IOP compared to other steroids.
    b. Lotemax 0.2% is available over the counter.
    c. Lotemax may prolong or exacerbate ophthalmic viral infections.
    d. Lotemax may be absorbed systemically and lead to HPA-axis suppression.

18. Which of the following prescriptions for Travatan Z is correct?

    a. Instill 1 drop into the affected eye(s) once daily in the evening.
    b. Instill 1 drop into the affected eye(s) twice a day, approximately 12 hours apart.
    c. Instill 2 drops into the affected eye(s) twice a day, approximately 12 hours apart.
    d. Instill 1 drop into the affected eye(s) four times a day.

19. Which of the following statements regarding brimonidine is true?

a. Brimonidine has been associated with a nonharmful darkening of the eyelid, eyelashes, and iris.

b. Brimonidine has been associated with a localized allergic-type reaction in 5–9% of patients.

c. Brimonidine has been associated with lowering of heart rate and CHF exacerbations.

d. Brimonidine has been associated with elevations in intraocular pressure when used for > 14 days.

20. A patient brings in a prescription for Ocuflox. You notice in her profile that she is allergic to Levaquin. Which of the following antibiotics could you recommend?

a. Ciloxan

b. Vigamox

c. Neosporin

d. Zymar

21. Which of the following is the generic name for Zaditor?

a. Erythromycin

b. Ketotifen

c. Tobramycin

d. Travoprost

22. Which of the following statements is true regarding allergic conjunctivitis?

a. Allergic conjunctivitis commonly occurs seasonally.

b. Mast cell stabilizers work quickly to treat acute allergy symptoms.

c. Agents used to treat allergic conjunctivitis are available by prescription only.

d. Topical antihistamines should only be used for 48–72 hours.

23. In order to prevent ophthalmia neonatorum due to *Neisseria gonorrhoeae*, all neonates should receive an ophthalmic preparation of which of the following?

a. Erythromycin

b. Gatifloxacin

c. Neosporin

d. TobraDex

24. Which of the following agents is *not* indicated for the treatment of glaucoma?

a. Brimonidine

b. Olopatadine

c. Timolol

d. Travoprost

25. Timoptic ophthalmic drops have been associated with all of the following adverse effects *except*:

a. bradycardia.

b. bronchospasm.

c. hypotension.

d. seizure.

26. In which of the following situations may loteprednol be recommended for use?

a. A 22-year-old woman with bacterial conjunctivitis

b. A 56-year-old woman with a fungal infection of the cornea

c. A 33-year-old man with inflammation of the iris, or iritis

d. A 78-year-old woman with a history of allergy to dexamethasone drops

27. Which of the following ophthalmic agents is the drug of choice when treating bacterial conjunctivitis in a patient who wears contact lenses?

a. Ketotifen

b. Moxifloxacin

c. Neomycin + loteprednol

d. Tobramycin + dexamethasone

28. Which of the following statements regarding ophthalmic ointments is true?

a. Ophthalmic ointments should be refrigerated when not in use.

b. Ophthalmic ointments are less effective than ophthalmic drops.

c. Ophthalmic ointments may be preferred in patients with poor administration technique.

d. Ophthalmic ointments do not have a risk of secondary infection.

29. Which of the following is a combination of both a steroid and an antibacterial agent?

a. Combigan

b. TobraDex

c. Neosporin

d. All of the above

30. Which of the following agents can be used for allergic conjunctivitis?

a. Ketotifen

b. Loteprednol

c. Olopatadine

d. All of the above

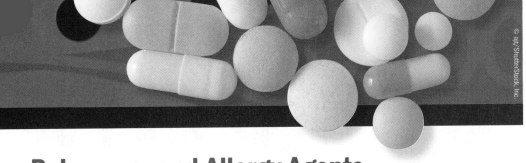

Pulmonary and Allergy Agents

Christina Rose, PharmD, BCPS

ANTICHOLINERGICS, INHALED

Introduction

Anticholinergic inhalers and nasal preparations are primarily used for chronic obstructive pulmonary disease (COPD), allergic and nonallergic rhinitis, and nasal cold symptoms. Long-acting anticholinergic inhalation preparations are not used in the chronic treatment of asthma. Ipratropium may be used during acute asthma exacerbation but only in combination with short-acting beta-adrenergic agonists. The most common adverse reaction associated with the inhalation preparations is dry mouth.

Mechanism of Action for the Drug Class

The drug class appears to produce bronchodilation by blocking acetylcholine at muscarinic receptors, therefore blocking the direct constrictor effects of acetylcholine on bronchial smooth muscle. Ipratropium blocks all muscarinic receptors. Tiotropium is a long-acting agent, selective to the M3 receptors. Local application to nasal mucosa inhibits mucous gland secretions.

Members of the Drug Class

In this section: Ipratropium, tiotropium
Others: None

⊙ Ipratropium

Brand Names
Atrovent, Atrovent HFA

Generic Name
Ipratropium

Rx Only

Dosage Forms
Aerosol for oral inhalation 17 µg/actuation, solution for nebulizer 0.02%, nasal spray 0.03% and 0.06%

Usage

Maintenance treatment of bronchospasm associated with COPD,* adjunct in asthma exacerbations, allergic and nonallergic rhinitis (nasal spray 0.03%), common cold (nasal spray 0.06%)

Pregnancy Category B

Dosing

- COPD:
  - 2 puffs inhaled by mouth four times a day (doses 6–8 hours apart)
  - Maximum dose: 12 puffs per day
- Solution for nebulizers:
  - 500 µg inhaled by mouth three to four times a day (doses 6–8 hours apart)
  - Maximum dose: 2 mg every 24 hours
- Acute asthma exacerbation (in combination with short-acting beta-adrenergic agonists):
  - Inhaler: 8 inhalations every 20 minutes as needed for up to or 3 hours
  - < 12 years: 4 inhalations every 20 minutes as needed for up to or 3 hours
  - Solution for nebulizer: 500 µg every 20 minutes for 3 doses then as needed
  - < 12 years: 250 µg every 20 minutes for 3 doses then as needed
- Allergic/nonallergic rhinitis, nasal spray 0.03%:
  - 2 puffs in each nostril two to three times a day
  - Maximum dose: 12 puffs every 24 hours
- Common cold, nasal spray 0.06%:
  - 2 puffs in each nostril three to four times a day
  - Maximum dose: 16 puffs every 24 hours

Adverse Reactions: Most Common

Cough, dry mouth, chest pain/palpitations, nausea, dizziness, headache, dyspepsia, urinary retention, nasal irritation (nasal spray), epistaxis (nasal spray), taste perversion

---

* Throughout the text, an asterisk (*) is used to indicate the most common uses of a drug.

Adverse Reactions: Rare/Severe/Important

Paradoxical bronchospasms; worsening of narrow-angle glaucoma/mydriasis; increased intraocular pressure (especially if sprayed into eyes); worsening of urinary retention

Major Drug Interactions

Drugs Affecting Ipratropium

Other anticholinergics or drugs that have anticholinergic properties: May potentiate effects

Counseling Points

- Use proper administration technique
- The Atrovent HFA inhalation aerosol does not have to be shaken before use
- Avoid spraying into eyes
- Directions for proper use of aerosol for oral inhalation:
  1. The inhaler must be "primed" two times before taking the first dose from a new inhaler or when the inhaler has not been used for > 3 days
  2. Insert the metal canister into the top of the mouthpiece and remove the protective dust cap from the mouthpiece
  3. Exhale deeply through your mouth
  4. Put the mouthpiece in your mouth and close your lips. Keep your eyes closed so the medicine will not spray into your eyes.
  5. Inhale slowly through your mouth and at the same time press firmly once on the canister, continuing to breathe deeply
  6. Hold your breath for 10 seconds or as long as you feel comfortable
  7. Exhale slowly
  8. Wait at least 15 seconds before repeating steps 1 through 7 for the next inhalation
  9. Replace the dust cap after use
  10. Keep the mouthpiece clean. Wash it at least once a week. Shake it to remove excess water and let it air dry.
- Mouthpiece cleaning instructions:
  1. Remove and set aside the canister and dust cap from the mouthpiece
  2. Wash the mouthpiece through the top and bottom with warm running water for at least 30 seconds. Do not use anything other than water to wash the mouthpiece.
  3. Dry the mouthpiece by shaking off the excess water and allow it to air dry
  4. When the mouthpiece is dry, replace the canister. Make sure the canister is fully and firmly inserted into the mouthpiece.
- If using more than the prescribed amount, contact your healthcare provider
- Use with a proper spacing device

Key Points

- Most commonly used for COPD
- Can be used for the treatment of acute bronchospasms in COPD and as an adjunct in asthmatic patients
- Most common adverse reaction is dry mouth and nasal irritation with nasal spray
- Use with caution in patients with glaucoma or urinary retention

◉ Tiotropium

Brand Name

Spiriva

Generic Name

Tiotropium

Rx Only

Dosage Forms

Capsule containing 18 µg powder for inhalation delivered via a special dry powder inhaler device (HandiHaler) for oral inhalation only

Usage

Long-term management of COPD*

Pregnancy Category C

Dosing

Contents of 1 capsule (18 µg) inhaled orally once daily using HandiHaler

Adverse Reactions: Most Common

Cough, dry mouth, dyspepsia, blurred vision, headache, sore throat, urinary retention

Adverse Reactions: Rare/Severe/Important

Worsening of narrow-angle glaucoma, worsening of urinary retention, paradoxical bronchospasms

Major Drug Interactions

Drugs Affecting Tiotropium

Other anticholinergics may potentiate effects

Counseling Points

- Capsule is for inhalation only via the HandiHaler device; do not swallow
- Should not be used to treat acute bronchospasms
- Directions for proper use of the HandiHaler device:
  1. Open the HandiHaler device. Pull the cap upward to expose the mouthpiece.
  2. Open the mouthpiece by pulling the mouthpiece ridge upward away from the base
  3. Remove the capsule from the blister pack. Do not open the capsule.

4. Insert the capsule into the center chamber of the HandiHaler device. It does not matter which end of the capsule you put in the chamber.
5. Close the mouthpiece until you hear a click, but leave the cap open
6. Hold the HandiHaler device with the mouthpiece upright
7. Press the green button until it is flat against the base and release
8. Breathe out completely. Do not exhale into the mouthpiece.
9. Hold the HandiHaler device by the gray base and raise the device to your mouth. Close your lips tightly around the mouthpiece.
10. Breathe in slowly and deeply so you hear or feel the capsule vibrate
11. Hold your breath as long as it is comfortable and at the same time take the inhaler out of your mouth

12. To get the full dose of the medication, you must breathe out completely and repeat steps 9–11. Do not press the green button again.
13. After you finish taking your daily dose, open the mouthpiece again. Tip out the used capsule and throw it away.
14. Close the mouthpiece cap for storage of your HandiHaler

Key Points
- Used for chronic treatment of COPD; tiotropium should not be used to treat acute bronchospasms
- Capsule should be inhaled via HandiHaler only and should not be swallowed
- Use with caution in patients with glaucoma or urinary retention

ANTIHISTAMINES, FIRST GENERATION, SEDATING

Introduction

The first-generation antihistamines are used primarily for hypersensitivity/allergic reactions, sleep disorders, and as antiemetics. They are not typically used chronically for allergic rhinitis due to the potential for sedation, but they are still used in some cases because many of these agents are available without a prescription. These agents are generally used on an as-needed basis, depending on the indication. Chronic use of these agents should be avoided in the elderly due to their sedative and anticholinergic effects. Sedation is the most common adverse reaction associated with these agents, and concomitant drugs that cause sedation should be avoided.

Mechanism of Action for the Drug Class

These agents reversibly, competitively antagonize H1 receptors peripherally and centrally, blocking the increased capillary permeability (edema/wheel formation) and itching caused by histamine release. Some agents (anticholinergics) block muscarinic receptors, resulting in antiemetic effects.

Adverse Reactions for the Drug Class: Most Common

Drowsiness, somnolence, fatigue, dizziness, headache, nausea, nervousness, tremor

Major Drug Interactions for the Drug Class
Drugs Affecting Antihistamines
- Alcohol and CNS depressants: Potentiate drowsiness
- Other anticholinergic drugs: Potentiate side effects

Members of the Drug Class

In this section: Diphenhydramine, hydroxyzine, promethazine
Others: Brompheniramine, chlorpheniramine, clemastine doxylamine

◉ Diphenhydramine

Brand Name
Benadryl

Generic Name
Diphenhydramine

Rx (Injectable) and OTC

Dosage Forms
Capsule, tablet, chewable tablet, liquid, injection, topical cream

Usage
Allergic dermatitis,* hypersensitivity reactions,* allergic reactions,* sleep disorders,* allergic rhinitis, antitussive, motion sickness, treatment of drug-induced extrapyramidal reactions

Pregnancy Category B

Dosing

- Children:
  - < 2 years: Use not recommended due to dosing errors and accidental ingestion
  - 2–6 years:
    - 6.25 mg PO every 4–6 hours
    - Maximum dose: 37.5 mg every 24 hours
  - 6–12 years:
    - 12.5–25 mg PO every 4–6 hours
    - Maximum dose: 150 mg every 24 hours
  - > 12 years: See adult dosing
- Adults:
  - 25–50 mg PO every 4–8 hours
  - Maximum dose: 300 mg every 24 hours

Adverse Reactions: Rare/Severe/Important

Excitation in young children

Major Drug Interactions

Diphenhydramine's Effect on Other Drugs

Tamoxifen, tramadol: May decrease effectiveness by inhibiting the metabolism of each drug to its active metabolite

Contraindications

Neonates or premature infants

Counseling Points

- Young children may experience a paradoxical excitation effect
- Tolerance to CNS effects may develop quickly; sedation will no longer be troublesome after a few days
- For motion sickness, take the dose 30 minutes to 1 hour before traveling

Key Points

- Diphenhydramine is commonly used for allergies, motion sickness, and sleep disorders
- Sedation is the most common adverse reaction
- Not recommended for use in children < 2 years of age
- May be inappropriate to use in the elderly due to sedative and anticholinergic effects

◉ Hydroxyzine

Brand Names

Atarax, Vistaril

Generic Name

Hydroxyzine

Rx Only

Dosage Forms

Tablet, capsule, syrup, oral suspension, IM injection

Usage

Pruritus,* sedation,* anxiety, motion sickness, nausea and vomiting

Pregnancy Category C

Dosing

- Pruritus:
  - Children:
    - 2–6 years:
      - 12.5 mg PO every 6 hours as needed
      - Maximum dose: 50 mg every 24 hours
    - 6–12 years:
      - 12.5–25 mg PO every 6 hours as needed
      - Maximum dose: 100 mg every 24 hours
    - > 12 years: See adult dosing
  - Adults:
    - 25 mg PO every 6–8 hours
    - Maximum dose: 400 mg every 24 hours
- Sedation:
  - Children:
    - 0.6 mg/kg PO as a single dose
    - Maximum dose: Not to exceed 50 mg as a single dose
  - Adults:
    - Oral: 50–100 mg as a single dose
    - IM injection: 50 mg as a single dose
- Hepatic dosage adjustment: Change dosing interval to every 24 hours in patients with primary biliary cirrhosis

Adverse Reactions: Common

None

Adverse Reactions: Rare/Severe/Important

None

Contraindications

Early pregnancy; intravenous, subcutaneous, or intra-arterial administration

Counseling Points

- Tolerance to CNS effects may develop quickly; sedation will no longer be troublesome after a few days
- Avoid use with other medications that cause sedation
- Can be used on an as-needed basis

Key Points

- Most commonly used as a sedative and antipruritic
- Sedation is the most common adverse reaction
- Hydroxyzine is a vesicant and should be administered as an IM injection only
- Use may be inappropriate in the elderly due to its sedative and anticholinergic effects

◉ Promethazine

Brand Name

Phenergan

Generic Name

Promethazine

Rx Only

Dosage Forms

Tablet, syrup, suppository, injection

Usage

Antiemetic,* motion sickness, treatment of allergic conditions, sedation, adjunct for pain

Pregnancy Category C

Dosing

- Oral, rectal, injection:
  - Children > 2 years:
    - Use with caution
    - Use the lowest effective dose
    - 0.1–1 mg/kg/dose every 6 hours
    - Maximum: 25–50 mg/dose (varies based on indication)
  - Adults:
    - 25–50 mg at bedtime *or*
    - 12.5–25 mg every 4–8 hours if needed
    - Maximum dose: 150 mg every 24 hours

Adverse Reactions: Rare/Severe/Important

Photosensitivity, blood dyscrasias, extrapyramidal symptoms, neuroleptic malignant syndrome, injection site reactions (IM is preferred route of parenteral administration; IV administration may cause severe tissue damage and is not recommended)

Contraindications

Allergy to phenothiazines, children < 2 years of age, intra-arterial or SUB-Q administration

Counseling Points

- Tolerance to CNS effects may develop quickly; sedation will no longer be troublesome after a few days
- Take with food, water, or milk to decrease GI upset
- For motion sickness take 30 minutes to 1 hour before traveling
- Use sugarless gum or candy, ice, or saliva substitute to decrease dry mouth

Key Points

- Most commonly used for hypersensitivity reactions, motion sickness, and as an antiemetic
- Promethazine is available in multiple dosage forms
- Contraindicated in patients < 2 years of age. Use with caution in children > 2 years of age. Use the lowest effective dose and avoid with other CNS/respiratory depressant medications.
- IV administration can cause severe tissue damage. Use IM route.

ANTIHISTAMINES, SECOND GENERATION, NONSEDATING

Introduction

The second-generation antihistamines are used for allergic rhinitis and urticaria. They are used to treat these chronic conditions due to the low risk of adverse events. These agents are more commonly used than the first-generation antihistamines because of the decreased risk of sedation. Sedation is most common with cetirizine. All of these agents are available in combination with pseudoephedrine. The combination products should not be used in patients < 12 years of age.

Mechanism of Action for the Drug Class

These agents reversibly, competitively antagonize H1 receptors peripherally, blocking the increased capillary permeability (edema/wheel formation) and itching caused by histamine release. They do not cross the blood–brain barrier, resulting in reduced sedation.

Usage for the Drug Class

Allergic rhinitis,* chronic urticaria

Adverse Reactions for the Drug Class: Most Common

Dizziness, dyspepsia, headache, nausea, xerostomia

Adverse Reactions for the Drug Class: Rare/Severe/Important

None

Members of the Drug Class

In this section: Fexofenadine, loratadine, cetirizine, levocetirizine
Others: Desloratadine, acrivastine (available with pseudoephedrine only)

⊙ Fexofenadine

Brand Names

Allegra, Allegra D 12 hour (60 mg fexofenadine/120 mg pseudoephedrine), Allegra D 24 hour (180 mg fexofenadine/240 mg pseudoephedrine)

Generic Name

Fexofenadine

OTC

Dosage Forms

Tablet, extended-release tablet, oral disintegrating tablet (ODT; contains phenylalanine)

Pregnancy Category C

Dosing

- Children:
  - Combination product with pseudoephedrine should not be used in children < 12 years of age
  - 6 months to < 2 years:
    - 15 mg twice daily
    - Maximum dose: 15 mg twice daily
  - 2–11 years:
    - 30 mg twice daily
    - Maximum dose: 30 mg twice daily
  - > 12 years:
    - 60 mg twice daily or 180 mg once daily
    - Maximum dose: 60 mg PO twice daily or 180 mg once daily
  - Renal dosage adjustment: If CrCl < 80 mL/min:
    - 6 months to < 2 years: Initial dose of 15 mg once daily
    - 2–11 years: Initial dose of 30 mg once daily
    - ≥ 12 years: Initial dose of 60 mg once daily
- Adults:
  - 60 mg twice daily or 180 mg once daily
  - Maximum dose: 60 mg twice daily or 180 mg once daily
  - Renal dosage adjustment: If CrCl < 80 mL/min, then initial dose of 60 mg once daily

Major Drug Interactions

Drugs Affecting Fexofenadine

- Ketoconazole and erythromycin: May increase levels (without evidence of QT prolongation)
- Concomitant use of aluminum- or magnesium-containing antacids: Decreases bioavailability

Counseling Points

- Take at regular intervals
- Avoid aluminum- or magnesium-containing antacids
- Shake suspension before each use
- ODT not recommended in children < 6 years of age
- ODT should be taken on an empty stomach and should not be chewed
- Avoid use of other CNS depressants and alcohol; concomitant use may cause excess drowsiness

Key Points

- Should not cause drowsiness
- Available with pseudoephedrine for patients > 12 years of age
- Patient should be counseled to shake suspension before use
- ODT should be taken on an empty stomach and should not be chewed

⦿ Loratadine

Brand Names

Alavert, Claritin, Claritin D 12 hour (5 mg loratadine/120 mg pseudoephedrine), Claritin D 24 hour (10 mg loratadine/240 mg pseudoephedrine)

Generic Name

Loratadine

OTC

Dosage Forms

Liquid gel capsule, orally disintegrating tablet (ODT), chewable tablet, syrup

Pregnancy Category B

Dosing

- Children:
  - 2–6 years:
    - 5 mg once daily
    - Maximum dose: 5 mg once daily
  - > 6 years:
    - 10 mg once daily
    - Maximum dose: 10 mg once daily
- Adults:
  - 10 mg once daily
  - Maximum dose: 10 mg once daily
- Renal dosage adjustment: If CrCl < 30 mL/min, use same dose but change the frequency to every other day
- Hepatic dosage adjustment: Use same dose but change the frequency to every other day

Major Drug Interactions

None

Counseling Points

- Take at regular intervals
- Redi-tabs are rapidly disintegrating tablets that dissolve on the tongue. They can be administered with or without water.

Key Points

- Available with pseudoephedrine for patients > 12 years of age
- Should not cause drowsiness

⦿ Levocetirizine

Brand Name

Xyzal

Generic Name

Levocetirizine

Rx Only

Dosage Forms

Tablet, oral solution

Pregnancy Category B

Dosing

- Children:
  - 6 months to 5 years: 1.25 mg once daily in the evening
  - 6–11 years: 2.5 mg once daily in the evening
  - > 12 years: 5 mg once daily in the evening
  - Renal dosage adjustment: Children 6 months to 11 years of age with renal impairment should not receive levocetirizine
- Adults:
  - 5 mg once daily in the evening
  - Renal dosage adjustment:
    - CrCl = 50–80 mL/min: 2.5 mg once daily
    - CrCl = 30–50 mL/min: 2.5 mg once every other day
    - CrCl = 10–30 mL/min: 2.5 mg twice weekly (administer once every 3 to 4 days)
    - CrCl < 10 mL/min: Do not use levocetirizine
    - Hemodialysis: Do not use levocetirizine

Adverse Reactions: Rare/Severe/Important

None

Major Drug Interactions

May have interactions similar to cetirizine

Counseling Point

May cause drowsiness or dizziness; observe caution when driving and avoid using with alcohol or other medications that cause sedation

Key Points

- Levocetirizine is the R-enantiomer of cetirizine
- Somnolence similar to cetirizine may occur
- Should be adjusted in renal impairment

◉ Cetirizine

Brand Names

Zyrtec, Zyrtec D 12 hour (5 mg cetirizine/120 mg pseudo-ephedrine), All Day Allergy

Generic Name

Cetirizine

OTC

Dosage Forms

Liquid gel capsule, tablet, syrup, chewable tablet

Pregnancy Category B

Dosing

- Children:
  - 6–12 months:
    - 2.5 mg once daily
    - Maximum dose: 2.5 mg once daily
  - 12–23 months:
    - 2.5 mg once daily
    - Maximum dose: 2.5 mg twice daily
  - 2–5 years:
    - 2.5 mg once daily
    - Maximum dose: 5 mg once daily *or* 2.5 mg twice daily
  - > 6 years:
    - 5–10 mg once daily
    - Maximum dose: 10 mg once daily
  - Renal dosage adjustment:
    - 6–11 years: < 2.5 mg once daily
    - ≥ 12 years:
      - CrCl = 11–31 mL/min or hemodialysis: 5 mg once daily
      - CrCl < 11 mL/min, not on dialysis: Cetirizine use not recommended
  - Hepatic dosage adjustment:
    - 6–11 years: < 2.5 mg once daily
    - ≥ 12 years: 5 mg once daily
- Adults:
  - 5–10 mg once daily
  - Maximum dose: 10 mg once daily
  - Renal dosage adjustment:
    - CrCl = 11–31 mL/min or hemodialysis: 5 mg once daily
    - CrCl < 11 mL/min, not on dialysis: Cetirizine use not recommended
  - Hepatic dosage adjustment: 5 mg once daily

Adverse Reactions: Rare/Severe/Important

None

Major Drug Interactions

Drug Affecting Cetirizine

- Ritonavir: May increase concentration and half-life
- Theophylline ≥ 400 mg: May decrease clearance
- Alcohol or CNS depressants: Avoid concomitant use; additional decrease in mental alertness may occur

Counseling Point

May cause drowsiness or dizziness; observe caution when driving or taking other medications that cause somnolence, avoid drinking alcohol while on this medication

Key Points

- Will cause more drowsiness compared with other agents in this class
- Available with pseudoephedrine for patients > 12 years of age

ANTITUSSIVE

Introduction

Antitussives are used in the treatment of nonproductive cough. Benzonatate is used for acute and chronic cough. Benzonatate is chemically related to anesthetic agents in the para-amino-benzoic acid class (e.g., procaine, tetracaine). Sedation and GI upset are the most common side effect seen with these agents. Benzonatate capsules should not be crushed or chewed.

Mechanism of Action for the Drug Class

Suppress cough through a peripheral action, anesthetizing the stretch or cough receptors of vagal afferent fibers. May suppress cough reflexes in the medulla by a central mechanism.

Members of the Drug Class

In this section: Benzonatate
Others: Carbetapentane (note that codeine, dextromethorphan, and hydrocodone are covered in the Combination Cough/Cold Products section)

◉ Benzonatate

Brand Name
Tessalon

Generic Name
Benzonatate

Rx Only

Dosage Form
Capsule

Usage
Symptomatic relief of nonproductive cough*

Pregnancy Category C

Dosing

- Adults and children > 10 years:
  - Usual dose (age > 10 years): 100–200 mg three times a day as needed
  - Maximum dose (age > 10 years): 600 mg every 24 hours

Adverse Reactions: Most Common

Sedation, GI upset, constipation, drowsiness, dizziness, headache, confusion

Adverse Reactions: Rare/Severe/Important

Oropharyngeal anesthesia if capsules are chewed or dissolved in mouth; burning sensation in eyes; hypersensitivity reactions (including bronchospasm, laryngospasm, cardiovascular collapse) related to local anesthesia from sucking or chewing the capsules; hallucinations

Contraindication

Patients with a history of a prior reaction to related anesthetic agents (e.g., tetracaine)

Major Drug Interactions

Drugs Affecting Benzonatate
Alcohol and CNS depressants: Potentiate drowsiness

Counseling Points

- Swallow whole; do not chew or dissolve capsule in mouth
- Report any persistent CNS changes or burning/numbness in mouth or chest to your healthcare provider

Key Points

- Most commonly used for cough
- Do not break or puncture capsule. Swallow whole.
- Patients should discontinue use if hallucinations or burning in chest occur.

BETA-2 AGONIST AND ANTICHOLINERGIC COMBINATION INHALER

Introduction

The primary use of these combination inhalers is for the chronic treatment of COPD when bronchospasms are still occurring despite treatment with a single bronchodilator. They also may be used for the treatment of bronchospasms or exacerbations associated with COPD and asthma. These agents can be used on a scheduled or on an as-needed basis, depending on the indication. The most common adverse events associated with these agents are dry mouth and nervousness. The Combivent brand product contains soya lecithin; patients with a history of soy or peanut allergy should avoid this product. The Combivent Respimat product does not contain soya lecithin.

Mechanism of Action for the Drug Class

The use of both drugs with different mechanisms of action may have a synergistic bronchodilator effect.

Anticholinergic Inhaler

The drug class appears to produce bronchodilation by blocking acetylcholine at muscarinic receptors, therefore blocking the direct constrictor effects of acetylcholine on bronchial smooth muscle. Ipratropium blocks all muscarinic receptors.

Beta-2 Agonist

Activation of the beta-2 receptors results in increases of cyclic AMP, which stimulates relaxation of the smooth airway. Beta-2 agonists also produce bronchodilation by inhibiting the release of inflammatory mediators from mast cells and preventing microvascular leakage into the bronchial mucosa.

Members of the Drug Class

In this section: Albuterol, ipratropium
Others: None

⊙ Albuterol and Ipratropium

Brand Names

Combivent, Combivent Respimat, DuoNeb

Generic Names

Albuterol and ipratropium

Rx Only

Dosage Forms

Metered-dose inhaler (MDI), solution for nebulization

Usage

Bronchospasms associated with COPD,* acute asthma exacerbations

Pregnancy Category C

Dosing

- Combivent:
  - 2 puffs inhaled orally four times a day; can be used on an as-needed basis
  - Maximum dose: 12 puffs every 24 hours
- Combivent Respimat:
  - 1 puff inhaled orally four times a day; can be used on an as-needed basis
  - Maximum dose: 6 puffs every 24 hours
- Solution for nebulization: 3 mL nebulized and inhaled orally every 4–6 hours

Adverse Reactions: Most Common

Dry mouth, cough, nervousness, respiratory tract infections, palpitations, tachycardia, tremor, headache, CNS stimulation

Adverse Reactions: Rare/Severe/Important

Hypokalemia, hypertension, worsening of narrow-angle glaucoma, mydriasis, increased intraocular pressure (especially if sprayed into eyes), worsening of urinary retention

Major Drug Interactions

Drugs Affecting Albuterol
None

Drugs Affecting Ipratropium
Other anticholinergics or drugs that have anticholinergic properties: May potentiate effects

Contraindication

Combivent: History of severe allergic reaction to soy or peanuts

Counseling Points

- Use proper administration technique:
  - Combivent:
    1. Shake inhaler for at least 10 seconds and remove the dust cap
    2. If this is the first time you are using the inhaler or if you have not used it for > 24 hours, shake the canister for 10 seconds and spray away from your eyes three times
    3. Exhale slowly and deeply
    4. Hold the inhaler upright and place the mouthpiece between your lips. Be careful not to block the opening with your tongue or teeth.
    5. Press down on the inhaler once as you start a slow, deep inhalation
    6. Continue to inhale slowly and deeply through your mouth. Try to inhale over at least 5 seconds.
    7. Hold your breath for 10 seconds or as long as you feel comfortable
    8. Exhale slowly
    9. Wait approximately 1–2 minutes before repeating steps 1–8 for the next inhalation
  - Combivent Respimat:
    1. Before using the inhaler for the first time, the Combivent Respimat cartridge must be inserted into the Combivent Respimat inhaler and then primed
    2. Priming is necessary when the inhaler is used for the first time or when the inhaler has not been used for > 3 days
       - When using the unit for the first time, actuate the inhaler toward the ground until an aerosol cloud is visible and then repeat the process three more times
       - If not used for > 3 days, actuate the inhaler once to prepare the inhaler for use
       - If not used > 21 days, actuate the inhaler until an aerosol cloud is visible and then repeat the process three more times to prepare the inhaler for use
    3. Hold the Combivent Respimat inhaler upright with the orange cap closed to avoid accidental release of dose
    4. Turn the clear base in the direction of the white arrows on the label until it clicks (half a

turn) and flip the orange cap until it snaps fully open

5. Breathe out slowly and fully and then close your lips around the end of the mouthpiece without covering the air vents. Point the Combivent Respimat inhaler to the back of your throat.

6. While taking in a slow, deep breath through your mouth, press the dose release button and continue to breathe in slowly for as long as you can. Hold your breath for 10 seconds or for as long as comfortable.

7. Close the orange cap until you use your iCombivent Respimat inhaler again.

- If using more than the prescribed amount, contact your healthcare provider

- Avoid contact with eyes
- Use with the proper spacing device
- Protect the nebulization solution from light

Key Points
- Commonly used in COPD
- Most common adverse effects are dry mouth and nervousness
- Use with caution in patients with glaucoma or urinary retention
- Combivent Respimat does not contain soya lecithin. Use the Combivent product with caution in patients with soy or peanut allergy.
- Usage instructions differ depending on the brand

BETA-2 AGONIST AND CORTICOSTEROID COMBINATION INHALER

Introduction

Beta-2 agonist/corticosteroid inhaler combinations are used for the chronic treatment of asthma and severe or very severe COPD. Different strengths of corticosteroids are available depending on the patient's asthma severity. It is important to counsel patients on the proper use of the inhaler and to rinse their mouth with water after each use. Patients should also be informed that these inhalers should not be used to treat acute bronchospasm or shortness of breath and that these agents need to be used regularly to achieve maximal effect. Coughing, dry mouth, and oral candidiasis are the most common adverse effects seen with these agents.

Mechanism of Action for the Drug Class

Beta-2 Agonist

Activation of the beta-2 receptors results in increases of cyclic AMP, which stimulates relaxation of the smooth airway. Beta-2 agonists also produce bronchodilation by inhibiting the release of inflammatory mediators from mast cells and preventing microvascular leakage into the bronchial mucosa.

Inhaled Corticosteroids

Inhaled corticosteroids do not directly affect airway smooth muscle. Inhaled corticosteroids decrease the number of inflammatory cells (basophils, mast cells, neutrophils, eosinophils, macrophages, and lymphocytes) and inflammatory mediators (histamines, leukotrienes, and cytokines), leading to decreased airway edema and hyperresponsiveness of smooth muscle. Steroids also inhibit mucus secretion in the airways.

Usage for the Drug Class
Chronic treatment of asthma,* COPD*

Adverse Reactions for the Drug Class: Most Common
Hoarseness, pharyngitis, dry mouth, coughing, headache, hypokalemia, oral candidiasis, palpitations, tachycardia, tremor

Adverse Reactions for the Drug Class: Rare/Severe/Important
Adrenal insufficiency, upper respiratory tract infections, pneumonia, decreases in bone mineral density, possible asthma-related death

Counseling Points for the Drug Class
- Rinse mouth out with water after each use
- Use every day
- Do not use for acute attacks. You must have a rescue inhaler available for breakthrough attacks.
- Use proper administration technique
- Do not discontinue abruptly

Key Points for the Drug Class
- Used in the chronic treatment of COPD and asthma
- Should not be used for treatment of exacerbations
- Use as prescribed to see maximal benefit
- It may take 1–4 weeks to see maximal benefit
- Rinse mouth out with each use to avoid oral candidiasis

Members of the Drug Class

In this section: Fluticasone and salmeterol, budesonide and formoterol
Others: Mometasone and formoterol

◉ Fluticasone and Salmeterol

Brand Names

Advair, Advair HFA

Generic Name

Fluticasone and salmeterol

Rx Only

Dosage Forms

Powder for inhalation via Diskus inhaler, CFC-free inhalation aerosol

Pregnancy Category C

Dosing

- Diskus:
  - Children, asthma:
    - 4–11 years: Initial dose is fluticasone 100 µg/salmeterol 50 µg, 1 puff inhaled orally every 12 hours (this is maximum dose)
    - > 12 years: Initial dose is fluticasone 100 µg/salmeterol 50 µg, 1 puff inhaled orally every 12 hours
  - Adults:
    - Asthma:
      - Initial dose: Fluticasone 100 µg/salmeterol 50 µg, 1 puff inhaled orally every 12 hours
      - Dosage adjustment: Titrate to the most effective dose that controls symptoms
      - Maximum dose: Fluticasone 500 µg/salmeterol 50 µg (2 inhalations daily)
    - COPD: Fluticasone 250 µg/salmeterol 50 µg, 1 puff inhaled orally every 12 hours (this is also the maximum dose in COPD)
- Inhalation aerosol:
  - 2 puffs inhaled orally every 12 hours
  - Maximum dose: Fluticasone 230 µg/salmeterol 21 µg per inhalation (4 inhalations/day)

Major Drug Interactions

Drugs Affecting Fluticasone

- Ketoconazole or CYP3A4 inhibitors: Increase levels (clinical effect unknown)
- Protease inhibitors: Decrease metabolism; reports of Cushing's syndrome developing from this combination have been found in the literature

Drugs Affecting Salmeterol

Inducers or inhibitors of CYP3A4: Affect salmeterol concentrations

Contraindication

Advair Diskus contains lactose. Avoid use in patients with severe hypersensitivity to milk proteins.

Counseling Points

- The dose indicator tells you how many doses are left
- Use proper administration technique:
  - Diskus:
    1. Activate the dry powder inhaler by sliding the activator. Every time the lever is pushed back, a dose is ready to be inhaled. Do not close or tilt the diskus after the lever is pushed back.
    2. Breathe out deeply
    3. Inhale the powder contents completely
  - Inhalation aerosol:
    1. Shake well for 5 seconds before each spray. Prime with 4 test sprays (into air and away from face) before using for the first time. If canister is dropped or not used for > 4 weeks, prime with 2 sprays.
    2. Take the cap off the mouthpiece and shake the inhaler for 5 seconds
    3. Put the mouthpiece in your mouth and seal lips around it
    4. Push the top of the canister all the way down while you breathe in deeply and slowly through your mouth. Hold your breath for 10 seconds or as long as you can.
    5. Wait 30 seconds, shake inhaler for 5 seconds again, and repeat steps 3 and 4

◉ Budesonide and Formoterol

Brand Name

Symbicort

Generic Name

Budesonide and formoterol

Rx Only

Dosage Form

Metered-dose inhaler (MDI)

Pregnancy Category C

Dosing

Children > 12 years and adults:

- Two inhalations by mouth twice daily
- Maximum dose: 4 inhalations/day

Major Drug Interactions

Drugs Affecting Budesonide

CYP3A4 inhibitors: May potentiate adverse effects

Counseling Point

Counsel on proper inhalation technique. Prior to first use the inhaler must be primed by releasing 2 test sprays into the air; shake well for 5 seconds before each spray. Inhaler must be reprimed if not used for > 7 days or if it has been dropped. Shake well for 5 seconds before each use.

BETA-2 AGONISTS, INHALED

Introduction

The inhaled beta-2 agonists are primarily used for the treatment and prevention of bronchospasms in patients with obstructive airway disease. They can be used chronically or in the treatment of an exacerbation of the disease. Short-acting beta-2 agonists are commonly used on an as-needed basis for shortness of breath. The inhaled preparation of albuterol is used more commonly than the systemic preparations. The tablets and syrup are associated with an increased frequency of adverse reactions and are no longer recommended for the treatment of asthma. Long-acting agents should only be used twice daily and not on an as-needed basis. Patients should be counseled on the proper use of these medications. The most common adverse reactions are palpitations, tachycardia, and tremor. Adverse reactions are more common with the short-acting beta-2 agonists than with the long-acting agents.

Mechanism of Action for the Drug Class

Activation of the beta-2 receptors results in increases of cyclic AMP, which stimulates relaxation of the smooth airway. Beta-2 agonists also produce bronchodilation by inhibiting the release of inflammatory mediators from mast cells and preventing microvascular leakage into the bronchial mucosa.

Adverse Reactions for the Drug Class: Most Common

Nervousness, palpitations, tachycardia, tremor, headache, CNS stimulation

Adverse Reactions for the Drug Class: Rare/Severe/Important

Paradoxical bronchospasms, hyperglycemia, hypokalemia, hypertension; use caution in patients with cardiac arrhythmias, uncontrolled hypertension, uncontrolled hyperthyroidism, or diagnosed or suspected pheochromocytoma because these agents may exacerbate the condition

Major Drug Interactions for the Drug Class

Drugs Affecting Beta-Agonists

Nonselective beta blockers (ophthalmic and systemic): May blunt the bronchodilating effects of albuterol

Beta-Agonists' Effect on Other Drugs
None

Members of the Drug Class

In this section: Albuterol, formoterol, levalbuterol, salmeterol
Others: Arformoterol, indacaterol, metaproterenol, pirbuterol, terbutaline

◉ Albuterol

Brand Names
Ventolin HFA, Proventil HFA, ProAir HFA

Generic Name
Albuterol

Rx Only

Dosage Forms
HFA inhaler, nebulizer solution, tablet, extended-release tablet, syrup

Usage
Relief and prevention of bronchospasm associated with asthma and COPD,* acute attacks of bronchospasm, exercise-induced bronchospasm,* treatment of acute hyperkalemia

Pregnancy Category C

Dosing

- Relief and prevention of bronchospasm:
  - HFA: Children age > 4 years and adults should take 2 puffs inhaled orally every 4–6 hours as needed
  - Nebulizer solution:
    - Children:
      - 2–12 years: 0.63–1.25 mg inhaled via nebulizer every 4–6 hours as needed (up to 2.5 mg/dose has been used)
      - > 12 years: See adult dosing
    - Adults: 1.25–2.5 mg inhaled via nebulizer every 4–8 hours as needed (up to 5 mg/dose has been used)
  - Oral tablets, syrup:
    - Children:
      - 2–6 years:
        - 0.1–0.2 mg/kg/dose every 8 hours
        - Maximum dose: 12 mg every 24 hours
      - 6–12 years:
        - 2 mg orally every 6–8 hours
        - Maximum dose: 24 mg every 24 hours
      - > 12 years: See adult dosing
    - Adults:
      - 2–4 mg orally every 6–8 hours
      - Maximum dose: 32 mg every 24 hours
  - Extended-release tablets:
    - Children:
      - 6–12 years:
        - 4 mg orally every 12 hours
        - Maximum dose: 24 mg every 24 hours
      - > 12 years: See adult dosing
    - Adults:
      - 4–8 mg orally every 12 hours
      - Maximum dose: 32 mg/24 hours
- Exercised-induced asthma: Usual MDI dose for age > 4 years and adults is 2 puffs inhaled orally 15–30 minutes before exercise

Counseling Points

- Use proper administration technique:
  1. Shake the inhaler well immediately before each use. Then remove the cap from the mouthpiece.
  2. Prime the inhaler before using it for the first time and when the inhaler has not been used for > 2 weeks. Prime by releasing 4 sprays into the air, away from your face.
  3. Breathe out fully from your mouth, expelling as much air from your lungs as possible. Place the mouthpiece fully into the mouth, holding the inhaler in its upright position and closing the lips around it.
  4. While breathing in deeply and slowly through the mouth, press the top of the metal canister with your index finger.
  5. Hold your breath as long as possible, up to 10 seconds. Before breathing out, remove the inhaler from your mouth and release your finger from the canister.
  6. If your physician has prescribed additional puffs, wait 1 minute, shake the inhaler again, and repeat steps 3–5. Replace the cap after use.
- If using more than the prescribed amount, contact your healthcare provider
- If using more than two times a week and not on any anti-inflammatory inhalers, check with your healthcare provider
- Swallow extended-release tablets whole; do not crush or chew

Key Points

- Albuterol is a short-acting beta-2 selective agonist
- The inhaled dosage forms are the most commonly recommended
- Oral tablets and syrup are not recommended for the immediate relief of bronchospasms or for the chronic treatment of asthma
- Use with caution in patients with cardiac arrhythmias, uncontrolled hypertension, uncontrolled hyperthyroidism, or diagnosed or suspected pheochromocytoma

◉ Formoterol

Brand Names

Foradil, Perforomist Solution for Nebulization

Generic Name

Formoterol

Rx Only

Dosage Forms

Powder for oral inhalation, solution for nebulization

Mechanism of Action

Formoterol is a long-acting beta-2 selective agonist that causes relaxation of bronchial smooth muscle

Usage

Chronic maintenance of asthma,* maintenance treatment of COPD,* prevention of exercise-induced bronchospasm

Pregnancy Category C

Dosing

- Asthma and COPD:
  - Oral powder for inhalation: 12 µg capsule inhaled by mouth twice daily
  - Solution for nebulization: 20 µg inhaled twice daily
- Exercise-induced asthma: 12 µg capsule inhaled by mouth 30 minutes before exercise

Adverse Reactions: Rare/Severe/Important

May increase the risk of asthma-related deaths

Contraindications

Use as monotherapy in asthma, history of severe allergic reaction to milk proteins (formulation contains lactose)

Counseling Points

- Capsules should be inhaled, not swallowed
- Do not use for acute attacks
- Do not use more frequently than the recommended dose
- Use the Aerolizer inhaler properly:
  1. Remove capsule from foil blister immediately before use.
  2. Place capsule in the capsule chamber in the base of the Aerolizer Inhaler.
  3. Press both buttons once only and then release. Keep inhaler in a level, horizontal position. Exhale fully. Do not exhale into the inhaler.
  4. Inhale quickly and deeply. Hold your breath for as long as possible. If any powder remains in capsule, exhale and inhale again. Repeat until capsule is empty. Throw away the empty capsule; do not leave it in inhaler.
- Do not use a spacer with the Aerolizer Inhaler

Key Points

- Formoterol is a long-acting beta-2 agonist
- It should only be used in combination with inhaled corticosteroids in asthma
- Patients should be counseled on proper administration technique
- The capsule should be inhaled only; do not swallow
- Adverse effects are minimal compared with short-acting beta-2 agonists

◉ Levalbuterol

Brand Names

Xopenex, Xopenex HFA

Generic Name

Levalbuterol

Rx Only

Dosage Forms

Metered dose inhaler (MDI), solution for nebulization

Usage

Treatment of bronchospasms in children and adults with asthma and adults with COPD*

Pregnancy Category C

Dosing

- HFA: Children age > 4 years and adults should take 2 puffs inhaled by mouth every 4–6 hours
- Solution for nebulization:
  - Children:
    - ≤ 4 years: 0.31–1.25 mg inhaled by nebulizer every 4–6 hours as needed
    - 5–11 years: 0.31–0.63 mg inhaled via nebulizer every 8 hours as needed
    - ≥ 12 years: 0.63–1.25 mg inhaled via nebulizer every 8 hours as needed
  - Adults: 0.63–1.25 mg inhaled via nebulizer every 8 hours as needed
- *Note:* May use higher doses in patients with asthma and COPD exacerbations

Counseling Points

- Use proper administration technique:
  1. Shake the inhaler well immediately before each use. Then remove the cap from the mouthpiece.
  2. Prime the inhaler before using it for the first time and when the inhaler has not been used for > 2 weeks. Prime by releasing 4 sprays into the air, away from your face.
  3. Breathe out fully from your mouth, expelling as much air from your lungs as possible. Place the mouthpiece fully into the mouth, holding the inhaler in its upright position and closing the lips around it.
  4. While breathing in deeply and slowly through the mouth, press the top of the metal canister with your index finger.
  5. Hold your breath as long as possible, up to 10 seconds. Before breathing out, remove the inhaler from your mouth and release your finger from the canister.
  6. If your physician has prescribed additional puffs, wait 1 minute, shake the inhaler again, and repeat steps 3–5. Replace the cap after use.
- If using more than the prescribed amount, contact your healthcare provider
- If using more than two times a week and not on any anti-inflammatory inhalers, check with your healthcare provider

Key Points

- Levalbuterol is the active R-isomer of albuterol
- Levalbuterol is a short-acting beta-2 agonist used to treat bronchospasms
- Ensure proper administration of the inhaler or procedure for nebulization
- Levalbuterol is thought to have fewer adverse reactions compared with albuterol, but this has not been proven in clinical studies
- Levalbuterol is commonly used in children due to the belief that there are fewer adverse reactions associated with its use

◉ Salmeterol

Brand Name

Serevent Diskus

Generic Name

Salmeterol

Rx Only

Dosage Forms

Powder for inhalation

Mechanism of Action

Salmeterol is a long-acting beta-2 agonist that produces bronchodilation by relaxing smooth muscles of the bronchioles

Usage

Chronic maintenance of asthma,* maintenance treatment of COPD,* prevention of exercise-induced bronchospasm

Pregnancy Category C

Dosing

- Asthma and COPD: 1 inhalation twice daily (morning and evening)
- Exercise-induced asthma: 1 inhalation 30 minutes before exercise

Adverse Reactions: Rare/Severe/Important

Anaphylaxis due to lactose component in oral inhalation powder may increase the risk of asthma-related deaths

Major Drug Interactions

Drugs Affecting Salmeterol

Inducers or inhibitors of CYP3A4: Affect salmeterol concentrations

Contraindications

Use as monotherapy in asthma, history of a severe allergic reaction to milk proteins (formulation contains lactose)

COMBINATION COLD AND COUGH PRODUCTS

Introduction

Combination cold and cough products contain guaifenesin, which acts as an expectorant, or an antihistamine, which alleviates upper respiratory cold symptoms, and a narcotic or narcotic derivative as a cough suppressant. These agents should be used short term to treat symptoms of a cough and cold. The preparations containing narcotics are scheduled controlled substances and have abuse potential. The most common adverse effect of these agents is sedation. Cough and cold preparations are no longer recommended in children < 2 years of age due to the potential for dosing errors. There is no evidence that cough-suppressant therapy can prevent coughing. These drugs do not resolve the underlying pathophysiology that is responsible for the coughing. In patients with cough due to upper respiratory infection, cough suppressants have limited efficacy and are not recommended for this use. In patients with chronic bronchitis, cough suppressants such as codeine and dextromethorphan are recommended for the short-term symptomatic relief of coughing. In patients with acute cough due to the common cold, OTC combination cold medications, with the exception of older antihistamine–decongestants, are not recommended due to the lack of supportive evidence. Expectorants have not been consistently shown to be effective either.

Members of the Drug Class

In this section: Guaifenesin and codeine, guaifenesin with dextromethorphan, hydrocodone and chlorpheniramine, promethazine with codeine,
Others: Benzonatate (covered in an earlier section), carbetapentane

◉ Guaifenesin and Codeine

Brand Names
Robitussin AC, Guaiatussin AC (multiple)

Generic Name
Guaifenesin and codeine

Rx Only
Schedule V (capsules, liquid) and Schedule III (tablet) controlled substance

Dosage Forms
Liquid, capsule, tablet

Mechanism of Action
Guaifenesin enhances the removal of mucus by decreasing its viscosity and surface tension. Codeine has a central mechanism of action on opioid receptors in the medullary cough center and may also have additional peripheral action on cough receptors in the proximal airways.

Usage
Temporary relief of cough and chest congestion*

Pregnancy Category C
Some liquid preparations may contain alcohol and can be teratogenic if consumed in large quantities during pregnancy

Dosing
- Children:
    - 6–11 years:
        - Guaifenesin 100–200 mg and codeine 5–10 mg every 4–6 hours as needed for cough
        - Maximum dose: Guaifenesin 1,200 mg/day and codeine 60 mg/day
    - ≥ 12 years: See adult dosing
- Adults:
    - Guaifenesin 200–400 mg and codeine 10–20 mg every 4–6 hours as needed for cough
    - Maximum dose: Guaifenesin 2,400 mg/day and codeine 120 mg/day

Adverse Reactions: Most Common
CNS depression, constipation, headache, respiratory depression, urinary retention

Adverse Reactions: Rare/Severe/Important

Excessive sedation, respiratory depression (codeine), urolithiasis

Major Drug Interactions

Drugs Affecting Guaifenesin with Codeine

- CNS depressants: May enhance the effect and increase adverse reactions
- CYP2D6 inhibitors: May decrease the effects of codeine by preventing the formation of its active metabolite

Counseling Points

- Avoid alcohol, which may increase the sedative effects
- Follow each dose with a full glass of water
- Sugar-free formulations are available

Key Points

- Schedule V controlled substance
- Using more than the recommended amount can cause CNS depressant effects and respiratory depression
- Should be administered under close supervision to individuals with a history of drug abuse or dependence
- Commonly used for cough

◉ Guaifenesin with Dextromethorphan

Brand Names

Mucinex DM, Coricidin HBP Chest Congestion and Cough, Vicks 44E, Robitussin Peak Cold Cough + Chest Congestion DM (multiple brands available)

Generic Name

Guaifenesin with dextromethorphan

OTC

Dosage Forms

Liquid, tablet, capsule, extended-release tablet

Mechanism of Action

Guaifenesin enhances the removal of mucus by decreasing its viscosity and surface tension. Dextromethorphan is the D-isomer of the codeine analog methorphan and has no analgesic or addictive properties. Dextromethorphan depresses the cough center in the medulla.

Usage

Temporary relief of cough and chest congestion*

Pregnancy Category C

Some liquid preparations may contain alcohol and can be teratogenic if consumed in large quantities during pregnancy

Dosing

- Guaifenesin 200–400 mg and dextromethorphan 10–20 mg every 4–6 hours as needed
- Maximum dose: Guaifenesin 2,400 mg and dextromethorphan 120 mg over 24 hours

Adverse Reactions: Most Common

Drowsiness, dizziness, headache, lightheadedness, confusion

Adverse Reactions: Rare/Severe/Important

None

Major Drug Interactions

Drugs Affecting Guaifenesin with Dextromethorphan

MAOIs and other serotonin modulators: May cause hypertension, hyperpyrexia, agitation, confusion, hallucinations (serotonin syndrome)

Contraindication

Use with or within 14 days of an MAOI

Counseling Points

- Follow each dose with a full glass of water
- Do not crush or chew extended-release preparations
- May cause sedation
- Do not take more than prescribed or indicated on product labeling

Key Points

- Multiple dosage forms and strengths available
- Available OTC
- May cause drowsiness and sedation
- Sugar-free formulations are available

◉ Hydrocodone and Chlorpheniramine

Brand Names

Tussionex, TussiCaps

Generic Name

Hydrocodone and chlorpheniramine

Rx Only

Schedule III controlled substance

Dosage Forms

Liquid, capsule

Mechanism of Action

Chlorpheniramine reversibly, competitively antagonizes H1 receptors peripherally. Hydrocodone depresses the cough center in the medulla.

Usage

Temporary relief of cough associated with allergy or a cold*

Pregnancy Category C

Dosing

- Children:
  - 6–12 years:
    - Capsule (5 mg/4 mg):
      - 1 capsule every 12 hours
      - Maximum dose: 2 capsules every 24 hours
    - Liquid:
      - 2.5 mL every 12 hours
      - Maximum dose: 5 mL every 24 hours
  - ≥ 12 years: See adult dosing
- Adults:
  - Capsule (10 mg/8 mg):
    - 1 capsule every 12 hours
    - Maximum dose: 2 capsules every 24 hours
  - Liquid:
    - 5 mL every 12 hours
    - Maximum dose: 10 mL every 24 hours

Adverse Reactions: Most Common

Drowsiness, constipation, dry mouth, headache, fatigue, dizziness, nausea

Adverse Reactions: Rare/Severe/Important

Physical dependence (hydrocodone component), respiratory depression (hydrocodone component)

Major Drug Interactions

Drugs Affecting Hydrocodone and Chlorpheniramine

Alcohol and CNS depressants: Potentiate drowsiness; other anticholinergic drugs potentiate side effects

Contraindication

Children < 6 years of age

Counseling Points

- Shake suspension well before using
- May cause drowsiness; use caution when driving
- Take only as prescribed

Key Points

- Schedule III controlled substance
- Should be administered under close supervision to individuals with a history of drug abuse or dependence

◉ Promethazine with Codeine

Brand Name
Phenergan with Codeine

Generic Name
Promethazine with codeine

Rx Only
Schedule V controlled substance

Dosage Form
Liquid

Mechanism of Action

Promethazine reversibly, competitively antagonizes H1 receptors peripherally. Codeine depresses the cough center in the medulla.

Usage

Temporary relief of cough and upper respiratory symptoms due to allergy and common cold*

Pregnancy Category C

Dosing

- Children:
  - 6–11 years:
    - 2.5–5 mL every 4–6 hours
    - Maximum dose: 30 mL every 24 hours
  - ≥ 12 years: See adult dosing
- Adults:
  - 5 mL every 4–6 hours
  - Maximum dose: 30 mL in 24 hours
- Renal dosage adjustment: Reduce dose in cases of renal impairment
- Hepatic dosage adjustment: Reduce dose in cases of hepatic impairment

Adverse Reactions: Most Common

Drowsiness, blurred vision, constipation, dry mouth, headache, fatigue, dizziness, nausea, photosensitivity (also see promethazine)

Adverse Reactions: Rare/Severe/Important

Physical dependence (codeine component), respiratory depression (codeine component) (also see promethazine)

Major Drug Interactions

Drugs Affecting Promethazine with Codeine

- Alcohol and CNS depressants: Potentiate drowsiness
- Other anticholinergic drugs: Potentiate side effects

Contraindication

Children < 6 years of age

Counseling Points

- May cause drowsiness; exercise caution when driving
- Take with food to reduce GI upset
- Avoid prolonged exposure to sunlight
- Take only as prescribed

Key Points

- Schedule V controlled substance
- Should be administered under close supervision to individuals with a history of drug abuse or dependence
- Use in children < 6 years of age is contraindicated due to risk of respiratory depression
- Not recommended for use in patients with chronic respiratory disease

CORTICOSTEROIDS, INHALED

Introduction

Inhaled corticosteroids are used for the chronic treatment of asthma. Their exact mechanism of action is unknown, but they are thought to decrease inflammatory cells and cause smooth muscle relaxation. The lowest possible dose should be used to avoid adverse reactions. The most common adverse reactions include hoarseness, dry mouth, and oral candidiasis. Patients should be counseled on the proper use of the inhalation devices, to rinse out their mouth after each use, and to use as directed. They should not be used as rescue inhalers.

Mechanism of Action for the Drug Class

Inhaled corticosteroids do not directly affect airway smooth muscle. Inhaled corticosteroids decrease the number of inflammatory cells (basophils, mast cells, neutrophils, eosinophils, macrophages, and lymphocytes) and inflammatory mediators (histamines, leukotrienes, cytokines), leading to decreased airway edema and hyperresponsiveness of smooth muscle. Steroids also inhibit mucus secretion in the airways.

Usage for the Drug Class

Chronic maintenance of asthma,* COPD

Rx Only for the Drug Class

Adverse Reactions for the Drug Class: Most Common

Hoarseness, pharyngitis, dry mouth, coughing, headache, oral candidiasis

Adverse Reactions for the Drug Class: Rare/Severe/Important

Adrenal insufficiency, growth suppression in children, cataracts, respiratory infection

Counseling Points for the Drug Class

- Rinse mouth with water after each use to prevent oral thrush
- It may take 1–4 weeks to see maximal benefit
- Use every day
- Do not use for acute attacks
- You must have a rescue inhaler available for breakthrough attacks
- Learn the proper administration technique for each inhalation device

Key Points for the Drug Class

- Used in the chronic treatment of asthma
- Should not be used for treatment of exacerbations
- It may take 1–4 weeks to see maximal benefit
- Rinse mouth after each use
- Fluticasone and budesonide should be avoided with CYP3A4 inhibitors, specifically protease inhibitors. Cushing's syndrome has been reported with concomitant use of these agents.

Members of the Drug Class

In this section: Beclomethasone, budesonide, fluticasone
Others: Ciclesonide, mometasone

◉ Beclomethasone

Brand Names

QVAR 40, QVAR 80

Generic Name

Beclomethasone

Dosage Forms

Metered-dose inhaler (MDI)

Pregnancy Category C

Dosing

- Children:
  - 5–11 years:
    - Usual daily dose: 40 µg inhaled by mouth twice daily
    - Maximum dose: 80 µg inhaled by mouth twice daily
  - ≥ 12 years: See adult dosing
- Adults:
  - Previous therapy of bronchodilators only:
    - Initial dose: 40–80 µg twice daily
    - Maximum dose: 320 µg twice day
  - Previous therapy of inhaled corticosteroids:
    - Initial dose: 40–160 µg twice daily
    - Maximum dose: 320 µg twice daily
  - Low dose: 40–120 µg inhaled twice daily
  - Medium dose: 120–240 µg inhaled twice daily
  - High dose: > 240 µg inhaled twice daily

Major Drug Interactions

None

Counseling Point

It is recommended to prime the QVAR inhaler before first use and when the inhaler has not been used for > 10 days. Prime by releasing two actuations into the air, away from your eyes and face.

◉ Budesonide

Brand Names

Pulmicort Flexhaler, Pulmicort Respules

Generic Name

Budesonide

Dosage Forms

Powder for oral inhalation (Flexhaler), suspension for nebulization (Pulmicort Respules)

Pregnancy Category B

Dosing

- Powder for oral inhalation (Flexhaler):
  - Children ages 6–17 years:
    - Initial dose: 180 µg twice daily (some patients may be initiated at 360 µg twice daily)
    - Maximum dose: 360 µg twice daily
    - Low dose: 90–200 µg inhaled twice daily
    - Medium dose: 200–400 µg inhaled twice daily
    - High dose: > 400 µg inhaled twice daily
  - Adults:
    - Initial dose: 360 µg twice daily (selected patients may be initiated at 180 µg twice daily)
    - Maximum dose: 720 µg twice daily
    - Low dose: 60–300 µg inhaled twice daily
    - Medium dose: 300–600 µg inhaled twice daily
    - High dose: > 600 µg inhaled twice daily
- Suspension for nebulization:
  - Children 12 months to 8 years:
    - Initial dose: 0.25 mg/day
    - Previous therapy of bronchodilators alone: 0.5 mg/day administered as a single dose or divided twice daily, up to a maximum daily dose of 0.5 mg
    - Previous therapy of inhaled corticosteroids: 0.5 mg/day administered as a single dose or divided twice daily, up to a maximum daily dose of 1 mg
    - Previous therapy of oral corticosteroids: 1 mg/day administered as a single dose or divided twice daily, up to a maximum daily dose of 1 mg

Contraindication

Severe hypersensitivity to milk proteins (Flexhaler)

Major Drug Interactions

Drugs Affecting Budesonide

CYP3A4 inhibitors: May potentiate adverse effects

Counseling Points

- Ensure proper use of the Flexhaler:
  1. Prime the inhaler before first use (you do not have to prime the inhaler ever again). Take off the cover, hold the inhaler in the middle, and twist the brown grip one way all the way it will go and then twist in the opposite direction (you will hear a click). Repeat.
  2. Load the dose. Take off the cover, hold the inhaler in the middle, and twist the brown grip one way all the way it will go and then twist in the opposite direction (you will hear a click).
  3. Inhale the dose. Exhale away from the inhaler (do not blow into the mouthpiece), place the mouthpiece to the mouth, and seal your lips around the mouthpiece. Inhale as deeply as possible. When inhale is complete, place the cover back on the inhaler.

- Do not immerse the inhaler in water. Wipe outside of inhaler with a dry tissue once weekly.
- Use Pulmicort Respules only with a jet nebulizer; do not mix with other inhaled medications in the nebulizer

◉ Fluticasone

Brand Names

Flovent HFA, Flovent Diskus

Generic Name

Fluticasone

Dosage Forms

Metered-dose inhaler (MDI) HFA, powder for oral inhalation (Flovent Diskus)

Pregnancy Category C

Dosing

- HFA/MDI:
  - Children:
    - 0–4 years:
      - Low dose: 88 µg inhaled twice daily
      - Medium dose: 88–176 µg inhaled twice daily
      - High dose: > 176 µg inhaled twice daily
    - 5–11 years:
      - Initial dose: 50 µg inhaled twice daily
      - Maximum dose: 100 µg inhaled twice daily
      - Low dose: 44–88 µg inhaled twice daily
      - Medium dose: 88–176 µg inhaled twice daily
      - High dose: > 176 µg inhaled twice daily
    - > 12 years: See adult dosing
  - Adults:
    - Previous therapy of bronchodilator alone:
      - Initial dose: 88 µg twice daily
      - Maximum dose: 440 µg twice daily
    - Previous therapy of inhaled corticosteroids:
      - Initial dose: 88–220 µg twice daily
      - Maximum dose: 440 µg twice daily
    - Previous therapy of oral corticosteroids (OCS):
      - Initial dose: 440 µg twice daily
      - Maximum dose: 880 µg twice daily
    - Low dose: 44–132 µg inhaled twice daily
    - Medium dose: 132–220 µg inhaled twice daily
    - High dose: > 220 µg inhaled twice daily
- Diskus:
  - Children:
    - 4–11 years:
      - Initial dose: 50 µg twice daily, up to a maximum of 100 µg twice daily
      - Low dose: 50–100 µg inhaled twice daily
      - Medium dose: 100–200 µg inhaled twice daily
      - High dose: > 200 µg inhaled twice daily
    - > 12 years: See adult dosing

- Adults:
  - Previous therapy of bronchodilator only:
    - Initial dose: 100 µg twice daily
    - Maximum dose: 500 µg twice daily
  - Previous therapy of inhaled corticosteroids:
    - Initial dose: 100–250 µg twice daily
    - Maximum dose: 500 µg twice daily
  - Previous therapy of oral corticosteroids:
    - Initial dose: 500–1,000 µg twice daily
    - Maximum dose: 1,000 µg twice daily
  - Low dose: 50–150 µg inhaled twice daily
  - Medium dose: 150–250 µg inhaled twice daily
  - High dose: > 250 µg inhaled twice daily

Major Drug Interactions

Drugs Affecting Fluticasone

- Ketoconazole or CYP3A4 inhibitors: Increase levels (clinical effect unknown)
- Protease inhibitors: Decrease metabolism; reports of Cushing's syndrome developing from this combination have been found in the literature

Counseling Points

- Aerosol inhalation: Flovent HFA must be primed before first use, when not used for 7 days or more, or if dropped. To prime the first time, release 4 sprays into the air. Shake well before each spray and spray away from face. If dropped or not used for 7 days or more, prime by releasing a single test spray. See the albuterol HFA for instructions on use.
- Flovent Diskus: Do not use with a spacer device. Do not exhale into the Diskus. Do not wash or take apart. Use in horizontal position. See Fluticasone/Salmeterol Diskus for instructions on use.

Key Points

- Instruct on proper use of inhalation device
- Dosage varies based on inhalation device
- Commonly used with asthma
- Monitor for drug interactions with CYP3A4 inhibitors and inducers. Drug therapy may need to be adjusted in patients with some drug interactions.

CORTICOSTEROIDS, INTRANASAL

Introduction

Intranasal corticosteroids are primarily used for rhinitis and occasionally for the prevention of nasal polyps. The maximal benefit of these agents may not be seen for 1–2 weeks. The most common adverse reactions include epistaxis and nasal irritation. All patients should be counseled on the proper administration technique of intranasal products and instructed to blow their nose before use.

Mechanism of Action for the Drug Class

Corticosteroids may decrease the number of inflammatory mediators. They may also reverse dilatation and increase vessel permeability in the area, resulting in decreased entry of cells to the sites of damage.

Usage for the Drug Class

Relief of symptoms of seasonal and perennial allergic rhinitis,* nonallergic rhinitis, prevention of nasal polyps, adjunct to antibiotics in the treatment of sinusitis

Rx Only for the Drug Class

Adverse Reactions for the Drug Class: Most Common

Headache, dizziness, epistaxis, throat discomfort, nasal irritation

Adverse Reactions for the Drug Class: Rare/Severe/Important

Nasal ulcerations, nasal candida infections, nasal septum perforations, glaucoma/cataracts

Major Drug Interactions for the Drug Class

None

Counseling Points for the Drug Class

- Blow your nose before each use
- Insert the applicator into the nostril. Keeping the bottle upright, tilt your head forward slightly and close off the other nostril. Breathe in through the nose. While inhaling, press pump to release spray. Do not spray directly onto the wall between the two nostrils (the septum).
- Avoid blowing your nose for 10–15 minutes after use
- Intranasal corticosteroids do not provide immediate relief of nasal symptoms. It may take 1–2 weeks to see maximal benefit.

Key Points for the Drug Class

- Most commonly used for seasonal and allergic rhinitis
- Do not provide immediate relief of symptoms
- Administer by nasal inhalation only
- Caution spraying into eyes

Members of the Drug Class

In this section: Beclomethasone, budesonide, fluticasone, mometasone, triamcinolone
Others: Ciclesonide, flunisolide

◉ Beclomethasone

Brand Names
Beconase AQ, Qnasl

Generic Name
Beclomethasone

Dosage Forms
Nasal inhalation

Pregnancy Category C

Dosing
- Children:
  - 6–12 years:
    - Beconase AQ: 1 spray into each nostril twice daily
    - Maximum dose: 8 sprays every 24 hours
  - > 12 years: See adult dosing.
- Adults:
  - Beconase AQ:
    - Initial dose: 1–2 sprays into each nostril twice daily
    - Maximum dose: 8 sprays every 24 hours
  - Qnasl:
    - Initial dose: 2 sprays in each nostril once daily
    - Maximum dose: 4 sprays every 24 hours

Counseling Points
- Beconase AQ: Shake well prior to each use. Prior to initial use, prime pump six times (or until fine spray appears); repeat priming if product not used for ≥ 7 days. Nasal applicator and dust cap may be washed in warm water and dried thoroughly.
- Qnasl: Shake well prior to each use. Prior to initial use, prime pump four times. If product not used for ≥ 7 days, prime pump two times.
- Spray in nostril(s); avoid spraying in eyes or mouth

◉ Budesonide

Brand Name
Rhinocort Aqua

Generic Name
Budesonide

Dosage Forms
Nasal inhalation

Pregnancy Category B

Dosing
- Children:
  - > 6 years: Usual dose of 1 spray into each nostril daily
  - 6–11 years: Maximum dose of 2 sprays into each nostril every 24 hours
  - > 12 years: Maximum dose of 4 sprays into each nostril every 24 hours
- Adults: Maximum dose of 4 sprays into each nostril every 24 hours

Major Drug Interactions
Drugs Affecting Budesonide
- Strong inhibitors of CYP3A4: May increase serum concentration
- Telaprevir: May increase concentration of budesonide nasal; concurrent use is not recommended

Counseling Points
- Shake the inhaler before each use
- Nasal inhaler must be primed before first use and if not used for more than 2 days in a row. To prime the inhaler before first use, remove the cap, shake gently and press down on the white collar eight times. If not used for more than 2 days in a row, prime the inhaler with one spray or until a fine mist appears.

◉ Fluticasone

Brand Names
Flonase, Veramyst

Generic Name
Fluticasone

Dosage Forms
Nasal inhalation, intranasal suspension (Flonase, Veramyst)

Pregnancy Category C

Dosing
- Flonase:
  - Children:
    - 4–12 years:
      - Usual dose: 1 spray into each nostril once daily
      - Maximum dose: 4 sprays every 24 hours
    - > 12 years: See adult dosing
  - Adults:
    - Usual dose: 2 sprays into each nostril once daily
    - Maximum dose: 4 sprays every 24 hours
- Veramyst:
  - Children:
    - 2–11 years:
      - Usual dose: 1 spray into each nostril once daily
      - Maximum dose: 4 sprays every 24 hours
    - > 11 years: See adult dosing
  - Adults:
    - Usual dose: 2 sprays into each nostril once daily
    - Maximum dose: 4 sprays every 24 hours

Major Drug Interactions
Drugs Affecting Fluticasone
- Use with ritonavir is not recommended due to the risk of systemic effects secondary to increased exposure to fluticasone
- Potent CYP3A4 inhibitors (e.g., ketoconazole): May increase systemic exposure to fluticasone, resulting in increased systemic effects

Counseling Points

- Shake contents before each use
- Flonase: Prime pump (press six times until fine spray appears) prior to first use or if spray unused for ≥ 7 days. Once a week the nasal applicator may be removed and rinsed with warm water to clean.
- Veramyst: Prime the spray (press mist release button six times or until fine mist appears) before first use, if spray is unused for > 30 days, or if the cap has been left off the bottle for ≥ 5 days

◉ Mometasone

Brand Name
Nasonex

Generic Name
Mometasone

Dosage Form
Nasal inhalation

Pregnancy Category C

Dosing
- Children:
  - 2–11 years: Usual dose is 1 spray into each nostril daily
  - ≥ 12 years: Usual dose is 2 sprays into each nostril once daily
- Adults: Usual dose is 2 sprays into each nostril once daily

Counseling Point
Before you use Nasonex for the first time prime the pump by pressing downward on the shoulders of the white nasal applicator 10 times or until a fine spray appears. If unused for more than 1 week, reprime by spraying two times or until a fine spray appears.

◉ Triamcinolone

Brand Name
Nasacort AQ

Generic Name
Triamcinolone

Dosage Form
Nasal inhalation

Pregnancy Category C

Dosing
- Children:
  - 2–5 years:
    - Usual dose: 1 spray into each nostril once daily
    - Maximum dose: 1 spray into each nostril once daily
  - 6–12 years:
    - Usual dose: 1 spray into each nostril once daily
    - Maximum dose: 4 sprays every 24 hours
  - > 12 years: See adult dosing
- Adults:
  - Usual dose: 2 sprays into each nostril once daily
  - Maximum dose: 4 sprays every 24 hours

Counseling Point
Prime prior to first use, discharging 5 sprays into the air. If product is not used for more than 2 weeks, reprime with 1 spray.

DECONGESTANT

Introduction
Topical decongestants are used for temporary relief of nasal congestion due to a cold or rhinitis. Sprays are preferable to drop preparations due to a decreased risk of systemic absorption. Oxymetazoline should not be used > 3 days due to the risk of rebound congestion. Patients with coronary heart disease and hypertension should use this agent with caution. The most common adverse effects include restlessness, nasal dryness, and sneezing.

Mechanism of Action for the Drug Class
Stimulate alpha-adrenergic receptors of vascular smooth muscle, resulting in relief of nasal congestion. Intranasal administration results in constriction of dilated blood vessels in the nasal mucosa, reducing blood flow to engorged edematous tissue. These effects promote drainage of the sinuses, relieving nasal stuffiness and improving nasal ventilation.

Members of the Drug Class
In this section: Oxymetazoline
Others: Naphazoline, phenylephrine, tetrahydrozoline

◉ Oxymetazoline

Brand Names
Afrin, Dristan

Generic Name
Oxymetazoline

OTC

Dosage Form
Intranasal solution, spray, drops

Usage
Temporary relief of nasal congestion due to common cold,* sinusitis, and allergies; adjunctive therapy for middle ear infections associated with acute or chronic rhinitis

Pregnancy Category C

Dosing
- Adults and children > 6 years, 0.05% solution:
  - Usual dose: 2–3 drops or sprays in each nostril up to twice daily for < 3 days
  - Maximum dose: 2 doses every 24 hours

Adverse Reactions: Most Common
Nasal dryness, nasal irritation, insomnia, nausea, sneezing

Adverse Reactions: Rare/Severe/Important
Rebound congestion, high blood pressure, palpitations

Major Drug Interactions
Drugs Affecting Oxymetazoline

Tricyclic antidepressants, MAOIs: Potentiate the pressor effects of oxymetazoline

Counseling Points
- Wipe the tip of the applicator clean after each use
- Do not share the container with another individual
- Prior to initial use of metered sprays, the nasal inhalers should be primed by pressing the pump several times
- Sprays should be pumped into each nostril with the head erect so that excess solution is not released
- Drops should be applied to the dependent (lower) nostril with the head tilted back. Remain in this position for 5 minutes, and then apply the solution to the other nostril in a similar manner. Drops may also be instilled while reclining with the head tilted back as far as possible.
- Do not use medication > 3 days without your healthcare provider's recommendation due to potential occurrence of rebound congestion

Key Points
- Sprays may be preferable to drops because of the decreased risk of swallowing the drug and resultant systemic absorption
- Use with caution in patients with coronary heart disease, angina, hypertension, enlarged prostate, glaucoma, and hyperthyroidism
- Do not use > 3 days unless prescribed by a healthcare provider

EXPECTORANT

Introduction
Expectorants are used to thin respiratory secretions to make a cough more productive. These agents should be used for short-term treatment of a cough. If a cough persists > 1 week, patients should be referred to a physician. Guaifenesin is commonly found in combination with decongestants and antihistamines. Adverse effects are rare with guaifenesin.

Mechanism of Action for the Drug Class
Enhances the removal of viscous mucus by reducing adhesiveness and surface tension

Members of the Drug Class
In this section: Guaifenesin
Others: None

◉ Guaifenesin
Brand Names
Humibid, Mucinex, Diabetic Tussin (multiple)

Generic Name
Guaifenesin

OTC

Dosage Forms
Tablet, extended-release tablet, syrup

Usage
Cough associated with common cold and bronchitis*

Pregnancy Category C

Dosing
- Tablet, syrup:
  - Children:
    - 6 months to 2 years:
      - Usual dose: 25–50 mg every 4 hours
      - Maximum dose: 300 mg every 24 hours
    - 2–6 years:
      - Usual dose: 50–100 mg every 4 hours
      - Maximum dose: 600 mg every 24 hours
    - 6–11 years:
      - Usual dose: 100–200 mg every 4 hours
      - Maximum dose: 1,200 mg every 24 hours
    - ≥ 12 years: See adult dosing

- Adults:
  - ◆ Usual dose: 200–400 mg every 4 hours
  - ◆ Maximum dose: 2,400 mg every 24 hours
- Extended-release tablets, adults:
  - Usual dose: 600–1,200 mg twice daily
  - Maximum dose: 2,400 mg every 24 hours

Adverse Reactions: Most Common

Diarrhea, drowsiness, dizziness, headache

Adverse Reactions: Rare/Severe/Important

Urolithiasis with large doses

Major Drug Interactions

None

Counseling Points

- Use caution with children < 2 years of age
- Follow each dose with a full glass of water
- Do not chew and crush extended-release formulations
- Sugar-free formulations are available

Key Points

- Supporting data are very limited and effectiveness is controversial
- Guaifenesin is usually used in combination with decongestants, antihistamines, and antitussives
- Use cautiously in children. Ensure that doses are correct to avoid an overdose.

LEUKOTRIENE INHIBITOR

Introduction

Leukotriene inhibitors are used in adults and children with chronic asthma. They are administered orally, which improves patient compliance with asthma therapy. These agents are not the preferred first-line treatment for persistent asthma. Montelukast is also used for allergic rhinitis. Montelukast may interact with drug therapies affecting the CYP2C9 and 3A4 enzyme systems. Adverse reactions are minor and include headache, nausea, and diarrhea. Serious reactions that have been reported include elevated liver enzymes, eosinophilia, and neuropsychiatric symptoms.

Mechanism of Action for the Drug Class

Leukotrienes are produced by arachidonic metabolism and are released by various cells, including eosinophils and mast cells. Leukotriene receptors are found in the airways, where they can cause airway edema and constriction, and on proinflammatory cells. Leukotriene inhibitors selectively block leukotriene receptors in airways, thereby decreasing airway edema, relaxing smooth muscles, and inhibiting inflammatory responses. They also block leukotrienes produced in nasal mucosa following allergen exposure.

Members of the Drug Class

In this section: Montelukast
Others: Zafirlukast

⊙ Montelukast

Brand Name

Singulair

Generic Name

Montelukast

Rx Only

Dosage Forms

Tablet, chewable tablet, oral granules (chewable tablets and granules contain phenylalanine)

Usage

Prophylaxis and chronic treatment of asthma,* second-line prevention of exercise-induced asthma, seasonal allergic rhinitis, perennial allergic rhinitis, chronic urticaria

Pregnancy Category B

Dosing

- Asthma or allergic rhinitis:
  - Children:
    - ◆ 12 months–5 years: 4 mg (chewable tablet or packet of granules) by mouth once daily in the evening
    - ◆ 6–14 years: 5 mg by mouth once daily in the evening
    - ◆ ≥ 15 years: See adult dosing
  - Adults: 10 mg by mouth once daily in the evening
- Exercise-induced asthma: 10 mg by mouth at least 2 hours before exercise. Additional doses should not be taken in the same 24 hours.

Adverse Reactions: Most Common

Headache, nausea, diarrhea, LFT abnormalities (asymptomatic)

Adverse Reactions: Rare/Severe/Important

Churg-Strauss syndrome (eosinophilic vasculitis), neuropsychiatric symptoms (agitation, aggression, hallucinations, suicidal behavior), increased bleeding/thrombocytopenia

Major Drug Interactions

Drugs Affecting Montelukast

CYP3A4 inducers (phenobarbital and rifampin): Decrease concentration by 40%

Counseling Points

- Not for acute attacks
- For control of asthma and allergic rhinitis, use every day
- Granules may be mixed with applesauce, formula, breast milk, ice cream. Opened packets should be used within 15 minutes.

Key Points

- Used as adjunct treatment for asthma
- Montelukast should not be used in patients with severe liver disease
- Doses may have to be adjusted when used with drugs that inhibit or induce CYP2C9 and 3A4 enzyme systems
- Monitor patients for neuropsychiatric symptoms

XANTHINE DERIVATIVE

Introduction

Theophylline has been used for the treatment of asthma and COPD for decades. Currently, the role of theophylline is limited for these indications due to the introduction of inhaled bronchodilators and the potential for serious adverse reactions with xanthine derivatives. Theophylline is now considered last-line or adjunct therapy for these indications. Different forms of theophylline have different bioavailability. Theophylline has a narrow therapeutic range, and changes in dosing should only occur after a serum concentration is obtained. Theophylline is metabolized by CYP1A2, 2E1, and 3A4 isoenzymes. Because of this, it may potentially interact with multiple medications. The most common adverse reactions are nausea and gastroesophageal reflux symptoms.

Mechanism of Action for the Drug Class

Exact mechanism is unknown. Theophylline is a nonselective phosphodiesterase (PDE) inhibitor. PDE inhibition and the concomitant elevation of cellular cAMP and cyclic guanosine monophosphate (cGMP) account for the bronchodilator action of theophylline. Several PDE isoenzymes have now been recognized; those important in smooth muscle relaxation include PDE3, PDE4, and PDE5. Theophylline is a weak inhibitor of all PDE isoenzymes. Theophylline may also have anti-inflammatory effects in asthma by inhibiting infiltration of eosinophils and CD4$^+$ lymphocytes into the airways after allergen exposure. May stimulate the medullary respiratory center and promote catecholamine release.

Members of the Drug Class

In this section: Theophylline
Others: Aminophylline

⊙ Theophylline

Brand Names
Theo-24, Elixophyllin

Generic Name
Theophylline

Rx Only

Dosage Forms

Extended-release tablet, extended-release capsule, oral solution, injection

Usage

Symptomatic treatment or prevention of bronchial asthma,* COPD (chronic bronchitis, or emphysema), apnea in infants

Pregnancy Category C

Dosing

- Dosing must be individualized based on age, weight, smoking history, evidence of heart failure, and liver function
- Loading doses may be given to obtain therapeutic concentrations quickly but are usually not needed for maintenance therapy
- Children ≥ 1 year and < 45 kg:
  - Initial dose: 10–14 mg/kg/day
  - Maximum dose: 300 mg/day
- Adults without risk factors for impaired theophylline clearance: Initial maintenance dose of 300–400 mg/day
- Hepatic dosage adjustment: Decrease dose by at least 50% in severe liver disease/cirrhosis

Adverse Reactions: Most Common

Gastroesophageal reflux, nausea, vomiting, headache, insomnia, nervousness

Adverse Reactions: Rare/Severe/Important

Seizures, cardiac arrhythmias, increased urination

Major Drug Interactions

Drugs Affecting Theophylline

- Carbamazepine, phenytoin, phenobarbital, rifampin, ketoconazole, cigarette smoking, St. John's wort: Decrease serum concentration
- Allopurinol, cimetidine, clarithromycin, ciprofloxacin, erythromycin, febuxostat, thyroid hormones, verapamil, zafirlukast: Increase serum concentration

Theophylline's Effect on Other Drugs
Lithium: Decreases levels

Essential Monitoring Parameters

Therapeutic blood concentration should be 5–15 µg/mL, with a target concentration of 10 µg/mL. Serum theophylline concentrations should be monitored prior to making dose changes, in the presence of signs or symptoms of toxicity, when changing medications, or in the event of illness. Age, smoking status, liver function, and evidence of heart failure can alter theophylline clearance; doses may need to be adjusted in these patients.

Counseling Points

- Do not break, chew, or crush extended-release formulations
- Capsules may be sprinkled on small amount of food and swallowed whole without chewing

- Avoid smoking. Smoking can change the metabolism of theophylline.
- Avoid dietary stimulants (coffee, tea, chocolate) that may increase adverse effects

Key Points

- Theophylline should only be used as an adjunctive treatment in COPD and asthma
- Dosing must be individualized based on age, organ function, smoking history, and concomitant drug therapy
- Dose adjustment should not be made without drug concentration monitoring
- Most patients achieve a therapeutic effect with low likelihood of adverse effects at concentrations of 10 µg/mL
- Theophylline interacts with drugs that inhibit or induce CYP2E1, 1A2, or 3A4

MISCELLANEOUS RESPIRATORY AGENT

Introduction

Omalizumab is a recombinant DNA-derived monoclonal antibody that selectively binds to human immunoglobulin E (IgE) on mast cells and basophils and limits the release of mediators of the allergic response. Omalizumab is used for persistent moderate to severe allergic asthma not controlled on corticosteroids. Omalizumab has been shown to decrease asthma exacerbations in these patients. It should be administered subcutaneously by a healthcare professional in a healthcare setting in order to monitor for anaphylaxis. The package labeling for omalizumab contains a black box warning for anaphylaxis and angioedema. A medication guide must be distributed to the patient before initiation of treatment.

Mechanism of Action for the Drug Class

Omalizumab inhibits the binding of IgE to the high-affinity IgE receptor on the surface of mast cells and basophils. Reduction in surface-bound on IgE on the receptor limits the release of mediators of the allergic response. Treatment with omalizumab also reduces the number of receptors on basophils in atopic patients.

Members of the Drug Class

In this section: Omalizumab
Others: None

◉ Omalizumab

Brand Name
Xolair

Generic Name
Omalizumab

Rx Only

Dosage Forms
Single-use injection, powder for reconstitution (150 mg)

Usage
Treatment of moderate to severe persistent allergic asthma (confirmed by a positive skin test or in vitro reactivity to a perennial aeroallergen) in adults and children ≥ 12 years of age) not controlled with inhaled corticosteroids. Severe allergic asthma inadequately controlled on a high-dose inhaled corticosteroid and inhaled long-acting beta-2 agonists.*

Pregnancy Category B
No well-controlled studies have been conducted in pregnant women, but a registry has been established to monitor outcomes in women exposed to omalizumab during pregnancy or within 8 weeks prior to pregnancy. Studies in monkeys have revealed no evidence of impaired fertility or harm to the fetus.

Dosing
- SUB-Q by healthcare provider only: 150–375 mg injection every 2–4 weeks
- Dose is based on pretreatment IgE serum levels (IU/mL) and body weight (kg). Dosing should not be adjusted based on IgE levels taken during treatment or < 1 year following discontinuation of therapy; doses should be adjusted during treatment for significant changes in body weight.

Adverse Reactions: Most Common
Arthralgia, fatigue, injection site reactions, pain, upper respiratory tract infections

Adverse Reactions: Rare/Severe/Important

Anaphylactic shock (majority occur after first dose, but may occur beyond 1 year after beginning treatment), urticaria, angioedema, malignancy, fever, arthralgia, rash, parasitic infections, thrombocytopenia

Major Drug Interactions

May enhance the toxic/immunosuppressant effects of other immunosuppressants

Essential Monitoring Parameters

Monitor IgE before initiation of therapy and > 1 year following discontinuation of therapy. IgE levels may be elevated up to a year after discontinuation. Watch for signs/symptoms of anaphylaxis after omalizumab administration.

Counseling Points

- Learn the signs and symptoms of anaphylaxis and seek medical care if such symptoms occur
- Do not abruptly discontinue systemic or inhaled corticosteroids upon initiation of omalizumab therapy

due to risk of eosinophilia or features of vasculitis consistent with Churg-Strauss syndrome
- Do not change or stop taking any asthma medication unless instructed to do so by your healthcare provider

Key Points

- Powder for reconstitution (150 mg): Reconstitute each vial with 1.4 mL of sterile water for injection. Keep unreconstituted vials refrigerated.
- Do not use to treat acute asthma symptoms or status asthmaticus
- Dosing is based on weight and baseline IgE concentrations
- Serum IgE can remain elevated up to 1 year after discontinuation of treatment and should not be checked until this time
- Patients should remain under healthcare observation after administration of omalizumab to monitor for anaphylactic symptoms
- A medication guide must be distributed to the patient before administration of omalizumab

---

REVIEW QUESTIONS

1. Which of the following is a long-acting inhaled anticholinergic agent?

    a. Albuterol
    b. Diphenhydramine
    c. Ipratropium
    d. Tiotropium

2. Which of the following is the most common adverse reaction associated with an Atrovent inhaler?

    a. Dry mouth
    b. Oral candidiasis
    c. Sedation
    d. Worsening glaucoma

3. Which of the following is a common use of Benadryl?

    a. Asthma
    b. Cough
    c. Fever
    d. Sleep disorders

4. Which of the following medications is considered a first-generation sedating antihistamine?

    a. Allegra
    b. Vistaril
    c. Xyzal
    d. Zyrtec

5. Which of the following would be an inappropriate antihistamine to prescribe to an elderly patient due to increased anticholinergic adverse events?

    a. Diphenhydramine
    b. Chlorpheniramine
    c. Hydroxyzine
    d. All of the above should be avoided in the elderly.

6. Which of the following would be the safest agent to use for motion sickness in a pregnant patient?

    a. Diphenhydramine
    b. Hydroxyzine
    c. Promethazine
    d. Tiotropium

7. Dosing of which of the following antihistamines should be changed in renal impairment?

    a. Allegra
    b. Claritin
    c. Xyzal
    d. All of the above

8. Which of the following antihistamines is *not* available in a liquid formulation?

    a. Cetirizine
    b. Levocetirizine
    c. Fexofenadine
    d. Loratadine

9. Benzonatate is commonly used to treat which of the following?

   a. Allergic rhinitis
   b. Asthma
   c. Cough
   d. Motion sickness

10. A patient with a severe allergy to tetracaine should avoid which of the following medications?

    a. Cetirizine
    b. Benzonatate
    c. Hydroxyzine
    d. Salmeterol

11. Which of the following inhaled medications is available in combination with albuterol?

    a. Budesonide
    b. Epinephrine
    c. Ipratropium
    d. Triamcinolone

12. Which of the following combination products contains a corticosteroid?

    a. Combivent
    b. Mucinex DM
    c. Symbicort
    d. Tussionex

13. Which of the following inhaled medications can be used to prevent exercise-induced bronchospasms?

    a. Albuterol
    b. Formoterol
    c. Salmeterol
    d. All of the above

14. Which of the following is considered a short-acting beta-2 agonist and can be used to treat acute bronchospasms?

    a. Formoterol
    b. Ipratropium
    c. Levalbuterol
    d. Salmeterol

15. Which of the following medications may decrease the effectiveness of Foradil and should be avoided when taking Foradil?

    a. Albuterol
    b. Aspirin
    c. Atenolol
    d. Propranolol

16. Which of the following inhalers is not commonly used in the chronic treatment of asthma?

    a. Advair
    b. Atrovent
    c. Symbicort
    d. Xopenex

17. Which of the following medications should be avoided with ketoconazole due to a potential drug interaction?

    a. Advair
    b. Proventil HFA
    c. Nasacort AQ
    d. Xopenex

18. Which of the following medications has a high potential for dosing errors in children < 2 years of age and is not recommended for use in this age group?

    a. Cetirizine
    b. Guaifenesin with codeine
    c. Levalbuterol
    d. Montelukast

19. Singulair belongs to which of the following drug classes?

    a. Anticholinergics
    b. Beta-2 agonists
    c. Leukotriene inhibitors
    d. Xanthine derivatives

20. Which of the following drugs acts by binding to human IgE on mast cells and basophils, limiting the release of inflammatory mediators?

    a. Albuterol
    b. Budesonide
    c. Montelukast
    d. Omalizumab

21. Which of the following medications should only be administered in a healthcare provider's office?

    a. Arformoterol
    b. Budesonide
    c. Omalizumab
    d. Theophylline

22. Which of the following adverse reactions should patients be monitored for immediately after administration with Xolair?

    a. Anaphylaxis
    b. Injection site reactions
    c. Pain
    d. Thrombocytopenia

23. Which of the following agents is only used for allergic asthma?

    a. Allegra
    b. Flovent
    c. Xolair
    d. Xyzal

24. The clearance of theophylline will be decreased due to which of the following patient-specific factors?

    a. Arrhythmias
    b. Cirrhosis
    c. Malignancy
    d. Smoking

25. A patient with a history of peptic ulcer disease and severe gastroesophageal reflux disease may have an increased risk of adverse reactions with which of the following medications?

    a. Albuterol
    b. Levalbuterol
    c. Ipratropium
    d. Theophylline

26. Which of the following medications may decrease the concentration of montelukast?

    a. Calcium carbonate
    b. Famotidine
    c. Phenobarbital
    d. Warfarin

27. Oxymetazoline is not recommended for long-term use due to which of the following adverse reactions?

    a. Angioedema
    b. Development of arrhythmias
    c. Rebound congestion
    d. Tachyphylaxis

28. Humibid belongs to which of the following drug classes?

    a. Anticholinergics
    b. Corticosteroid nasal inhalers
    c. Cough suppressants
    d. Expectorants

29. Which of the following indications is Beconase AQ used to treat?

    a. Allergic rhinitis
    b. Chronic urticaria
    c. COPD
    d. Exercise-induced bronchospasms

30. Which of the following inhaled medications should be primed prior to the first use?

    a. Combivent Respimat
    b. Flovent HFA
    c. ProAir HFA
    d. All of the above

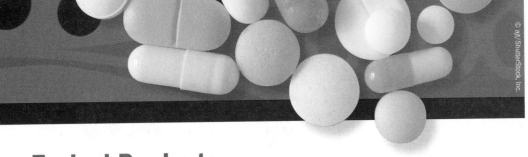

Topical Products

Susan Kent, PharmD, CGP

ANALGESICS

Introduction

Capsaicin induces the release of substance P from peripheral sensory neurons. Substance P is the primary mediator of pain impulses from the periphery to the CNS; after repeated application, capsaicin depletes the neuron of substance P and prevents reaccumulation. The lidocaine topical patch offers a unique option for chronic pain syndromes. Systemic adverse reactions with appropriate use are unlikely, due to the small dose absorbed.

Mechanism of Action for the Drug Class

Although the exact mechanism of action has not been fully elucidated, capsaicin is a neuropeptide-active agent that affects the synthesis, storage, transport, and release of substance P. In addition to mediating pain impulses, substance P has also been shown to be released into joint tissues, where it activates inflammatory intermediates that are involved with the development of rheumatoid arthritis. Capsaicin renders skin and joints insensitive to pain by depleting and preventing reaccumulation of substance P in peripheral sensory neurons. With the depletion of substance P in the nerve endings, local pain impulses cannot be transmitted to the brain. Lidocaine is an amide-type local anesthetic agent. It has been suggested that it stabilizes neuronal membranes by inhibiting the ionic fluxes required for the initiation and conduction of impulses, producing an analgesic effect.

Members of the Drug Class

In this section: Capsaicin, lidocaine topical patch
Others: Benzyl alcohol, capsaicin (topical patch), lidocaine (jelly, spray, gel, cream, ointment), methyl salicylate and menthol, trolamine, zucapsaicin

◉ Capsaicin

Brand Name
  Capzasin-P

Generic Name
  Capsaicin

OTC

Dosage Forms
  Topical cream, gel, lotion

Usage
  Temporary treatment of minor muscle and joint pain due to backache, strains, sprains, bruises, cramps, or arthritis*; temporary relief of pain associated with diabetic neuropathy; treatment of pain associated with psoriasis and intractable pruritus; potential use as topical agent in burning mouth syndrome and oral mucositis

Pregnancy Category B

Dosing
  Apply to affected area three to four times a day; efficacy may be decreased if used less than three times a day. Best results are seen after 2–4 weeks of continuous use.

Adverse Reactions: Most Common
  Application site reactions of erythema, pain, rash, pruritus. Nausea and nasopharyngitis may also occur.

Adverse Reactions: Rare/Severe/Important
  Transient hypertension (reported with transdermal product only)

Major Drug Interactions
  None

Counseling Points
  - For external use only. Avoid contact with eyes or mucous membranes.
  - Wear gloves to apply. Wash hands with soap and water after applying to avoid spreading to eyes or other sensitive areas of the body.

---

* Throughout the text, an asterisk (*) is used to indicate the most common uses of a drug.

- Do not apply to broken or irritated skin. Do not expose treated area to heat or direct sunlight. Do not apply a bandage to the affected area.
- Transient burning may occur and generally disappears after several days; discontinue use if severe burning develops
- Stop use and consult your healthcare provider if redness or irritation develops, symptoms get worse, or symptoms resolve and then recur

Key Points
- Efficacy may be decreased if used less than three times a day. Best results seen after 2–4 weeks of continuous use.
- Mild burning may occur with initial use but should resolve after several days. Discontinue use if severe burning develops.

⊚ Lidocaine Topical Patch

Brand Names
Lidoderm, Lido Patch

Generic Name
Lidocaine

Rx and OTC

Dosage Forms
Rx: Extended-release 5% topical patch
OTC: Extended-release topical patch containing 3.99% lidocaine and 1% menthol

Usage
Relief of chronic pain in postherpetic neuralgia (PHN)*; treatment of pain and other chronic pain syndromes, often in an effort to avoid or minimize use of opioid agents and related adverse effects*; relief of allodynia (painful hypersensitivity); temporary relief of localized pain (Lido Patch)*

Pregnancy Category B

Dosing
- PHN: Apply patch to most painful area after removal from protective envelope. Up to 3 patches may be applied in a single application. Patch may remain in place for up to 12 hours in any 24-hour period. It should only be applied to intact skin.
- Localized pain: Apply OTC patch to painful area. Patch may remain in place for up to 12 hours in a 24-hour period. No more than 1 patch should be used in a 24-hour period.
- Renal dosage adjustment: Lidocaine is rapidly metabolized in the liver to various metabolites and is excreted by the kidneys. Smaller areas of treatment are recommended in a debilitated patient or a patient with impaired elimination.

- Hepatic dosage adjustment: Lidocaine is rapidly metabolized in the liver to various metabolites and is excreted by the kidneys. Smaller areas of treatment are recommended in a debilitated patient or a patient with impaired elimination.

Adverse Reactions: Most Common
Application site reactions are generally mild and transient, resolving within minutes to hours

Adverse Reactions: Rare/Severe/Important
Allergic and anaphylactoid reactions associated with lidocaine, although rare, can occur. Transdermal patch may contain conducting metal (e.g., aluminum); remove patch before MRI to avoid burns.

Major Drug Interactions
Local anesthetics: When lidocaine is used concomitantly with other products containing local anesthetic agents, the amount absorbed from all formulations must be considered

Drugs Affecting Lidocaine
- Class III antiarrhythmics, beta blockers, conivaptan, CYP1A2/3A4 inhibitors: Increase effect
- CYP1A2/3A4 inducers, herbs with 3A4 induction properties: Decrease effect

Lidocaine's Effect on Other Drugs
Class III antiarrhythmics, prilocaine: Increases effect; toxic effects are additive and potentially synergistic

Contraindications
Hypersensitivity to another amide-type local anesthetic. Avoid concomitant use with conivaptan.

Essential Monitoring Parameters
Renal and hepatic function

Counseling Points
- Apply to intact skin only
- Patches may be cut into smaller sizes with scissors before removal of the release liner
- If irritation or a burning sensation occurs during application, remove the patch and do not reapply until the irritation subsides
- Wash hands after handling lidocaine and avoid eye contact
- Store and dispose of patches out of the reach of children, pets, and others; do not reuse
- Patches should not be tightly bandaged, used in conjunction with heating pads, or applied to open wounds or sensitive skin
- Report irritation, pain, persistent numbness, tingling, swelling, restlessness, dizziness, acute weakness, blurred vision, ringing in ears, or respiratory difficulty to your healthcare provider

ANTIBIOTIC, METRONIDAZOLE

Introduction

Topical metronidazole is a member of the imidazole class of antibacterial agents and is used in the treatment of inflammatory lesions of acne rosacea and bacterial vaginosis

Mechanism of Action for the Drug Class

Metronidazole is classified as an antiprotozoal and antibacterial agent that is active against susceptible organisms. After diffusing into an organism, metronidazole interacts with DNA to cause a loss of helical DNA structure and strand breakage, resulting in inhibition of protein synthesis and cell death in susceptible organisms.

Members of the Drug Class

In this section: Metronidazole
Others: Tinidazole (nitroimidazole)

◉ Metronidazole

Brand Names

MetroGel, MetroCream, MetroGel-Vaginal, MetroLotion, Noritate, Rosadan, Vandazole

Generic Name

Metronidazole

Rx Only

Dosage Forms

Topical cream, gel, and lotion; vaginal gel

Usage

Treatment of inflammatory papules, pustules, and erythema of acne rosacea*; treatment of bacterial vaginosis (BV)*

Pregnancy Category B

Dosing

- Topical 0.75%: Apply and rub a thin film twice daily to entire affected area
- Topical 1%: Apply thin film to affected area once daily
- Vaginal: One applicatorful (~37.5 mg metronidazole) intravaginally once or twice daily for 5 days. Apply once in morning and evening if using twice daily; if daily, use at bedtime.

Adverse Reactions: Most Common

Burning, skin irritation, dryness, headache; vulva/vaginal irritation, vaginal discharge, fungal infection, ocular burning and irritation

Adverse Reactions: Rare/Severe/Important

Redness, leukopenia

Major Drug Interactions

Drugs Affecting Metronidazole

Mebendazole: Enhances adverse/toxic effects

Metronidazole's Effect on Other Drugs

- Ethyl alcohol, disulfiram, ritonavir, tipranavir: Enhances adverse/toxic effects
- Warfarin: Oral metronidazole has been reported to potentiate the anticoagulant effect of warfarin, resulting in a prolongation of prothrombin time. The effect of topical metronidazole on prothrombin time is not known.

Contraindications

Vaginal gel: Alcohol use during and for at least 3 days after metronidazole use, concomitant use with or within the last 2 weeks of disulfiram, and hypersensitivity to parabens

Essential Monitoring Parameters

CBC with total and differential leukocyte counts before and after therapy

Counseling Points

- For external use only. Avoid contact with eyes or mouth.
- Wash hands and affected areas before application; wash hands after applying
- Cosmetics may be used after application of topical metronidazole
- Do not engage in vaginal intercourse or use other vaginal products (tampons, douches) during the entire course of therapy with metronidazole vaginal gel. Vaginal intercourse or vaginal products could reduce the efficacy of the gel.
- Discontinue use and notify your healthcare provider at first sign of skin rash or allergic reaction

Key Points

- Follow instructions carefully for topical and vaginal products. Apply thin layer to affected areas; use vaginal applicator as directed by physician; cleanse areas to be treated before topical and vaginal application.
- Avoid contact with eyes
- Monitor for skin rash or allergic reaction

- Disulfiram-like reaction to ethanol may occur with the vaginal gel; consider avoidance of alcoholic beverages during therapy with vaginal gel. Do not administer the vaginal gel to patients who have taken disulfiram within the past 2 weeks.
- Metronidazole is a nitroimidazole and should be used with care in patients with evidence of, or history of, blood dyscrasia

ANTIBIOTIC, MUPIROCIN

Introduction

Mupirocin is an antibiotic produced from *Pseudomonas fluorescens* that is structurally unrelated to any other topical or systemic antibiotics. Mupirocin is used topically in the treatment of impetigo caused by *Staphylococcus aureus* and beta-hemolytic streptococci, including *Streptococcus pyogenes*. Mupirocin is considered a drug of choice for treatment of impetigo, especially when limited numbers of lesions are present.

Mechanism of Action for the Drug Class

Mupirocin reversibly and specifically binds to bacterial isoleucyl transfer RNA synthetase, thereby inhibiting bacterial protein and RNA synthesis. DNA synthesis and cell wall formation are affected to a lesser extent. This agent does not demonstrate in vitro cross-resistance with other classes of antimicrobial agents. Mupirocin is bacteriostatic at low concentrations and bactericidal at high concentrations.

Members of the Drug Class

In this section: Mupirocin
Others: None

◉ Mupirocin

Brand Names

Bactroban, Bactroban Nasal, Centany

Generic Name

Mupirocin

Rx Only

Dosage Forms

Topical cream, ointment; intranasal ointment

Usage

Eradication of nasal colonization with MRSA in adult patients and healthcare workers (intranasal),* treatment of impetigo or secondary infected traumatic skin lesions due to *S. aureus* and *S. pyogenes* (topical)*

Pregnancy Category B

Dosing

- Impetigo: Apply topical ointment to affected area three times a day
- Secondary skin infections: Apply topical cream to affected area three times a day for 10 days
- Elimination of MRSA colonization: Approximately one-half of the intranasal ointment from the single-use tube should be applied into one nostril and the other half into the other nostril twice daily for 5 days
- Renal dosage adjustment: Use with caution in cases of renal impairment

Adverse Reactions: Most Common

Burning, stinging, pruritus, pain, erythema

Adverse Reactions: Rare/Severe/Important

Secondary wound infections

Major Drug Interactions

Drugs Affecting Mupirocin

None

Mupirocin's Effect on Other Drugs

Live attenuated typhoid vaccine: May decrease level/effect

Essential Monitoring Parameters

Reevaluate patients who have not shown a clinical response within 3–5 days of starting therapy (cream or ointment). Watch for evidence of sensitization or severe local irritation.

Counseling Points

- For external use only. Avoid contact with eyes or mouth.
- Use caution in patients with extensive burns or open wounds, because the polyethylene glycol contained in some topical products may be absorbed percutaneously
- Use proper administration technique

- Treated areas may be covered with gauze dressings, if desired
- Notify your healthcare provider of any local side effects, if no improvement is seen in 3–5 days, or if signs/symptoms of infection develop
- Patients using the intranasal form should not use other intranasal products concomitantly
- When applied intranasally, drug may cause headache, pharyngitis, or rhinitis

Key Points
- Effective for the treatment of skin lesions due to *S. aureus* and *S. pyogenes* (topical cream) and impetigo (topical ointment) and eradication of nasal MRSA colonization (intranasal ointment)
- Follow appropriate dosing and duration of treatment depending on indication
- Be aware of sound-alike/look-alike issues with Bactrim, bacitracin, and baclofen

ANTIBIOTIC, CHLORHEXIDINE GLUCONATE

Introduction

Chlorhexidine gluconate is used topically as an anti-infective skin cleanser for surgical hand antisepsis, preoperative skin preparation, routine hand hygiene in healthcare personnel, and skin wound and general skin cleansing. It is active against gram-positive and gram-negative organisms, facultative anaerobes, aerobes, and yeast.

Mechanism of Action for the Drug Class

The bactericidal effect of chlorhexidine gluconate is a result of the binding of the cationic molecule to negatively charged bacterial cell walls and extramicrobial complexes. At low concentrations, this causes an alteration of bacterial cell osmotic equilibrium and leakage of potassium and phosphorous, resulting in a bacteriostatic effect. At high concentrations, the cytoplasmic contents of the bacterial cell precipitate, resulting in cell death.

Members of the Drug Class

In this section: Chlorhexidine gluconate
Others: Benzalkonium chloride, hexachlorophene

◉ Chlorhexidine Gluconate

Brand Names

Avagard, BactoShield, Betasept, ChloraPrep, Chlorascrub, Dyna-Hex, Hibiclens, Hibistat, Operand Chlorhexidine Gluconate

Generic Name

Chlorhexidine gluconate

OTC

Dosage Forms

Liquid, lotion, solution, sponge/brush, sponge, swab, wipe

Usage

Skin cleanser for line placement, skin wounds, preoperative skin preparation*; germicidal hand rinse*

Pregnancy Category B or C

Depends on the manufacturer

Dosing
- Surgical scrub: Scrub 3 minutes and rinse thoroughly; wash for an additional 3 minutes
- Hand sanitizer (Avagard): Dispense 1 pumpful in palm of one hand; dip fingertips of opposite hand into solution and work it under nails. Spread remainder evenly over hand and just above elbow, covering all surfaces. Repeat on other hand. Dispense another pumpful in each hand and reapply to each hand up to the wrist. Allow to dry before gloving.
- Hand wash: Wash for 15 seconds and rinse
- Hand rinse: Rub 15 seconds and rinse

Adverse Reactions: Most Common

Skin erythema, roughness, and/or dryness; sensitization

Adverse Reactions: Rare/Severe/Important

Allergic reactions, anaphylaxis, chemical injury to cornea (with accidental exposure)

Major Drug Interactions

None

Counseling Points
- Keep out of eyes, ears, and mouth
- Avoid use in children < 2 months of age due to increased absorption and/or irritation
- May stain fabrics
- Do not apply to wounds that involve more than superficial layers of skin
- Avoid contact with meninges (do not use on lumbar puncture sites)
- Solutions may be flammable (contain isopropyl alcohol); avoid exposure to open flame and/or ignition sources until completely dry
- Avoid application to hairy areas, which may significantly delay drying time

- Note that if used as a disinfectant before midstream urine collection, a false-positive urine protein may result (with dipstick method based on pH indicator color change)

- Chlorhexidine gluconate is used topically as an anti-infective skin cleanser
- Active against gram-positive and gram-negative organisms, facultative anaerobes, aerobes, and yeast
- Follow specific washing times per product for adequate skin cleansing and eradication of bacteria

ANTIBIOTIC, CLINDAMYCIN PHOSPHATE

Introduction

Clindamycin is a semisynthetic derivative of lincomycin and is categorized as a lincosamide antibiotic. It is used topically for the treatment of inflammatory acne vulgaris and intravaginally for the treatment of bacterial vaginosis (BV).

Mechanism of Action for the Drug Class

Clindamycin appears to inhibit protein synthesis in susceptible organisms by binding to 50S ribosomal subunits. The exact mechanism by which clindamycin reduces lesions of acne vulgaris is not fully understood; however, the effect appears to be related to the antibacterial activity of the drug. The drug inhibits the growth of susceptible organisms on the surface of the skin and reduces the concentration of free fatty acids in sebum. Free fatty acids are comedogenic and are believed to be a possible cause of the inflammatory lesions of acne. Clindamycin may be bacteriostatic or bactericidal in action, depending on the concentration of the drug attained at the site of infection and the susceptibility of the infecting organism. Clindamycin phosphate is inactive until hydrolyzed to free clindamycin; phosphatases on the skin rapidly hydrolyze the drug following topical application.

Members of the Drug Class

In this section: Clindamycin phosphate
Others: Benzoyl peroxide, metronidazole, lincomycin

⊙ Clindamycin Phosphate

Brand Names

Cleocin, Cleocin-T, Cleocin Vaginal Ovules, Clinda-Derm, Clindagel, ClindaMax, Clindets Pledgets, Clindesse, Evoclin

Generic Name

Clindamycin phosphate

Rx Only

Dosage Forms

Topical gel, lotion, foam, solution, pledget, vaginal suppository/cream

Usage

Treatment of severe acne (*Propionibacterium acnes*)*; treatment of bacterial vaginosis (*Gardnerella vaginalis*)*; treatment of susceptible bacterial infections, mainly those caused by anaerobes, streptococci, pneumococci, and staphylococci

Dosing

- Gel (Cleocin T, ClindaMax), pledget, lotion, solution: Apply a thin film twice daily
- Foam (Clindagel, Evoclin): Apply once daily
- Suppositories: Insert 1 ovule (100 mg clindamycin) daily into vagina at bedtime for 3 days
- Vaginal cream:
  - Cleocin: 1 applicatorful inserted intravaginally once daily before bedtime for 3 or 7 consecutive days in nonpregnant patients or for 7 consecutive days in pregnant patients
  - Clindesse: 1 applicatorful inserted intravaginally as a single dose at any time during the day in nonpregnant patients

Adverse Reactions: Most Common

Dryness, burning, itching, scaliness, erythema, or peeling of skin; oily skin; headache; vaginal candidiasis, vaginitis, pruritus, vaginal pain

Adverse Reactions: Rare/Severe/Important

Pseudomembranous colitis, diarrhea, abdominal pain, hypersensitivity reactions, atrophic vaginitis, local edema, menstrual disorders, pyelonephritis, urinary tract infection

Major Drug Interactions

Neuromuscular blocking agents: Clindamycin has been shown to have neuromuscular blocking properties that may enhance the neuromuscular blocking action of other agents. Use with caution in patients receiving such agents, because clindamycin can be absorbed systemically following intravaginal application.

Contraindications

Previous *C. difficile*–associated diarrhea, regional enteritis, ulcerative colitis

Counseling Points

- Topical gel, lotion, or solution: Wash hands thoroughly before applying or wear gloves. Apply thin film of gel, lotion, or solution to affected area. Wash hands thoroughly. Wait 30 minutes before shaving or applying makeup. Shake lotion well prior to use.
- Solution or pledget: Avoid contact with eyes, mouth, or other mucous membranes. Solution/pledget contains an alcohol base; if inadvertent contact with mucous membranes occurs, rinse with liberal amounts of water. Remove pledget from foil immediately before use; discard after single use. May use more than one pledget for each application to cover area.
- Topical foam: Do not dispense directly onto hands or face. Pick up small amounts of foam with fingertips and gently massage into affected areas until foam disappears. Wash hands thoroughly. Wait 30 minutes before shaving or applying makeup.
- Vaginal: Wash hands before using. At bedtime: If using applicator, gently insert full applicator into vagina and expel cream. Wash applicator with soap and water following use. If using suppository, remove foil and insert high into vagina. Remain lying down for 30 minutes following administration. Avoid intercourse during therapy. Vaginal products may weaken condoms or contraceptive diaphragms. Barrier contraceptives are not recommended concurrently or for 3–5 days following treatment (depends on the product).
- Report persistent burning, swelling, itching, excessive dryness, or worsening of condition to your healthcare provider.

Key Points

- Clindamycin is active against *Gardnerella vaginalis* and *Propionibacterium acnes* and is effective in the treatment of bacterial vaginosis and acne vulgaris
- Wash hands thoroughly before applying product or wear gloves

ANTIFUNGALS, IMIDAZOLES

Introduction

Ketoconazole and miconazole, synthetic azole antifungal agents, are imidazole derivatives and active against both dermatophytes and *Candida* species. These agents are structurally related to other imidazole-derivative azole antifungal agents.

Mechanism of Action for the Drug Class

These agents alter cell membranes, resulting in increased cell wall permeability, secondary metabolic effects, and growth inhibition. The fungistatic activity of these drugs may result from interference with ergosterol synthesis.

Members of the Drug Class

In this section: Ketoconazole, miconazole
Others: Butoconazole, clotrimazole, econazole, oxiconazole, sulconazole, tioconazole

◉ Ketoconazole

Brand Names

Extina, Nizoral, Xolegel, Nizoral A-D (OTC)

Generic Name

Ketoconazole

Rx and OTC

Dosage Forms

Cream, foam, gel, shampoo

Usage

Treatment of a variety of cutaneous fungal infections, including cutaneous candidiasis,* tinea pedis, tinea cruris, and tinea corporis;* dandruff;* seborrheic dermatitis;* tinea versicolor*

Pregnancy Category C

Dosing

- Fungal infections:
  - Tinea infections: Rub cream gently into the affected area once daily for duration of treatment:
    - Tinea corporis: 2 weeks
    - Tinea cruris: 2 weeks
    - Tinea pedis: 6 weeks
  - Tinea versicolor (pityriasis): Apply 2% shampoo to damp skin, lather, leave on 5 minutes, and rinse (one application should be sufficient)
- Seborrheic dermatitis:
  - Cream: Rub gently into the affected area twice daily for 4 weeks
  - Foam: Apply to affected area twice daily for 4 weeks
  - Gel: Rub gently into the affected area once daily for 2 weeks
  - 1% shampoo: Apply twice weekly for up to 8 weeks with at least 3 days between each shampoo

Adverse Reactions: Most Common

Severe skin irritation, pruritus, burning sensation

Adverse Reactions: Rare/Severe/Important

Painful allergic reactions (local swelling and inflammation), contact dermatitis

Counseling Points

- For external use only; not for ophthalmic, oral, or intravaginal use
- Although improvement and symptom relief usually occur within the first week of therapy, tinea corporis and cruris should be treated for 2 weeks
- Tinea pedis should be treated for 6 weeks; cutaneous candidiasis for 2 weeks
- Do not wash topical application sites for at least 3 hours after drug is applied
- Ketoconazole 2% gel or foam is used only for the treatment of seborrheic dermatitis; the safety and efficacy of the foam or gel for the treatment of fungal infections have not been established
- Contact your healthcare provider if severe or persistent adverse effects occur or if condition worsens

Key Points

- Apply exactly as directed
- Wash hands thoroughly before and after applying
- Keep away from eyes or mouth

◉ Miconazole

Brand Names

Lotrimin AF, Micatin, Baza Antifungal, Carrington Antifungal, Micaderm, DiabetAid Antifungal Foot Bath, Micro-Guard

Generic Name

Miconazole

OTC

Dosage Forms

Aerosol powder/spray, cream, lotion, ointment, powder, tincture

Usage

Treatment of a variety of cutaneous fungal infections, including cutaneous candidiasis,* tinea pedis, tinea cruris, tinea corporis,* tinea versicolor*

Pregnancy Category C

Dosing

- Tinea corporis: Apply aerosol powder/spray, cream, lotion, ointment, powder, or tincture to affected area twice daily for 4 weeks
- Tinea pedis:
  - Apply aerosol powder/spray, cream, lotion, ointment, powder, or tincture to affected area twice daily for 4 weeks
  - Effervescent tablet: Dissolve 1 tablet in 1 gallon of water; soak feet for 15–30 minutes; pat dry

- Tinea cruris: Apply aerosol powder/spray, cream, lotion, ointment, powder, or tincture to affected area twice daily for 2 weeks
- Tinea versicolor (pityriasis):
  - Apply to affected area once daily
  - Clinical and mycologic clearing usually occurs after 2 weeks of treatment

Adverse Reactions: Most Common

Burning, irritation, maceration

Adverse Reactions: Rare/Severe/Important

Allergic contact dermatitis

Major Drug Interactions

Drugs Affecting Miconazole

St. John's wort: May decrease levels

Miconazole's Effect on Other Drugs

- Warfarin: Potential for increased plasma concentrations with intravaginal miconazole; potential for interaction with miconazole applied topically to skin is unknown
- Oral sulfonylureas: May inhibit metabolism

Essential Monitoring Parameter

Diabetic patients should test blood glucose regularly; miconazole may inhibit the metabolism of oral sulfonylureas

Counseling Points

- Wash and dry area before applying medication; apply thinly
- For topical use only; do not get in or near eyes
- If diabetic, test blood glucose regularly; miconazole may inhibit the metabolism of oral sulfonylureas
- Tincture: Patients with diabetes, circulatory problems, or renal or hepatic dysfunction should contact their healthcare provider prior to self-medication
- Cutaneous candidiasis and tinea cruris should be treated for 2 weeks and tinea corporis and pedis for 1 month to reduce the possibility of recurrence
- Miconazole powder or aerosol powder are not recommended for use on the scalp or nails
- Report persistent burning, itching, or irritation to your healthcare provider

Key Points

- Apply exactly as directed
- Wash hands thoroughly before and after applying
- Keep away from eyes

Introduction

Terbinafine is a synthetic allylamine antifungal agent that is structurally and pharmacologically related to naftifine. Compared to azole antifungal agents, terbinafine is more active against dermatophytes and less active against *Candida* species.

Mechanism of Action for the Drug Class

Drugs in this class inhibit squalene epoxidase, a key enzyme in sterol biosynthesis in fungi. This results in a deficiency in ergosterol within the fungal cell wall, resulting in cell death. Terbinafine may be fungicidal or fungistatic in action, depending on the concentration of the drug and the specific fungus tested.

Members of the Drug Class

In this section: Terbinafine
Others: Naftifine

⊙ Terbinafine

Brand Name
Lamisil AT

Generic Name
Terbinafine

Rx and OTC

Dosage Forms
Cream, gel, solution

Usage
Treatment of a variety of cutaneous fungal infections, including cutaneous candidiasis*; tinea pedis; tinea cruris; tinea corporis*; tinea versicolor*

Pregnancy Category B

Dosing
- Cutaneous candidiasis: Apply to affected area once or twice daily for 7–14 days
- Tinea pedis: Apply to affected area once daily for at least 1 week, not to exceed 4 weeks
- Tinea corporis:
  - OTC cream: Apply to affected area once daily for at least 1 week, not to exceed 4 weeks
  - OTC gel: Apply to affected area once daily for 7 days
  - OTC solution: Apply to affected area once daily for 7 days
- Tinea cruris:
  - OTC cream: Apply to affected area once daily for at least 1 week, not to exceed 4 weeks
  - OTC gel: Apply to affected area once daily for 7 days
  - OTC solution: Apply to affected area once daily for 7 days

- Tinea versicolor:
  - OTC cream: Apply to affected area once daily for at least 1 week, not to exceed 4 weeks
  - Rx cream: Apply to affected area once or twice daily for 2 weeks
  - OTC gel: Apply to affected area once daily for 7 days
  - Rx solution: Apply to affected area once or twice daily for 2 weeks

Adverse Reactions: Most Common

Burning, dryness, irritation, pruritus, rash, stinging, tingling

Adverse Reactions: Rare/Severe/Important

Contact dermatitis, exfoliation

Major Drug Interactions

None

Counseling Points

- Cream, gel, and spray are for topical use only; avoid contact with eyes, nose, or mouth
- Wash and dry area thoroughly before applying; apply to affected areas exactly as directed
- Do not use occlusive dressings
- Wash hands after touching the affected areas so that the infection is not spread to other areas of the body or to other individuals
- Do not to use spray solution on the face. If accidental contact with eyes occurs, rinse eyes thoroughly with running water and consult a clinician if symptoms persist.
- Tinea pedis: Wear well-fitting, ventilated shoes and change socks at least once daily
- Report irritation or development of rash to your healthcare provider
- Women of childbearing age should inform their healthcare provider of plans to become pregnant or breast-feed

Key Points

- Apply to affected areas exactly as directed; avoid contact with eyes, nose, mouth, or other mucous membranes
- Thoroughly wash hands before and after application
- Clinical improvement usually is evident within the first week of therapy, and patients usually show continued improvement for several weeks after completion of treatment. Reevaluate diagnosis if no improvement within 2–6 weeks of completing therapy.

14

Topical Products

ANTIFUNGAL, TRIAZOLE

Introduction

Terconazole, a triazole derivative, is a synthetic azole antifungal agent used intravaginally for the treatment of vulvovaginal candidiasis. Terconazole is structurally similar to imidazole-derivative antifungal agents; however, triazoles have three nitrogens in the azole ring. Terconazole is active against dermatophytes and *Candida* species. At high concentrations, the drug also has in-vitro activity against some gram-positive and gram-negative bacteria.

Mechanism of Action for the Drug Class

Terconazole exhibits fungicidal activity against *Candida albicans* by disrupting normal fungal cell membrane permeability

Members of the Drug Class

In this section: Terconazole
Others: Butoconazole, clotrimazole, miconazole, nystatin, tioconazole

⊙ Terconazole

Brand Names
Terazol 3, Terazol 7

Generic Name
Terconazole

Rx Only

Dosage Forms
Vaginal cream, suppository

Usage
Treatment of uncomplicated vulvovaginal candidiasis*

Pregnancy Category C

Dosing
- Vaginal cream 0.4%: Insert 1 applicatorful vaginally at bedtime for 7 consecutive days
- Vaginal cream 0.8%: Insert 1 applicatorful vaginally at bedtime for 3 consecutive days
- Vaginal suppositories: Insert 1 suppository vaginally at bedtime for 3 consecutive days

Adverse Reactions: Most Common
Headache, vulvar/vaginal burning, irritation, or itching

Adverse Reactions: Rare/Severe/Important
Abdominal pain, dysmenorrhea, chills, fever, allergic reactions

Major Drug Interactions
None

Counseling Points
- For vaginal use only
- Open applicator just before administration to prevent contamination
- Clean applicator after use with mild soap solution and rinse with water
- Complete full course of therapy as directed
- Refrain from intercourse during period of treatment; sexual partner may experience penis irritation
- Suppositories may cause breakdown of rubber/latex products such as condoms and diaphragms; avoid concurrent use
- Inform prescriber of intent to become pregnant or breast-feed
- Report persistent vaginal burning, itching, irritation, or rash to your healthcare provider

Key Points
- Terconazole is a topical azole antifungal agent used intravaginally for the treatment of vulvovaginal candidiasis
- Advise patients to finish complete course, even if symptoms have resolved
- Microbiological studies should be repeated in patients not responding to terconazole to confirm the diagnosis and rule out other pathogens
- Efficacy of intravaginal terconazole is not affected by concomitant use of oral contraceptives
- Administration of intravaginal terconazole does not appear to affect estradiol or progesterone concentrations in women receiving low-dose oral contraceptives

Introduction

Docosanol 10% cream should be used *only* for symptomatic treatment of herpes labialis, such as perioral herpes, cold sores, and fever blisters in immunocompetent adults and children ≥ 12 years of age. The drug is not indicated for preventive therapy.

Mechanism of Action for the Drug Class

Docosanol is a naturally occurring 22-carbon saturated aliphatic alcohol with antiviral activity against various Herpesviridae, including herpes simplex virus types 1 and 2 (HSV-1, HSV-2). The mechanism of action of docosanol in the treatment of herpes labialis lesions does not involve direct virucidal activity against HSV. Docosanol reduces viral replication and activity by effectively inhibiting the fusion between the plasma membrane and the herpes simplex virus envelope.

Members of the Drug Class

In this section: Docosanol
Others: Acyclovir

⊙ Docosanol

Brand Name
Abreva

Generic Name
Docosanol

OTC

Dosage Form
Topical cream

Usage
Topical treatment of recurrent herpes labialis in adults and children ≥ 12 years of age (perioral herpes, cold sores, fever blisters)*

Pregnancy Category
Studies have not been conducted, thus fetal risk cannot be ruled out. Consult clinician before use.

Dosing

Herpes simplex (face/lips): Apply topical cream five times a day to affected area of face or lips. Start at first sign of cold sore or fever blister and continue until healed.

Adverse Reactions: Most Common

Application site reactions (burning, stinging), headache

Major Drug Interactions

None

Counseling Points

- Wash hands before and after applying docosanol
- Rub in gently to cover affected area completely; avoid contact with eyes
- Use only to treat oral/facial herpes simplex on the lips and face. Do not use on genital herpes lesions.
- May cause application site reactions or headache
- For best results, cosmetics should be removed from the affected areas prior to applying or reapplying docosanol cream
- Cosmetics may be applied to the lips or skin after docosanol cream is applied. To avoid spreading the HSV infection, a separate applicator should be used to apply cosmetics or sunscreen over unhealed lesions.
- Topical docosanol should be discontinued if lesions are not healed after 10 days of treatment. An updated diagnosis and additional treatment may be indicated.
- Women of childbearing age should inform their healthcare provider of plans to become pregnant or breast-feed

Key Points

- Initiate therapy at the earliest sign or symptom (tingling, pruritus, redness, presence of a bump) of herpes labialis
- Docosanol is only for symptomatic treatment of herpes labialis. It is not indicated for preventive therapy.
- Remove makeup or other cosmetic products from affected areas prior to docosanol application
- Secondary bacterial infection may be present if lesions do not heal within 7–10 days

14

Topical Products

COMBINATION ANTIBIOTIC, BACITRACIN, NEOMYCIN, AND POLYMYXIN B

Introduction

Neosporin is a combination antibiotic composed of bacitracin, neomycin, and polymyxin B. Bacitracin is active against many gram-positive organisms, such as staphylococci, streptococci, anaerobic cocci, corynebacteria, and *Clostridia*. It is also active against gonococci, meningococci, and fusobacteria, but not against most other gram-negative organisms. Neomycin is active against many aerobic gram-negative bacteria and some aerobic gram-positive bacteria. The drug is inactive against fungi, viruses, and most anaerobic bacteria. Polymyxin B is a polypeptide antibiotic that has bactericidal activity against nearly all strains of gram-negative bacilli, excluding the *Proteus* group. It is not active against gram-positive bacteria, fungi, gram-negative cocci, *Neisseria gonorrhoeae*, and *Neisseria meningitidis*.

Mechanism of Action for the Drug Class

Bacitracin is a polypeptide antibiotic produced by *Bacillus subtilis*. It inhibits bacterial cell wall synthesis by preventing transfer of mucopeptides into the growing cell wall. Neomycin is an aminoglycoside antibiotic obtained from cultures of *Streptomyces fradiae*. Neomycin is usually bactericidal in action and appears to inhibit protein synthesis in susceptible bacteria by irreversibly binding to 30S ribosomal subunits. Polymyxin B binds to phospholipids and exerts its effect by increasing bacterial cell membrane permeability. In combination, these agents are used for the prevention or treatment of superficial infections of the skin caused by susceptible bacteria.

Members of the Drug Class

In this section: Bacitracin, neomycin, polymyxin B
Others: This combination plus hydrocortisone or pramoxine

⊙ Bacitracin, Neomycin, and Polymyxin B

Brand Names

Neosporin, Neosporin Neo To Go

Generic Names

Bacitracin, neomycin, polymyxin B

OTC

Dosage Forms

Topical ointment, spray

Usage

Prevention of infection in minor cuts, scrapes, and burns*

Pregnancy Category C

Dosing

Apply one to three times a day to the infected area; may cover with sterile bandage if necessary

Adverse Reactions: Most Common

Erythema, itching, swelling, irritation

Adverse Reactions: Rare/Severe/Important

Allergic contact dermatitis, failure to heal, anaphylaxis

Major Drug Interactions

Drugs Affecting Bacitracin, Neomycin, and Polymyxin B
- Amphotericin B, cephalosporin antibiotics, cisplatin, loop diuretics, NSAIDs, and vancomycin: Increase levels/effects
- Penicillin: Decrease levels/effects

Bacitracin, Neomycin, and Polymyxin B's Effect on Other Drugs
Colistimethate, cyclosporine, neuromuscular blocking agents, vitamin K antagonists: Increase levels/effects

Contraindications

Epithelial herpes simplex keratitis, mycobacterial or fungal infections

Counseling Points

- For external use only. Keep out of mouth, nose, and eyes. Wash hands before and after use.
- Should not be used for self-medication on deep or puncture wounds, animal bites, or serious burns; not for application to large areas of the body
- Clean affected area before use and dry well; apply a thin layer to affected skin and rub in gently; may cover with dressing if needed
- Notify healthcare provider if needed for > 1 week

Key Points

- Used for the prevention and treatment of superficial dermal infections; may also minimize appearance of scars
- Wash hands before and after use; not for use in mouth, nose, or eyes
- Do not use > 1 week

COMBINATION ANTIBIOTIC, ERYTHROMYCIN AND BENZOYL PEROXIDE

Introduction

Erythromycin and benzoyl peroxide is a combination topical antibiotic product used for the treatment of acne vulgaris

Mechanism of Action for the Drug Class

Erythromycin is a macrolide antibiotic that is active against strains of susceptible organisms. Erythromycin inhibits RNA-dependent protein synthesis at the chain-elongation step; it binds to the 50S ribosomal subunit, resulting in blockage of transpeptidation. Benzoyl peroxide is an antibacterial and keratolytic agent that releases free-radical oxygen and oxidizes bacterial proteins in the sebaceous follicles, decreasing the number of anaerobic bacteria and irritating-type free fatty acids.

Members of the Drug Class

In this section: Erythromycin and benzoyl peroxide
Others: Clindamycin and benzoyl peroxide, benzoyl peroxide and hydrocortisone

◉ Erythromycin and Benzoyl Peroxide

Brand Names

Benzamycin, Benzamycin Pak

Generic Names

Erythromycin, benzoyl peroxide

Rx Only

Dosage Form

Gel

Usage

Treatment of mild to moderate acne vulgaris*

Pregnancy Category C

Dosing

Adults and children ≥ 12 years of age: Apply to affected area twice daily, morning and evening

Adverse Reactions: Most Common

Peeling, erythema, edema, dry skin, urticaria

Adverse Reactions: Rare/Severe/Important

Sunburn, bleaching of hair and colored fabric, abdominal pain, cramps, diarrhea

Counseling Points

- For external use only; avoid contact with eyes and mouth
- Do not use any other topical acne preparation unless otherwise directed by your healthcare provider
- Report any adverse effects or if condition worsens
- Benzamycin Pak: Mix together the two compartments of one foil pouch in the palm of the hand immediately prior to use
- Keep topical gel refrigerated after reconstitution; discard after 3 months

Key Points

- Clean skin before use; apply twice daily to affected area
- Patients should not use any other topical acne preparation concomitantly
- Benzamycin may bleach hair or colored fabric
- Follow manufacturer's reconstitution and storage recommendations

---

COMBINATION ANTIFUNGAL AND CORTICOSTEROID

Introduction

The combination of clotrimazole and betamethasone is used to treat fungal skin infections, such as athlete's foot, jock itch, and ringworm

Mechanism of Action for the Drug Class

Clotrimazole is a synthetic antifungal agent that is active against most strains of dermatophytes. Clotrimazole binds to phospholipids in the fungal cell membrane, altering cell wall permeability, which results in the loss of essential intracellular elements. Betamethasone is a synthetic corticosteroid used to relieve redness, swelling, itching, and other discomforts of fungal infections. Betamethasone controls the rate of protein synthesis; depresses the migration of polymorphonuclear leukocytes and fibroblasts; and reverses capillary permeability and lysosomal stabilization at the cellular level to prevent or control inflammation.

Members of the Drug Class

In this section: Clotrimazole and betamethasone dipropionate
Others: Nystatin/triamcinolone

⊙ Clotrimazole and Betamethasone Dipropionate

Brand Name

Lotrisone

Generic Name

Clotrimazole and betamethasone dipropionate

Rx Only

Dosage Forms

Cream, lotion

Usage

Treatment of symptomatic inflammatory tinea pedis, tinea cruris, and tinea corporis*; allergic or inflammatory diseases

Pregnancy Category C

Dosing

- Adults ≥ 17 years of age: Massage into affected area twice daily, morning and evening
- Do not exceed application of 45 g of cream per week or 45 mL of lotion per week

Adverse Reactions: Most Common

Itching, skin irritation, dry skin, paresthesia

Adverse Reactions: Rare/Severe/Important

Erythema, drug-induced adrenocortical insufficiency, HPA-axis suppression

Major Drug Interactions

Potential pharmacologic interaction with other corticosteroid-containing preparations

Essential Monitoring Parameters

Periodic HPA-axis suppression tests, especially with prolonged use, use under occlusive dressings, or use over large surface area

Counseling Points

- For external use only. Avoid contact with eyes and mouth.
- Shake lotion well before use
- Use for the full treatment duration, even if symptoms have improved
- Notify your healthcare provider if there is no improvement after 1 week for tinea cruris or tinea corporis or after 2 weeks for tinea pedis
- Do not bandage, cover, or wrap the treated area
- Do not use on open wounds

Key Points

- Clinical improvement usually seen within 1 week for tinea cruris and tinea corporis and within 2 weeks for tinea pedis
- Follow recommended duration of treatment
- This medication should not be used > 2 weeks for tinea corporis or tinea cruris or > 4 weeks for tinea pedis
- This medication is not recommended for the treatment of diaper dermatitis

CORTICOSTEROID, CLOBETASOL PROPIONATE

Introduction

Clobetasol propionate is a very high-potency synthetic fluorinated corticosteroid

Mechanism of Action for the Drug Class

Following topical application, corticosteroids produce anti-inflammatory, antipruritic, and vasoconstrictor actions. The activity of this class is thought to result at least in part from binding with a steroid receptor that controls the rate of protein synthesis. It depresses the migration of polymorphonuclear leukocytes and fibroblasts and reverses capillary permeability and lysosomal stabilization at the cellular level to prevent or control inflammation.

Members of the Drug Class

In this section: Clobetasol propionate
Others: Betamethasone dipropionate 0.05%, fluocinonide 0.1%, halobetasol 0.05%

⊙ Clobetasol Propionate

Brand Names

Clobevate, Clobex, Cormax, Embeline, Olux, Temovate

Generic Name

Clobetasol propionate

Rx Only

Dosage Forms

Aerosol (foam), cream, gel, lotion, ointment, shampoo, solution

Usage

Short-term relief of the inflammatory and pruritic manifestations of moderate to severe corticosteroid-responsive dermatoses, including plaque psoriasis and scalp psoriasis*; oral mucosal inflammation (unlabeled)

Pregnancy Category C

Dosing

- Apply to affected area twice daily, morning and evening, for up to 2 weeks
- Total dose should not exceed 50 g per week (or 50 mL per week)
- Scalp psoriasis: Apply thin film of shampoo to *dry* scalp once daily; leave in place for 15 minutes; then add water, lather, and rinse thoroughly

Adverse Reactions: Most Common

Skin burning, tingling, cracking, pruritus, folliculitis, alopecia, headache

Adverse Reactions: Rare/Severe/Important

Acneiform eruptions, allergic contact dermatitis

Contraindication

Primary scalp infections

Essential Monitoring Parameters

Periodic HPA-axis suppression tests, especially with prolonged use, use under occlusive dressings, or use over large surface area

Counseling Points

- For external use only; follow specific product directions
- Apply the smallest amount that will cover the affected area. Do not apply to face, groin, or axilla areas. Total dose should not exceed 50 g per week (or 50 mL per week).
- Foam: Turn can upside down and spray a small amount (golf-ball size) of foam into the cap or another cool surface. If fingers are warm, rinse with cool water and dry before handling (foam will melt on contact with warm skin). Massage foam into affected area.
- Spray: Spray directly onto affected area of skin. Gently and completely rub into skin after spraying.

Key Points

- For external use only
- Do not apply to face, axilla, or groin areas
- Discontinue when control achieved; treatment beyond 2 consecutive weeks is not recommended. Total dosage should not exceed 50 g per week (50 mL per week).
- The treated skin area should not be bandaged or wrapped unless directed by a physician
- Adverse systemic effects including hyperglycemia, fluid and electrolyte changes, and HPA-axis suppression may occur when used on large surface areas, for prolonged periods, or with an occlusive dressing

CORTICOSTEROID, FLUOCINONIDE

Introduction

Fluocinonide is a high-potency fluorinated topical corticosteroid.

Members of the Drug Class

In this section: Fluocinonide
Others: Betamethasone dipropionate/valerate, desoximetasone, triamcinolone acetonide

⊙ Fluocinonide

Brand Names

Lidex, Lidex E, Vanos

Generic Name

Fluocinonide

Rx Only

Dosage Forms

Very high potency: 0.1% cream; high potency: 0.05% cream, gel, ointment, solution

Usage

Atopic dermatitis,* corticosteroid-responsive dermatoses,* plaque psoriasis,* epidermolysis bullosa, oral lichen planus

Pregnancy Category C

Dosing

- Pruritus and inflammation (0.05%): Apply thin layer to affected area two to four times daily depending on the severity of the condition
- Plaque-type psoriasis (0.1%): Apply a thin layer once or twice daily to affected areas for maximum of 2 consecutive weeks or 60 g per week total exposure

Adverse Reactions: Most Common

Dry skin, pruritus, sensation of burning of skin, headache, nasal congestion

Adverse Reactions: Rare/Severe/Important

Cushing's syndrome, hyperglycemia, adrenal suppression, allergic contact dermatitis

Contraindications

Untreated bacterial infection; skin lesions caused by tuberculosis, fungal, or viral agents, including herpes simplex, vaccinia, and varicella

Essential Monitoring Parameters

HPA-axis suppression should be tested periodically when fluocinonide is applied to large or occluded areas or used on altered skin barriers. It should also be tested in those patients receiving prolonged therapy or concomitant steroids or in those with liver failure.

Counseling Points

- For external use only. Avoid exposure to eyes, mucous membranes, or open wounds.
- Topical (0.1% cream): Affected area should be limited to < 10% of body surface area. Not recommended for use > 2 weeks or > 60 g per week total exposure.
- Use exactly as directed and for no longer than the period prescribed

- Before using, wash and dry area gently. Apply in a thin layer.
- Do not use occlusive dressing unless advised by prescriber. Avoid prolonged or excessive use around sensitive tissues or the genital or rectal areas.
- Avoid exposing treated area to direct sunlight
- Inform your healthcare provider if condition worsens or fails to improve

Key Points

- Therapy should be discontinued when control is achieved. If no improvement is seen, reassessment of diagnosis may be necessary.
- Not for ophthalmic use (0.05% cream, ointment)
- The 0.1% formulation should not be used on the face, groin, or axilla
- Use of the 0.1% formulation for > 2 weeks is not recommended

CORTICOSTEROID, HYDROCORTISONE

Introduction

Hydrocortisone is a low-to-medium potency corticosteroid used for the relief of inflammatory and pruritic manifestations of corticosteroid-responsive dermatoses

Members of the Drug Class

In this section: Hydrocortisone
Others: Desonide, fluocinolone acetonide, mometasone (low to medium potency)

◉ Hydrocortisone

Brand Names

Various (Anusol-HS, Cortaid, Cortenema, Dermacort, Hytone, Proctocort, Westcort)

Generic Name

Hydrocortisone

Rx and OTC

Dosage Forms

Topical cream, gel, lotion, ointment, paste, solution, foam; rectal cream, foam, suppository, suspension enema

Usage

Minor skin irritations*; itching and rash due to eczema, dermatitis, insect bites, poison ivy, poison oak, poison sumac, soaps, detergents, cosmetics, or jewelry*; late phase of allergic contact dermatitis*; scalp dermatitis*; seborrheic or atopic dermatitis*; psoriasis*; adjunctive treatment of ulcerative colitis*; anogenital pruritus*; proctitis*; inflamed hemorrhoids*; oral lesions

Pregnancy Category C

Dosing

- Skin dermatoses: Apply appropriate product sparingly one to four times daily; apply aerosol foam to affected area two to four times daily
- Scalp dermatoses: Part the hair and apply small amount of lotion or solution directly to the affected area; rub gently into scalp. Maintain usual hair care, but do not wash out lotion immediately after application. Alternatively, apply aerosol to dry scalp after shampooing.
- Oral lesions: Press a small amount of paste to the lesion without rubbing until a thin film develops two or three times daily after meals and at bedtime

Adverse Reactions: Most Common

Eczema, pruritus, stinging, dry skin, folliculitis, acneiform eruptions, hypertrichosis

Adverse Reactions: Rare/Severe/Important

Allergic contact dermatitis, burning, HPA-axis suppression, hypopigmentation, skin atrophy, secondary infection, perioral dermatitis, metabolic effects

Contraindications

Rectal enema is contraindicated with systemic fungal infections and ileocolostomy during the immediate or early postoperative period. Cortifoam is also contraindicated with obstruction, abscess, perforation, peritonitis, fresh intestinal anastomoses, extensive fistulas, and sinus tracts (other enemas are labeled to be used with caution).

Essential Monitoring Parameters

HPA-axis suppression should be tested periodically when hydrocortisone is applied to large or occluded areas or used on altered skin barriers. It should also be tested in those patients receiving prolonged therapy or concomitant steroids.

Counseling Points

- For dermatologic use only; avoid contact with eyes
- Hydrocortisone and its acetate, buteprate, butyrate, and valerate esters are applied topically
- Nonprescription preparations should not be used for self-medication for > 7 days
- If the condition worsens or symptoms persist, discontinue and consult your healthcare provider
- Before applying, wash area gently and thoroughly; apply a thin film to cleansed area and rub in gently until medication vanishes
- Reserve occlusive dressings for severe or resistant dermatoses as directed by your healthcare provider
- Avoid exposing affected area to sunlight

Key Points

- Consider location of the lesion and the condition being treated when choosing a dosage form
- Creams are suitable for most dermatoses, but ointments may also provide some occlusion and are usually used for the treatment of dry, scaly lesions
- Lotions are best for treatment of weeping eruptions, especially in areas subject to chafing. Lotions, gels, and aerosols may be used on hairy areas, particularly the scalp.
- Patients applying a topical corticosteroid to a large surface area and/or to areas under occlusion should be evaluated periodically for evidence of HPA-axis suppression

CORTICOSTEROID, MOMETASONE FUROATE

Introduction

Mometasone furoate is a synthetic, nonfluorinated, medium-potency topical corticosteroid that has anti-inflammatory, antipruritic, and vasoconstrictive properties. Mometasone is a derivative of prednisolone and differs structurally from beclomethasone. The structural differences are thought to enhance the topical anti-inflammatory activity of mometasone.

Members of the Drug Class

In this section: Mometasone furoate
Others: Hydrocortisone butyrate 0.1%, hydrocortisone valerate 0.2%, betamethasone valerate 0.1% cream; fluocinolone acetonide 0.025% (medium potency)

◉ Mometasone Furoate

Brand Name
Elocon

Generic Name
Mometasone furoate

Rx Only

Dosage Forms
Cream, lotion, ointment

Usage
Relief of inflammatory and pruritic manifestations of corticosteroid-responsive dermatoses*

Pregnancy Category C

Dosing

Apply a thin film (cream, ointment) or a few drops (lotion) to affected areas once daily

Adverse Reactions: Most Common

Burning, pruritus, stinging/tingling

Adverse Reactions: Rare/Severe/Important

Dryness, irritation, skin atrophy, bacterial skin infection, skin depigmentation

Essential Monitoring Parameters

HPA-axis suppression should be tested periodically when mometasone furoate is applied to large or occluded areas

Counseling Points

- For external use only. Avoid contact with eyes, mouth, and open wounds.
- Avoid prolonged or excessive use around sensitive tissues, underarms, or the genital or rectal areas
- Wash and dry affected area gently before applying product
- Report severe or persistent adverse effects or if no improvement in 2 weeks to your healthcare provider
- Discontinue use and notify your healthcare provider at the first sign of allergic reaction or skin rash
- The treated skin area should not be covered with any occlusive dressing

Key Points

- Topical mometasone furoate products are applied sparingly in thin films and are rubbed into the affected area, usually once daily
- The treated skin area should not be covered with any occlusive dressing because this can increase percutaneous penetration of mometasone

CORTICOSTEROID, TRIAMCINOLONE ACETONIDE

Introduction

Triamcinolone acetonide is a medium- to high-potency synthetic fluorinated corticosteroid that has anti-inflammatory, antipruritic, and vasoconstrictive properties.

Members of the Drug Class

In this section: Triamcinolone acetonide
Others: Betamethasone valerate, hydrocortisone valerate, fluocinolone acetonide

◉ Triamcinolone Acetonide

Brand Names

Aristocort, Flutex, Kenalog, Kenalog in Orabase, Oralone, Triderm

Generic Name

Triamcinolone acetonide

Rx Only

Dosage Forms

Aerosol, cream, lotion, ointment, paste

Usage

Inflammatory dermatoses responsive to steroids, including contact/atopic dermatitis*; adjunctive treatment and temporary relief of symptoms associated with oral inflammatory lesions and ulcerative lesions resulting from trauma

Pregnancy Category C

Dosing

- Cream, ointment:
  - 0.025% or 0.05%: Apply thin film to affected areas two to four times a day
  - 0.1% or 0.5%: Apply thin film to affected areas two to three times a day
- Spray: Apply to affected area three to four times a day
- Oral topical: Press a small dab (about 0.25 inch) to the lesion without rubbing until a thin film develops; apply at bedtime and, if necessary, two or three times daily after meals

Adverse Reactions: Most Common

Dryness, burning, itching, irritation, folliculitis

Adverse Reactions: Rare/Severe/Important

Acneiform eruptions, allergic contact dermatitis, secondary skin infection, skin atrophy

Contraindications

Fungal, viral, or bacterial infections of the mouth or throat (oral topical formulation)

Essential Monitoring Parameters

Periodic HPA-axis suppression tests, especially with prolonged use, use under occlusive dressings, or use over large surface area

Counseling Points

- For external use only. Do not apply to eyes, mucous membranes, or open wounds.
- Oral topical (Kenalog in Orabase): Apply at bedtime or after meals if applications are needed throughout the day. Do not use if fungal, viral, or bacterial infections of the mouth or throat are present. If lesion has not improved in 7 days, notify your healthcare provider.
- Ointment: Apply a thin film sparingly. Do not use on open skin or wounds. Do not occlude area unless directed.
- Spray: Avoid eyes and do not inhale if spraying near face. Occlusive dressing may be used if instructed. Monitor for infection.

Key Points

- Follow specific product directions for application; for external use only
- Triamcinolone acetonide 0.5% cream and 0.1% ointment: high-range potency
- Triamcinolone acetonide 0.1% cream and 0.1% lotion: medium-range potency
- Generally most effective in acute or chronic dermatoses (seborrheic or atopic dermatitis, localized neurodermatitis, anogenital pruritus, psoriasis, late phase of allergic contact dermatitis, inflammatory phase of xerosis)
- Avoid eyes, mucous membranes, or open wounds
- Avoid prolonged or excessive use around sensitive tissues or the genital or rectal areas
- Inform your healthcare provider if condition worsens (skin irritation/contact dermatitis) or fails to improve

Introduction

Permethrin, a pyrethroid, is active against a broad range of pests, including lice, ticks, fleas, mites, and other arthropods. Permethrin is active against *Pediculus humanus var. capitis* (the head louse) and its nits (eggs); *Phthirus pubis* (the pubic or crab louse) and its nits; and *Sarcoptes scabiei*, the causative parasite of scabies. Permethrin has the advantages of a low potential for toxicity and good ovicidal activity; however, widespread resistance to permethrin has been reported in other countries and the prevalence of resistance to the drug in the United States is unclear.

Mechanism of Action for the Drug Class

Like natural pyrethrins, permethrin acts as a neurotoxin by depolarizing the nerve cell membranes of parasites. The drug disrupts the sodium channel current by which membrane repolarization is regulated. Delayed repolarization results in paralysis of the nerves in the exoskeletal respiratory muscles of the parasite, leading to death. At a concentration of 1%, permethrin is pediculicidal; concentrations of 5% also are scabicidal. Permethrin is rapidly metabolized by ester hydrolysis to inactive metabolites, which are excreted primarily in the urine.

Members of the Drug Class

In this section: Permethrin
Others: Benzyl alcohol, benzyl benzoate, crotamiton, ivermectin, lindane, malathion, pyrethrins/piperonyl butoxide, spinosad

◉ Permethrin

Brand Names

A200 Lice, Acticin, Elimite, Nix Complete Lice Treatment System, Nix Creme Rinse Lice Treatment, Nix Creme Rinse, Nix Lice Control Spray, Rid

Generic Name

Permethrin

Rx and OTC

Dosage Forms

Rx: 5% topical cream; OTC: 0.25–1% topical liquid, lotion, solution

Usage

Single-application treatment of infestation with *Pediculus humanus var. capitis* (head louse) and its nits or *Sarcoptes scabiei* (scabies)*; indicated for prophylactic use during epidemics of lice

Pregnancy Category B

The amount of permethrin available systemically following topical application is ≤ 2%. No adequate, controlled studies using topical permethrin in pregnant women have been conducted; thus, use during pregnancy only when clearly needed. The CDC considers permethrin 5% a drug of choice for the treatment of pediculosis or scabies in pregnant or lactating women. Pregnant women should be advised to consult their healthcare provider before self-medicating with topical permethrin.

Dosing

- Head lice in adults and children > 2 months of age: Shampoo hair and rinse with water, towel dry, apply permethrin to scalp, leave on 10 minutes, rinse; remove nits with nit comb; repeat application if live lice or nits present 7 days after initial treatment.
- Scabies:
  - Apply a generous amount of cream from head to feet, leave on for 8–14 hours, wash with soap/water
  - Repeat application if living mites are present 14 days after initial treatment
  - For infants, also apply on the hairline, neck, scalp, temple, and forehead

Adverse Reactions: Most Common

Pruritus, erythema, rash, stinging, tingling, numbness or scalp discomfort, edema

Major Drug Interactions

None

Contraindication

Permethrin lotion is contraindicated for use in infants < 2 months of age

Counseling Points

- For external use only. Do not apply to face and avoid contact with eyes or mucous membranes.
- Clothing and bedding must be washed in hot water or dry cleaned to kill nits. May need to treat all members of household and all sexual contacts concurrently. Wash all combs and brushes with permethrin and rinse thoroughly.
- Because scabies and lice are so contagious, use caution to avoid spreading or infecting oneself; wear gloves when applying
- Apply a sufficient volume of creme rinse to saturate the hair and scalp; also apply behind the ears and at the base of the neck. Shake cream rinse well before using.

- Contact your healthcare provider if pruritus, edema, erythema, or stinging or burning of skin occurs; if condition persists; or if skin becomes infected
- Pregnant women should be advised to consult their healthcare provider before self-medicating with topical permethrin

Key Points

- Follow proper application technique, depending on affected body site
- Wear gloves when applying to avoid spreading or becoming infected
- Consider treatment for all household members and sexual contacts
- Wash clothes, bedding, and personal items in hot, soapy water to prevent reinfection

---

REVIEW QUESTIONS

1. Which of the following is *not* part of Neosporin?
   a. Polymyxin B
   b. Bacitracin
   c. Erythromycin
   d. Neomycin

2. Which of the following is used to treat bacterial vaginosis?
   a. Cleocin
   b. Nizoral
   c. Benzamycin
   d. Vanos

3. Which of the following is *not* a dosage form of clindamycin phosphate?
   a. Topical gel
   b. Pledget
   c. Vaginal suppository
   d. Anal suppository

4. Which of the following is *not* a brand name of clindamycin phosphate?
   a. Evoclin
   b. Cleoget
   c. Clindesse
   d. Cleocin

5. Nizoral is *not* used for which of the following infections?
   a. Tinea pedis
   b. Tinea cruris
   c. Tinea capitis
   d. Tinea corporis

6. Which of the following is *not* a common adverse reaction with Benzamycin?
   a. Diarrhea
   b. Peeling
   c. Edema
   d. Erythema

7. Lotrisone can be used to treat which of the following?
   a. Diaper dermatitis
   b. Tinea cruris
   c. Acne vulgaris
   d. Plaque psoriasis

8. Clobetasol propionate is also known as which of the following?
   a. Vanos
   b. Temovate
   c. Kenalog
   d. Elocon

9. A patient comes to your pharmacy with a new prescription for Vanos. Which of the following is *not* a counseling point?
   a. Do not use in eyes, mucous membranes, or open wounds.
   b. Avoid exposing treated area to direct sunlight.
   c. Wash and dry the area gently before application.
   d. Always use occlusive dressing after application.

10. Which of the following may be considered a low-potency topical corticosteroid?
    a. Elocon
    b. Vanos
    c. Olux
    d. Proctocort

11. Hydrocortisone is indicated for all of the following, *except*:

    a. acne rosacea.
    b. oral lesions.
    c. psoriasis.
    d. seborrheic dermatitis.

12. Which of the following is the correct dosing of Elocon?

    a. Apply thin film to affected area twice daily.
    b. Apply thin film to affected area once daily.
    c. Apply thick layer to affected area twice daily.
    d. Apply thick layer to affected area once daily.

13. A pregnant female comes to the pharmacy complaining of cracked, peeling skin between her toes for 3 weeks. This skin irritation started after she joined a local gym, and it has not resolved. You recognize these symptoms as tinea pedis, or athlete's foot. Which of the following should you recommend?

    a. Lotrisone cream: Massage into affected area every morning and evening.
    b. Nizoral 200 mg PO daily for 14 days.
    c. No treatment is necessary; counsel her to wear flip-flops at the gym shower.
    d. Lamisil AT 1% cream applied daily for 1 week.

14. Which of the following statements regarding terbinafine is *false*?

    a. Terbinafine is structurally and pharmacologically related to naftifine.
    b. Terbinafine is more active against *Candida* species compared to azole antifungal agents.
    c. Terbinafine may be fungistatic or fungicidal in action depending on the drug concentration and type of fungus.
    d. Terbinafine inhibits squalene epoxidase, an important enzyme in fungal sterol synthesis.

15. Which of the following is true of Abreva?

    a. It is most effective as a preventative regimen for HSV-1.
    b. It is safe in patients < 12 years of age.
    c. It should be applied five times daily to the affected area.
    d. It is recommended for use with genital herpes lesions.

16. Which of the following is indicated for the treatment of herpes labialis?

    a. Capsaicin
    b. Docosanol
    c. Mupirocin
    d. Terbinafine

17. Which of the following is a key counseling point for patients using miconazole?

    a. Intravaginal miconazole may increase plasma warfarin concentrations.
    b. St. John's wort is safe to use concurrently with miconazole.
    c. Tinea corporis should be treated for 2 weeks.
    d. All of the above.

18. Tinea versicolor is caused by *Pityrosporum ovale* and is most common in adolescent and young adult males. The main symptom is patches of discolored skin with sharp edges and fine scales. The most common sites are the back, underarms, upper arms, chest, and neck. Which of the following can be used to treat this condition?

    a. Abreva
    b. Lotrimin AF
    c. Avagard
    d. Lotrisone

19. Which of the following drug information points is correct regarding Benzamycin?

    a. It is indicated for the treatment of mild to moderate acne rosacea.
    b. It is available over the counter.
    c. It contains a macrolide antibiotic.
    d. All of the above.

20. Which of the following is indicated for the treatment of vulvovaginal candidiasis?

    a. Clindesse
    b. Terazol 3
    c. MetroGel
    d. Extina

21. Which of the following is correct for terconazole vaginal products?

    a. Insert one suppository vaginally at bedtime for 7 days.
    b. Vaginal 0.4% cream: Insert one applicatorful at bedtime for 3 days
    c. Vaginal 0.8% cream: Insert one applicatorful at bedtime for 3 days.
    d. All of the above.

22. Which of the following Neo to Go drug information points is *incorrect*?

    a. It contains an aminoglycoside antibiotic.
    b. It is recommended for the treatment of topical fungal infections.
    c. Do not self-medicate with this product for > 1 week.
    d. Proper use may reduce the appearance of scars.

23. Which of the following is a medium-potency cortico-steroid?

   a. Clobetasol
   b. Mometasone
   c. Fluocinonide
   d. Betamethasone

24. Fluocinonide is contraindicated in which of the following conditions?

   a. Presence of untreated bacterial infection
   b. Skin lesions caused by fungal infections
   c. Skin lesions caused by herpes simplex
   d. All of the above

25. Clobetasol is usually prescribed for up to how many weeks?

   a. 2 weeks
   b. 1 week
   c. 4 weeks
   d. As needed for skin irritation

26. Which of the following is *not* an available dosage form for clotrimazole plus betamethasone dipropionate?

   a. Cream
   b. Lotion
   c. Gel
   d. All of the above formulations are available.

27. Which of the following is recommended for the treatment of tinea pedis?

   a. Lotrisone
   b. Lidex
   c. Elocon
   d. Westcort

28. Which of the following products does *not* contain permethrin?

   a. Nix Complete Lice Treatment System
   b. Rid
   c. A200 Lice
   d. Lindane

29. What pregnancy category is Nix?

   a. Pregnancy category B
   b. Pregnancy category C
   c. Pregnancy category D
   d. Pregnancy category X

30. Which of the following is *not* an appropriate counseling point for triamcinolone?

   a. Avoid eyes, mucous membranes, and open wounds.
   b. Apply a thin film sparingly.
   c. For oral topical triamcinolone, notify prescriber if lesion is not improved in 48 hours.
   d. All of the above are appropriate counseling points.

Natural Products, Dietary Supplements, and Nutrients

Patrick McDonnell, PharmD

GENERAL STATEMENT: NATURAL PRODUCTS, DIETARY SUPPLEMENTS, AND NUTRIENTS

Herbs and botanicals have been used for centuries for the treatment and prevention of disease. Egyptian papyruses, as well as Babylonian stone tablets, list "prescriptions" for certain herbals remedies.

These products, defined legally as *dietary supplements* in the United States and referred to as *natural health products* in the United States and Canada, consist of single or many ingredients. Under the Food and Drug Administration's (FDA) 1994 Dietary Supplement Health and Education Act, a *dietary supplement* is defined as a product taken by mouth that contains a "dietary ingredient" intended to supplement the diet. The dietary ingredients in these products may include vitamins, minerals, herbs or other botanicals, amino acids, and substances such as enzymes, organ tissues, glandulars, and metabolites. Although far from complete, data on the safety and efficacy of individual ingredients are more comprehensive for nutrients, such as vitamins, than for herbals and other botanicals. Note that in the United States these products, which number in the thousands, are marketed with limited regulatory oversight. For example, these products are not monitored for product safety, efficacy, or quality. However, the FDA does regulate the labeling and types of claims made on these products.

This chapter presents some of the most commonly used dietary supplement ingredients. The products available that contain each ingredient are too numerous to list beyond a few examples from the U.S. marketplace. Indications listed are common uses and are not necessarily supported by clinical evidence. Dosing ranges for nutrients are based on the highest Dietary Reference Intake (DRI) level for nonpregnant, nonlactating adults. Dosing for other ingredients is based more on current usage than on dose-finding trials. Additionally, dosing of an ingredient may differ between the products containing them and may not necessarily be well supported in the literature. Although generally well tolerated, dietary supplement products can produce adverse effects and interactions. These are based predominantly on case reports and may be reflective of the ingredient itself or the quality of the product it is delivered in. Dietary supplement ingredients do not receive formal pregnancy category ratings, and in most cases they have not been evaluated in pregnancy or lactation. Patients should always consult with their healthcare provider before taking any nonprescription medication or herbal/dietary supplement.

NATURAL SUPPLEMENT, CHAMOMILE

Introduction

Chamomile is a popular herbal supplement most often associated with teas, but it has also been used and touted as a "calmative" and gastrointestinal antispasmodic. It is also used for skin inflammation and other indications. Clinical trials supporting any use of chamomile for medical conditions are very limited.

Mechanism of Action for the Drug Class

It is thought that the anti-inflammatory effects are related to several chemical constituents of chamomile, namely bisbolol and flavonoids, which have demonstrated antispasmodic effects in animals. Its use as a calmative in some animal models is attributed to apigenin, a chamomile extract, that affects benzodiazepine binding sites in the brain.

---

* Throughout the text, an asterisk (*) is used to indicate the most common uses of a drug.

◉ Chamomile

Brand Names

Generics only

Generic Names

Chamomile, *Matricaria recutita, Chamaemelum nobile*

OTC

Dosage Forms

Tablet, capsule, liquid extract, tea, topical cream

Usage

GI antispasmodic,* calmative, anti-inflammatory

Pregnancy Category

Poorly documented adverse reactions have been reported (e.g., abortifacient effects, menstrual cycle irregularities, uterine stimulation with excessive use). Well-documented information regarding safety and efficacy in pregnancy is lacking. However, because it may possess weak estrogenic activity, avoid use in pregnancy.

Dosing

- Typical oral dose: 9–15 g daily
- See specific manufacturers' labels for other dosage forms (topicals, teas)
- Renal dosage adjustment: None

Adverse Reactions: Most Common

Patients who are sensitive to ragweed or who get hay fever have been known to "cross-react" when exposed to chamomile-containing products

Adverse Reactions: Rare/Severe/Important

None

Major Drug Interactions

Chamomile's Effect on Other Drugs

Warfarin: May increase effect (case reports of bleeding with warfarin)

Counseling Point

If you are allergic to ragweed or flowers such as chrysanthemums and asters, avoid use of chamomile-containing products

Key Points

- Best to avoid during pregnancy and lactation due to purported estrogenic effects
- Gargles of chamomile flowers used as a natural treatment for chemotherapy-induced mucositis were no more effective than placebo in a clinical trial

NATURAL SUPPLEMENT, CHONDROITIN

Introduction

Derived from animal cartilage, chondroitin is a popular and relatively safe natural supplement used to reduce the pain of osteoarthritis

Mechanism of Action for the Drug Class

This mixture of polysulfated glycosaminoglycans (e.g., chondroitin-4-SO_4, chondroitin-6-SO_4) serves as a substrate for cartilage synthesis and may inhibit leukocyte elastase and improve joint mobility

◉ Chondroitin

Brand Names

Cosamin, Cosamin DS, Cosamin Protek, others

Generic Name

Chondroitin

OTC

Dosage Forms

Tablet, capsule, liquid extract

Usage

Pain relief from osteoarthritis,* maintenance of joint cartilage

Pregnancy Category

Information regarding safety and efficacy in pregnancy is lacking. Avoid use.

Dosing

- 200–400 mg two to three times daily
- Maximum dose: 1,200 mg daily
- Renal dosage adjustment: Not known

Adverse Reactions: Most Common

Nausea, diarrhea, mild epigastric pain, headache

Adverse Reactions: Rare/Severe/Important

Myelosuppression (very rare)

Major Drug Interactions

Theoretical interaction with anticoagulants because chondroitin's structure is similar to heparinoid compounds

Counseling Points

- Animal sources of chondroitin (e.g., bovine, porcine, shark) may pose risk of transmitting infectious agents; use products from trusted manufacturers
- Often found in combination products with glucosamine, although frequently in amounts lower than label claims

- Multi-ingredient products containing manganese may provide doses of this mineral above the tolerable upper limit for adults (11 mg)

Key Point

Best to avoid during pregnancy and lactation until safety data are available

---

NATURAL SUPPLEMENT, CINNAMON

Introduction

Best known as an aromatic and spice, cinnamon has been used in some cultures for GI disorders and as an antimicrobial, an antidiarrheal, and a dysmenorrheal. However, limited scientific data support these uses. In addition, claims have been made of cinnamon's antidiabetic properties, but data are also lacking to support this use.

Mechanism of Action for the Drug Class

Cinnamon bark and essential oils of cinnamon have been shown to have in vitro activity against some bacterial endotoxins, as well as fungal aflatoxins. Prostaglandin inhibition has been demonstrated with cinnamon, leading to its use as an anti-inflammatory. Polyphenols isolated from cinnamon have been shown to demonstrate some insulin-like activity.

◉ Cinnamon

Brand Name
Cinnulin PF

Generic Name
Cinnamon

OTC

Dosage Forms
Tablet, capsule, ground cinnamon

Usage
Antimicrobial,* antidiabetic agent,* antioxidant

Pregnancy Category
Information regarding safety and efficacy in pregnancy is lacking. Generally recognized as safe when used in food.

Dosing

- Cinnulin: 250 mg twice daily before meals
- Ground powder: 1.0–1.5 g per day
- Renal dosage adjustment: None

Adverse Reactions: Most Common
None. The FDA gives cinnamon GRAS status (generally recognized as safe).

Adverse Reactions: Rare/Severe/Important
When cinnamon is ingested in large quantities in bark or oil form, increases in heart rate, breathing, GI motility, and perspiration have been noted

Major Drug Interactions
Theoretical synergistic effect with antidiabetic agents

Counseling Points

- Avoid ingestion of large quantities of bark or oil due to unwanted adverse effects
- Do not use as the sole agent to self-treat diabetes. Research has demonstrated no significant effect on cinnamon's ability to lower blood glucose or glycohemoglobin.

Key Point

- 500 mg of Cinnulin aqueous extract is equivalent to approximately 10 g of cinnamon powder
- If pregnant, avoid doses above those found in food, because safety and efficacy have not been proven

---

NATURAL SUPPLEMENT, CO-ENZYME Q

Introduction

Co-enzyme Q is a popular antioxidant that consumers use to promote "heart health."

Mechanism of Action for the Drug Class

Co-enzyme Q, a mitochondrial enzyme synthesized endogenously and containing 10 isoprenoid subunits, is involved in electron transport and ATP generation

⊙ Co-enzyme Q

Brand Names

Heart Actives, Heart Support, Pure CoQ-10, Q-Gel, Q-Sorb, others

Generic Names

Co-enzyme Q, co-enzyme-Q_{10}, CoQ, CoQ_{10}, ubiquinone, ubidecarenone

OTC

Dosage Forms

Tablet, capsule, liquid extract

Usage

Antioxidant activity for several disorders, particularly cardiovascular disease (e.g., cardiomyopathy, heart failure, hypertension),* HIV, and Parkinson's disease; prevention of statin-induced myopathy

Pregnancy Category

Information regarding safety and efficacy in pregnancy is lacking. Avoid use.

Dosing

- Usual dose: 50–200 mg daily
- Heart failure: 50 mg twice daily
- Hypertension: 60 mg twice daily
- Angina: 50 mg three times daily
- HIV: 200 mg daily
- Parkinson's disease: Up to 1,200 mg daily
- Prevention of statin-induced myopathy: 150–250 mg daily
- Renal dosage adjustment: Not known

Adverse Reactions: Most Common

Anorexia, nausea, vomiting

Adverse Reactions: Rare/Severe/Important

Headache, dizziness, fatigue, maculopapular rash, thrombocytopenia, elevated liver function tests, hypotension

Major Drug Interactions

Drugs Affecting Co-enzyme Q

HMG-CoA reductase inhibitors and beta blockers: Reduce serum concentration

Co-enzyme Q's Effect on Other Drugs

Warfarin: Decreases effect (theoretical only)

Counseling Points

- Use only with medical supervision for cardiovascular disorders
- Take with food

Key Points

- Supplied exogenously through many foods and also synthesized endogenously (sharing some synthetic pathways with cholesterol), but significance of source to co-enzyme Q status not yet clear
- Best to avoid during pregnancy and lactation until safety data are available

NATURAL SUPPLEMENT, CREATINE

Introduction

Popular among younger consumers, creatine supplements are widely used to enhance muscle strength and athletic performance

Mechanism of Action for the Drug Class

Synthesized endogenously and stored predominantly in skeletal muscle as creatine-phosphate. It serves as a high-energy phosphate source during anaerobic metabolism.

⊙ Creatine

Brand Names

CRE Active, Creatine Blast, Creatine Fuel, Creatine Powder, CreaVATE, others

Generic Names

Creatine, creatine monohydrate, N-amidinosarcosine, N- (amino-imino-methyl)-N-methylglycine

OTC

Dosage Forms

Capsule, powder

Usage

Improves muscle strength, athletic performance, and recovery during exercise*

Pregnancy Category

Information regarding safety and efficacy in pregnancy is lacking. Avoid use.

Dosing

- Initial or loading dose of 5 g four times daily for 2–5 days followed by 2–5 g daily for 1–5 weeks
- May be supplied in varying doses as an ingredient in different exercise or "body-building" supplements
- Renal dosage adjustment: Not known, but avoid use in renal dysfunction

Adverse Reactions: Most Common

Nausea, abdominal pain, diarrhea

Adverse Reactions: Rare/Severe/Important

Renal failure

Major Drug Interactions

Use with other drugs that may affect renal hemodynamics (NSAIDs, ACE inhibitors/angiotensin receptor blockers, and/or diuretics) can increase the risk of renal failure

Counseling Points

- Maintain adequate hydration (at least 2,000 mL of water daily)
- Avoid use in combination with caffeine and ephedra
- Products may contain an impurity from processing (dicyandiamide)

Key Points

- Average diet supplies about 2 g creatine daily as well as the amino acid precursors for endogenous synthesis
- Best to avoid during pregnancy and lactation until safety data are available

NATURAL SUPPLEMENT, ECHINACEA

Introduction

Echinacea is primarily used as an immune "booster" and is usually derived from the *Asteraceae* genus of plants. This genus includes the purple coneflower, which is the most common botanical source.

Mechanism of Action for the Drug Class

A number of polysaccharides, alkylamides, caffeic acid esters (echinacosides), and other constituents, which vary among species and plant parts, possess nonspecific immunomodulatory activity. It is thought that these constituents alter cell surface binding (T lymphocytes, macrophages) and increase cytokine production.

◉ Echinacea

Brand Names

EchinaGuard, Echinaforce, Esberitox, Echinacea, others

Generic Names

Echinacea, *Echinacea purpurea*, *Echinacea angustifolia*, *Echinacea pallida*, black-eyed susan, coneflower, hedgehog, Indian head, purple coneflower, snakeroot

OTC

Dosage Forms

Tablet, capsule, liquid extract

Usage

Treatment of the common cold,* prevention and treatment of minor upper respiratory infections

Pregnancy Category

Information regarding safety and efficacy in pregnancy is lacking. Avoid use.

Dosing

- 900 mg three times daily of portions of *E. purpurea* standardized to 4% phenolics
- Because preparations vary, always refer to specific manufacturer's instructions for dosing
- 0.25–1.0 mL three times daily of a liquid extract (1:1 in 45% ethanol)
- Renal dosage adjustment: Not known

Adverse Reactions: Most Common

GI complaints (altered taste, nausea, vomiting); neurologic complaints (transient tiredness, somnolence, dizziness, headache); dermatologic reactions (allergic skin reaction, eczema); asthma exacerbation; anaphylaxis

Adverse Reactions: Rare/Severe/Important

Hepatotoxicity with long-term chronic use and or use with other known hepatotoxins

Contraindications

Patients on immunosuppressant therapy should avoid use of echinacea because of a theoretical interaction with concurrent use. Patients with autoimmune disorders (e.g., rheumatoid arthritis, lupus) should avoid the use of this dietary supplement.

Major Drug Interactions

Echinacea's Effect on Other Drugs

- Immunomodulating agents: Potential interference with (theoretical)
- CYP3A4 or P-glycoprotein: May inhibit levels of CYP3A4 or P-glycoprotein substrates (low risk)

Counseling Points

- Limit continuous use to 2–8 weeks
- Value for treatment may exceed that for prevention of upper respiratory infections
- Avoid use if you have a history of allergy to ragweed, daisy, sunflower, and/or chrysanthemum, because they are likely to cross-react with echinacea

Key Points

- Contraindicated for patients with autoimmune diseases and/or on immunosuppressant agents
- Best to avoid during pregnancy and lactation until safety data are available

NATURAL SUPPLEMENT, FEVERFEW

Introduction

Feverfew is one of the more commonly used herbal supplements because of it purported anti-inflammatory and analgesic effects. It is sometimes favored as a natural product for migraine sufferers.

Mechanism of Action for the Drug Class

Various metabolites, including parthenolide, inhibit prostaglandin synthesis, platelet aggregation, and leukotriene synthesis

⊙ Feverfew

Brand Names

Feverfew Extract, Herbal Sure Feverfew, Mygrafew, NuVeg Feverfew Leaf, Premium Feverfew Leaf

Generic Names

Feverfew, *Tanacetum parthenium*

OTC

Dosage Forms

Tablet, capsule, liquid extract

Usage

Pain and inflammation;* headache, including migraine treatment and prophylaxis*

Pregnancy Category

Information regarding safety and efficacy in pregnancy is lacking. Avoid use. Based on the antiprostaglandin effect of this dietary supplement, fetal toxicity may be expected to be similar to what one may see with nonsteroidal anti-inflammatory drugs (NSAIDs), including premature closure of the ductus arteriosus and fetal nephro- and cardiotoxicity.

Dosing

- 200–250 mg daily
- Renal dosage adjustment: Not known; however, use with caution in patients with renal impairment due to expected effects on renal prostaglandins

Adverse Reactions: Most Common

Avoid skin contact due to high potential for sensitization, transient tachycardia, bruising, bleeding, GI ulceration, abdominal pain, diarrhea

Adverse Reactions: Rare/Severe/Important

Renal failure, hepatotoxicity

Contraindications

Based on the antiprostaglandin effect of feverfew, fetal toxicity can be expected similar to what one may see with nonsteroidal anti-inflammatory drugs (NSAIDs), including premature closure of the ductus arteriosus and fetal nephro- and cardiotoxicity

Major Drug Interactions

Drugs Affecting Feverfew

NSAIDs: Concurrent use can increase risk of GI toxicities (dyspepsia, GI ulceration) and nephrotoxicity

Feverfew's Effect on Other Drugs

- Antiplatelet agents and anticoagulants: May increase risk of bleeding
- Use caution with drugs that can negatively impact renal hemodynamics, such as diuretics, ACE inhibitors/angiotensin receptor blockers, NSAIDs, methotrexate, lithium

Counseling Points

- Monitor for signs and symptoms of bleeding, especially if using concurrent therapies such as anticoagulants, NSAIDs, and antiplatelet therapy
- Discontinue 7–10 days before elective surgery
- Monitor for any changes in renal function particularly if using concurrent NSAIDs, ACE inhibitors, angiotensin receptor blockers, and/or diuretics

Key Points

- Avoid in patients with severe renal disease
- Avoid during pregnancy, particularly the third trimester, due to inhibition of prostaglandins on fetal cardiac physiology

NATURAL SUPPLEMENT, GARLIC

Introduction

Garlic, a popular botanical, is believed to have many pharmacologic effects, leading to its use as an antiseptic, antihypertensive, antilipemic, and expectorant. It is thought that most of garlic's benefits are derived from the raw garlic clove versus commercially prepared products.

Mechanism of Action for the Drug Class

Alliins are the most active substances in garlic. It is thought that garlic alliins block adenosine triphosphate citrate lyases, an important enzymatic step in the process of converting carbohydrates to fat. Another substance in garlic, ajoene, seems to demonstrate antimicrobial properties. It is believed, however, that any pharmacologic effect with garlic is seen with the use of freshly prepared products versus commercialized capsules, tablets, and powders.

⊙ Garlic

Brand Names

Garlicin, Garlique, Garlic Oil, Triple Garlic, Kyolic-Branded Products, High Allicin Garlic, Odor-Free Concentrated Garlic

Generic Names

Garlic, *Allium sativum*, allium, clove garlic

OTC

Dosage Forms

Tablet, capsule, liquid extract, dried powder, raw garlic clove

Usage

Treatment of hyperlipidemia* and high blood pressure;* antiseptic agent*

Pregnancy Category

Information regarding safety and efficacy in pregnancy is lacking. Avoid use.

Dosing

- Hyperlipidemia: Total daily dose of 600–900 mg of garlic powder (standardized to 1.3% of alliin content)
- Hypertension: 200–300 mg three times daily
- Antiseptic: Fresh garlic can be applied to the skin as an antimicrobial dressing for a few hours; prolonged contact may lead to skin irritation/burns
- Renal dosage adjustment: Not known

Essential Monitoring Parameter

Due to potential antiplatelet effects, monitor for any marked bruising or bleeding, particularly in patients taking drugs that increase bleeding risk

Adverse Reactions: Most Common

Headache, fatigue, myalgias, skin reactions/burns with prolonged application of fresh garlic preparations to skin, dyspepsia, body odor, halitosis, lacrimation

Adverse Reactions: Rare/Severe/Important

Increases bleeding risk, particularly when combined with antiplatelet agents and/or anticoagulants

Major Drug Interactions

Garlic's Effects on Other Drugs

Antiplatelets, NSAIDs, warfarin, anticoagulants: Increases bleeding risk

Counseling Points

- Increased bleeding risk when used with antiplatelets, NSAIDs, warfarin, and anticoagulants; monitor accordingly
- Discontinue 7–10 days before elective surgery
- Best therapeutic results are seen with freshly prepared garlic

Key Points

- Increased bleeding risk when used with antiplatelets, NSAIDs, warfarin, and anticoagulants; monitor accordingly
- Avoid use during pregnancy and lactation

NATURAL SUPPLEMENT, GINGER

Introduction

The folk remedy of drinking ginger ale for nausea seems to have some validity. More recent interest in ginger centers on its use to prevent and manage nausea due to a variety of causes. Some other uses for ginger, mainly for arthritic pain, have been explored, but the data are insufficient to support this use.

Mechanism of Action for the Drug Class

Ginger's antiemetic properties are believed to be related to both enhanced GI transport and its anti-5-hydroxytryptamine effects

Ginger

Brand Name

Generics only

Generic Names

Ginger, ginger root, *Zingiberis rhizoma*

OTC

Dosage Forms

Tablet, capsule, liquid extract

Usage

Treatment and management of nausea,* motion sickness,* chemotherapy-related nausea, postoperative nausea, pregnancy-related nausea

Pregnancy Category

Although studied for pregnancy-related nausea ("morning sickness"), the trials provided no data on fetal outcomes. Without this data, reasons for caution exist, thus avoid use until safety is established.

Dosing

- Nausea: 250 mg to 1 g; repeat three to four times daily
- Motion sickness: 250 mg to 2 g per dose; repeat three to four times daily
- Postoperative nausea: 1 g dose
- Renal dosage adjustment: Not known

Adverse Reactions: Most Common

Heartburn, diarrhea, mouth irritation

Adverse Reactions: Rare/Severe/Important

Case report of arrhythmia

Major Drug Interactions

The interaction reported with warfarin may be "over-hyped" due to the fact that pharmacokinetic studies demonstrated that warfarin kinetics were unchanged when coadministered with ginger, with no changes in protein binding or INR. Extra monitoring may be advised only in patients with high ginger intake.

Counseling Point

If nausea persists after several days with self-treatment with ginger, contact your healthcare provider

Key Point

Best to avoid during pregnancy and lactation until safety data are available

NATURAL SUPPLEMENT, GINKGO

Introduction

Supplements derived from *Ginkgo biloba* are used by those who believe it can improve memory and cognitive function

Mechanism of Action for the Drug Class

The leaf extract contains terpene lactones (ginkgolides, bilobalide), flavonoids, and amino acids that contribute to antiplatelet, vasodilatory, and free-radical scavenging activity to improve circulatory flow. Ginkgolide B inhibits platelet-activating factors.

Ginkgo

Brand Names

Ginkai, Ginkgold, Ginkgo

Generic Names

Ginkgo, *Ginkgo biloba*, bai guo ye, fossil tree, kew tree, maidenhair tree, salisburia, yinshing

OTC

Dosage Forms

Tablet, capsule, tincture

Usage

Memory enhancer,* cerebrovascular insufficiency (dementia, memory impairment),* vertigo, tinnitus, peripheral vascular disease (intermittent claudication)

Pregnancy Category

Information regarding safety and efficacy in pregnancy is lacking. Avoid use.

Dosing

- 40–80 mg three times daily of a leaf extract standardized to 22–27% flavone glycosides and 5–7% terpenes
- Refer to the product labeling for dosing recommendations
- Renal dosage adjustment: Not known

Adverse Reactions: Most Common

Nausea, vomiting, diarrhea, headache, dizziness, restlessness, palpitations, bleeding

Adverse Reactions: Rare/Severe/Important

Allergic skin reaction, Stevens-Johnson syndrome

Ginkgo's Effect on Other Drugs

- Antiplatelets and anticoagulants: Increases effects
- Antiepileptics: Decreases effects if excessive amounts of natural contaminant from ginkgo seeds are present

Counseling Points

- May require at least 4 weeks and possibly 6–8 weeks of treatment for full effect
- Report any skin rashes, unusual bruising, or bleeding to your healthcare provider

- Use caution if combined with other products that may possess antiplatelet or anticoagulant effects
- Discontinue 2 weeks before surgery to reduce bleeding risk
- May be taken without regard to meals or food intake

Key Points

- Avoid during pregnancy and lactation
- Increases the effect of antiplatelets and anticoagulants

NATURAL SUPPLEMENT, GINSENG

Introduction

Ginseng (*Panax* spp.) is a very popular natural supplement worldwide. It is used as a general tonic to improve well-being and increase energy levels.

Mechanism of Action for the Drug Class

The mature root contains numerous triterpenoid saponins (ginsenosides) of varying composition and concentration between species, as well as flavonoids and vitamins, that may contribute to CNS stimulation/suppression, hypertension/hypotension, immunomodulation, and antioxidant and anti-inflammatory activities. These effects may occur through an effect on the hypothalamic-pituitary-adrenal (HPA) axis and neurotransmitter pathways.

⊙ Ginseng

Brand Names

Ginsana, G-115, Ginseng

Generic Names

Ginseng, Asian ginseng (*Panax ginseng*), Chinese ginseng, Japanese ginseng, Korean ginseng, jintsan, red ginseng, ninjin, ren shen, seng, American ginseng (*Panax quinquefolius*), anchi ginseng, red berry, ren shen, sang, tienchi ginseng

OTC

Dosage Forms

Tablet, capsule, tincture

Usage

Improved well-being,* energy boost,* stress relief

Pregnancy Category

Information regarding safety and efficacy in pregnancy is lacking. Avoid use.

Dosing

- 200–600 mg daily of root extract standardized to 4–5% ginsenoside
- Renal dosage adjustment: Not known

Adverse Reactions: Most Common

Headache, transient nervousness, insomnia, cerebral arteritis, mydriasis, disturbance of accommodation, hypertension, hypotension, hypoglycemia

Adverse Reactions: Rare/Severe/Important

Dermatologic reactions such as Stevens-Johnson syndrome, postmenopausal vaginal bleeding, breast tenderness

Major Drug Interactions

Ginseng's Effect on Other Drugs

- Warfarin: May decrease anticoagulant effect
- Antiplatelet agents: May increase bleeding risk
- Caffeine and products that contain natural guarana: May increase effects
- Monoamine oxidase inhibitors (MAOIs): May increase stimulant effect

Counseling Points

- Avoid doses > 3 g daily
- Take within 2 hours of a meal to avoid potential hypoglycemia
- Limit continuous use to < 3 months
- Siberian ginseng (*Eleutherococcus senticosus*) contains no ginsenosides and is actually a different botanical product called eleuthera

Key Point

Avoid use during pregnancy and lactation

NATURAL SUPPLEMENT, GLUCOSAMINE

Introduction

Glucosamine, a very popular supplement for joint health, is used alone or in conjunction with chondroitin. Studies have shown mixed results on the benefits of glucosamine; however, it remains a favorite of consumers and has a relatively good safety record.

Mechanism of Action for the Drug Class

This hexosamine sugar is a substrate for glycoproteins, glycolipids, glycosaminoglycans, proteoglycans, and hyaluronic acid, all of which are required for cartilage synthesis

◉ Glucosamine

Brand Names

Cosamin, Cosamin DS, Cosamin Protek, others

Generic Name

Glucosamine

OTC

Dosage Forms

Tablet, capsule, liquid extract

Usage

Pain relief from osteoarthritis,* maintenance of joint function*

Pregnancy Category

Information regarding safety and efficacy in pregnancy is lacking. Avoid use.

Dosing

- 500 mg orally three times daily
- Renal dosage adjustment: Not known

Adverse Reactions: Most Common

Altered taste, nausea, vomiting, constipation, flatulence, abdominal bloating, cramps, diarrhea, headache, allergic reactions (may cross-react in patients with severe shellfish allergies)

Adverse Reactions: Rare/Severe/Important

None reported

Contraindication

Patients with severe shellfish allergy should avoid using glucosamine. Although derived from the shells of these animals, some glucosamine products may contain shellfish protein, which could lead to an allergic reaction.

Major Drug Interactions

Glucosamine's Effects on Other Drugs

Insulin and oral antidiabetic agents: May decrease sensitivity to these agents. This is of primary concern in patients with hard to manage glycemic control (i.e., those with "brittle diabetes").

Counseling Point

Those with shellfish allergies should select products carefully because some formulations are derived from marine exoskeletons

Key Points

- Glucosamine sulfate has been studied more frequently than other salts
- Multi-ingredient products containing manganese may provide doses of this mineral above the tolerable upper limit for adults (11 mg)

NATURAL SUPPLEMENT, GOLDENSEAL

Introduction

Goldenseal (*Hydrastis canadensis*) is native to the eastern United States. American Indians used goldenseal root as a stimulant, a diuretic, and even as an insect repellant. Today, people claim the usefulness of goldenseal in cold and flu preparations and eyewashes and as a treatment for topical infections and diarrhea.

Mechanism of Action for the Drug Class

Alkaloids of goldenseal have shown modest antimicrobial activity in vitro. In addition, it may also have a sodium-sparing diuretic effect, as well as immunostimulatory properties; however, the mechanism has not been well described.

⊚ Goldenseal

Brand Names
Many different brands are available

Generic Names
Goldenseal, *Hydrastis canadensis*, yellowroot, orangeroot, eyeroot, goldenroot, jaundice root, yellow puccon, Indian tumeric, sceau d'or

OTC

Dosage Forms
Tablet, capsule, liquid extract

Usage
Antimicrobial,* antidiarrheal, diuretic, eye ailments

Pregnancy Category
Do not use during pregnancy. Goldenseal is a known uterine stimulant.

Dosing
- Varies considerably from 250 mg to 1 g three times daily, some labeling suggests doses as high as 3,420 mg daily
- Extracts used for cold and influenza: 10 to 30 drops of the extract two to four times daily
- Renal dosage adjustment: Not known

Adverse Reactions: Most Common
Anorexia, nausea, vomiting

Adverse Reactions: Rare/Severe/Important
Photosensitivity; very high doses may induce vomiting, nausea, anxiety, and/or seizures

Major Drug Interactions
Use with caution with cardiovascular agents, because goldenseal causes vasodilation and hypotension

Counseling Points
- Use of high doses or doses not consistent with labeling increases the risk for serious adverse effects
- Use caution when self-treating eye ailments with goldenseal. It is better to seek medical attention from a specialist.

Key Points
- Goldenseal is a known uterine stimulant. Do not use during pregnancy.
- Although goldenseal has been touted as an "eye tonic" and eyewash, reports of ophthalmic phototoxicity with lens damage have been reported

NATURAL SUPPLEMENT, KAVA

Introduction
Kava, or kava-kava, is a popular botanical derived from *Piper methysticum* that is used for anxiety relief. However, it is a potentially dangerous herbal supplement. Warnings from the FDA have highlighted hepatotoxicity from this product. The sale of kava is banned in the United Kingdom, Germany, Switzerland, France, Canada, and Australia due to the risk of liver damage.

Mechanism of Action for the Drug Class
Kava lactones/pyrones have muscle-relaxing, anticonvulsive, and antispasmodic effects. Kava also has hypnotic, analgesic, and psychotropic properties. It also can inhibit cyclo-oxygenase 2.

⊚ Kava

Brand Names
Pharma Kava, Kava Kava Premium

Generic Names
Kava, *Piper methysticum*, kava-kava, ava, ava pepper, intoxicating pepper, tonga, kew

OTC

Dosage Forms
Capsule, tincture, tea

Usage
Anxiety, stress, tension, agitation*

Pregnancy Category
Information regarding safety and efficacy in pregnancy is lacking. Avoid use.

Dosing
- Capsules of kava root extract: 150–300 mg twice daily
- Tincture: 30 drops with water three times daily
- Renal dosage adjustment: Not known

Adverse Reactions: Most Common

CNS complaints of dizziness, headache, pupillary dilation

Adverse Reactions: Rare/Severe/Important

Case reports of hepatotoxicity, with some being irreversible and fatal. Kava dermopathy is a reversible darkening or yellowing of the skin with whitish scaly flakes.

Major Drug Interactions

Kava's Effect on Other Drugs

- Antiplatelets, NSAIDs, and anticoagulants: Increases bleeding risk; monitor accordingly
- Drugs metabolized by CYP1A2, 2C9, 2C19, 3A4: In vitro inhibition; exercise caution with concomitant use
- Centrally acting agents (benzodiazepines, barbiturates, opiates, ethanol): Increases CNS toxicities
- Dopaminergic agents (levodopa): Decreases effectiveness

Contraindications

Concurrent use of hepatotoxins or MAOIs

Counseling Points

- Increased bleeding risks when used with antiplatelets, NSAIDs, and anticoagulants; monitor accordingly
- Discontinue 7–10 days before elective surgery
- Avoid use with concurrent hepatotoxins; monitor for signs and symptoms of liver toxicity
- Food enhances absorption
- Notify your physician and pharmacist if self-initiating due to numerous drug interactions
- This product should be avoided because of the risk of liver toxicity

Key Points

- Avoid during pregnancy and lactation
- Avoid use with concurrent hepatotoxins; monitor for signs and symptoms of liver toxicity. Note FDA warning concerning kava.

NATURAL SUPPLEMENT, MELATONIN

Introduction

Melatonin is noted for its effects on the sleep cycle and use as a sleep aid. Consumers who travel use melatonin to help allay feelings of tiredness from jet lag.

Mechanism of Action for the Drug Class

This pineal gland hormone is involved in regulating several functions, including the sleep–wake cycle (circadian rhythm). Melatonin is synthesized endogenously from serotonin.

◉ Melatonin

Brand Names

Melatonex, Melatonin, Melatonin Forte, Melatonin PM Complex

Generic Names

Melatonin, N-acetyl-5-methoxytryptamine

OTC

Dosage Forms

Tablet, capsule

Usage

Promotion of sleep,* prevention of symptoms of jet lag,* treatment of insomnia*

Pregnancy Category

Information regarding safety and efficacy in pregnancy is lacking. Avoid use.

Dosing

- Sleep aid: 0.3–3 mg at bedtime
- Jet lag: Up to 5 mg daily for 3 days before and 3 days after air travel
- Renal dosage adjustment: Not known

Adverse Reactions: Most Common

Neurologic complaints, including migraines, daytime drowsiness, and depression

Adverse Reactions: Rare/Severe/Important

Hypothermia, hypertension, retinopathy, seizure, infertility

Major Drug Interactions

Potentially additive effects with CNS depressants (e.g., narcotics, benzodiazepines)

Counseling Points

- Do not drive or operate machinery or engage in other skilled activities for several hours after taking melatonin
- Use only for short durations; do not use chronically
- Select immediate- over sustained-release products
- Select products containing synthetic melatonin over those derived from animal pineal glands

Key Point

Avoid during pregnancy, with breastfeeding, or if trying to conceive

NATURAL SUPPLEMENT, MILK THISTLE

Introduction

Milk thistle is best known as a "liver tonic" due to its purported hepatoprotective effects. It has been used for centuries in the treatment of hepatobiliary disease.

Mechanism of Action for the Drug Class

The main active constituent of milk thistle, silymarin, inhibits the peroxidation of lipids within hepatic cells. The other active constituent, silibinin, decreases synthesis of cholesterol in the liver. In addition, silymarin may inhibit inflammatory and cytotoxic mediators. Both silymarin and silibinin are also known to be free-radical scavengers, hence its antioxidant activity.

⊙ Milk Thistle

Brand Names
Generics only

Generic Names
Milk thistle, holy thistle, lady's thistle, marian thistle, Mary thistle, St. Mary thistle, silybum

OTC

Dosage Forms
Tablet, capsule, liquid extract, crude milk thistle seed

Usage
Hepatoprotectant for hepatitis, cirrhosis, and other liver diseases; treatment of toxicity due to *Amanita* mushroom poisoning

Pregnancy Category
Information regarding safety and efficacy in pregnancy is lacking. Avoid use.

Dosing
- 420–600 mg daily in two divided doses
- Crude milk thistle seed has been used at 12–15 g per day for hepatitis and other liver conditions
- Renal dosage adjustment: Not known

Adverse Reactions: Most Common
Anorexia, nausea, vomiting, bloating

Adverse Reactions: Rare/Severe/Important
None reported

Major Drug Interactions
- Inactivates CYP3A4 and 2C9. Clinical significance of this is not well defined. Use caution when using high-dose milk thistle with substrates of these enzymes with narrow therapeutic indices.
- Potent selective inhibitor of the enzyme UGT1A1. Clinical importance of this interaction is unknown.

Counseling Point
Do not self-treat liver conditions with milk thistle without proper diagnosis and medical management

Key Point
Best to avoid during pregnancy and lactation until safety data are available

NATURAL SUPPLEMENT, PROBIOTICS

Introduction

Lactobacillus acidophilus is a normal gut flora bacterium and is one of the most commonly used probiotics. According to the World Health Organization (WHO), a *probiotic* is a supplement that contains live microorganisms that when administered in adequate amounts confer a health benefit on the host. In addition to *L. acidophilus*, *Bifidobacterium bifidum* and *Saccharomyces* derived from yeast also are found in probiotic supplements as well as yogurt. Sufficient clinical trials have been conducted to enable meta-analyses to be conducted for several clinical conditions. Evidence exists to support the use of probiotics in the treatment of bacterial vaginosis, diarrhea (acute infectious, antibiotic associated, and persistent), irritable bowel syndrome (IBS), necrotizing enterocolitis in neonates, and ventilator-associated pneumonia. Meta-analyses have shown no effect of probiotics on Crohn's disease, eczema, pancreatitis, or ulcerative colitis or in patients in intensive care.

Mechanism of Action for the Drug Class

Live gut microorganisms that when ingested in food products or supplements help to maintain or reestablish the normal bowel or vaginal flora.

⊙ Probiotics

Brand Names

These products may contain one or more of the previously mentioned bacteria, consult product specific labeling for details: Align, Bacid Caplets, Bulgaricum IB, DDS-Acidophilus, FLORAjen, Acidophilus Extra Strength, Intestinex, Kyo-Dophilus, Lactinex, Lactinex Granules, Probiata, ProBiotic Restore, Superdophilus

OTC

Dosage Forms

Capsule, powder, tablet

Usage

Treatment of uncomplicated diarrhea, particularly that caused by modification of intestinal flora by antibiotic therapy;* diarrhea due to infections; ulcerative colitis; patients with colostomies with diarrhea or constipation; spastic diarrhea;* bacterial vaginosis*

Pregnancy Category

No adequate and well-controlled studies have been conducted in pregnant women. Pregnant women should only use *L. acidophilus* under medical supervision.

Dosing

Products vary from manufacturer to manufacturer and among batches produced by one manufacturer. Because it is often not clear what the product's active component(s) is, standardization may not be possible, making it difficult to compare the clinical effects of different brands. Dosing varies based on the particular product and dosage form. See individual product labels/instructions for dosing.

Adverse Reactions: Most Common

Flatulence with initial use

Adverse Reactions: Rare/Severe/Important

Case reports of fatal *Lactobacillus* septicemia in markedly immunocompromised patients who have used acidophilus/probiotic products

Contraindication

Patients with severe lactose intolerance/allergy should not use probiotics containing *L. acidophilus*

Major Drug Interactions

Antibiotics: Although often prescribed together with antibiotics to help prevent antibiotic-related diarrhea, these same antibiotics can be bacteriocidal to the *Lactobacillus,* rendering the probiotic ineffective. Probiotics are best used when a course of antibiotic therapy is completed.

Counseling Points

- Expect an increase in flatulence with initiation of probiotics
- It is best to wait to start to use probiotics until after the course of antibiotics has been completed
- When self-treating diarrhea with probiotics, seek out medical attention if there is no clear-cut benefit after 2 days of therapy or if fever develops

Key Point

Patients who are immunocompromised or taking immunosuppressant therapy should avoid the use of *L. acidophilus* and other probiotics

---

NATURAL SUPPLEMENT, RED YEAST RICE

Introduction

Red yeast rice, which is derived from *Monascus purpureu,* is the natural source of mevinolin, the active ingredient in lovastatin. Its primary use is as a natural supplement to treat hyperlipidemia.

Mechanism of Action for the Drug Class

Red yeast rice forms naturally occurring HMG-CoA reductase inhibitors. The major active ingredient is monacolin K, which is also known as mevinolin/lovastatin. Inhibition of this enzyme is the rate-limiting step in the production of cholesterol.

⊙ Red Yeast Rice

Brand Name

Cholestin

Generic Names

Red yeast rice, *Monascus purpureu,* monascus, red mold, red rice yeast, rotschimmelreis (Europe); zhitai, hon-chi, xuezhikang (China); red-koji, beni-koji (Japan)

OTC

Dosage Forms

Capsule

Usage

Treatment of high cholesterol*

Pregnancy Category

Contraindicated in pregnancy because it is a form of lovastatin. Prescription lovastatin is a Category X drug. Do not use red yeast rice if pregnant or planning to become pregnant.

Dosing

- 1,200 mg twice daily
- Renal dosage adjustment: None

Adverse Reactions: Most Common

Nausea, anorexia, diarrhea

Adverse Reactions: Rare/Severe/Important

Myopathies and rhabdomyolysis, increased liver function tests

Major Drug Interactions

Drugs Affecting Red Yeast Rice

- Cyclosporine: Increases serum concentrations. Case reports have documented rhabdomyolysis with concomitant use.

- Grapefruit juice: Increases blood levels of the active ingredients in red yeast rice, leading to greater adverse reactions and potential liver damage
- CYP3A4 inhibitors: Theoretically will increase the active lovastatin-like ingredient in red yeast rice

Red Yeast Rice's Effects on Other Drugs

Statins: Do not use with prescription statins. Concomitant use can lead to serious adverse reactions, including myopathies/rhabdomyolysis and hepatotoxicity.

Counseling Points

- Avoid self-treatment of lipid disorders without first being properly diagnosed by a healthcare provider
- Report any signs or symptoms of unexplained muscle aches, dark or tea-colored urine, yellowing of the skin/sclera, changes in urine output, or unexplained abdominal pain to your healthcare provider
- Use only with medical supervision for proper diagnosis of cardiovascular and lipid disorders
- Take with food

Key Point

- Contraindicated in women who are pregnant or planning to become pregnant
- Do not use red yeast rice with prescription statins

NATURAL SUPPLEMENT, SAW PALMETTO

Introduction

Saw palmetto (*Serenoa repens* and *S. serrulata*) is touted for prostate health, although recent randomized prospective controlled trials have shown little benefit for this indication. Nonetheless, it remains a popular product among consumers.

Mechanism of Action for the Drug Class

The lipid fraction (fatty acids, sterols) in saw palmetto inhibits 5-alpha-reductase activity and possesses antiandrogenic, antiproliferative, and anti-inflammatory properties.

◉ Saw Palmetto

Brand Names

Nutrilite, PROST Active, PROST Active Plus, Sabal Select, Solaray

Generic Names

Saw palmetto, *Serenoa repens*, *Serenoa serrulata*, American dwarf palm tree, cabbage palm, sabal fructus

OTC

Pregnancy Category

Information regarding safety and efficacy in pregnancy is lacking. Avoid use.

Dosage Forms

Tablet, capsule

Usage

Symptoms of benign prostatic hypertrophy (BPH)*

Dosing

- 160 mg twice daily *or* 320 mg daily of a liposterolic extract of ripe fruit, standardized to 85–95% fatty acids/sterols
- Renal dosage adjustment: Not known

Adverse Reactions: Most Common

Nausea, vomiting, constipation, diarrhea, headache, insomnia, dizziness, estrogenic effects (primarily manifested as breast tenderness and gynecomastia in men, decreased libido)

Adverse Reactions: Rare/Severe/Important

None

Major Drug Interactions

None

Counseling Points

- Before use, see healthcare provider to rule out prostate cancer
- May require at least 4–6 weeks and as long as 3–6 months for full effect, although the benefit is questionable

Key Points

- Avoid during pregnancy and lactation; not intended for women
- Does not seem to alter prostate size; questionable benefit, as demonstrated by randomized prospective controlled trials

NATURAL SUPPLEMENT, ST. JOHN'S WORT

Introduction

St. John's wort (*Hypericum perforatum*) is widely touted for depression and is quite popular in Europe as well as in the United States and Canada for this indication. Clinical trials have demonstrated its effectiveness as an antidepressant for mild depression.

Mechanism of Action for the Drug Class

Extract from the flower contains naphthodianthrones (hypericins), flavonoids (hyperoside), phloroglucinols (hyperforin), and other constituents that probably have an inhibitory action on central serotonin, norepinephrine, dopamine, and gamma-aminobutyric acid reuptake.

⊙ St. John's Wort

Brand Names

St. John's Wort (from various manufacturers)

Generic Names

St. John's wort, *Hypericum perforatum*, goat weed, hypericum, John's wort, Klamath weed, millepertuis, tipton weed

OTC

Dosage Forms

Tablet, capsule, liquid

Usage

Mild to moderate depression*

Dosing

- 300 mg three times daily or 450 mg twice daily of a flower extract standardized to 0.3% dianthrones (or total hypericins) or 2–6% hyperforin
- Renal dosage adjustment: Not known

Adverse Reactions: Most Common

Dry mouth, nausea, vomiting, constipation, abdominal pain, bloating, diarrhea, headache, dizziness, insomnia, fatigue, restlessness, anxiety, hypomania, serotonin syndrome, allergic skin reaction, photosensitivity, anorgasmia

Adverse Reactions: Rare/Severe/Important

Serotonin syndrome, hypertensive crisis

Major Drug Interactions

St. John's Wort's Effects on Other Drugs

- Benzodiazepines, cyclosporine, digoxin, estrogens/oral contraceptives, irinotecan, protease inhibitors, simvastatin, tacrolimus, theophylline, warfarin: Increases clearance because it is a strong enzyme inducer (CYP3A4, CYP2D6, CYP1A2, P-glycoprotein) through pregnane X receptor binding
- Antidepressants: Additive effects
- Serotoninergic-acting drugs (e.g., antidepressants, tramadol, meperidine, "triptans" for migraines): Additive effects
- Drugs known to be photosensitizers (i.e., amiodarone, methotrexate, tetracyclines): Increases phototoxicity

Counseling Points

- Requires at least 2–3 weeks of treatment for effect
- Take in the morning if you experience insomnia
- Limit sun exposure or use sunscreen
- Avoid alcohol
- Do not use with prescription antidepressants without the approval of a medical psychiatric professional

Key Points

- Avoid use during pregnancy and lactation
- Review any medications (prescription and nonprescription) the patient is taking because St. John's wort has numerous drug interactions
- Concomitant use with protease inhibitors or oral contraceptives is not recommended

NATURAL SUPPLEMENT, VALERIAN

Introduction

Valerian (*Valeriana officinalis*) in the form of teas and capsules is used as a sleep aid. However, these same sedative effects can pose a risk to those using other CNS depressants.

Mechanism of Action for the Drug Class

Valerianic acid components have been shown to decrease the degradation of gamma-aminobutyric acid (GABA) with an increase of GABA at the synaptic cleft via inhibition of reuptake and an increase in secretion. This increase of available GABA may be one factor responsible for the sedative effects of valerian.

⊙ Valerian

Brand Names

Herbal Sure Valerian Root, NuVeg Valerian Root, Quanterra Sleep, Natural Herbal Valerian Root, Nature's Root Nighttime

Generic Names

Valerian, *Valeriana officinalis*, valerian root, capon's tail, heliotrope, vandal root

OTC

Dosage Forms

Tea/teabag, extract, tablet, capsule

Usage

Sleep aid,* insomnia caused by anxiety,* restlessness

Pregnancy Category

Information regarding safety and efficacy in pregnancy is lacking. Avoid use.

Dosing

- Restlessness: 220 mg of extract three times daily
- Sleep aid: 400–900 mg 30 minutes before bedtime
- Renal dosage adjustment: Not known

Adverse Reactions: Most Common

Nausea, vomiting, constipation, diarrhea, headache, insomnia, dizziness

Adverse Reactions: Rare/Severe/Important

Reports of hepatotoxicity (rare)

Major Drug Interactions

Valerian's Effects on Other Drugs

- Antiplatelet agents and anticoagulants: Increases risk of bleeding
- Barbiturates, benzodiazepines, ethanol, opiates: Increases CNS depression
- Hepatotoxins: May elevate transaminases; use with caution
- Iron: Binds with oral iron salts, leading to malabsorption; separate administration time by 1–2 hours
- Loperamide: Paradoxical delirium and confusion

Counseling Points

- Avoid driving or working with heavy equipment when starting therapy due to sedative effects
- Avoid use with alcohol or other sedatives
- Monitor for signs and symptoms of hepatotoxicity (dark amber urine, skin or eye jaundice/yellowing, right upper quadrant abdominal pain)

Key Point

Avoid use during pregnancy and lactation

NUTRIENTS AND VITAMINS

Introduction

Vitamins are macronutrients essential for life. They regulate metabolism and assist in different biochemical processes, such as the formation of hormones, blood cells, nervous system chemicals, and genetic material. They differ in their physiologic actions. The fat-soluble vitamins include vitamins A, D, E, and K. These are generally consumed along with fat-containing foods. The water-soluble vitamins include the B vitamins and vitamin C. These cannot be stored by the body and must be consumed frequently, usually every day. The only vitamin manufactured in our bodies is vitamin D. All others must be derived from the diet. Deficiencies in vitamin intake can cause different health problems.

DIETARY SUPPLEMENT, BETA-CAROTENE

Introduction

Beta-carotene is one of several hundred carotenoids. Activity varies depending on the isomer. It is converted, in part, to vitamin A (retinol) at the GI tract and may contribute some antioxidant activity.

◉ Beta-Carotene

Brand Names

Various

Generic Names

Beta-carotene, all-*trans*-beta-carotene, vitamin A

Dosage Forms

Tablet, capsule

OTC

Usage

Meet vitamin A intake requirement;* reduce risk of cardiovascular disease, cancer, age-related macular degeneration, and cataracts*

Pregnancy Category

Pregnancy category X (dose dependent). Excessive vitamin A during pregnancy may cause craniofacial malformations, as well as CNS, heart, and thymus abnormalities. Doses of > 6,000 units/day have not been established to be safe in pregnant women and should be avoided.

Dosing

- RAE = Retinol activity equivalent; 1 RAE = retinol 1 µg or dietary beta-carotene 12 µg; Retinol 1 µg = 3.33 units of vitamin A

- Recommended dietary allowance (RDA):
  - Children 1–3 years: 300 µg/day (1,000 units/day)
  - Children 4–8 years: 400 µg/day (1,330 units/day)
  - Children 9–13 years: 600 µg/day (2,000 units/day)
  - Males > 13 years: 900 µg/day (3,000 units/day)
  - Females > 13 years: 700 µg/day (2,330 units/day)
  - Pregnant females 14–18 years: 750 µg/day (2,500 units/day)
  - Lactating females 14–18 years: 1,200 µg/day (4,000 units/day)
- Renal dosage adjustment: Not known

Adverse Reactions: Rare/Severe/Important

High doses may cause hepatotoxicity, carotenoderma (orange/yellow skin discoloration)

Major Drug Interactions

Drugs Affecting Beta-Carotene

Cholestyramine, mineral oil, orlistat, and proton pump inhibitors: Reduce absorption

Beta-Carotene's Effect on Other Drugs

- Carotenoids: Decreases bioavailability (e.g., lutein)
- Oral retinoins (e.g., isotretinoin): Increases risk of vitamin A toxicities

Counseling Point

Dietary content of beta-carotene is approximately 3 mg daily

Key Point

Doses of > 6,000 units/day have not been established to be safe in pregnant women and should be avoided

---

DIETARY SUPPLEMENT, CALCIUM

Introduction

Calcium has a structural role in bone and teeth. It also has important roles in vascular, neuromuscular, and glandular function.

◉ Calcium

Brand Names

Calcium (Various), Cal-Lac, Caltrate, Calsorb, Citracal, Os-Cal, Tums

Generic Names

Calcium, calcium salts, calcium carbonate, citrate, etc.

OTC

Dosage Form

Tablet

Usage

Prevention or treatment of calcium deficits,* management of osteoporosis,* hypertension, premenstrual syndrome, reduction of risk of colon cancer

Pregnancy Category

Not assigned for most common oral forms of calcium, such as calcium carbonate; refer to dosing for pregnant women

Dosing

- 500 mg of elemental calcium two to three times daily
- 14–18 years:
  - 1,300 mg daily
  - Pregnant or lactating: 1,300 mg daily
- 19–50 years:
  - 1,000 mg daily
  - Pregnant or lactating: 1,000 mg daily
- > 50 years: 1,200 mg daily
- Tolerable upper intake level: 2,500 mg daily from all sources
- Renal dosage adjustment: Not known

Adverse Reactions: Most Common

Nausea, constipation, flatulence

Adverse Reactions: Rare/Severe/Important

Renal insufficiency, nephrolithiasis, hypercalcemia

Major Drug Interactions

Drugs Affecting Calcium

- Corticosteroids: Decrease calcium status
- Loop diuretics: Increase urinary calcium loss
- Thiazide diuretics: Increase renal calcium reabsorption

Calcium's Effect on Other Drugs

- Etidronate, levothyroxine, oral fluoroquinolones, oral tetracyclines, iron, magnesium, levothyroxine, zinc: Decreases absorption; separate dosing by at least 2 hours to avoid this interaction
- Tamoxifen: Increases hypercalcemia risk

Counseling Points

- Avoid the following sources of calcium because of potential contaminants: Bone meal, dolomite, oyster shells (may be of risk in patients with severe shellfish allergy)
- Dose in terms of elemental calcium (see **Table 15-1**)
- Maximize calcium absorption by dividing doses (500 mg/dose maximum)
- Take with meals

TABLE 15-1 Dosing in Terms of Elemental Calcium

Calcium Salt	Elemental Calcium	Calcium (mg)/ Salt (g)
Calcium carbonate	40%	400
Dibasic calcium phosphate	23%	230
Calcium citrate	21%	210
Calcium lactate	13%	130
Calcium gluconate	9%	90

DIETARY SUPPLEMENT, CYANOCOBALAMIN

Introduction

Cyanocobalamin, or vitamin B_{12}, is essential in the maintenance of cellular integrity, particularly in disease states such as anemia, pregnancy, thyrotoxicosis, malignancy, liver, neurologic disorders, or kidney disease

⊙ Cyanocobalamin

Brand Names

CaloMist, Nascobal, Twelve-Resin

Generic Names

Cyanocobalamin, vitamin B_{12}

OTC

Dosage Forms

Tablet, injection, lozenge, intranasal solution

Usage

Prevention and treatment of vitamin B_{12} deficiency,* treatment of pernicious anemia*

Pregnancy Category

Pregnancy category A when using at the RDA or recommended dose for pregnant women; Category C at higher doses and intranasal dosage form

Dosing

- Recommended intake:
  - Adults: 2.4 µg/day
  - Pregnant women: 2.6 µg/day
  - Lactating women: 2.8 µg/day
- Vitamin B_{12} deficiency dosing:
  - Intranasal:
    - Nascobal: 500 µg in one nostril once weekly
    - CaloMist: Maintenance therapy (following correction of vitamin B_{12} deficiency) is 25 µg in each nostril daily; if suboptimal response, 25 µg in each nostril twice daily
  - Oral: 250 µg/day
  - IM, deep SUB-Q:
    - Initial dose: 30 µg/day for 5–10 days
    - Maintenance dose: 100–200 µg/month

- Pernicious anemia:
  - IM, deep SUB-Q:
    - Initial dose: 100 µg/day for 6–7 days; if improvement noted, administer the same dose on alternating days for seven doses, then every 3–4 days for 2–3 weeks
    - Maintenance dose: 100 µg/month
    - Alternative dosing: 1,000 µg/day for 5 days followed by a maintenance dose of 500–1,000 µg/month
  - Maintenance dose for a hematologic remission/correction of pernicious anemia:
    - Intranasal (Nascobal): 500 µg in one nostril once weekly
    - Oral: 1,000–2,000 µg/day
    - IM, deep SUB-Q: 100–1,000 µg/month
  - Renal dosage adjustment: None

Adverse Reactions: Most Common

Injection site reactions/redness with IM and deep SUB-Q injections

Adverse Reactions: Rare/Severe/Important

Congestive heart failure, polycythemia vera, paresthesias, pulmonary edema

Major Drug Interactions

Drugs Affecting Cyanocobalamin

Chloramphenicol: May diminish effect

Cyanocobalamin's Effects on Other Drugs

Alcohol: Heavy use/consumption > 2 weeks can impair absorption

Counseling Point

Use exactly as prescribed

DIETARY SUPPLEMENT, ERGOCALCIFEROL

Introduction

Ergocalciferol, a vitamin D analog, is essential in the maintenance of vitamin D levels, particularly in women to prevent osteoporosis and in patients with chronic kidney disease.

Mechanism of Action for the Drug Class

Ergocalciferol stimulates calcium and phosphorous absorption from the small intestine and promotes secretion of calcium from bone to blood; it also promotes renal tubule resorption of phosphorous.

◉ Ergocalciferol

Brand Name

Drisdol

Generic Name

Ergocalciferol

OTC

Pregnancy Category

Category A when used at RDA; Category C at higher doses

Dosage Forms

Capsule, liquid, tablet (Note: 1 µg = 40 international units [IU])

Usage

Prevention and treatment of vitamin D deficiency,* treatment of refractory rickets, treatment of hypophosphatemia and hypoparathyroidism

Dosing

- Recommended intake:
  - 18–50 years: 5 µg/day
  - 51–70 years: 10 µg/day
- Osteoporosis prevention and treatment for adults age ≥ 50 years: 10 µg/day
- Vitamin D deficiency/insufficiency in patients with chronic kidney disease (CKD) (Kidney Disease Outcomes Quality Initiative guidelines for stage 3–4 CKD):
  - Serum 25-hydroxyvitamin D level < 5 ng/mL: 50,000 IU/week for 12 weeks, then 50,000 IU/month
  - Serum 25-hydroxyvitamin D level 5–15 ng/ml: 50,000 IU/week for 4 weeks, then 50,000 IU/month
  - Serum 25-hydroxyvitamin D level 16–30 ng/mL: 50,000 IU/month
- Hypoparathyroidism: 625 µg to 5 mg/day orally
- Nutritional rickets and osteomalacia:
  - Adults with normal absorption: 25–125 µg/day
  - Adults with malabsorption: 250–7,500 µg/day
- Renal dosage adjustment: None

Adverse Reactions: Most Common

Nausea, metallic taste in mouth, dry mouth

Adverse Reactions: Rare/Severe/Important

None

Major Drug Interactions

None

Counseling Point

Use exactly as prescribed

Key Point

For osteoporosis, adequate calcium supplementation is required with vitamin D analog supplementation

Introduction

Ferrous sulfate is one of the most widely used iron supplements. It is widely used in the treatment of iron deficiency anemia.

Mechanism of Action for the Drug Class

These supplements replace the iron found in hemoglobin, myoglobin, and other enzymes

◉ Ferrous Sulfate

Brand Names

Feosol, Fer-Gen-Sol, Fer-in-Sol, Fer-Iron, Feratab, Slow-Fe

Generic Name

Ferrous sulfate

OTC

Pregnancy Category

Not assigned an FDA pregnancy risk category; assess risk versus benefit of therapy during pregnancy

Dosage Forms

Elixir, liquid, tablet, extended-release tablet

Usage

Prevention and treatment of iron deficiency anemia*

Dosing

- Treatment of iron deficiency anemia:
  - Immediate-release formulations: 300 mg two to four times daily
  - Extended-release formulations: 250 mg one to two times daily
- Prophylaxis of iron deficiency: 300 mg daily
- Renal dosage adjustment: None

Adverse Reactions: Most Common

Constipation, dark stools, GI irritation, nausea, stomach cramping, vomiting, staining of teeth with liquid preparations

Adverse Reactions: Rare/Severe/Important

None

Major Drug Interactions

Drugs Affecting Iron

- Antacids: May decrease absorption of iron salts; consider therapy modification
- H2-receptor antagonists: May decrease absorption of iron salts

Iron's Effect on Other Drugs

- Bisphosphonates: May decrease absorption
- Cefdinir: May decrease concentration, forming an insoluble cefdinir–iron complex. This may be objectively noted by a red-appearing, nonbloody stool. Avoid this combination if possible; if not possible, separate doses by several hours to minimize interaction.
- Dimercaprol: Contraindicated with iron salts because it may enhance nephrotoxicity
- Fluoroquinolone antibiotics (oral), tetracycline derivatives (oral): May decrease absorption of these antibiotics; separate doses by 2–4 hours to avoid this interaction
- Levodopa, methyldopa, levothyroxine, pancrelipase, phosphate supplements: May decrease absorption; separate doses by 2–4 hours to lessen this interaction

Counseling Points

- Take between meals for maximal absorption; try to take on empty stomach. Do not take with milk or antacids.
- Use exactly as prescribed
- Keep out of reach of children; iron toxicity is one of the leading accidental drug poisonings seen in young children
- Stool may turn black; this is important to recognize, particularly when you are on anticoagulants and/or antiplatelet agents. Be aware that black stool can also be an indication of blood in stool. Contact your healthcare provider if this occurs while taking anticoagulants or antiplatelet agents with iron supplements.
- If constipation occurs, try increasing fluids and foods with fruit and fiber. If constipation lasts > 3–4 days, contact your healthcare provider.

Key Points

- Foods, particularly grains, dietary fiber, tea, coffee, eggs, milk, and wines with tannins, may decrease oral iron salt absorption. Counsel patients to take on empty stomach if possible.
- The elemental iron content of ferrous sulfate is 20%; 324 mg of ferrous sulfate tablet contains 65 mg of elemental iron. Therefore, with special-formulated preparations (exsiccated), such as Feosol, a 200-mg tablet contains 65 mg of elemental iron. Slow-Fe, an oral exsiccated and time-released tablet, has 50 mg of elemental iron in a 160 mg tablet.
- Oral solution and elixir prescriptions should never be written in only volume (milliliters) because different concentrations of iron exist; use dosages in milligrams
- Use with caution in patients receiving multiple blood transfusions to prevent accidental iron overload/toxicity

15

Natural Products, Dietary Supplements, and Nutrients

DIETARY SUPPLEMENT, FLUORIDE

Introduction

With more and more communities removing fluorides from drinking water, patients, particularly parents with young children, need to rely on oral fluoride supplementation to prevent dental caries.

Mechanism of Action for the Drug Class

Ionic forms of fluorine (fluorides) are cariostatic, inhibiting the bacteria implicated in causing dental cavities/caries. They also strengthen dental enamel.

◉ Oral Fluorides

Brand Names

ACT, APF, CaviRinse, CavityShield, ControlRx, Duraphat Varnish, EtheDent, Fluor-A-Day, Fluorabon Drops, Fluorinse, Fluoritab, Fluorofoam, Flura-Drops, Gel-Kam, Gel-Kam DentinBloc, Just for Kids, Minute-Foam, Neutra-Foam, NeutraCare, OMNI, OrthoWash, PerioMed, Phos-Flur, PreviDent 5000 Plus, PreviDent, PreviDent Varnish, SF 5000 Plus, SF, Stop, Vanish Varnish

Generic Names

Sodium fluoride, tin fluoride, stannous fluoride

OTC

Dosage Forms

Lozenge, solution, chewable tablet, cream, foam, gel, oral rinse

Usage

Prevention of dental caries*

Pregnancy Category B

Safe when taken per instructions of individual dental products. Tolerable upper daily limit is 10 mg; however, the American Dental Association (ADA) does not recommend supplemental fluoride during pregnancy.

Dosing

- Varies widely per product and dosage form; refer to label and instructions for individual products

- Table 15-2 lists the oral dosage of supplemental fluoride (as a lozenge, chewable tablet, or solution) for children living in areas with drinking water that has insufficient quantities of fluoride (expressed in terms of fluoride ion)

Adverse Reactions: Most Common

Staining or pigmentation (e.g., yellow, brown, brown-black) of the teeth may result from topical application of concentrated solutions or gels of stannous fluoride, particularly in patients with poor oral hygiene

Adverse Reactions: Rare/Severe/Important

Consuming excessive amounts of fluorides can result in fluorosis (hypocalcification and hypoplasia) and osseous changes in children < 8 years of age, especially at levels of water fluoridation > 0.6 ppm. Dyspnea has occurred in asthmatic children using a 5% sodium fluoride solution. Hypersensitivity reactions.

Major Drug Interactions

Drugs Affecting Fluoride

Drugs/supplements that contain aluminum hydroxide, calcium salts, and magnesium hydroxide: May decrease bioavailability of oral fluorides. Do not take at the same time; separate by at least 2 hours.

Counseling Points

- Dairy products can reduce bioavailability of oral fluorides; do not ingest at the same time
- Follow instructions per product labeling
- Children in locations with adequate fluoride concentrations in the drinking water (> 0.6 ppm) do not need supplemental fluorides

Key Point

- Children in locations with adequate fluoride concentrations in the drinking water (> 0.6 ppm) do not need supplemental fluorides
- Although safe for pregnant women, the ADA does not recommend fluoride supplementation during pregnancy

TABLE 15-2 Fluoride Dosing for Children Based on Fluoride Concentration in Drinking Water

Age	Fluoride Ion Concentration in Drinking Water		
	< 0.3 ppm	0.3–0.6 ppm	> 0.6 ppm
0–6 months	None	None	None
6 months to 3 years	0.25 mg	None	None
3–6 years	0.5 mg	0.25 mg	None
6–16 years	1 mg	0.5 mg	None

DIETARY SUPPLEMENT, FOLIC ACID

Introduction

Folic acid is a water-soluble B vitamin. Supplementation of folic acid in women who are pregnant or planning to become pregnant has significantly reduced the number of infants born with neural tube defects.

Mechanism of Action for the Drug Class

Folic acid is necessary for the formation of numerous enzymes and coenzymes in many metabolic systems, particularly in the formation of DNA and RNA bases (purines and pyrimidines). It is also required for the maintenance of red blood cell production.

◉ Folic Acid

Brand Names

Folvite, Folacin-800

Generic Name

Folic acid

OTC

Dosage Forms

Tablet, injectable

Pregnancy Category A

Usage

Treatment of megaloblastic (macrocytic) anemia due to folic acid deficiency,* antenatal dietary supplement to prevent fetal neural tube defects*

Dosing

- Treatment of folic acid deficiency: 0.4 mg daily
- Prevention of fetal neural tube defects in pregnant women: 0.4–0.8 mg daily. Women at high risk should receive 4 mg daily.

Adverse Reactions

Rare

Major Drug Interactions

Drugs Affecting Folic Acid

Methotrexate, trimethoprim, chloramphenicol, phenytoin, phenobarbital: Decrease effectiveness

Folic Acid's Effect on Other Drugs

Phenytoin, phenobarbital, primidone: Decreases effects

Contraindication

Treatment with folic acid in other megaloblastic anemias (pernicious anemia and vitamin B_{12} deficiency) without proper diagnosis can mask these anemias and lead to progression that can include irreversible nerve damage

Counseling Point

Take folic acid replacement only with the recommendation of a healthcare provider

Key Point

Decreases the incidence of fetal neural tube defects by > 50%; critical nutrient in prenatal care

---

DIETARY SUPPLEMENT, VITAMIN C

Introduction

Vitamin C is an important vitamin. Many consumers take vitamin C supplements to reduce the severity and duration of the common cold.

Mechanism of Action for the Drug Class

Vitamin C is an essential cofactor in numerous biochemical reactions. It indirectly provides electrons to enzymes that require prosthetic metal ions in reduced form for their activity. It is an antioxidant in aqueous environments. It is a cofactor in the synthesis of carnitine, neurotransmitters, and collagen. Vitamin C exists in both reduced and oxidized forms.

◉ Vitamin C

Brand Names

Ascorbate-C, C Aspa Scorb, Ester-C, Vicks Vitamin C, others

Generic Names

Vitamin C, L-ascorbic acid

OTC

Dosage Forms

Tablet, chewable tablet, capsule, powder

Natural Products, Dietary Supplements, and Nutrients

Pregnancy Category A (at RDA Levels) and C (at High Doses)

Usage

Improves wound healing,* reduces symptoms of the common cold (unproven; anecdotal),* prevents and treats scurvy, improves dietary iron absorption

Dosing

- RDA:
  - Men: 90 mg daily
  - Women: 75 mg daily
  - Smokers: Increase RDA by 35 mg
- Renal dosage adjustment: Lower doses recommended in renal insufficiency

Adverse Reactions: Most Common

Nausea, abdominal cramps, flatulence, diarrhea

Adverse Reactions: Rare/Severe/Important

Renal consequences, including hyperoxaluria, risk of nephrolithiasis

Major Drug Interactions

Drugs Affecting Vitamin C

- Aspirin, ethanol: Reduce tissue saturation of vitamin C
- Oral contraceptives, tobacco smoke exposure: Increase clearance

Vitamin C's Effect on Other Drugs

- Co-trimoxazole: Increases bioavailability
- Estradiol/levonorgestrel: Increases clearance
- Warfarin: Decreases effect

Counseling Points

- Intestinal absorption and renal reabsorption are saturable processes, so doses > 200 mg should be divided to limit GI discomfort
- Tolerable upper intake level set at 2,000 mg daily from all sources
- Chronic use of chewable vitamin C products may increase the risk of dental erosions and caries
- No difference in bioavailability or activity exists between natural and synthetic vitamin C

Key Points

- High daily doses may interfere with laboratory tests, but may be assay-dependent:
  - Serum aspartate aminotransferase, bilirubin, creatinine, carbamazepine: False increase
  - Serum lactate dehydrogenase, uric acid, vitamin B_{12}, theophylline: False decrease
  - Guaiac test for occult blood: False negative
- Use with caution in patients with glucose-6-phosphate dehydrogenase deficiency
- For pregnant women, daily limits from all sources should be no greater than 2,000 mg of vitamin C

DIETARY SUPPLEMENT, VITAMIN D

Introduction

Vitamin D is essential for promoting calcium absorption in the gut and maintaining adequate serum calcium and phosphate concentrations

⊙ Cholecalciferol

Brand Names

Vitamin D, D_3

Generic Name

Cholecalciferol

Rx and OTC

Dosage Forms

Capsule, tablet

Usage

Dietary supplement, treatment or prophylaxis of vitamin D deficiency,* osteoporosis prevention and treatment*

Pregnancy Category

When doses are consistent with the RDA, vitamin D analogs are pregnancy category A. Doses should not exceed the RDA in pregnant women. Doses greater than the RDA are considered to be pregnancy category C.

Dosing

- 18–50 years: 200 IU/day
- 51–70 years: 400 IU/day
- > 70 years: 600 IU/day

Contraindications

Hypercalcemia, hypersensitivity

Adverse Reactions: Most Common

None

Adverse Reactions: Rare/Severe/Important

Hypervitaminosis D is a severe adverse reaction. Signs and symptoms include hypercalcemia resulting in headache, nausea, vomiting, lethargy, confusion, sluggishness, abdominal pain, bone pain, polyuria, polydipsia, weakness, cardiac arrhythmias (e.g., QT shortening, sinus tachycardia), soft tissue calcification, calciuria, and nephrocalcinosis.

Major Drug Interactions

Drugs Affecting Vitamin D

Mineral oil, orlistat, bile acid sequestrants: May decrease absorption of vitamin D analogs; separate dosing by 2–4 hours to lessen this interaction

Vitamin D's Effect on Other Drugs

Aluminum hydroxide and sucralfate: Increases serum concentrations; avoid concomitant use or separate by 2–4 hours to lessen this effect

Counseling Point

Take as directed

DIETARY SUPPLEMENT, VITAMIN E

Introduction

Vitamin E is an important vitamin that protects cell membranes from oxidative damage, inhibits proliferation of smooth muscle, and decreases adhesion of platelets, leukocytes, and endothelial cells.

◉ Vitamin E

Brand Name

None

Generic Names

Vitamin E, tocopherols (alpha, beta, gamma, and delta), tocotrienols (alpha, beta, gamma, and delta)

OTC

Dosage Forms

Tablet, capsule

Usage

Vitamin E deficiency,* prevention of cardiovascular disease morbidity and mortality (not labeled/approved)*, slowing progression of neurologic disorders (e.g., dementia, Parkinson's disease [not labeled/approved])

Pregnancy Category A (at RDA) and C (at Higher Doses)

Vitamin E crosses the placenta. Maternal serum concentrations of alpha-tocopherol increase with lipid concentrations as pregnancy progresses; however, placental transfer remains constant. Additional supplementation is not needed in pregnant women without deficiency.

Dosing

- RDA: 15 mg daily of alpha-tocopherol
- Tolerable upper intake: 1,000 mg daily from all alpha-tocopherol sources
- Renal dosage adjustment: None

Adverse Reactions: Most Common

GI upset

Adverse Reactions: Rare/Severe/Important

Increased risk of bleeding and hemorrhagic stroke, thrombocytopenia

Major Drug Interactions

Drugs Affecting Vitamin E

- Cholestyramine, orlistat, mineral oil: Decrease absorption
- Fish oil: Increases vitamin E requirements

Vitamin E's Effect on Other Drugs

Warfarin, antiplatelet agents, insulin, digoxin: Increases effects

Counseling Point

Take as prescribed

Key Points

- The predominant form of vitamin E in the diet is gamma-tocopherol. In the body it is alpha-tocopherol. Select a product containing both forms.
- Bioavailability is enhanced in the presence of food containing some dietary fat
- Use a water-miscible formulation in patients with malabsorptive disorders
- Although IUs are no longer recognized as a dosing unit for vitamin E, it is still found in product labeling; this requires conversion to milligram alpha-tocopherol for comparison to dosing recommendations:
  - mg = IU all-*rac*-alpha-tocopherol as acetate/succinate/2.2
  - mg = IU RRR-alpha-tocopherol as acetate/succinate/1.5

REVIEW QUESTIONS

1. Which of the following herbal supplements is touted for its cholesterol-lowering capabilities, mainly because it possesses pharmacologic properties similar to lovastatin?
   a. St. Johns wort
   b. Chondroitin
   c. Valerian
   d. Red yeast rice

2. Which of the following dietary supplements is derived from cattle trachea or shark cartilage?
   a. Coenzyme-Q
   b. Creatine
   c. Glucosamine
   d. Chondroitin

3. Which of the following herbal supplements is used as a calmative or sleep aid?
   a. Valerian
   b. Feverfew
   c. Echinacea
   d. Digitalis

4. Q-sorb products contain which of the following natural supplements?
   a. Co-enzyme Q
   b. Tocopherol
   c. Asian ginseng
   d. Siberian ginseng

5. Ginseng is popularly used to:
   a. treat mild to moderate depression.
   b. adjust sleep and mood cycles.
   c. increase energy.
   d. All of the above

6. Patients with severe shellfish allergy are advised to avoid using products that contain which of the following dietary supplements?
   a. Glucosamine
   b. Chondroitin
   c. Ginger
   d. None of the above

7. Kava should be avoided due to its risk of:
   a. liver toxicity.
   b. CYP450 drug interactions.
   c. memory loss.
   d. All of the above

8. Which of the following dietary supplements is used as a sleep aid?
   a. Melatonin
   b. Valerian
   c. Chamomile
   d. All of the above

9. Iron salts in dietary supplements may decrease the absorption of which of the following if taken concomitantly?
   a. Levothyroxine
   b. Oral ciprofloxacin
   c. Pancreatic lipase enzymes
   d. All of the above

10. Pernicious anemia results from a deficiency of which of the following?
    a. Vitamin A
    b. Vitamin B_{12}
    c. Vitamin C
    d. Vitamin K

11. Interactions with which of the following may increase therapeutic failure with drugs such as cyclosporine and protease inhibitors?
    a. Gingko biloba
    b. Glucosamine
    c. Valerian
    d. St. John's wort

12. A kidney transplant patient is being administered cyclosporine. Which of the following dietary supplements should this patient avoid or use only after consultation with the appropriate healthcare provider?
    a. St. John's wort
    b. Echinacea
    c. Probiotics that contain *Lactobacillus acidophilus*
    d. All of the above

13. Although vitamins are generally safe during pregnancy, which of the following should be taken in a higher amount than the RDA to lessen the chance of fetal neural tube malformations?
    a. Vitamin C
    b. Thiamine
    c. Folic acid
    d. Vitamin B_{12}

14. Patients with significant ragweed allergy may react unfavorably to which of the following dietary supplements?
    a. Chamomile
    b. Valerian
    c. Ginseng
    d. All of the above

15. Which of the following dietary supplements has been taken in conjunction with cholesterol-lowering drugs, such as simvastatin and lovastatin, to lessen the risk of myopathies?
    a. Garlic
    b. Aloe
    c. Ginseng
    d. Co-enzyme Q

16. Diabetics sometimes use _____ to help with glycemic control, even though the clinical data do not support this use.

    a. cinnamon
    b. nutmeg
    c. valerian
    d. vanilla bean

17. Which of the following dietary supplements is used primarily as an anti-inflammatory agent?

    a. Horse chestnut
    b. Ma huang
    c. Feverfew
    d. Milk thistle

18. Which of the following increases the risk of bleeding if taken with anticoagulants and/or antiplatelet agents?

    a. Horse chestnut
    b. Garlic
    c. Chamomile
    d. All of the above

19. Which of the following is the most commonly reported adverse effect seen in patients who regularly use ginger supplements?

    a. Flatulence
    b. Heartburn
    c. Constipation
    d. Asymptomatic prolonged QTc interval

20. Although touted as an eye tonic, which of the following may causes ophthalmic phototoxicity with actual lens damage?

    a. Chamomile tea
    b. Valerian root
    c. Goldenseal
    d. Milk thistle

21. Which of the following dietary supplements is a form of a pineal gland hormone?

    a. Melatonin
    b. Acidophilus
    c. Chondroitin
    d. Glucosamine

22. Silymarin and silibinin are the active botanical ingredients in which of the following dietary supplements?

    a. Creatine
    b. Kava kava
    c. Ma huang
    d. Milk thistle

23. Ingesting large quantities of grapefruit juice may increase toxicities with which of the following dietary supplements?

    a. Red yeast rice
    b. Horse chestnut
    c. Iron salts
    d. Both A and B

24. Which of the following dietary supplements was widely thought to help men with prostate issues until recently disproven in a clinical trial to have such benefit?

    a. Creatine
    b. Saw palmetto
    c. St. John's wort
    d. None of the above

25. *Hypericum,* goat weed, Klamath weed, and tipton weed are references to which of the following dietary supplements?

    a. Yohimbe
    b. St. John's wort
    c. Goldenseal
    d. Ginseng

26. Ingestion of excessive amounts _____ during pregnancy can lead to teratogenic effects in the fetus and at high doses is considered to be an FDA pregnancy category X drug.

    a. vitamin A
    b. vitamin C
    c. folic acid
    d. vitamin B_{12}

27. Tums contains primarily what mineral/dietary supplement?

    a. Iron
    b. Aluminum
    c. Vitamin E
    d. Calcium

28. Which calcium salt contains the highest percentage of elemental calcium?

    a. Glucobionate
    b. Gluconate
    c. Citrate
    d. Carbonate

29. Ergocalciferol is an analog of which of the following vitamins?

    a. Vitamin A
    b. Vitamin B_6
    c. Vitamin C
    d. Vitamin D

30. Consistent ingestion of which of the following vitamins can cause false negative results on the guaiac test used to detect hidden blood in the stool/feces?

    a. Vitamin A
    b. Vitamin C
    c. Vitamin E
    d. Vitamin D

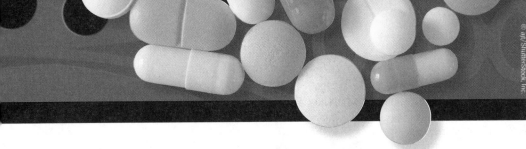

Biologic and Immunologic Agents

Jane F. Bowen, PharmD, BCPS
Carol Holtzman, PharmD, MS

VACCINES

Introduction

Vaccines are one of the most effective methods of disease prevention available. Vaccines contain the same antigens or parts of antigens that cause diseases, but are either killed or greatly weakened. They are produced and used for diseases that tend to cause premature deaths or have a costly impact, such as increased physician visits or hospitalizations. Vaccines are available for a variety of infections, including polio, measles, diphtheria, pertussis (whooping cough), rubella (German measles), mumps, tetanus, and *Haemophilus influenzae* type b (Hib), *Streptococcus pneumoniae*, varicella zoster, and influenza. The main adverse effect of vaccines is a local injection site reaction (erythema, tenderness, pain, swelling, hematoma, and pruritus). Allegations of vaccine-related autism have been shown to be false, but the fear has led many people to avoid vaccines that would otherwise benefit them. As a result, some vaccine-preventable illnesses have begun to reemerge in developed countries.

Mechanism of Action for the Drug Class

Vaccines contain the same antigens or parts of antigens that cause diseases. These antigens are either killed (inactivated) or greatly weakened (live attenuated). This produces an antibody response that results in immunity to the disease.

Members of the Drug Class

In this section: Influenza virus vaccine, pneumococcal polysaccharide vaccine, zoster vaccine
Others: Numerous others

◉ Influenza Virus Vaccine

Brand Names
Inactivated: Fluarix, Fluzone, Afluria, FluLaval, Fluvirin, Flucelvax
Live attenuated: FluMist

Generic Name
Influenza virus vaccine

Rx Only

Dosage Forms
Injection (inactivated), intranasal solution (live attenuated)

Usage
Provision of active immunity for the prevention of infections caused by influenza virus subtype A and B strains contained in the vaccine

Pregnancy Category B (Inactivated) and C (Live Attenuated)

Dosing
- Inactivated: 45 µg/0.5 mL IM
- Live attenuated: 0.1 mL intranasal in each nostril

Adverse Reactions: Most Common
Inactivated: Pain and redness at the injection site, muscle aches, fatigue, headache
Live attenuated: Runny nose or nasal congestion in all ages, fever in children 2–6 years of age, sore throat in adults

Adverse Reactions: Rare/Severe/Important
Life-threatening allergic reactions (very rare)

Major Drug Interactions
Drugs Affecting Influenza Virus Vaccine
Immunosuppressive therapies: May reduce immune response to the vaccine

Influenza Virus Vaccine's Effect on Other Drugs
Aspirin-containing products: Avoid aspirin-containing therapy in children and adolescents during the first 4 weeks after vaccination with the live attenuated vaccine due to risk of Reye's syndrome

---

* Throughout the text, an asterisk (*) is used to indicate the most common uses of a drug.

Essential Monitoring Parameter

For individuals who report a history of egg allergy but for whom it was determined that the inactivated vaccine can be used, observe for at least 30 minutes after receipt of vaccine. This is not an issue with Flucelvax, which is not cultured from eggs.

Contraindications

With live attenuated vaccine, avoid concomitant use of antiviral agents active against influenza A or B viruses. All formulations except Flucelvax cannot be used in patients with severe allergic reactions to egg proteins (worse than hives). Do not use the live attenuated vaccine in children 2–17 years of age receiving aspirin therapy.

Counseling Points

- Get vaccinated every year as soon as the flu season vaccine becomes available in your community
- Consult your healthcare provider before receiving the flu vaccine if you have an egg allergy, a history of Guillain-Barré syndrome, or are pregnant. If you have egg allergies worse than hives, then you should not receive the influenza vaccination with most available formulations of the flu vaccine.

Key Points

- Because the dominant influenza strains change each year, annual vaccination is required
- Everyone who is at least 6 months of age should get a flu vaccine in the absence of a contraindication
- Three different injectable flu vaccines and one nasal spray flu vaccine are available and are approved for different ages:
  - Regular flu shot: Approved for use in people ≥ 6 months of age
  - Flucelvax: Approved for use in people ≥ 18 years of age
  - High-dose flu shot (Fluzone High dose): Approved for use in people ≥ 65 years of age
  - Intradermal flu (Fluzone Intradermal) shot: Approved for use in people 18–64 years of age
  - Intranasal flu vaccine (FluMist): Approved for people 2–49 years of age
- Avoid use of intranasal flu vaccine (live attenuated) in pregnant or immunosuppressed patients
- People with a history of Guillain-Barré syndrome should consult with their healthcare provider before receiving the flu vaccine

◉ Pneumococcal Polysaccharide Vaccine

Brand Name

Pneumovax 23

Generic Name

Pneumococcal polysaccharide vaccine

Rx Only

Dosage Form

Injection

Usage

Provision of active immunity for the prevention of pneumococcal diseases caused by the 23 serotypes contained in the vaccine

Pregnancy Category C

Dosing

0.5 mL IM or SUB-Q

Adverse Reactions: Most Common

Injection site reactions (e.g., pain, tenderness, swelling, erythema), asthenia and fatigue, myalgia, headache

Adverse Reactions: Rare/Severe/Important

Fever, severe local reactions

Major Drug Interactions

Zoster vaccine: Separate administration by 4 weeks to prevent reduced immune response to the zoster vaccine

Counseling Point

Tell your healthcare provider immediately if you experience wheezing, difficulty breathing, rash, or hives

Key Points

- The following populations should receive the pneumococcal polysaccharide vaccine:
  - All adults aged ≥ 65 years of age
  - Children and adults 2–64 years of age who:
    - Have a long-term health problem (e.g., heart disease, lung disease, diabetes)
    - Are immunocompromised (e.g., malignancies such as leukemia or lymphoma, HIV infection, or damaged spleen)
    - Are taking immunosuppressive therapy (e.g., long-term steroids)
  - Adults 19–64 years of age who smoke or have asthma
- Not approved for children < 2 years of age
- Should not be confused with the pneumococcal conjugate vaccine (PVC-13), which is often given to children < 2 years of age and does not provide immunity to as many serotypes as the pneumococcal polysaccharide vaccine

◉ Zoster Vaccine

Brand Name

Zostavax

Generic Name

Zoster vaccine

Rx Only

Dosage Form

Injection

Usage

Prevention of herpes zoster (shingles)

Pregnancy Category

Use during pregnancy is contraindicated

Dosing

Single 0.65 mL dose SUB-Q

Adverse Reactions: Most Common

Injection site reactions, headache

Major Drug Interactions

Drugs Affecting the Zoster Vaccine

- Pneumococcal polysaccharide vaccine: Separate administration by 4 weeks to prevent reduced immune response to the zoster vaccine
- Acyclovir, famciclovir, valacyclovir: Discontinue these medications at least 24 hours before administration of zoster vaccine, if possible

Contraindications

History of anaphylactic/anaphylactoid reaction to gelatin, neomycin, or any other component of the vaccine; immunosuppression or immunodeficiency; pregnancy

Counseling Point

Injection site reactions and headache are common adverse reactions

Key Points

- The zoster vaccine is a live attenuated vaccine
- The zoster vaccine is a one-time vaccination
- The zoster vaccine is not a substitute for the varicella vaccine and should not be used in patients < 50 years of age. The varicella vaccine is indicated for the prevention of chickenpox. Its dosing and composition are distinct from the zoster vaccine.
- Although the FDA approved it for use in those ≥ 50 years of age, the Center for Disease Control and Prevention recommends use in people ≥ 60 years of age
- Even if patients have had shingles previously, they can still receive the shingles vaccine to help prevent future occurrences of the disease
- The zoster vaccine is not recommended for persons of any age who have received the varicella vaccine

IMMUNOSUPPRESSANT AGENTS, CALCINEURIN INHIBITORS

Introduction

Calcineurin inhibitors are the backbone of organ transplant immunosuppression. They are used in combination with other immunosuppressant agents to prevent organ rejection after transplant. They can also be used for the treatment of other immunologic conditions, but usually not as first-line therapy. These medications require therapeutic drug monitoring of trough concentrations and have many drug interactions.

Mechanism of Action for the Drug Class

Inhibit interleukin-2 production, and subsequently T cell differentiation and proliferation, thus preventing allograft rejection

Members of the Drug Class

In this section: Cyclosporine, tacrolimus

◉ Cyclosporine

Brand Names

Gengraf, Neoral, Restasis, Sandimmune

Generic Name

Cyclosporine

Rx Only

Dosage Forms

Capsule, oral solution, injection, eye drops

Usage

Prevention of organ transplant rejection,* prevention and treatment of graft-versus-host disease, rheumatoid arthritis, psoriasis, severe ulcerative colitis; increase tear production (Restasis only)

Pregnancy Category C

Dosing

- Prevention of organ transplant rejection:
  - Oral: 7–15 mg/kg in two divided doses depending on type of transplant. Subsequent doses are adjusted based on serum concentrations.
  - IV: One-third of the oral dose infused over 2–6 hours
- Rheumatoid arthritis:
  - 2.5 mg/kg per day in two divided doses; dose is titrated based on response
  - Maximum dose: 4 mg/kg per day
- Psoriasis:
  - 2.5 mg/kg per day in two divided doses; dose is titrated based on response
  - Maximum dose: 4 mg/kg per day
- Severe ulcerative colitis:
  - Oral: 5–10 mg/kg per day in two divided doses
  - IV: 2–4 mg/kg per day infused continuously over 24 hours
- Increase tear production: 1 drop in each eye every 12 hours
- Renal dosage adjustment: Adjust dose to maintain lower cyclosporine blood trough concentrations

Pharmacokinetic Monitoring

Monitor trough levels. Therapeutic range is based on the organ transplanted, time after transplant, and organ function. Typical range is 25–200 ng/mL.

Adverse Reactions: Most Common

Oral, IV: Edema, hirsutism, gingival hyperplasia, headache, tremor, increased triglycerides. Ophthalmic: Burning, stinging

Adverse Reactions: Rare/Severe/Important

Oral, IV: hypertension, nephrotoxicity, hyperkalemia, hypomagnesemia, hyperuricemia, hepatotoxicity, coma, encephalopathy, leukoencephalopathy, seizure, hemolytic uremic syndrome, infectious disease, lymphoma

Major Drug Interactions

Drugs Affecting Cyclosporine

- CYP3A4 inducers (i.e., phenytoin, phenobarbital, carbamazepine, rifampin, nevirapine, St. John's wort): Decrease blood concentrations
- CYP3A4 inhibitors (i.e., azole antifungals, amiodarone, macrolide antibiotics, diltiazem, verapamil, ritonavir, grapefruit juice): Increase toxicity
- Allopurinol: Increases toxicity
- Vancomycin, aminoglycosides, ACE inhibitors, colchicine, NSAIDs: May potentiate renal dysfunction
- ACE inhibitors, potassium-sparing diuretics: May enhance hyperkalemic effect

Cyclosporine's Effects on Other Drugs

- HMG-CoA reductase inhibitors: Increases HMG-CoA reductase inhibitor concentrations, placing patients at an increased risk of rhabdomyolysis
- Digoxin: Increases levels
- Dabigatran: Increases concentrations of dabigatran's active metabolites

Contraindications

- IV formulation contraindicated in patients with hypersensitivity to polyoxyethylated castor oil
- Rheumatoid arthritis and psoriasis: Abnormal renal function, uncontrolled hypertension, malignancies
- Psoriasis: Concomitant treatment with PUVA or UVB therapy, methotrexate, other immunosuppressive agents, coal tar, or radiation therapy
- Ophthalmic cyclosporine is contraindicated in patients with ocular infections

Essential Monitoring Parameters

Trough levels, renal function, potassium, magnesium, liver function, blood pressure, lipids, uric acid. Therapeutic range is based on the organ transplanted, time after transplant, and organ function; typical range is 25–200 ng/mL.

Counseling Points

- Take prescribed dose at the same time each day with meals
- When administering the solution, mix with water or orange juice in a glass, not plastic, container, then stir and drink all at once
- Avoid grapefruit and grapefruit juice, which can affect the metabolism of cyclosporine
- Avoid live vaccines while on therapy or within 3 months of discontinuing therapy
- Frequent laboratory monitoring will be needed

Key Points

- Cyclosporine modified (Neoral, Gengraf) and nonmodified (Sandimmune) products are not bioequivalent and therefore are not interchangeable
- Bioavailability of nonmodified (Sandimmune) oral solution is 30% of the IV solution
- Nonmodified (Sandimmune) capsules and oral solution have decreased bioavailability compared with modified (Neoral) formulations. Cyclosporine blood trough concentrations should be monitored frequently (every 4–7 days until stable blood trough levels are achieved) when switching between products.
- Cyclosporine dose adjustments should be made in small increments (about a 25% change at any one time)

⊙ Tacrolimus

Brand Names

Prograf, Protopic

Generic Name

Tacrolimus

Rx Only

Dosage Forms

Capsule, ointment, injection

Usage

Prevention of organ transplant rejection,* prevention and treatment of graft-versus-host disease, moderate to severe atopic dermatitis

Pregnancy Category C

Dosing

- Prevention of organ transplant rejection:
  - Oral: 0.075–0.2 mg/kg per day in two divided doses depending on type of transplant
  - IV: 0.01–0.05 mg/kg per day as a continuous infusion
    - Renal dosage adjustment for oral and IV: Adjust dose to maintain lower tacrolimus blood trough concentrations
    - Hepatic dosage adjustment for oral and IV: In cases of severe hepatic impairment, lower doses may be required. Monitor tacrolimus blood trough concentrations and adjust dose based on levels.
- Atopic dermatitis: Apply thin layer of topical formulation to affected area twice daily

Pharmacokinetic Monitoring

Trough levels should be monitored. Therapeutic range is based on the organ transplanted, time after transplant, and organ function. Typical range is 5–20 ng/mL.

Adverse Reactions: Most Common

Oral, IV: Alopecia, pruritus, rash, constipation, diarrhea, nausea, vomiting, anemia, leukocytosis or leukopenia, thrombocytopenia, headache, insomnia, paresthesia, tremor. Topical: skin burning, pruritus, erythema, paresthesia.

Adverse Reactions: Rare/Severe/Important

Hypertension, prolonged QT interval, diabetes mellitus, hypomagnesemia, hyperkalemia, anaphylaxis, infectious disease, lymphoma, seizure, leukoencephalopathy, nephrotoxicity, hepatotoxicity

Major Drug Interactions

Drugs Affecting Tacrolimus

- Potent CYP3A4 inhibitors (i.e., azole antifungals, amiodarone, macrolide antibiotics, diltiazem, verapamil, ritonavir, grapefruit juice): Increase toxicity
- Potent CYP3A4 inducers (i.e., phenytoin, phenobarbital, carbamazepine, rifampin, nevirapine, St. John's wort): Decrease concentration
- QT-prolonging drugs (i.e., haloperidol, methadone, amiodarone, sotalol, erythromycin, clarithromycin): Increase risk of QT prolongation

- Vancomycin, aminoglycosides, ACE inhibitors, colchicine, NSAIDs: May potentiate renal dysfunction
- Proton pump inhibitors: Increase concentration
- ACE inhibitors, potassium-sparing diuretics: May enhance hyperkalemic effect

Tacrolimus' Effect on Other Drugs

Dabigatran: Increases concentrations of dabigatran's active metabolites

Contraindication

IV formulation contraindicated in patients with hypersensitivity to polyoxyethylated castor oil

Essential Monitoring Parameters

Trough levels, renal function, potassium, magnesium, liver function, blood pressure, blood glucose. Therapeutic range is based on the organ transplanted, time after transplant, and organ function; typical range is 5–20 ng/mL.

Counseling Points

- Take prescribed dose at the same time each day. Tacrolimus may be taken with or without food as long as you are consistent.
- Avoid grapefruit or grapefruit juice, which can affect the metabolism of tacrolimus
- Avoid live vaccines while on therapy or within 3 months of discontinuing therapy
- Frequent laboratory monitoring will be needed

IMMUNOSUPPRESSANT AGENTS, IMPDH INHIBITORS

Introduction

IMPDH inhibitors are used concomitantly with other immunosuppressant medications, such as steroids and a calcineurin inhibitor, to prevent organ transplant rejection. Like the calcineurin inhibitors, they can also be used to treat other immunologic conditions. Unlike calcineurin inhibitors, trough levels are not monitored.

Mechanism of Action of the Drug Class

IMPDH inhibitors inhibit inosine monophosphate dehydrogenase (IMPDH), an enzyme that is essential for T and B cell proliferation

Members of the Drug Class

In this section: Mycophenolic acid

◉ Mycophenolic Acid

Brand Names
CellCept, Myfortic

Generic Names
Mycophenolic acid, mycophenolate mofetil

Rx Only

Dosage Forms
Capsule, tablet, oral suspension, injection

Usage
Prevention of organ transplant rejection,* moderate to severe psoriasis, prevention and treatment of graft-versus-host disease, lupus nephritis, myasthenia gravis

Pregnancy Category D

Dosing

Prevention of organ transplant rejection:

- Oral:
  - CellCept: 2–3 g per day in two divided doses
  - Myfortic: 1,440 mg per day in two divided doses
- IV: CellCept 2–3 g per day in two divided doses

Adverse Reactions: Most Common

Edema, hyper- or hypotension, headache, insomnia, leucopenia or leukocytosis, hyperglycemia, thrombocytopenia, hypercholesterolemia, weakness, tremor, nausea, vomiting, diarrhea, constipation, hypomagnesemia, hyper- or hypokalemia

Adverse Reactions: Rare/Severe/Important

Infectious disease, lymphoma, neutropenia, anemia, nephrotoxicity, hepatotoxicity, gastrointestinal ulcers/bleeding

Major Drug Interactions

Drugs Affecting Mycophenolic Acid

- Antacids, cholestyramine, sevelamer: Decrease absorption
- Probenecid: Increases concentrations
- Rifamycins: Decrease concentrations

Mycophenolic Acid's Effect on Other Drugs

Contraceptives: Decreased concentration of contraceptives (estrogens and progestins)

Contraindication

IV formulation contraindicated in patients with hypersensitivity to polysorbate 80

Essential Monitoring Parameters

Renal function, liver function, complete blood count

Counseling Points

- Women of childbearing age must have a negative urine or serum pregnancy test within 1 week prior to starting therapy
- Two forms of contraceptives should be used 4 weeks prior to starting mycophenolic acid, unless abstinence is the chosen method. Continue contraceptives for 6 weeks after stopping therapy.
- Breastfeeding is not recommended during therapy or for 6 weeks after completing therapy
- Oral dosage forms should be taken on an empty stomach to avoid variability in absorption
- Delayed-release tablets (Myfortic) should not be crushed, cut, or chewed
- Avoid live vaccines while on therapy or within 3 months of discontinuing therapy

Key Points

- CellCept and Myfortic dosage forms are not interchangeable due to differences in absorption
- Because mycophenolic acid commonly causes leukopenia, it may mask leukocytosis in patients with infections

---

TUMOR NECROSIS FACTOR INHIBITORS

Introduction

Tumor necrosis factor (TNF) inhibitors are genetically engineered protein molecules that block the proinflammatory cytokine TNF-alpha. These medications are used in the treatment of autoimmune disorders such as rheumatoid arthritis, ankylosing spondylitis, Crohn's disease, plaque psoriasis, and psoriatic arthritis when other options fail to achieve adequate response. These agents are expensive and have many adverse effects.

Mechanism of Action for the Drug Class

Block TNF effects by binding to it and blocking its action, preventing inflammatory processes

Adverse Reactions for the Drug Class: Most Common

Injection site reaction, headache, rhinitis, upper respiratory infection

Adverse Reactions for the Drug Class: Rare/Severe/Important

Heart failure; malignancies; serious infections, including *Legionella* pneumonia; listeriosis; tuberculosis; erythema multiforme; Stevens-Johnson syndrome; epidermal necrolysis; anemia; leucopenia; pancytopenia; autoimmune hepatitis; sepsis; multiple sclerosis; optic neuritis

Major Drug Interactions for the Drug Class

TNF Inhibitors' Effects on Other Drugs

- Disease-modifying antirheumatic drugs (DMARDs; abatacept, anakinra, natalizumab) and other concomitant immunosuppressive agents: Increase risk of toxicities and immunosuppression
- Live vaccines: Increase risk of developing vaccinial infections

Contraindications for the Drug Class

Patients with sepsis and/or active infections (chronic or acute)

Counseling Points for the Drug Class

- Stop medication and contact your healthcare provider immediately if you experience stomach pain or cramping, unusual bruising or bleeding, persistent fever, rash, night sweats, significant weight loss, muscle weakness, and/or signs of respiratory infections
- Avoid receiving immunizations during therapy and for at least 3 months after therapy with TNF inhibitors
- For agents given subcutaneously, rotate injection sites; new injections should be given at least 1 inch from an old site

Key Points for the Drug Class

- Patients should be evaluated for latent tuberculosis infection with a tuberculin skin test before therapy
- Use caution in patients with chronic infections. If a patient develops an acute serious infection or sepsis, the medication should be discontinued.
- Rare reactivation of hepatitis B has occurred while receiving these agents. Evaluate before initiation and during treatment.
- Use caution in patients with heart failure because exacerbations may occur

Members of the Drug Class

In this section: Etanercept, infliximab, adalimumab
Others: Certolizumab pegol, golimumab

◉ Etanercept

Brand Name
Enbrel

Generic Name
Etanercept

Rx Only

Dosage Form
Injection

Usage
Treatment of moderate to severe active RA,* moderate to severe active polyarticular JIA, psoriatic arthritis, active ankylosing spondylitis, moderate to severe chronic plaque psoriasis, hidradenitis suppurativa

Pregnancy Category B

Dosing
- Rheumatoid arthritis, psoriatic arthritis, ankylosing spondylitis:
  - 25 mg SUB-Q twice weekly *or*
  - 50 mg SUB-Q once weekly
- Plaque psoriasis: 50 mg SUB-Q twice weekly for 3 months, then 50 mg SUB-Q once weekly

◉ Infliximab

Brand Name
Remicade

Generic Name
Infliximab

Rx Only

Dosage Form
Injection

Usage
RA,* Crohn's disease*, ulcerative colitis, ankylosing spondylitis, psoriatic arthritis, plaque psoriasis, hidradenitis suppurativa, JIA

Dosing
- Crohn's disease and ulcerative colitis: 5 mg/kg IV at 0, 2, and 6 weeks, followed by 5 mg/kg every 8 weeks thereafter
- RA (in combination with methotrexate): 3 mg/kg IV at 0, 2, and 6 weeks, then every 8 weeks thereafter

Counseling Point
Common adverse reactions include abdominal pain, nausea, and rash

Key Points
- Contraindicated in patients with moderate to severe heart failure
- Must be given intravenously

◉ Adalimumab

Brand Name
Humira

Generic Name
Adalimumab

Rx Only

Dosage Form
Injection

Usage
Moderate to severe RA,* severe Crohn's disease,* plaque psoriasis, psoriatic arthritis, ankylosing spondylitis, severe JIA, ulcerative colitis

Pregnancy Category B

Dosing
- RA: 40 mg SUB-Q once every other week
- Crohn's disease: 160 mg SUB-Q (given as four injections on day 1 or as two injections per day over 2 consecutive days), then 80 mg 2 weeks later. Maintenance: 40 g every other week beginning day 29.

SELECTIVE COSTIMULATOR BLOCKERS

Introduction

Selective costimulator blockers block the stimulation of T cells, thus decreasing the immune response. Abatacept is a biologic disease modifying antirheumatic drug (DMARD) used in the treatment of rheumatoid arthritis, whereas belatacept is used to prevent kidney transplant rejection. These medications suppress the immune system and put patients at higher risk for infection. Therefore, patients need to be screened for latent TB infection prior to initiation.

Mechanism of Action for the Drug Class

Bind to the surface of antigen-presenting cells and prevent them from activating T cells. This inhibits the immune response, thus preventing joint tissue destruction (abatacept) or organ transplant rejection (belatacept).

Members of the Drug Class

In this section: Abatacept
Other: Belatacept

⊙ Abatacept

Brand Name
Orencia

Generic Name
Abatacept

Rx Only

Dosage Form
Injection

Usage
Moderate to severe juvenile idiopathic arthritis (JIA) and adult rheumatoid arthritis (RA)*

Pregnancy Category C

Dosing
- IV: Infused over 30 minutes. Total dose is based on weight. Doses are given at weeks 0, 2, and 4 and then every 4 weeks thereafter:
  - < 60 kg: 500 mg
  - 60–100 kg: 750 mg
  - > 100 kg: 1,000 mg
- SUB-Q: 125 mg within 24 hours of the IV infusion, then 125 mg SUB-Q once weekly. Can initiate SUB-Q dosing weekly if patient is unable to get first dose as IV infusion.

Adverse Reactions: Most Common
Acute exacerbation of chronic obstructive pulmonary disease (COPD), headache, nausea

Adverse Reactions: Rare/Severe/Important
Infection, including reactivation of hepatitis B and tuberculosis; anaphylaxis; malignancy (lymphoma and lung cancer)

Major Drug Interactions
Other immunosuppressive agents: Increase toxic effects of both immunosuppressive agents and increase risk of serious infection

Counseling Points
- Store in the refrigerator and protect from light
- SUB-Q administration: Allow prefilled syringe to warm to room temperature (30–60 minutes) prior to administration. Inject into the front of the thigh (preferred), abdomen (except for 2-inch area around the navel), or the outer area of the upper arms. Rotate injection sites (≥ 1 inch apart) and do not administer into tender, bruised, red, or hard skin.
- This drug increases susceptibility to infections; report any signs of infection to your healthcare provider
- Avoid live vaccines while on therapy or within 3 months of discontinuing therapy

Key Points
- Screen patients for latent TB infection prior to initiating therapy
- Screen patients for viral hepatitis prior to initiating therapy
- IV must be infused through a 0.2–1.2 micron low protein–binding filter
- Powder for injection contains maltose, which may falsely increase serum glucose readings on the day of infusion if using a glucose dehydrogenase pyrroloquinolinequinone (GDH-PQQ) glucose test
- Patients can develop antibodies to this product. The clinical significance of this is unknown.

SUPPRESSOR T CELL ACTIVATORS

Introduction

Glatiramer is used in the treatment of relapsing remitting multiple sclerosis (MS). Like the interferons, it should be used early in the disease, because it has been shown to modify disease progression and reduce relapse rates.

Mechanism of Action of the Drug Class

Induces and activates suppressor T cells in the periphery, thus modifying the immune process occurring against the nerves in the pathogenesis of MS.

Member of the Drug Class

In this section: Glatiramer acetate

◉ Glatiramer Acetate

Brand Name

Copaxone

Generic Name

Glatiramer acetate

Rx Only

Dosage Form

Injection

Usage

Multiple sclerosis*

Pregnancy Category B

Dosing

Inject 20 mg SUB-Q once daily

Adverse Reactions: Most Common

Transient chest pain post injection, vasodilation, injection site reaction, pain, weakness

Adverse Reactions: Rare/Severe/Important

Infections, anaphylaxis, injection site necrosis

Major Drug Interactions

Other immunosuppressive agents: May increase toxic effects of both immunosuppressive agents and increase risk of serious infection

Contraindication

Hypersensitivity to mannitol

Essential Monitoring Parameters

Postinjection reaction (flushing, chest pain, dyspnea, urticaria)

Counseling Points

- Store in the refrigerator
- Prior to use, let the syringe stand at room temperature for 20 minutes to allow solution to warm to room temperature
- Syringes are single-use only; any unused portion should be discarded
- For SUB-Q administration in the arms, abdomen, hips, or thighs, rotate injection sites to prevent lipoatrophy
- May cause reaction after injection, including flushing, chest tightness, dyspnea, or palpitations. Seek medical assistance if symptoms last more than a few minutes or are intense.
- Report any signs of infection
- Avoid live vaccines while on therapy or within 3 months of discontinuing therapy

Key Point

Because this is a biologic agent, neutralizing antibodies (IgG) can form in patients. The clinical significance of this is unknown.

INTERFERONS

Introduction

Interferons are proteins that are released in response to the presence of pathogens such as viruses, bacteria, parasites, or tumor cells. Synthetic interferons have been made to resemble naturally occurring interferons and to treat viral infections, such as chronic hepatitis B and chronic hepatitis C; neoplasms, such as hairy cell leukemia, lymphoma, malignant melanoma, Kaposi's sarcoma, and condylomata acuminata; and autoimmune diseases, such as multiple sclerosis. The most common adverse effects are flulike effects, such as fatigue, headache, fever, and rigors and injection-site reactions. Antibodies can form against the synthetic interferons, decreasing their effectiveness.

Mechanism of Action for the Drug Class

Synthetic interferons trigger the immune system to eradicate pathogens and neoplasms. This occurs through a multitude of different effects, including the inhibition of growth of some cells, changes in cell surface antigen expression, and induction of lymphocytic cytotoxicity. For some indications, the mechanism of action is not well established.

Members of the Drug Class

In this section: Interferon beta-1a, interferon beta-1b, peginterferon alfa-2a

Others: Interferon alfa-2b, interferon alpha-n3, interferon alfacon-1, interferon gamma-1b, peginterferon alfa-2b

◉ Interferon Beta-1a

Brand Names

Avonex, Rebif

Generic Name

Interferon Beta-1a

Rx Only

Dosage Form

Injection

Usage

Multiple sclerosis, relapsing forms* or clinically isolated syndrome

Pregnancy Category C

Dosing

- Avonex:
  - 30 µg IM once weekly *or*
  - 7.5 µg IM week 1, then increase dose by 7.5 mg each week until 30 µg once weekly is reached
- Rebif:
  - Target dose is 44 µg three times per week. Start with 8.8 µg SUB-Q three times per week for weeks 1 and 2, then increase to 22 µg SUB-Q three times per week for weeks 3 and 4, then increase to 44 µg SUB-Q three times per week.
  - Target dose is 22 µg three times per week. Start with 4.4 µg SUB-Q three times per week for weeks 1 and 2, then increase to 11 µg SUB-Q three times per week for weeks 3 and 4, then increase to 22 µg SUB-Q three times per week.

Adverse Reactions: Most Common

Flulike symptoms (chills, fever, myalgias, asthenia), injection site reactions

Adverse Reactions: Rare/Severe/Important

Depression and suicide; severe liver injury, including hepatic failure; pancytopenia; thrombocytopenia; autoimmune disorders; seizures; congestive heart failure

Essential Monitoring Parameters

Thyroid function tests every 6 months in patients with a history of thyroid dysfunction or as clinically indicated. CBC with differential 1, 3, and 6 months after initiation of therapy, then periodically. Liver function tests 1, 3, and 6 months after initiation of therapy, then periodically.

Counseling Points

- Injections:
  - Rotate areas of injection with each dose to minimize the likelihood of injection site reactions
  - Do not inject in area of the body where the skin is irritated, reddened, bruised, infected, or scarred
  - Check the injection site after 2 hours for redness, swelling, or tenderness
  - Contact your healthcare provider if you have a skin reaction that does not clear up in a few days
- Inform your healthcare provider immediately if you feel depressed or have suicidal thoughts; have chest pain or palpitations; experience pain, swelling, or redness at the injection site; or have seizures

Key Points

- Rebif is given SUB-Q and Avonex is given IM
- Pretreatment with analgesics or antipyretics on injection days may decrease flulike symptoms

◉ Interferon Beta-1b

Brand Names

Betaseron, Extavia

Generic Name

Interferon Beta-1b

Rx Only

Dosage Form

Injection

Usage

Multiple sclerosis*

Pregnancy Category C

Dosing

Inject 0.0625 mg SUB-Q every other day. Gradually increase dose by 0.0625 mg every 2 weeks, to a maximum dose of 0.25 mg every other day.

Adverse Reactions: Most Common

Flulike symptoms, including headache, fever, chills, malaise, diaphoresis, and myalgia; injection site reactions; edema; dizziness; insomnia; rash

Adverse Reactions: Rare/Severe/Important

Leukopenia, lymphopenia, neutropenia, anaphylaxis, hepatotoxicity, infection, injection site necrosis, neuropsychiatric conditions (psychosis, mania, depression, suicidal behavior), hyper- or hypothyroid

Contraindications

History of hypersensitivity to albumin or *E. coli*–derived products

Essential Monitoring Parameters

Complete blood count, thyroid function test, liver function tests

Counseling Points

- Solution for injection needs to be reconstituted. To reconstitute, inject 1.2 mL of the diluent provided into the vial of drug powder and gently swirl to dissolve. Do not shake. Reconstituted solution provides 0.25 mg/mL.
- Sites for self-injection include outer surface of the arms, abdomen, hips, and thighs. Rotate SUB-Q injection site.
- Use product immediately or within 3 hours of reconstitution if refrigerated and discard unused portion
- Flulike symptoms are a common side effect and usually decrease over time (average duration about 1 week)
- Immediately report any changes in mood or thoughts of suicide to your healthcare provider

Key Points

- Flulike symptoms are reported in up to 60% of patients on treatment days. These symptoms usually improve with time (~1 week). Analgesics or antipyretics may be used for patients with flulike symptoms.
- Patients can develop neutralizing antibodies to this product. The clinical significance of this is unknown.

⊙ Peginterferon Alfa-2a

Brand Name

Pegasys

Generic Name

Peginterferon Alfa-2a

Rx Only

Dosage Form

Injection

Usage

Chronic hepatitis C,* chronic hepatitis B

Pregnancy Category C

The combination with ribavirin is pregnancy category X

Dosing

- Chronic hepatitis C:
  - Combination therapy with ribavirin: 180 µg SUB-Q once weekly with ribavirin for 24 weeks (genotype 2 or 3) or 48 weeks (genotype 1 or 4 or coinfected with HIV)
  - Monotherapy: 180 µg SUB-Q once weekly for 48 weeks
- Chronic hepatitis B: 180 µg SUB-Q once weekly for 48 weeks

- Renal dosage adjustment: If CrCl < 30 mL/min, including hemodialysis, then 135 µg SUB-Q once weekly
- Hepatic dosage adjustment: If ALT > 5 × ULN or progressively rising above baseline, then 135 µg SUB-Q once weekly
- Dosage adjustments for lab abnormalities:
  - ANC < 700 cells/mm^3: 135 µg SUB-Q once weekly
  - ANC < 500 cells/mm^3: Discontinue treatment until ANC values return to > 1,000 cells/mm^3. Reinstitute at 90 µg and monitor ANC.
  - Platelet < 50,000 cells/mm^3: 135 µg SUB-Q once weekly
  - Platelet < 525,000 cells/mm^3: Discontinue treatment
- Dosage adjustment for depression:
  - Moderate depression: 135 µg SUB-Q once weekly (in some cases dose reduction to 90 µg may be needed)
  - Severe depression: Discontinue permanently

Adverse Reactions: Most Common

Flulike side effects (fatigue, headache, fever, and rigors), myalgias, headaches, GI intolerance, alopecia, psychiatric side effects (depression, irritability, and insomnia), injection site reactions, neutropenia, anemia

Adverse Reactions: Rare/Severe/Important

Neuropsychiatric (depression, emotional lability, mood disorders, frank psychosis, suicidal ideation, actual suicide, and homicide), pancytopenia, cardiovascular (supraventricular arrhythmias, chest pain, and myocardial infarction), autoimmune disorders, infections, pancreatitis, colitis, hepatic decompensation, ischemic and hemorrhagic cerebrovascular events, ophthalmic (decrease or loss of vision, retinopathy including macular edema, retinal artery or vein thrombosis, retinal hemorrhages and cotton wool spots, optic neuritis, papilledema and serous retinal detachment)

Major Drug Interactions

Peginterferon afla-2a can increase concentrations of theophylline and methadone

Contraindications

Autoimmune hepatitis, hepatic decompensation in cirrhotic patients before treatment, neonates, infants

Essential Monitoring Parameters

CBC at 2 and 4 weeks, then periodically thereafter; serum chemistries (including liver function tests) at 1, 2, 4, 6, and 8 weeks, then every 4–6 weeks thereafter; renal function; pregnancy test monthly and for 6 months after discontinuation of therapy (if on ribavirin); TSH and T4 every 12 weeks; mental health at every visit

Counseling Points

- If you are taking peginterferon alfa-2a with ribavirin, you or your sexual partner must not be pregnant throughout treatment and until 6 months after discontinuation of treatment
- Peginterferon alfa-2a is given by injection once a week under the skin (SUB-Q injection)
- Take your prescribed dose of peginterferon alfa-2a on the same day each week and at approximately the same time
- Do not switch to another brand of peginterferon without talking to your healthcare provider
- Avoid drinking alcohol to reduce the chance of further liver injury
- Call your healthcare provider right away if you experience any of the following problems while taking peginterferon alfa-2a:
  - New or worsening mental health problems, such as thoughts of hurting yourself or others
  - Feeling cold or hot all the time
  - Unusual bleeding or bruising
  - Nausea, vomiting, diarrhea, or abdominal pain
  - Changes in vision or changes to your eyes
  - Trouble breathing or chest pain
  - Any new weakness, loss of coordination, or numbness
  - Symptoms of infection, including fever, chills, burning or pain with urination, urinating often, tiredness, or coughing up yellow or pink mucus (phlegm)

Key Points

- Peginterferon alfa-2a monotherapy is not recommended for treatment of chronic hepatitis C unless a significant contraindication or intolerance to ribavirin is present
- Because peginterferon alfa-2a is often given with ribavirin for chronic hepatitis C, refer to ribavirin use before administering peginterferon alfa-2a
- Do not confuse peginterferon alfa-2a with peginterferon alfa-2b (PEG-INTRON), which differs in dosing
- Teach patient proper technique and placement of injections

IMMUNE GLOBULINS

Introduction

Immune globulin G (IgG) is collected during blood donation and pooled for administration as a separate product for patients with a variety of medical needs. These products, widely referred to as IVIG, are used for a wide variety of indications in which acquisition of antibodies is needed. These include instances of antibody deficiency, as well as in the treatment of autoimmune and inflammatory conditions. Because these are blood product derivatives, patients can develop infusion reactions while they are being administered.

Mechanism of Action of the Drug Class

Immune globulins replace native antibodies in patients with antibody deficiencies, provide passive immunity by increasing antibody titers, and suppress inflammatory and/or autoimmune processes

Members of the Drug Class

In this section: Immune globulin
Others: Antithymocyte globulin, botulism immune globulin, cytomegalovirus immune globulin, hepatitis B immune globulin, rabies immune globulin, $Rh_o(D)$ immune globulin, tetanus immune globulin, vaccinia immune globulin, varicella-zoster immune globulin

◉ Immune Globulin

Brand Names

Carimune, Flebogamma, GamaSTAN, Gammagard, Gammaked, Gammaplex, Gamunex, Hizentra, Octagam, Privigen, Vivaglobin

Generic Name

Immune globulin (IG)

Rx Only

Dosage Form

Injection

Usage

Replacement for primary or secondary immunodeficiencies,* treatment of acute or chronic immune (idiopathic) thrombocytopenia purpura (ITP),* prevention of bacterial infections in transplant patients with severe hypogammaglobulinemia,* prevention of renal transplant rejection, chronic inflammatory demyelinating polyneuropathy (CIDP), Guillain-Barré syndrome, remitting relapsing MS, myasthenia gravis, sepsis, Kawasaki disease

Pregnancy Category C

Dosing

- ITP:
  - Carimune: 400 mg/kg per day IV for 2–5 days as initial dose, then 400 mg/kg as needed to maintain platelet count ≥ 30,000/mm and/or control significant bleeding. Can increase dose if inadequate response to 800–1,000 mg/kg IV as single dose.
  - Gammagard: 1,000 mg/kg IV, can be repeated for up to three additional doses to be given on alternate days
  - Gammaked, Gamunex, Privigen: 1,000 mg/kg per day IV for 2 consecutive days
- Primary immunodeficiency:
  - IV: Dosing depends on product being used; 200–800 mg/kg IV infusion every 3–4 weeks
  - SUB-Q: Weekly SUB-Q infusion beginning 1 week after IV dose; initial weekly dose (grams) = [1.37 × IGIV dose (grams)] divided by [IV dose interval (weeks)]; adjust doses based on clinical response and trough serum IgG levels
  - IM: GamaSTAN 0.66 mL/kg (at least 100 mg/kg) IM every 3–4 weeks, double dose given at onset of therapy
- Renal dosage adjustment:
  - Administer IV and SUB-Q infusion at minimum infusion rate possible in patients with renal impairment
  - CrCl < 10 mL/min: Avoid IV use

Pharmacokinetic Monitoring

For SUB-Q infusion, monitor IgG trough levels every 2–3 months before and after conversion from IV

Adverse Reactions: Most Common

Infusion reaction with hypotension, tachycardia, fever, chills, nausea, vomiting; injection site reaction; myalgia; headache

Adverse Reactions: Rare/Severe/Important

Anaphylaxis/hypersensitivity reaction, hyperproteinemia, transfusion-related acute lung injury, acute renal failure, aseptic meningitis syndrome, hemolytic anemia, thrombotic events

Major Drug Interactions

Immune Globulin's Effect on Other Drugs
Live vaccines: May diminish therapeutic effect

Contraindications

Severe thrombocytopenia or any coagulation disorder that would contraindicate IM injections, IgA deficiency with antibodies against IgA

Essential Monitoring Parameters

Renal function, hemoglobin and hematocrit, platelet count (in ITP), volume status, neurologic symptoms for aseptic meningitis

Counseling Points

- Immune globulin is made from human plasma and may have viruses that can cause disease. This drug is screened, tested, and treated to decrease the chance that it carries an infection.
- Report any signs of infection
- Monitoring will be required during IV or SUB-Q infusion. Report any chills, chest pain or tightness, rapid heartbeat, back pain, or difficulty breathing to your healthcare provider.

Key Points

- Live vaccines should be withheld for up to 6 months following immune globulin administration. Live vaccine given immediately prior to immune globulin administration may require repeat vaccination.
- Octagam contains maltose and can falsely elevate blood glucose levels if measured using the glucose dehydrogenase pyrroloquinolinequinone (GDH-PQQ) methods
- Storage varies based on product. Some formulations require refrigeration.
- Dosing varies based on product used
- IV administration: Initial rate of administration and titration is specific to each IV IG product
- SUB-Q administration: Appropriate injection sites include the abdomen, thigh, upper arm, lower back, and/or lateral hip. Dose may be infused into multiple sites (spaced ≥ 2 inches apart) simultaneously. Rotate sites weekly.
- IM administration: Appropriate injection sites include anterolateral aspects of the upper thigh or deltoid muscle of the upper arm. Avoid gluteal region due to risk of injury to sciatic nerve. Divide doses > 10 mL and inject in multiple sites.

REVIEW QUESTIONS

1. Which of the following is a brand of cyclosporine?

   a. Gengraf
   b. Prograf
   c. CellCept
   d. Myfortic

2. Which of the following statements about cyclosporine is true?

   a. Formulations are bioequivalent and interchangeable.
   b. Patients should avoid concomitant grapefruit juice.
   c. It is commonly used in the treatment of multiple sclerosis.
   d. It is contraindicated in patients with a history of hypersensitivity to albumin.

3. Therapeutic drug concentrations should be monitored for which of the following medications?

   a. Etanercept
   b. Mycophenolate
   c. Tacrolimus
   d. Glatiramer acetate

4. Which of the following is a serious adverse effect of tacrolimus?

   a. Nephrotoxicity
   b. Injection site necrosis
   c. Chest pain
   d. Seizures

5. Betaseron is used for which of the following indications?

   a. Treatment of rheumatoid arthritis
   b. Treatment of multiple sclerosis
   c. Prevention of organ transplant rejection
   d. Prevention of immunodeficiency

6. Which of the following is the most common adverse effect of Betaseron?

   a. Hepatotoxicity
   b. Lymphoma
   c. Flulike symptoms
   d. Infection

7. Betaseron is administered by which of the following methods?

   a. Orally
   b. Intravenously
   c. Intramuscularly
   d. Subcutaneously

8. Which of the following is a common adverse reaction of immune globulin?

   a. Reactivation of latent TB
   b. Infusion reaction
   c. Electrolyte abnormalities
   d. Depression

9. Which of the following is true of immune globulin?

   a. It activates T suppressor cells.
   b. It inhibits production of tumor necrosis factor.
   c. It promotes B cell proliferation.
   d. It contains antibodies directed toward specific antigens.

10. Which of the following is *false* with regard to glatiramer acetate?

   a. Patients may develop antibodies of unknown clinical significance.
   b. Injection reaction may include symptoms of chest tightness.
   c. Women need a negative pregnancy test prior to starting therapy.
   d. It should be stored in the refrigerator.

11. Which of the following is an acceptable dose for Copaxone?

   a. 125 mg SUB-Q once weekly
   b. 20 mg SUB-Q once daily
   c. 1,000 mg PO twice daily
   d. 5 mg/kg PO once daily

12. Orencia is the brand name for which of the following?

   a. Abatacept
   b. Etanercept
   c. Interferon beta-1a
   d. Infliximab

13. Prior to initiating abatacept, patients should be screened for which of the following?

   a. Pregnancy
   b. Presence of antibodies
   c. Diabetes
   d. Viral hepatitis

14. Concomitant use of which of the following will lead to the decreased absorption of mycophenolate?

   a. Antacids
   b. Statins
   c. Digoxin
   d. Colchicine

15. Which of the following is an important counseling point for a patient taking mycophenolic acid?

    a. The CellCept and Myfortic formulations are interchangeable.
    b. Two forms of contraception should be used.
    c. Change in mood, including depression and thoughts of suicide, is a rare but serious side effect.
    d. Drug levels will need to be monitored periodically.

16. Which of the following is a live attenuated vaccine?

    a. Influenza virus injectable vaccine
    b. Pneumococcal polysaccharide vaccine
    c. Zoster vaccine
    d. Tetanus vaccine

17. Which of the following is the major adverse reaction associated with vaccines?

    a. Guillain-Barré syndrome
    b. Autism
    c. Injection site reactions
    d. Anaphylactic reactions

18. Who should receive the flu vaccine?

    a. People > 65 years
    b. Only people with specific comorbid conditions
    c. People between 6 months and 5 years of age
    d. Every person > 6 months of age

19. Which of the following is a reason why a patient between the ages of 2 and 64 should *not* receive the pneumococcal polysaccharide vaccine?

    a. The patient is a smoker.
    b. The patient has a long-term health problem (e.g., heart disease, lung disease, diabetes).
    c. The patient is immunocompromised (e.g., malignancies such as leukemia or lymphoma, HIV infection, or damaged spleen).
    d. The patient is taking immunosuppressive therapy (e.g., long-term steroids).

20. The zoster vaccine prevents which of the following?

    a. Herpes genitalia
    b. Herpes labialis
    c. Shingles
    d. Chickenpox

21. Which of the following is *not* a contraindication to the zoster vaccine?

    a. History of anaphylactic reaction to neomycin
    b. Severe allergic reactions to egg proteins
    c. Immunosuppression or immunodeficiency
    d. Pregnancy

22. Which vaccine should be received on a yearly basis?

    a. Zoster vaccine
    b. Influenza virus vaccine
    c. Pneumococcal polysaccharide vaccine
    d. Rubella vaccine

23. Which of the following is a common side effect of TNF inhibitors?

    a. Upper respiratory infection
    b. Congestive heart failure
    c. Sepsis
    d. Stevens-Johnson syndrome

24. Which of the following drugs does *not* interact with TNF inhibitors?

    a. Abatacept
    b. Zoster vaccine
    c. Tacrolimus
    d. Influenza virus vaccine

25. Which of the following is *not* a TNF inhibitor?

    a. Etanercept
    b. Infliximab
    c. Adalimumab
    d. Glatiramer

26. Which of the following is the *most* common adverse effect of interferons?

    a. Pancytopenia
    b. Flulike symptoms
    c. Suicide
    d. Hepatic failure

27. Interferons can be used for the treatment of all of the following, *except*:

    a. chronic hepatitis C.
    b. chronic hepatitis A.
    c. multiple sclerosis.
    d. neoplasms.

28. All of the following are serious adverse effects associated with interferons, *except*:

    a. renal failure.
    b. psychiatric disorders.
    c. hepatotoxicity.
    d. leukopenia.

29. Which of the following is *not* a contraindication to peginterferon alfa-2a?

    a. Neonates
    b. Pancytopenia
    c. Autoimmune hepatitis
    d. Hepatic decompensation in cirrhotic patients

30. When used in combination with ribavirin, peginterferon alfa-2 is pregnancy category:

    a. B.
    b. C.
    c. D.
    d. X.

Answer Key

Chapter 1

1.	A	11.	A	21.	D
2.	D	12.	C	22.	D
3.	C	13.	A	23.	B
4.	C	14.	B	24.	C
5.	D	15.	C	25.	B
6.	B	16.	A	26.	B
7.	A	17.	C	27.	C
8.	C	18.	C	28.	C
9.	C	19.	D	29.	D
10.	C	20.	C	30.	B

Chapter 2

1.	B	11.	A	21.	A
2.	C	12.	D	22.	A
3.	A	13.	B	23.	D
4.	D	14.	C	24.	C
5.	C	15.	C	25.	C
6.	B	16.	B	26.	A
7.	B	17.	B	27.	C
8.	A	18.	C	28.	C
9.	C	19.	B	29.	D
10.	C	20.	C	30.	C

Chapter 3

1.	C	11.	A	21.	B
2.	D	12.	B	22.	B
3.	D	13.	D	23.	A
4.	C	14.	C	24.	B
5.	B	15.	C	25.	B
6.	C	16.	B	26.	C
7.	C	17.	C	27.	C
8.	B	18.	B	28.	B
9.	C	19.	C	29.	A
10.	B	20.	A	30.	C

Chapter 4

1.	B	11.	D	21.	A
2.	C	12.	B	22.	B
3.	C	13.	A	23.	B
4.	A	14.	A	24.	C
5.	D	15.	D	25.	A
6.	A	16.	D	26.	C
7.	B	17.	A	27.	B
8.	C	18.	C	28.	C
9.	A	19.	A	29.	C
10.	C	20.	B	30.	C

Chapter 5

1.	C	11.	D	21.	A
2.	B	12.	C	22.	B
3.	A	13.	B	23.	A
4.	D	14.	A	24.	A
5.	D	15.	A	25.	C
6.	C	16.	B	26.	D
7.	C	17.	D	27.	D
8.	B	18.	C	28.	B
9.	A	19.	B	29.	C
10.	D	20.	C	30.	C

Chapter 6

1.	B	11.	D	21.	C
2.	A	12.	B	22.	A
3.	D	13.	A	23.	B
4.	B	14.	A	24.	A
5.	A	15.	D	25.	D
6.	C	16.	B	26.	B
7.	C	17.	A	27.	B
8.	C	18.	D	28.	C
9.	B	19.	D	29.	D
10.	C	20.	B	30.	D

Chapter 7

1.	A	11.	C	21.	B
2.	B	12.	D	22.	B
3.	A	13.	C	23.	B
4.	D	14.	B	24.	A
5.	B	15.	D	25.	D
6.	C	16.	B	26.	A
7.	D	17.	A	27.	B
8.	D	18.	B	28.	B
9.	A	19.	D	29.	C
10.	D	20.	C	30.	D

Chapter 8

1.	B	11.	B	21.	D
2.	C	12.	D	22.	C
3.	C	13.	A	23.	C
4.	D	14.	D	24.	B
5.	C	15.	C	25.	A
6.	D	16.	B	26.	D
7.	C	17.	C	27.	D
8.	D	18.	C	28.	A
9.	D	19.	B	29.	D
10.	B	20.	B	30.	D

Chapter 9

1.	A	11.	D	21.	A
2.	B	12.	C	22.	D
3.	A	13.	A	23.	C
4.	C	14.	B	24.	B
5.	B	15.	B	25.	D
6.	C	16.	A	26.	B
7.	D	17.	D	27.	C
8.	C	18.	A	28.	A
9.	B	19.	C	29.	A
10.	A	20.	B	30.	D

Chapter 10

1.	C	11.	D	21.	D
2.	D	12.	D	22.	D
3.	B	13.	A	23.	A
4.	A	14.	C	24.	A
5.	A	15.	B	25.	C
6.	D	16.	A	26.	A
7.	C	17.	B	27.	D
8.	B	18.	D	28.	A
9.	A	19.	A	29.	D
10.	C	20.	D	30.	B

Chapter 11

1.	B	11.	C	21.	C
2.	D	12.	A	22.	B
3.	A	13.	B	23.	C
4.	A	14.	C	24.	D
5.	C	15.	A	25.	C
6.	B	16.	D	26.	D
7.	B	17.	A	27.	A
8.	D	18.	D	28.	A
9.	D	19.	C	29.	C
10.	B	20.	B	30.	A

Chapter 12

1.	C	11.	B	21.	B
2.	C	12.	C	22.	A
3.	A	13.	A	23.	A
4.	C	14.	D	24.	B
5.	C	15.	D	25.	D
6.	D	16.	D	26.	C
7.	D	17.	C	27.	B
8.	C	18.	A	28.	C
9.	B	19.	B	29.	B
10.	C	20.	C	30.	D

Chapter 13

1.	D	11.	C	21.	C
2.	A	12.	C	22.	A
3.	D	13.	D	23.	C
4.	B	14.	C	24.	B
5.	D	15.	D	25.	D
6.	A	16.	B	26.	C
7.	D	17.	A	27.	C
8.	C	18.	B	28.	D
9.	C	19.	C	29.	A
10.	B	20.	D	30.	D

Chapter 14

1.	C	11.	A	21.	C
2.	A	12.	B	22.	B
3.	D	13.	D	23.	B
4.	B	14.	B	24.	D
5.	C	15.	C	25.	A
6.	A	16.	B	26.	C
7.	B	17.	A	27.	A
8.	B	18.	B	28.	D
9.	D	19.	C	29.	A
10.	D	20.	B	30.	C

Chapter 15

1.	D	11.	D	21.	A
2.	D	12.	D	22.	D
3.	A	13.	C	23.	A
4.	A	14.	A	24.	B
5.	C	15.	D	25.	B
6.	A	16.	A	26.	A
7.	A	17.	C	27.	D
8.	D	18.	D	28.	D
9.	D	19.	B	29.	D
10.	B	20.	C	30.	B

Chapter 16

1.	A	11.	B	21.	B
2.	B	12.	A	22.	B
3.	C	13.	D	23.	A
4.	A	14.	A	24.	D
5.	B	15.	B	25.	D
6.	C	16.	C	26.	B
7.	D	17.	C	27.	B
8.	B	18.	D	28.	A
9.	D	19.	A	29.	B
10.	C	20.	C	30.	D

Index

Dulcolax, 193
duloxetine, 135
DuoNeb, 281–282
Duraclon, 88–89
Duragesic, 4–5
Dyazide, 112
Dyna-Hex, 307–308

echinacea, 329–330
Echinaforce, 329–330
EchinaGuard, 329–330
Ecotrin, 14
Edluar, 155
EEMT, 174
EES (erythromycin), 43
efavirenz, 56
Effexor, Effexor XR, 135–136
Effient, 214
Efudex, 68
Elavil, 140–141
electrolyte supplements, 248–249
eletriptan, 115–116
Elimite, 321–322
Elixophyllin, 297–298
Elocon, 319
Eloxatin, 76–77
Embeline, 316–317
Emetrol, 204–205
emtricitabine, 54
Emtriva, 54
E-Mycin, 43
Enablex, 249
enalapril, 93–94
enalapril/HCTZ, 112
Enbrel, 359
Endocet, 11
endocrine agents
    alendronate, 170
    bisphosphonates, overview, 169
    calcitonin-salmon, 171
    conjugated estrogen, 173
    conjugated estrogen/medroxyprogesterone
        acetate, 174
    esterified estrogens and methyltestosterone,
        174
    estradiol, 172–173
    estradiol transdermal system, 173
    glucocorticoids, overview, 179–180
    ibandronate, 170
    medroxyprogesterone, 174
    oral contraceptives, biphasic, 176
    oral contraceptives, monophasic, 175–176
    oral contraceptives, progestin-only, 178
    oral contraceptives, triphasic, 177
    parathyroid hormone analogs, 181
    risedronate, 170
    selective estrogen receptor modulators
        (SERMs), 178–179
    sex hormones, overview, 172
    thyroid hormones, 182
    vaginal ring, 177–178
    zoledronic acid, 170–171
enoxaparin, 218–219
Epiklor, 248–249
epinephrine, 90–91
EpiPen, 90–91
Epitol, 123–124
Epivir, 53–54
Epivir-HBV, 53–54
epoetin alfa, 216
Epogen, 216
eprosartan/HCTZ, 112
Epzicom, 53–54, 55

Equetro, 123–124
Erbitux, 73
erectile dysfunction agents
    overview, 251–252
    tadalafil, 252–253
    vardenafil, 253
ergocalciferol, 344
erlotinib, 81
EryPed, 43
Ery-Tab, 43
erythromycin, 43
    erythromycin and benzoyl peroxide
        combination, 315
    ophthalmic products, 260–261
erythropoietins
    darbepoetin alfa, 216
    epoetin alfa, 216
    overview, 215
Esberitox, 329–330
escitalopram oxalate, 137
Eskalith, Eskalith CR, 143
esomeprazole, 200–201
Ester-C, 347–348
Estrace, 172–173
Estraderm, 173
estradiol, 172–173
estradiol transdermal system, 173
estrogens. See also oral contraceptives;
        selective estrogen receptor modulators
        (SERMs)
    conjugated estrogen, 173
    conjugated estrogen/medroxyprogesterone
        acetate, 174
    esterified estrogens and methyltestosterone,
        174
    estradiol, 172–173
    estradiol transdermal system, 173
    medroxyprogesterone, 174
    oral contraceptives, monophasic, 175–176
    overview, 172
    raloxifene, 178–179
    vaginal ring, 177–178
eszopiclone, 155–156
etanercept, 359
etodolac, 15
etoposide, 78–79
Evista, 178–179
Evoclin, 308–309
Exalgo, 5
Excedrin, 14
Excedrin IB, 15–16
Exelon, 150–151
ex-lax, 193
expectorant, 295–296
Extavia, 362
Extina, 309–310
ezetimibe, 230–231
ezetimibe/simvastatin, 233–234

factor XA inhibitors, 210–211
famotidine, 197–198
felodipine, 105
Femara, 72
fenofibrate, 228–229
Fenoglide, 228–229
fentanyl, 4–5
Fentora, 4–5
Feosol, 345
Feratab, 345
Fer-Gen-Sol, 345
Fer-in-Sol, 345
Fer-Iron, 345
ferrous sulfate, 345

feverfew, 330
Fexmid, 157–158
fexofenadine, 277–278
Fiberall, 191
fibric acid derivatives
    fenofibrate, 228–229
    gemfibrozil, 228
    overview, 227–228
filgrastim, 214–215
finasteride, 237
Fioricet, 2–3
Flagyl, 44
Flebogamma, 364–365
Flector, 14–15
Fleet Bisacodyl, 193
Flexeril, 157–158
Flomax, 88
Flonase, 293–294
Flovent Diskus, 291–292
Flovent HFA, 291–292
Fluarix, 353–354
fluconazole, 49–50
FluLaval, 353–354
flumazenil, 244–245
fluocinonide, 317–318
fluoride, 346
fluoroquinolones
    ciprofloxacin, 38–39
    levofloxacin, 39
    moxifloxacin, 39
    ophthalmic products, 261–262
    overview, 38
5-fluorouracil, 68
fluoxetine, 138
Flutex, 320
fluticasone, inhaled, 291–292
fluticasone, intranasal, 293–294
fluticasone and salmeterol, 283
fluvastatin, 225–227
Fluvirin Live attenuated: FluMist, 353–354
Fluzone, 353–354
Folacin-800, 347
folic acid, 347
folic acid synthesis inhibitors, 44–45
Folvite, 347
Foradil, 285
formoterol, 285
formoterol and budesonide, 283
Formula EM, 204–205
Fortamet, 21
Forteo, 181
Fortical, 171
Fosamax, Fosamax Plus D, 170
fosinopril, 94
fosinopril/HCTZ, 112
Fragmin, 218
5-FU, 68
Fungizone, 48
furosemide, 106–107

gabapentin, 125
Gablofen, 156–157
GamaSTAN, 364–365
Gammagard, 364–365
Gammaked, 364–365
Gammaplex, 364–365
Gamunex, 364–365
Garamycin, 31–32
garlic, 331
gastrointestinal agents
    antacids, 187–188
    anticholinergic/antispasmodic agents,
        202–203

parathyroid analogs, 181
Parcopa, 152
Parkinson's disease treatment, 151–153,
        241–242
paroxetine, 138–139
Pataday, 269
Patanol, 269
PediaCare, 92
pediculicide, 321–322
Pegasys, 363–364
pegfilgrastim, 215
peginterferon alfa-2a, 363–364
pemetrexed, 71
penicillins
        amoxicillin, 34–35
        amoxicillin/clavulanate, 35
        overview, 34, 35
Pennsaid, 14–15
Pen-VK, 35
Pepcid, 197–198
Pepcid AC, 197–198
Pepcid Complete, 197–198
Pepto-Bismol, 188–189
Percocet, 11
Perforomist Solution for Nebulization, 285
permethrin, 321–322
Pexeva, 138–139
Phazyme, 190
phenazopyridine, 255–256
Phenergan, 276–277
Phenergan with Codeine, 289
phenobarbital, 127–128
phenothiazine, 203–204
phentermine, 118–119
phenylalkylamines, 105–106
phenylephrine, 92
Phenytek, 128–129
phenytoin, 128–129
phosphodiesterase enzyme inhibitors, 108–109
phosphodiesterase inhibitors
        overview, 251–252
        sildenafil, 252
        tadalafil, 252–253
        vardenafil, 253
phosphorated carbohydrate solutions, 204–205
phosphoric acid/dextrose/fructose, 204–205
pioglitazone, 27
Piper methysticum, 335–336
Pitressin, 100–101
Plaquenil, 239–240
Platinol, Platinol-AQ, 75–76
platinum compounds
        carboplatin, 75
        cisplatin, 75–76
        overview, 74
        oxaliplatin, 76–77
Plavix, 213
Plendil, 105
pneumococcal polysaccharide vaccine, 354
Pneumovax 23, 354
polyenes
        amphotericin B, 48
        nystatin, 48–49
        overview, 48
polyethylene glycol 3350, 194
polymyxin B, bacitracin, neomycin
        combination, 314
potassium chloride, 248–249
Pradaxa, 220–221
prasugrel, 214
Pravachol, 225–227
pravastatin, 225–227

prednisone, 179–180
pregabalin, 129
Premarin, 173
Prevacid, 201
Prevalite, 232–233
Prezista, 58–59
Prilosec, 201
Primacor, 109
Prinzide, 112
Privigen, 364–365
ProAir HFA, 284–285
probiotics, 337–338
Procardia, Procardia XL, 105
prochlorperazine, 203–204
Procrit, 216
Proctocort, 318–319
Prodium, 255–256
progesterone. *See also* oral contraceptives
        conjugated estrogen/medroxyprogesterone
                acetate, 174
        medroxyprogesterone, 174
        vaginal ring, 177–178
progestin. *See also* oral contraceptives
        oral contraceptives, monophasic, 175–176
        progestin-only oral contraceptives, 178
Prograf, 356–357
prokinetic agents, 199
promethazine, 276–277
        promethazine with codeine, 289
Propecia, 237
propranolol, 103
propranolol/HCTZ, 112
Proscar, 237
protease inhibitors
        atazanavir, 58
        darunavir, 58–59
        lopinavir/ritonavir, 57–58
        overview, 56
        ritonavir, 57
Protonix, 201–202
proton pump inhibitors (PPIs)
        esomeprazole, 200–201
        lansoprazole, 201
        omeprazole, 201
        overview, 200
        pantoprazole, 201–202
        rabeprazole, 202
Protopic, 356–357
Proventil HFA, 284–285
Provera, 174
Provigil, 164
Prozac, 138
Prudoxin, 141–142
psyllium, 191
Pulmicort Flexhaler, 290–291
Pulmicort Respules, 290–291
pulmonary agents
        albuterol, 284–285
        anticholinergics, overview, 273
        antihistamines, overview, 275, 277
        antitussives, 280
        beclomethasone, 290, 293
        beta-2 agonist and anticholinergic inhalers,
                280–282
        beta-2 agonist and corticosteroid inhaler,
                282–283
        beta-2 agonists, inhaled, 284–287
        budesonide, inhaled, 290–291
        budesonide, intranasal, 293
        budesonide and formoterol, 283
        cetirizine, 279
        corticosteroids, inhaled, 290–292
        corticosteroids, intranasal, 292–294

cough and cold agents, overview, 287
decongestant, 294–295
diphenhydramine, 275–276
expectorant, 295–296
fexofenadine, 277–278
fluticasone, 293–294
fluticasone, inhaled, 291–292
fluticasone and salmeterol, 283
formoterol, 285
guaifenesin and codeine, 287–288
guaifenesin with dextromethorphan, 288
hydrocodone and chlorpheniramine,
        288–289
hydroxyzine, 276
ipratropium, 273–274
leukotriene inhibitor, 296–297
levalbuterol, 285–286
levocetirizine, 278–279
loratadine, 278
mometasone, 294
montelukast, 296–297
omalizumab, 298–299
promethazine, 276–277
promethazine with codeine, 289
salmeterol, 286–287
theophylline, 297–298
tiotropium, 274–275
xanthine derivative, 297–298
Pure CoQ-10, 328
Purinethol, 69
Pyridium, 255–256

Q-Gel, 328
Qnasl, 293
Q-Sorb, 328
Questran, 232–233
Questran Light, 232–233
quetiapine, 146
quinapril, 94
quinapril/HCTZ, 112
QVAR 40 and 80, 290

rabeprazole, 202
raloxifene, 178–179
raltegravir, 59
ramipril, 94
ramipril/HCTZ, 112
Ranexa, 96
ranitidine, 198
ranolazine, 96
Rebif, 362
Reclast, 170–171
red yeast rice, 338–339
Reglan, 199
Reguloid, 191
Relafen, 17–18
Relpax, 115–116
Remeron, Remeron Sol Tabs, 132–133
Remicade, 359
Reprexain, 11
Requip, Requip XL, 152–153
Restasis, 355–356
retinoic acid derivatives, 238–239
Revatio, 252
Revlimid, 83–84
Reyataz, 58
Rheumatrex, 69–71
Rhinocort Aqua, 293
Rid, 321–322
Rifadin, 33–34
rifampin, 33–34
Rimactane, 33–34
Riomet, 21

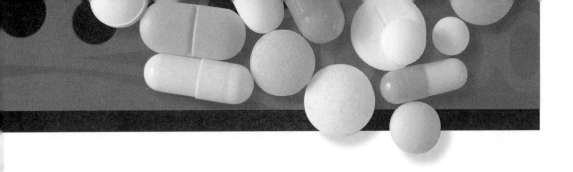

FREQUENTLY PRESCRIBED MEDICATIONS

Drugs You Need to Know

Second Edition

Michael A. Mancano, PharmD
Chair, Department of Pharmacy Practice
Clinical Professor of Pharmacy Practice
Temple University School of Pharmacy
Philadelphia, Pennsylvania

Jason C. Gallagher, PharmD, BCPS
Clinical Associate Professor of Pharmacy Practice
Temple University School of Pharmacy
Philadelphia, Pennsylvania

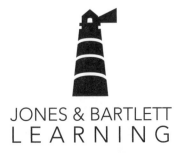

JONES & BARTLETT
L E A R N I N G

World Headquarters
Jones & Bartlett Learning
5 Wall Street
Burlington, MA 01803
978-443-5000
info@jblearning.com
www.jblearning.com

Jones & Bartlett Learning books and products are available through most bookstores and online booksellers. To contact Jones & Bartlett Learning directly, call 800-832-0034, fax 978-443-8000, or visit our website, www.jblearning.com.

Substantial discounts on bulk quantities of Jones & Bartlett Learning publications are available to corporations, professional associations, and other qualified organizations. For details and specific discount information, contact the special sales department at Jones & Bartlett Learning via the above contact information or send an email to specialsales@jblearning.com.

Production Credits

Publisher: William Brottmiller
Senior Acquisitions Editor: Katey Birtcher
Associate Editor: Teresa Reilly
Editorial Assistant: Sean Fabery
Production Editor: Jessica Steele Newfell
Marketing Manager: Grace Richards
VP, Manufacturing and Inventory Control: Therese Connell
Composition: Paw Print Media
Interior Design: Shawn Girsberger
Cover Design: Kristin E. Parker
Cover and Title Page Image: © ajt/ShutterStock, Inc.
Printing and Binding: Edwards Brothers Malloy
Cover Printing: Edwards Brothers Malloy

Library of Congress Cataloging-in-Publication Data
Frequently prescribed medications : drugs you need to know / [edited] by Michael A. Mancano and Jason C. Gallagher. — 2nd ed.
   p. ; cm.
 Includes bibliographical references and index.
 ISBN 978-1-4496-9884-3 — ISBN 1-4496-9884-0
 I. Mancano, Michael A. II. Gallagher, Jason C.
 [DNLM: 1. Pharmaceutical Preparations—Handbooks. QV 39]
 RM301.12
 615′.1—dc23
                    2013003927

6048

Printed in the United States of America
17 16 15 14 13   10 9 8 7 6 5 4 3 2 1